Geriatrics for Specialists

John R. Burton • Andrew G. Lee • Jane F. Potter

Editors

Geriatrics for Specialists

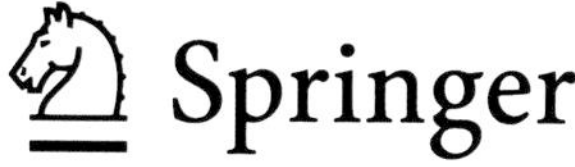
Springer

Editors
John R. Burton
Professor of Medicine
Johns Hopkins University School of Medicine
The Johns Hopkins Bayview Medical Center
Baltimore, MD, USA

Jane F. Potter
Harris Professor of Geriatric Medicine
Chief, Division of Geriatrics and Gerontology
Director, Home Instead Center for Successful
  Aging
Department of Internal Medicine
University of Nebraska Medical Center
Omaha, NE, USA

Andrew G. Lee
Chair of Ophthalmology
Blanton Eye Institute
Houston Methodist Hospital
Houston, TX, USA

Professor of Ophthalmology,
  Neurology, and Neurosurgery
Weill Cornell Medicine
New York, NY, USA

Clinical Professor
UTMB (Galveston) and the UTMD
  Anderson Cancer Center
Houston, TX, USA

Adjunct Professor
Baylor College of Medicine
Houston, TX, USA

Adjunct Professor
University of Iowa Hospitals and Clinics
Iowa City, IA, USA

Adjunct Professor
The University of Buffalo
Buffalo, NY, USA

ISBN 978-3-319-31829-5   ISBN 978-3-319-31831-8   (eBook)
DOI 10.1007/978-3-319-31831-8

Library of Congress Control Number: 2016941325

Printed on acid-free paper

This Springer imprint is published by Springer Nature
The registered company is Springer International Publishing AG Switzerland

This book is dedicated to the many scholars and teachers who launched this effort to develop on sound principles the field of specialty geriatric practice and those who continue its growth.

John R. Burton dedicates this book to all of his mentors and colleagues in geriatrics and the specialties who so profoundly inspired him to spread geriatric concepts broadly to all health professionals.

Andrew G. Lee dedicates this book to his children, Rachael and Virginia Lee, who will hopefully one day become part of the next generation of Lee physicians to care for elderly patients, and he also recognizes and thanks his wife, Hilary A. Beaver, MD, who has been a constant source of inspiration, love, patience, wisdom, and grounding.

Jane F. Potter dedicates this book to Dennis Jahnigen who provided her with encouragement to pursue a career as a mentor to students, David Solomon who provided her the opportunity to join the Geriatrics for Specialists Initiative, and Jeff Silverstein whose wit and wisdom made this project fun as well as rewarding.

Preface

Reasons for This Book

Over the last two decades, medical and surgical specialists have collaborated to bring together individual advances for geriatric populations within their specialties. This has resulted in a robust body of knowledge that now guides the standards of care for older people, the research agenda for the future, and the innovations in geriatric education among specialty trainees. This book is intended to fill the void of a single source of knowledge concerning these advances in specialty care.

Intended Audience

This book is designed to be a resource to the following major audiences:

(a) Specialty clinicians caring for seniors.
(b) Researchers with interest in the geriatric aspects of specialty fields. Chapters include description of the limits on knowledge and propose next research questions.
(c) Academicians who create and deliver content on aging within the clinical graduate and postgraduate specialty training programs.
(d) Geriatricians seeking in-depth knowledge of specialty care for older patients.
(e) Members of the interprofessional teams that are so critical to clinical care and research within geriatrics, including nursing, social work, pharmacy, physical and occupational therapies, and others.
(f) Policy makers seeking to understand the strength of evidence concerning quality care for older patients provided by specialists and their associates.

The Approach Used in Developing the Book

This text is divided into three parts: crosscutting issues, medical specialties, and surgical and related specialties.

Part I: The first part deals with the crosscutting issues and addresses concepts of critical importance to all specialist providers who conduct research for and about and who also care for older patients. These chapters are cross-referenced heavily throughout Parts II and III. This has reduced repetition within individual chapters on critical concepts such as frailty, assessment tools, delirium, dementia, pharmacology, perioperative care, etc., while allowing authors to describe in detail where these concepts fit specifically within that discipline and relevant related literature.

Parts II and III: The surgical (Part II) and medical (Part III) sections of the text are a series of chapters addressing the major selected surgical and medical disciplines; important related specialties (e.g., rehabilitation) are included in the surgical section.

The editors developed the table of contents reflecting the state of knowledge and then recruited specialty authors who are active in clinical care, teaching, and research in geriatrics. At least two editors and often all three reviewed each chapter and worked with the authors to ensure that the focus of the text was practical, timely, and clear so it could be a reliable resource in everyday practice.

Background

The editors acknowledge the work of many over two decades and in particular the inspiration of the late Drs. Dennis Jahnigen and T. Franklin Williams. Dr. Jahnigen initiated the geriatric surgical and related specialties movement in the 1990s, and Dr. Williams inspired much of the work to embed geriatric principles into the subspecialties of internal medicine. Both of these individuals were prominent geriatricians: Dr. Jahnigen was a past president of the American Geriatrics Society (AGS), and Dr. Williams was a past director of the National Institute on Aging. While Drs. Jahnigen and Williams initiated this work, the major developments that followed fell to their successors. The surgical and related specialty work was initiated within the AGS and was led by the late Dr. David Solomon and Dr. John Burton who was joined by Dr. Andrew Lee and others including Dr. Jane F. Potter, both of whom serve in leadership positions in the program. The work related to the development of geriatrics in the medical specialties was led by Drs. William Hazzard and Kevin High and became a program of the Association of Specialty Professors (ASP). The editors are grateful to Dr. High who participated fully as an editor in the early development of this book before other professional demands precluded his continuing involvement.

The strategy behind this collaborative effort was to recruit and nurture promising young faculty and trainees in the geriatric aspects of their specialty. This investment over the last two decades in medical and surgical specialists is a unique national success and has resulted in a robust body of knowledge related to specialty care of seniors.

Critical to the success of this effort was the AGS staff (including Janis Eisner succeeded by Marianna Drootin and Erin Obrusniak and others) and leadership (notably Nancy Lundebjerg, whose dedication and hard work have moved the inspiration of its founders into a growing focus within the American Geriatrics Society and in American medicine). None of this work would have been possible without the continuing encouragement and support of the John A. Hartford Foundation and its president until 2015, Corinne H. Rieder, EdD. The program director, Christopher Langston, and senior project officers (Laura Robbins, Donna Regenstrief, and Marcus Escobedo) of the John A. Hartford Foundation for the two programs (surgical and related specialties within the AGS and the medical specialties within the ASP) were full partners throughout the development and operation of these programs. Their dedication, vision, and commitment ensured success and inspired all involved in the projects. Collectively they formed a critical force behind the work that made this book possible. Within the AGS, the effort became known as the Geriatrics for Specialists Initiative (GSI). The GSI has evolved into an active group of physician specialists, geriatricians, and health professionals from other disciplines. The GSI fosters geriatric principles in education and research broadly in medical centers and within specialty societies and governing and regulatory bodies. The sustained effort within the AGS of the GSI has evolved into the Section for Enhancing Geriatric Understanding and Expertise Among Surgical and Medical Specialists (SEGUE). The leadership of SEGUE is now entirely specialists. This book is a natural succession of the work of the GSI and SEGUE within the AGS and the geriatrics program of the ASP. The career development programs, originally sponsored by the specialty organizations, were subsumed by the National Institute on Aging with the initiation of their program in 2011: Grants for Early Medical and Surgical Specialists Transitioning to Aging Research (GEMSSTAR). Many of the chapters are written by the new cohort of geriatric specialty scholars and their mentors and trainees associated with the GSI/SEGUE program of the AGS and the geriatrics program of the ASP.

Baltimore, MD, USA
Houston, TX, USA
Omaha, NE, USA

John R. Burton
Andrew G. Lee
Jane F. Potter

Contents

Contributors

Kristina L. Bailey, MD Pulmonary, Critical Care, Sleep, and Allergy Division, Department of Internal Medicine, University of Nebraska Medical Center, Omaha, NE, USA

Hilary A. Beaver, MD Methodist Eye Associates, Jack S. Blanton Eye Institute, Houston Methodist Hospital, Houston, TX, USA

Susan P. Bell, MBBS, MSCI Division of Cardiovascular and Geriatric Medicine, Department of Medicine, Vanderbilt University School of Medicine, Center for Quality Aging, Nashville, TN, USA

C. Barrett Bowling, MD, MSPH Atlanta VA Medical Center, Birmingham/Atlanta VA Geriatric Research, Education and Clinical Center, Decatur, GA, USA

Nicole J. Brandt, PharmD, MBA, BCPP, CGP, FASCP Department of Pharmacy Practice and Science, University of Maryland, School of Pharmacy, Baltimore, MD, USA

John R. Burton, MD Professor of Medicine, Johns Hopkins University School of Medicine, The Johns Hopkins Bayview Medical Center, Baltimore, MD, USA

Joseph C. Cleveland Jr, MD Division of CT Surgery, University of Colorado Anscutz Medical Center, Aurora, CO, USA

Elizabeth L. Cobbs, MD Division of Geriatrics and Palliative Medicine, George Washington University, Washington, DC, USA

Geriatrics, Extended Care and Palliative Care, Washington DC Veterans Affairs Medical Center, Washington, DC, USA

JoAnn Coleman, DNP, ACNP, ANP, AOCN, GCN Center for Geriatric Surgery, Department of Surgery, Sinai Hospital, Baltimore, MD, USA

Deborah J. Culley, MD Department of Anesthesiology, Perioperative and Pain Medicine, Brigham and Women's Hospital, Boston, MA, USA

William Dale, MD, PhD Section of Geriatrics and Palliative Medicine, Specialized Oncology Care & Research in the Elderly (SOCARE) Clinic, University of Chicago Medicine, Chicago, IL, USA

Stacie Deiner, MS, MD Department of Anesthesiology, The Icahn School of Medicine at Mount Sinai, New York, NY, USA

Danielle J. Doberman, MD, MPH Division of Geriatrics and Palliative Medicine, George Washington University, Washington, DC, USA

Kelly L. Dunn, MD Melbourne, FL, USA

David R. Ellington, MD, FACOG Division of Urogynecology and Pelvic Reconstructive Surgery, Department of Obstetrics and Gynecology, University of Alabama at Birmingham, Birmingham, AL, USA

Mindy J. Fain, MD Department of Medicine, Arizona Center in Aging, University of Arizona College of Medicine, Tucson, AZ, USA

Hermes Florez, MD, MPH, PhD Division of Epidemiology & Population Health, Department of Public Health Sciences, Miami VA Medical Center, Geriatrics Research, Education and Clinical Center (GRECC), University of Miami, Miami, FL, USA

Tomas L. Griebling, MD, MPH Department of Urology, The Landon Center on Aging, The University of Kansas School of Medicine, Kansas City, KS, USA

Karen E. Hall, MD, PhD Division of Gastroenterology, Department of Internal Medicine, University of Michigan Healthcare System, Ann Arbor, MI, USA

Rasheeda K. Hall, MD, MBA, MHS Medicine, Duke University Medical Center, Durham, NC, USA

Ahmed Hassan, MD Department of Surgery, The University of Arizona, Tucson, AZ, USA

Kevin P. High, MD, MS Department of Administration, Wake Forest Baptist Health, Medical Center Boulevard, Winston-Salem, NC, USA

Teresita M. Hogan, MD Department of Medicine, Section of Emergency Medicine, and Section of Geriatrics & Palliative Care, University of Chicago Medicine & Biological Sciences, Chicago, IL, USA

Jana D. Illston, MD Division of Urogynecology and Pelvic Reconstructive Surgery, Department of Obstetrics and Gynecology, University of Alabama at Birmingham, Birmingham, AL, USA

Jason Johanning, MD, MS Department of Surgery, University of Nebraska Medical Center, Nebraska Western Iowa VA Medical Center, Omaha, NE, USA

Bellal Joseph, MD, FACS Department of Surgery, The University of Arizona, Tucson, AZ, USA

Matthew Kashima, MD, MPH Department of Otolaryngology Head and Neck Surgery, Johns Hopkins Bayview Medical Center, Baltimore, MD, USA

Stephen L. Kates, MD Department of Orthopaedic Surgery, Virginia Commonwealth University, West Hospital, Richmond, VA, USA

Mark R. Katlic, MD, MMM Center for Geriatric Surgery, Department of Surgery, Sinai Hospital, Baltimore, MD, USA

Thuy T. Koll, MD Geriatric Medicine, University of Nebraska Medical Center, Omaha, NE, USA

Derek A. Kruse, MD Pulmonary, Critical Care, Sleep, and Allergy Division, Department of Internal Medicine, University of Nebraska Medical Center, Omaha, NE, USA

Andrew G. Lee, MD Chair of Ophthalmology, Blanton Eye Institute, Houston Methodist Hospital, Houston, TX, USA

Professor of Ophthalmology, Neurology, and Neurosurgery, Weill Cornell Medicine, New York, NY, USA

Clinical Professor, UTMB (Galveston) and the UTMD Anderson Cancer Center, Houston, TX, USA

Adjunct Professor, Baylor College of Medicine, Houston, TX, USA

Adjunct Professor, University of Iowa Hospitals and Clinics, Iowa City, IA, USA

Adjunct Professor, The University of Buffalo, Buffalo, NY, USA

Jason E. Liebowitz, MD Department of Internal Medicine, Johns Hopkins Bayview, Baltimore, MD, USA

Jason S. Lipof, MD Department of Orthopaedic Surgery and Rehabilitation, University of Rochester Medical Center, Rochester, NY, USA

Joseph M. Malek, MD Division of Urogynecology and Pelvic Reconstructive Surgery, Department of Obstetrics and Gynecology, University of Alabama at Birmingham, Birmingham, AL, USA

Rebecca L. Manno, MD, MHS Department of Internal Medicine, Division of Rheumatology, Johns Hopkins University, Baltimore, MD, USA

Marc S. Piper, MD Division of Gastroenterology, Department of Internal Medicine, University of Michigan Healthcare System, Ann Arbor, MI, USA

Jane F. Potter, MD Harris Professor of Geriatric Medicine, Chief, Division of Geriatrics and Gerontology, Director, Home Instead Center for Successful Aging, Department of Internal Medicine, University of Nebraska Medical Center, Omaha, NE, USA

Michael W. Rich, MD Department of Medicine, Division of Cardiology, Washington University School of Medicine, St. Louis, MO, USA

Holly E. Richter, PhD, MD, FACOG, FACS Division of Urogynecology and Pelvic Reconstructive Surgery, Department of Obstetrics and Gynecology, University of Alabama at Birmingham, Birmingham, AL, USA

Thomas N. Robinson, MD, MS Department of Surgery, Denver VA Medical Center, Denver, CO, USA

Robert Roca, MD, MPH, MBA Sheppard Pratt Health System, Inc., Baltimore, MD, USA

Thomas Spiegel, MD, MBA, MS Department of Medicine, Section of Emergency Medicine, University of Chicago Medicine & Biological Sciences, Chicago, IL, USA

Anna Stepczynski, MD, BSc Division of Geriatrics, General Internal Medicine and Palliative Medicine, Department of Medicine, University of Arizona College of Medicine, Tucson, AZ, USA

Dale C. Strasser, MD Department of Rehabilitation Medicine, Emory University Medical School, Emory Rehabilitation Hospital, Atlanta, GA, USA

Nicole T. Townsend, MD, MS Department of Surgery, School of Medicine, University of Colorado, Aurora, CO, USA

Willy Marcos Valencia, MD, MSc Division of Epidemiology & Population Health, Department of Public Health Sciences, Miami VA Medical Center, Geriatrics Research, Education and Clinical Center (GRECC), University of Miami, Miami, FL, USA

Tejo K. Vemulapalli, MD Division of Inpatient Medicine, Department of Medicine, University of Arizona College of Medicine, Tucson, AZ, USA

Jeremy D. Walston, MD Department of Medicine/Geriatrics, Johns Hopkins Asthma and Allergy Center, Johns Hopkins University, Baltimore, MD, USA

Susan E. Wozniak, MD, MBA Center for Geriatric Surgery, Department of Surgery, Sinai Hospital, Baltimore, MD, USA

Part I

Cross-Cutting Issues

Frailty

Jeremy D. Walston

1.1 Introduction

Frailty is a condition frequently observed in older adults that is a warning sign for high risk of adverse health outcomes. Although exact definitions and screening methods vary, approximately 15 % of the US population over age 65 and living in the community are considered frail, and therefore at significantly higher risk of adverse health outcomes and mortality than more resilient older adults. Clinicians from surgical and medical specialties are increasingly interested in frailty because of its potential to identify those individuals at highest risks for complications related to procedures and medical interventions. This chapter provides an overview of frailty definitions, epidemiology, etiologies, and consequences. In addition, the chapter is meant to provide guidelines as to how best identify and mange frail older adults, and highlight how frailty research can lead to better health care guidelines for the future.

1.2 Conceptualizing and Defining Frailty

Frailty is often conceptualized as a condition of late life decline characterized by weakness, weight loss, fatigue, decline in activity, and accumulating comorbidities [1–4]. It is considered a geriatric syndrome that is associated with aging and characterized by loss of biologic reserve that results in increased vulnerability to a host of adverse outcomes including disability, hospitalization, and death [5, 6]. A 2004 American Geriatrics Society/National Institute on Aging conference on frailty in older adults gave this

definition further specificity as it describes frailty as "a state of increased vulnerability to stressors due to age-related declines in physiologic reserve across neuromuscular, metabolic, and immune systems" [7].

Although many frailty measurement tools have been developed over the past 20 years, two commonly cited conceptual approaches have emerged that have greatly informed and facilitated the development of additional assessment tools (Fig. 1.1). Fried et al proposed a physical/phenotypic approach that conceptualized frailty as a deeply biologic process that results in a syndrome of weakness, weight loss, and slowness [1, 8]. A cycle of physiological decline was hypothesized that included interrelated and reinforcing declines in metabolism, nutrition utilization, and skeletal muscle that in sum drove worsening vulnerability. Triggers of this cycle of decline included acute illnesses, some medications, and aging related biological changes. Importantly, the authors maintain that although this cycle is often related to disability and disease, it can develop independently from disease states and disability because of its hypothesized biological origin. This model was operationalized into a clinical assessment tool for ambulatory older adults that included measures of weight loss, energy levels, muscle strength walking speed, and physical activity. Those who met cut-off criteria in 3, 4, or 5 of these measurements were considered frail. This methodology was validated in many large population cohorts as highly predictive of adverse outcomes. This conceptual basis and assessment approach has been widely adapted by many investigators to develop other physical frailty screening or assessment tools. In addition, many components of the biological underpinnings of frailty have been identified, and intervention strategies have been developed based on this assessment methodology.

Another major theoretical construct for frailty comes from Rockwood et al., who conceptualized frailty as an aggregate of illnesses, disability measures, cognitive and functional declines that has been termed deficit-driven frailty [9]. According to this model, the more deficits or conditions that an individual has, the more frail the individual is. In this

J.D. Walston, MD (✉)
Department of Medicine/Geriatrics, Johns Hopkins Asthma
and Allergy Center, Johns Hopkins University,
5501 Hopkins Bayview Circle, Rm 1.62, Baltimore,
MD 21224, USA
e-mail: jwalston@jhmi.edu

© Springer International Publishing Switzerland 2017
J.R. Burton et al. (eds.), *Geriatrics for Specialists*, DOI 10.1007/978-3-319-31831-8_1

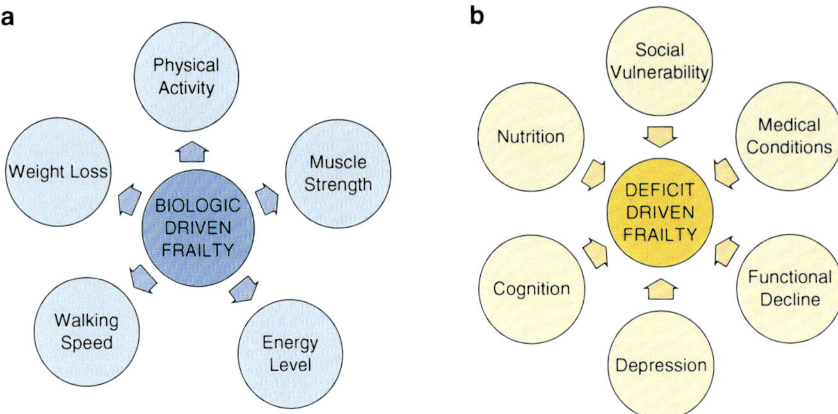

Fig. 1.1 Two conceptualizations of frailty. (**a**) Phenotypic frailty. Phenotypic frailty is conceptualized as a clinical syndrome driven by age-related biologic changes that drive physical characteristics of frailty and eventually, adverse outcomes. (**b**) Deficit accumulation frailty. The deficit model of frailty proposes that frailty is driven by the accumulation of medical, functional, and social deficits, and that a high accumulation of deficits represents accelerated aging. An important distinction between these two conceptualizations of frailty is that biologic driven frailty causes the physical characteristics of frailty (*arrows pointed outward*). In contrast, deficit accumulation frailty is caused by accumulated abnormal clinical characteristics (*arrows pointed inward*) (Adapted from Journal of the American College of Surgeons, Volume 221, Issue 6, Robinson TN, Walston JD, Brummel NE et al., Frailty for Surgeons: Review of a National Institute on Aging Conference on Frailty for Specialists, 1083–1092, Copyright 2015, with permission from Elsevier.)

agnostic approach, almost any conditions or deficits are interchangeable in index tools. This conceptual basis has also been widely utilized to develop risk assessment tools that tally a broad range of comorbid illnesses, mobility and cognitive measures, and environmental factors to capture frailty. Although this concept of deficit-driven frailty has been utilized in many population studies to assess risk for mortality and other adverse health outcomes, biological and intervention studies have been more difficult because of non-specificity in the hypothetical origin in this measure of frailty [10].

Beyond these two approaches, over 70 frailty measurement tools have been cited in the literature [11]. Most have been developed and validated in research population databases. Many have been developed through adaptations to either the phenotypic/physical frailty approach or the index/deficit approach or combinations of the two. Others have been developed to have a cognitive focus. Despite the proliferation of assessment tools in the literature, acceptance of a standardized definition for frailty in clinical practice has been slowed by the broad heterogeneity in measures that include medical, social, cognitive, psychological, and educational factors [12, 13]. Considerations related to chronological age, comorbidities, and disability, while associated with frailty, have also led to lack of consensus of frailty measurement [1, 13–15]. Despite this, many tools are usable for risk assessment and many are being developed for use in disease specific populations such as chronic kidney disease, transplantation candidates, or vascular surgery.

Finally, given the high prevalence of cognitive decline later in life, it is important to consider its potential role in frailty. Frailty is highly associated with an increased risk of mild cognitive impairment and an increased rate of cognitive decline with aging [16, 17]. Conversely, the presence of cognitive impairment increases the likelihood of adverse health outcomes in older adults who meet criteria for physical frailty. Hence, it may be considered an additive risk factor to frailty in those older adults with both conditions.

1.3 Frailty Prevalence, Epidemiology, and Risk

Dozens of population studies of frailty have been developed in the past 15 years [11]. Many have used physical/syndromic frailty or index/deficit type of frailty measures or derivatives to determine the demographics and epidemiology of frailty. Although the prevalence of frailty varies with the tool used to define frailty and with the population studied, most population studies performed in the USA and Canada have estimated that the prevalence of frailty lies between 4 and 16 % in men and women aged 65 and older [1, 18–21]. A large review study using physical frailty measured in 15 studies that included 44,894 participants identified a prevalence of frailty of 9.9 %; when psychosocial aspects were included in the definition, prevalence was 13.6 % among eight studies that included 24,072 participants [22]. Prefrail individuals, generally identified with a physical frailty type tool, are more common in these population studies, with prevalence ranging from 28 to 44 % [1, 20, 21].

As to clinical transition towards frailty, most of the studies have been performed using the physical frailty phenotype.

For example, in a study in the USA of nearly 6000 community-dwelling men aged 65 and older, at an average follow-up of 4.6 years, 54.4% of men who were robust at baseline remained robust, 25.3% became prefrail, and 1.6% became frail. The remaining subjects were accounted for by 5.7% mortality and the remaining 13% were lost to follow-up [21]. Of those individuals who were prefrail, over 10% went on to become frail over the next 3 years.

Demographic associations with frailty include older age [20], lower educational level [20], smoking, unmarried status, depression, and African American or Hispanic ethnicity [10, 21, 23]. A number of chronic disease states, including most especially congestive heart failure, diabetes mellitus, hypertension, and peripheral artery disease [14, 24, 25] are also significantly associated with physical frailty.

Frailty has been widely utilized as a mortality risk assessment tool. Several studies have compared the most commonly utilized screening tools and found that these indices were comparable in predicting risk of adverse health outcomes and mortality [18, 26, 27]. A 2013 consensus conference also referenced tools that can be easily utilized to diagnose frailty [28]. In most studies of physical frailty, the increasing mortality in models adjusted for disease, age, and socioeconomic factors ranges from 2.24 at 3 years in the Cardiovascular Health Study to 6.03 in the Women's Health and Aging Studies 1 and II [1, 19]. In the longitudinal Women's Health Initiative Observational Study, mortality risk was increased over 3 years in those with baseline frailty (HR 1.71; 95% CI 1.48–1.97) [20]. In a study in men, mortality was twice as high for frail, compared with robust, men (HR 2.05; 95% CI 1.55–2.72) [21]. Mortality prediction was demonstrated to be similar across 8 scales of frailty developed within previously collected data in the Survey of Healthy, Aging and Retirement in Europe (SHARE), with death rates three to five times higher in cases classified as frail compared with those not classified as frail in all tools studied [29]. This collective evidence suggests that those who are frail have a 2–6 fold risk of mortality in the subsequent 3 years compared to their robust counterparts.

In addition to mortality, frailty status is predictive of a host of adverse health outcomes. After adjustment for comorbidities, frailty predicted hip fractures (HR 1.74 (1.37–2.22) and disability (HR 5.44 (4.54–6.52) over 3 years in the participants of the Women's Health Initiative [20]. Frailty also predicted adverse outcomes related to renal transplantation, general surgery interventions, and trauma [30, 31].

In surgical populations, frailty predicts adverse outcomes as well. Using a frailty phenotype tool to ascertain frailty, this group measured frailty in a preoperative assessment and found that the frail individuals were at increased risk of postoperative complications (OR 2.54; 95% (I 1.12–5.77), increased length of stay (incidence ratio 1.69; 95% (I 1.28–2.23), and a markedly increased risk of discharge to an institutional care setting such as rehabilitation or nursing home (OR 20.48; 95% (I 5.54–75.68).

1.4 Pathophysiology

There is increasing evidence that dysregulated immune, endocrine, stress, and energy response systems are important to the development of physical frailty. The basis of this dysregulation likely relates to molecular changes associated with aging, genetics, and specific disease states, leading to physiologic impairments and clinical frailty (Fig. 1.2) [7]. Sarcopenia, or age-related loss of skeletal muscle and muscle strength, is a key component of physical frailty. Decline in skeletal muscle function and mass is driven in part by age-related hormonal changes [32–35] and increases in inflammatory pathway activation [36].

Multiple age-related hormonal changes have been associated with frailty. Decreased growth hormone and insulin-like growth factor-1 levels in later life (IGF-1) [32, 37, 38] are associated with lower strength and decreased mobility in a cohort of community-dwelling older women [39]. Decreased levels of the adrenal androgen dehydroepiandrosterone sulfate (DHEA-S) [32] are also lower in frail older adults. DHEA-S plays an important role in maintaining muscle mass and indirectly prevents the activation of inflammatory pathways that also are a component of frailty [40]. Chronically increased cortisol levels [41], especially in the afternoon, are common in frailty and likely impact skeletal muscle and immune system function. Evidence is mixed that lower levels of the reproductive hormones estrogen and testosterone contribute to frailty [42–45]. However, there is stronger evidence that links decreased 25(OH) vitamin D [46] levels to frailty [47, 48].

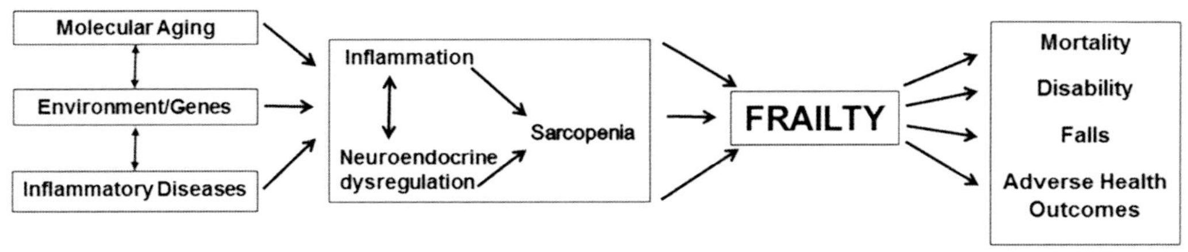

Fig. 1.2 Potential biological etiologies that drive physical frailty and the vulnerability to adverse health outcomes

There is strong evidence linking chronic inflammatory pathway activation to frailty. Serum levels of the proinflammatory cytokine IL-6 and C-reactive protein (CRP), as well as white blood cell and monocyte counts, are elevated in community-dwelling frail older adults [32, 46, 49, 50]. IL-6 acts as a transcription factor and signal transducer that adversely impacts skeletal muscle, appetite, adaptive immune system function, and cognition [51] and contributes to anemia [52, 53]. Immune system activation may trigger the clotting cascade, with a demonstrated association between frailty and clotting markers (factor VIII, fibrinogen, and D-dimer) [49]. Further, there is evidence linking a senescent immune system to chronic CMV infection and frailty [54]. Frail older adults are also less likely to mount an adequate immune response to influenza vaccination, suggesting a biological driver of frailty [55].

Vaccine failure may contribute to the increased vulnerability to influenza and higher levels of influenza infection observed in frail older adults. Finally, there is increasing evidence linking dysregulation in stress response systems to frailty beyond the inflammatory and cortisol component detailed above. For example, dysregulation of the autonomic nervous system [56] and age-related changes in the renin-angiotensin system and in mitochondria likely impact sarcopenia and inflammation, important components of frailty [57]. This dysregulation in stress response systems may be especially relevant to patients undergoing stress surgical procedures, and likely contributes to markedly increased risk of adverse outcomes in frail patients.

1.5 Clinical Assessment of Frailty

Clinical practitioners are increasingly interested in frailty, its definitions, and most importantly how it can be utilized to reduce risk of adverse outcomes and to improve the healthcare of older adults. Although no gold standard has emerged to measure frailty or on how best to use information on frailty once it is obtained, many research and clinical practice groups are moving toward incorporation of frailty measurements into clinical practice. Indeed, the identification of frailty in any clinical practice settings may be helpful in highlighting the need for additional assessment and the need for individualized treatment plans that reduce risk. As part of a movement to incorporate frailty measures into clinical practice, a consensus group of delegates from international and United States societies related to Geriatrics and Gerontology recently recommended that all persons over age 70, those adults with multiple chronic disease states or weight loss exceeding 5 % over a year should be screened for frailty. No one tool was recommended for frailty screen, although several currently available tools described below were highlighted for potential use [58].

1.6 Choosing a Specific Frailty Tool

Few guidelines exist on how to best choose a frailty assessment tool, although a recent publication outlines how most tools have been utilized to date [11]. This is in part because most frailty assessment tools have not been extensively validated or utilized across populations, and few comparison studies have been done that show clear benefit of using one tool over the other. In addition, different tools may or may not be good matches to the intended use. For example, a brief screening tool may be appropriate for risk stratification and decision making related to whether or not to pursue a treatment option. However, a more formal frailty assessment tool that includes physical measurements such as walking speed or grip strength might be required to better define potentially helpful preoperative interventions.

Given the wide array of tools and the wide variety of populations in which the tools may need to be implemented, the choice of which assessment tool to use should be tailored to a clinical situation and clinical need. Choosing a tool that has been previously used in a variety of populations and that has demonstrated predictive validity in several settings should also influence the choice of tools. Considerations of available time in a busy clinical practice may also drive the decision process.

Although not yet available, the development of discipline-specific frailty assessment tools, along with specific clinical guidelines of how best to manage frail older adults after they are identified is of crucial importance as older and more frail individuals are considered for medical and surgical interventions. A recent NIA conference on frailty in clinical practice has helped to formalize recommendations in a variety of clinical settings. The following list of frailty measurement tools, used mostly in the past for risk assessment in population studies, and rationale for their use was recently reviewed by Robinson et al. [59].

1.6.1 Single Item Surrogate Frailty Assessments (2–3 min)

Because of the need for quick and efficient frailty ascertainment in a busy clinical setting, single item measurement tools have been proposed to stand in for a more formal frailty measurement. For example, gait speed measured over a 4 m distance, one of the five measured factors in the physical frailty phenotype assessment discussed below, is recognized as a highly reliable single measurement tool that predicts adverse outcomes [60, 61]. The inability to rise from a chair, walk 10 feet, turn around, and return to sitting in the chair in ≥ 15 s, often termed the timed up and go test, is closely related to both postoperative complications and 1-year mortality [59]. Some of these single measures are components of

Table 1.1 Frail scale questions[a]

Fatigue	Are you fatigued?
Resistance	Can you climb 1 flight of stairs?
Ambulation	Can you walk 1 block?
Illnesses	Greater than 5
Loss of weight	Greater than 5 %

[a]Each question is assigned one point if affirmative. Frailty is considered with three or more points

both the frailty index and frailty phenotype approaches, and although they can be easy to use and predictive of adverse outcomes, they lack sensitivity and specificity of the full frailty assessment tools.

1.6.2 Frail Scale and Study of Osteoporotic Fractures (SOF) Frailty Tool (<5 min)

The Frail Scale was developed as a quick screening tool for frailty and is loosely based on the physical frailty phenotype construct with an additional comorbidity question [62–64]. The Geriatric Advisory Panel of the International Academy of Nutrition and Aging advocates this approach for develop frailty as a case-finding tool [60]. It requires asking five questions and scoring a one for each yes (Table 1.1). Those who are frail score 3, 4, and 5; those who are robust score 0 [63]. The assessment is easy to perform and score, requires no extra measuring device, and has been found to identify those at most risk for adverse outcomes in populations.

Another easy to use screening tool for quick risk assessment is the Study of Osteoporotic Fractures (SOF) frailty tool [26]. Frailty is determined when individuals have two of the following three components.

- Weight loss of 5 % in the last year
- Inability to rise from a chair five times without the use of arms, or
- A "no" response to the question "Do you feel full of energy?"

Both of these tools can be readily deployed in a clinical setting as a way to find high risk patients who may need further assessment.

1.6.3 Physical or Phenotypic Frailty (10 min)

Phenotypic or physical frailty is widely used by frailty researchers and has been widely adapted to measure frailty in many clinical and research settings. As described above in the conceptual basis of frailty, it was designed around the concept of an aggregate loss of function across physiological systems, which is in turn manifested by specific signs and symptoms in frail older adults [1, 8]. This was then operationalized into a clinical exam described below. The tool has been widely validated to predict risk for adverse health outcomes as well as most frailty assessment tools in many different research and clinical settings. It has been especially prominent in the study of the biological basis of frailty, and in the development of interventions focused on the specific components of frailty [65, 66]. This frailty assessment tool was 1 of 2 strategies recognized by the American College of Surgeons/American Geriatric Society's optimal preoperative assessment of the older adult [67]. Although the tool requires a questionnaire, a hand-held dynamometer, and a stopwatch in order to assess for frailty, it takes less than 10 min to perform by a trained clinician/technician. The recent development of comprehensive instructions and a web-based calculator for this tool has made it easier to use and has further reduced the time that it takes to get a frailty score. Access to needed measurement equipment, training guides, and the web-based calculator is available at http://hopkinsfrailtyassessment.org (December 23, 2015).

This clinical phenotype has five components that can be assessed using readily available measurement equipment and a web-based frailty calculator as described below. The score is determined on a 0–5 scale with 0 being not frail; 1–2 prefrail; and 3–5 frail. The severity of the risk is linear.

The major measurement domains include:

1. *Shrinking* (greater than 5 % loss of body weight in the last year).
2. *Weakness* (grip strength of the dominant hand in the lowest 20 % of the age and body mass index (BMI).
3. *Poor endurance* (self-reported exhaustion).
4. *Slowness* (lower 25 % of population average measures 4 m walking time).
5. *Low activity* (assessed by activity questions that identify weekly energy expenditure of less than 383/270 Kcals for males and females, respectively).

1.6.4 Deficit Accumulation or Frailty Index

The most widely recognized deficit accumulation method to measure frailty was developed from the Canadian Health and Aging Study [68].

Between 21 and 70 deficits or comorbidities have been published and recommended for use in this assessment [68, 69]. Although considerable time may be needed to gather information on individual patients and set up an algorithm in a medical record, a frailty index score can be quickly and automatically generated once the electronic record is in place. The frailty index score is calculated as the number of characteristics that are abnormal (or "deficits") divided by the total number of characteristics measured. Scoring has mostly been done by summing the total deficits and comparing to a published cut-off score, or by calculating a ratio between deficits and total number of characteristics. This tool can be accessed in a series of references [69–71] or through the link biomedgerontology.oxfordjournals.org/content/62/7/722.long (December 23, 2015).

1.6.5 Frailty Index Adaptations

Recent adaptations of index-type tools for risk assessment in a variety of clinical settings have been developed. These uses include risk assessment in older trauma patients and in HIV infected individuals [72, 73]. Given that no physical measurements are necessary to calculate an index score, hospitalized and non-ambulatory patients can be assessed using historical data gathered from medical records and perhaps family members. This makes these tools especially valuable for prognostication, and risk assessment for outcomes. Strength of these types of tools includes the fact that each is more specificity related to the condition than other more general tools, which in turn may allow for improved risk assessment and eventually guideline development. However, screening for frailty after acute illness or injury does not facilitate prehabilitation or other risk reduction techniques that may predate hospitalization.

1.6.6 Additional Tools

There are many additional published measures of frailty but to date are not as well studied or as broadly validated [74]. A recent review article identifies dozens and articulates their specific uses over the past decade [11]. Some of these validated tools with specific purposes (clinical risk assessment, intervention prevention) may be identified in select situations.

Chapter 8—Office Tools for Geriatric Assessment contains information on many commonly used instruments.

1.7 Management of Frail Older Adults

Once a frail or prefrail patient is identified there are no succinct guidelines on how to best mange them. However, tenets of the practice of Geriatric Medicine, which include comprehensive geriatric assessment, risk mitigation, advanced planning and delirium prevention should be put in place. Building on these recommendations, and on the frail patient history should focus on energy levels and excessive fatigue, the ability to perform or maintain physical activities like stair climbing, and the ability to get out of the home and walk at least one block.

When considering the diagnosis of frailty, it is crucial to develop a differential diagnosis list and rule out underlying medical or psychological issues that may be driving signs and symptoms of frailty. There are many conditions to be considered in older patients with signs and symptoms of frailty that may in fact be driving the frailty phenotype (Table 1.2).

In addition to the usual tenets of disease focused physical examination, a frailty focused assessment may include an assessment of the patient's ability to rise from a stable, heavy chair five times without the use of arms, and the ability to walk across the room.

1.7.1 Laboratory Testing

When evaluating a frail patient for the first time, laboratory testing should be undertaken in order to rule out treatable conditions. A suggested initial screen, based on the differential diagnosis, might include:

Complete blood count, basic metabolic panel, liver biochemical tests, including albumin, vitamin B12, vitamin D, and TSH.

1.7.2 Establishing Goals of Care

Once a frail older adult is identified goal setting with patients and their families is crucial in providing care, establishing individual priorities, weighing risks and benefits of interventions

Table 1.2 Diseases with symptoms consistent with frailty phenotype that must be ruled out when evaluating a frail patient

Depression	
Cognitive decline	
Malignancy	Lymphoma, multiple myeloma, occult solid tumors
Rheumatologic disease	Polymyalgia rheumatica, vasculitis, rheumatoid arthritis
Endocrinologic disease	Thyroid abnormalities, diabetes mellitus
Cardiovascular disease	Hypertension, heart failure, coronary artery disease, peripheral vascular disease
Renal disease	Renal insufficiency
Hematologic disease	Myelodysplasia, iron deficiency, and pernicious anemia
Nutritional deficits	Vitamin D and other vitamin deficiencies
Neurologic disease	Parkinson disease, vascular dementia, serial lacunar infarcts

and making decisions regarding aggressiveness of care. As the older adult progresses along the frailty spectrum and develops more severe disease and/or disability, it becomes increasingly important to tailor medical care and interventions to the needs of these most vulnerable patients. Potential interventions (see below) that might be beneficial along the continuum of frailty are exercise, nutritional supplementation, comprehensive geriatric assessment, prehabilitation, and reduction treatments.

For robust older patients, the medical practitioner should appropriately treat known chronic diseases, manage intermittent acute illness and events, and assure age-appropriate screening measures and preventive care [75]. In the moderately-to-severely frail patient, a less aggressive approach is often indicated as aggressive screening or intervention for non-life-threatening conditions may be rife with complications. Procedures or hospitalizations may bring about unnecessary burden and decreased quality of life to a patient who already has a high risk of morbidity and mortality [76]. Hence careful conversation and very clear articulation of potential risk is in order for frail patients and their families.

1.8 Interventions

While it is believed that interventions to maximize functional status for older adults in general, such as exercise, can reasonably be applied to patients with frailty, data on specific exercise interventions designed to improve outcomes in patients with frailty are limited. In one trial conducted in community-dwelling frail and prefrail individuals, interventions aimed at cognitive skills (weekly training for 12 weeks followed by fortnightly "booster" sessions for 12 weeks), physical exercise (supervised group exercises 2 days per week for 12 weeks), and nutrition (supplemental iron, calcium, vitamins, and calories), individual or combination interventions improved frailty scores at 3 and 6 months, but did not impact patient-meaningful secondary outcomes (hospitalizations, falls, or performance of activities of daily living) [65]. Another study showed that frail older adults may benefit from interventions targeting specific components of their physical frailty exam. Finally, frail older adults may benefit from an additional comprehensive geriatric assessment where social, psychological, cognitive, functional, and medical issues are identified and proactively addressed [66, 77].

1.8.1 Prehabilitation

In surgical settings, prehabilitation is being developed in order to reduce adverse outcome risk for all patients. Frail patients may benefit the most given their high risk status. Exercise is believed to be the most effective intervention in older adults to improve quality of life and functionality.

The demonstrated benefits of exercise in older adults include increased mobility, enhanced performance of activities of daily living (ADL), improved gait, decreased falls, improved bone mineral density, and increased general well-being. Studies suggest that even the frailest oldest adults are likely to benefit from physical activity at almost any level that can be safely tolerated. For example, a program of resistance training in octogenarian nursing home residents doubled muscle strength, and increased lower extremity muscle size and gait velocity [78] as well as increased mobility and spontaneous physical activity. In another study of resistance training, benefit was reported for exercise activity on as few as 2 days per week [79]. Even simple interventions can be helpful. For example, walking as little as a mile in a 1-week period was associated with a slower progression of functional limitations over a follow-up period of 6 months [80].

While functionally limited or frail individuals may never be able to meet minimum recommended activity levels, even modest activity and muscle strengthening can impact the progression of functional limitations. For these individuals a recommendation of walking for 5 min twice a day as a starting point is reasonable. The identification of a set of key activities the patient feels capable of doing helps incorporate self-efficacy into the physical activity recommendation and makes it more likely to succeed [81].

1.8.2 Nutritional Supplementation

For patients with weight loss as a component of frailty, attention should be focused on medication side effects, depression, difficulties with chewing and swallowing, dependency on others for eating, and the use of unnecessary dietary restrictions (low salt/low fat). In treatment of weight loss, oral nutritional supplements between meals (low-volume, high caloric drinks or puddings) may be helpful in adding protein and calories. A meta-analysis of studies of nutritional supplements showed that providing nutritional supplements to older undernourished adults yielded small gains in weight (2.2 %) [82]. Vitamin D supplementation for those with low serum vitamin D levels is effective for fall prevention, improving balance, and preserving muscle strength [83] and may play a role in preventing or treating frailty. In one report, lower serum levels of 25-hydroxyvitamin D (<20.0 ng/mL) were associated with a higher prevalence of frailty at baseline in a group of 1600 men over age 65, but did not predict greater risk for developing frailty at 4.6 years [84]. Given that vitamin D appears to play an important role in both muscle and nervous tissue maintenance with aging, assessment and supplementation are often indicated. In a recent intervention study that combined protein and vitamin D supplementation, those taking leucine-enriched whey protein plus vitamin D had significant improvement in physical frailty related measurements [85].

1.8.3 Medication Review

Periodic evaluation of a patient's drug regimen is especially important for patients who are prefrail or frail. Such a review may indicate the need for eliminating certain prescription drugs that may be contributing to symptoms of frailty. Changes may include discontinuing a therapy prescribed for an indication that no longer exists, discontinuing therapy with side effects that may be contributing to frailty symptoms, substituting a therapy with a potentially safer agent, changing drug dosage, or adding a new medication. In reviewing medications, it is important to focus on the established goals of care with the patient and caregivers. Chapter 5—Medication Management, provides details on the subject.

1.9 Summary

Frailty is an increasingly recognized clinical state of vulnerability with inherent increased risk for adverse health outcomes, including functional decline and mortality. Although there is no gold standard for diagnosing frailty, there are many tools that are validated and can be used for screening depending on the purpose. The physical frailty and deficit accumulative frailty tools are predominate in the literature. An international consensus group has recommended that all persons over age 70 and adults with chronic disease or weight loss exceeding 5 % over a year be screened for frailty. The Frail Scale is one tool that can be readily incorporated into history-taking and used for a quick risk assessment. However, multiple other validated screening tools have been developed and may be better for subspecialties and for biologic or intervention research. Physical examination should include assessment of the patient's ability to rise from a firm chair five times without the use of arms, and the ability to walk across the room.

Goal setting with patients and their families is crucial in providing care for the frail individual, establishing individual priorities, weighing risks and benefits of interventions and making decisions regarding aggressiveness of care. Exercise and activity interventions have been shown to have a positive impact on even the frailest older adults. To date, no biological or pharmaceutical interventions are recommended for frailty per se, although biologically targeted interventions may play a role in the future.

References

1. Fried LP, Tangen C, Walston J, et al. Frailty in older adults: evidence for a phenotype. J Gerontol. 2001;56A(3):M1–11.
2. Ferrucci L, Guralnik JM, Studenski S, Fried LP, Cutler Jr GB, Walston JD. Designing randomized, controlled trials aimed at preventing or delaying functional decline and disability in frail, older persons: a consensus report. J Am Geriatr Soc. 2004;52(4): 625–34.
3. Chin APM, Dekker JM, Feskens EJ, Schouten EG, Kromhout D. How to select a frail elderly population? A comparison of three working definitions. J Clin Epidemiol. 1999;52(11):1015–21.
4. Cigolle CT, Ofstedal MB, Tian Z, Blaum CS. Comparing models of frailty: the Health and Retirement Study. J Am Geriatr Soc. 2009;57(5):830–9.
5. Clegg A, Young J, Iliffe S, Rikkert MO, Rockwood K. Frailty in elderly people. Lancet. 2013;381(9868):752–62.
6. Rodriguez-Manas L, Feart C, Mann G, et al. Searching for an operational definition of frailty: a Delphi method based consensus statement: the frailty operative definition-consensus conference project. J Gerontol A Biol Sci Med Sci. 2013;68(1):62–7.
7. Walston J, Hadley EC, Ferrucci L, et al. Research agenda for frailty in older adults: toward a better understanding of physiology and etiology: summary from the American Geriatrics Society/National Institute on Aging Research Conference on Frailty in Older Adults. J Am Geriatr Soc. 2006;54(6):991–1001.
8. Fried LP, Walston J. Frailty and failure to thrive. In: Hazzard W, editor. Principles of geriatric medicine and gerontology. New York: McGraw Hill 1998. p. 1387–402.
9. Song X, Mitnitski A, Rockwood K. Prevalence and 10-year outcomes of frailty in older adults in relation to deficit accumulation. J Am Geriatr Soc. 2010;58(4):681–7.
10. Bandeen-Roche K, Seplaki CL, Huang J, et al. Frailty in older adults: a nationally representative profile in the United States. J Gerontol A Biol Sci Med Sci. 2015;70(11):1427–34.
11. Buta B, Walston J, Godino J, et al. Frailty assessment instruments: systematic characterization of the uses and contexts of highly-cited instruments. Ageing Res Rev. 2015;26:53–61.
12. Sternberg SA, Wershof SA, Karunananthan S, Bergman H, Mark CA. The identification of frailty: a systematic literature review. J Am Geriatr Soc. 2011;59(11):2129–38.
13. Hamerman D. Toward an understanding of frailty. Ann Intern Med. 1999;130(11):945–50.
14. Newman AB, Gottdiener JS, Mcburnie MA, et al. Associations of subclinical cardiovascular disease with frailty. J Gerontol A Biol Sci Med Sci. 2001;56(3):M158–66.
15. Walston J. Frailty – the search for underlying causes. Sci Aging Knowledge Environ. 2004;2004(4):e4.
16. Boyle PA, Buchman AS, Wilson RS, Leurgans SE, Bennett DA. Physical frailty is associated with incident mild cognitive impairment in community-based older persons. J Am Geriatr Soc. 2010;58(2):248–55.
17. Robertson DA, Savva GM, Coen RF, Kenny RA. Cognitive function in the prefrailty and frailty syndrome. J Am Geriatr Soc. 2014;62(11):2118–24.
18. Kiely DK, Cupples LA, Lipsitz LA. Validation and comparison of two frailty indexes: the MOBILIZE Boston Study. J Am Geriatr Soc. 2009;57(9):1532–9.
19. Bandeen-Roche K, Xue Q, Ferrucci L, et al. Phenotype of frailty: characterization in the Women's Health and Aging Studies. J Gerontol. 2006;61(3):260–1.
20. Woods NF, LaCroix AZ, Gray SL, et al. Frailty: emergence and consequences in women aged 65 and older in the Women's Health Initiative Observational Study. J Am Geriatr Soc. 2005;53(8): 1321–30.
21. Cawthon PM, Marshall LM, Michael Y, et al. Frailty in older men: prevalence, progression, and relationship with mortality. J Am Geriatr Soc. 2007;55(8):1216–23.
22. Collard RM, Boter H, Schoevers RA, Oude Voshaar RC. Prevalence of frailty in community-dwelling older persons: a systematic review. J Am Geriatr Soc. 2012;60(8):1487–92.
23. Lakey SL, LaCroix AZ, Gray SL, et al. Antidepressant use, depressive symptoms, and incident frailty in women aged 65 and older

from the Women's Health Initiative Observational Study. J Am Geriatr Soc. 2012;60(5):854–61.

24. Kalyani RR, Varadhan R, Weiss CO, Fried LP, Cappola AR. Frailty status and altered glucose-insulin dynamics. J Gerontol A Biol Sci Med Sci. 2011;67(12):1300–6.

25. Blaum CS, Xue QL, Tian J, Semba RD, Fried LP, Walston J. Is hyperglycemia associated with frailty status in older women? J Am Geriatr Soc. 2009;57(5):840–7.

26. Ensrud KE, Ewing SK, Taylor BC, et al. Comparison of 2 frailty indexes for prediction of falls, disability, fractures, and death in older women. Arch Intern Med. 2008;168(4):382–9.

27. Ensrud KE, Ewing SK, Cawthon PM, et al. A comparison of frailty indexes for the prediction of falls, disability, fractures, and mortality in older men. J Am Geriatr Soc. 2009;57(3):492–8.

28. Evenhuis HM, Hermans H, Hilgenkamp TI, Bastiaanse LP, Echteld MA. Frailty and disability in older adults with intellectual disabilities: results from the healthy ageing and intellectual disability study. J Am Geriatr Soc. 2012;60(5):934–8.

29. Theou O, Brothers TD, Mitnitski A, Rockwood K. Operationalization of frailty using eight commonly used scales and comparison of their ability to predict all-cause mortality. J Am Geriatr Soc. 2013;61(9): 1537–51.

30. Makary MA, Segev DL, Pronovost PJ, et al. Frailty as a predictor of surgical outcomes in older patients. J Am Coll Surg. 2010; 210(6):901–8.

31. Garonzik-Wang JM, Govindan P, Grinnan JW, et al. Frailty and delayed graft function in kidney transplant recipients. Arch Surg. 2012;147(2):190–3.

32. Leng SX, Cappola AR, Andersen RE, et al. Serum levels of insulin-like growth factor-I (IGF-I) and dehydroepiandrosterone sulfate (DHEA-S), and their relationships with serum interleukin-6, in the geriatric syndrome of frailty. Aging Clin Exp Res. 2004;16(2):153–7.

33. Valenti G, Denti L, Maggio M, et al. Effect of DHEAS on skeletal muscle over the life span: the InCHIANTI study. J Gerontol A Biol Sci Med Sci. 2004;59(5):466–72.

34. Wang H, Casaburi R, Taylor WE, Aboellail H, Storer TW, Kopple JD. Skeletal muscle mRNA for IGF-IEa, IGF-II, and IGF-I receptor is decreased in sedentary chronic hemodialysis patients. Kidney Int. 2005;68(1):352–61.

35. Morley JE, Baumgartner RN, Roubenoff R, Mayer J, Nair KS. Sarcopenia. J Lab Clin Med. 2001;137(4):231–43.

36. Schaap LA, Pluijm SM, Deeg DJ, et al. Higher inflammatory marker levels in older persons: associations with 5-year change in muscle mass and muscle strength. J Gerontol A Biol Sci Med Sci. 2009;64(11):1183–9.

37. Nass R, Thorner MO. Impact of the GH-cortisol ratio on the age-dependent changes in body composition. Growth Horm IGF Res. 2002;12(3):147–61.

38. Lanfranco F, Gianotti L, Giordano R, Pellegrino M, Maccario M, Arvat E. Ageing, growth hormone and physical performance. J Endocrinol Invest. 2003;26(9):861–72.

39. Cappola AR, Xue QL, Ferrucci L, Guralnik JM, Volpato S, Fried LP. Insulin-like growth factor I and interleukin-6 contribute synergistically to disability and mortality in older women. J Clin Endocrinol Metab. 2003;88(5):2019–25.

40. Schmidt M, Naumann H, Weidler C, Schellenberg M, Anders S, Straub RH. Inflammation and sex hormone metabolism. Ann N Y Acad Sci. 2006;1069:236–46.

41. Varadhan R, Walston J, Cappola AR, Carlson MC, Wand GS, Fried LP. Higher levels and blunted diurnal variation of cortisol in frail older women. J Gerontol A Biol Sci Med Sci. 2008;63(2):190–5.

42. Poehlman ET, Toth MJ, Fishman PS, et al. Sarcopenia in aging humans: the impact of menopause and disease. J Gerontol A Biol Sci Med Sci. 1995;50:73–7.

43. O'Donnell AB, Araujo AB, McKinlay JB. The health of normally aging men: the Massachusetts Male Aging Study (1987–2004). Exp Gerontol. 2004;39(7):975–84.

44. Travison TG, Nguyen AH, Naganathan V, et al. Changes in reproductive hormone concentrations predict the prevalence and progression of the frailty syndrome in older men: the concord health and ageing in men project. J Clin Endocrinol Metab. 2011; 96(8):2464–74.

45. Mohr BA, Bhasin S, Kupelian V, Araujo AB, O'Donnell AB, McKinlay JB. Testosterone, sex hormone-binding globulin, and frailty in older men. J Am Geriatr Soc. 2007;55(4):548–55.

46. Puts MT, Visser M, Twisk JW, Deeg DJ, Lips P. Endocrine and inflammatory markers as predictors of frailty. Clin Endocrinol (Oxf). 2005;63(4):403–11.

47. Halfon M, Phan O, Teta D. Vitamin D: a review on its effects on muscle strength, the risk of fall, and frailty. Biomed Res Int. 2015;2015:953241.

48. Pabst G, Zimmermann AK, Huth C, et al. Association of low 25-hydroxyvitamin D levels with the frailty syndrome in an aged population: results from the KORA-age Augsburg study. J Nutr Health Aging. 2015;19(3):258–64.

49. Walston J, McBurnie MA, Newman A, et al. Frailty and activation of the inflammation and coagulation systems with and without clinical morbidities: results from the Cardiovascular Health Study. Arch Intern Med. 2002;162:2333–41.

50. Leng SX, Xue QL, Tian J, Huang Y, Yeh SH, Fried LP. Associations of neutrophil and monocyte counts with frailty in community-dwelling disabled older women: results from the Women's Health and Aging Studies I. Exp Gerontol. 2009;44(8):511–6.

51. Ershler WB, Keller ET. Age-associated increased interleukin-6 gene expression, late-life diseases, and frailty. Annu Rev Med. 2000;51:245–70.

52. Ershler WB. Biological interactions of aging and anemia: a focus on cytokines. J Am Geriatr Soc. 2003;51(3 Suppl):S18–21.

53. Leng S, Chaves P, Koenig K, Walston J. Serum interleukin-6 and hemoglobin as physiological correlates in the geriatric syndrome of frailty: a pilot study. J Am Geriatr Soc. 2002;50(7):1268–71.

54. Wang GC, Kao WH, Murakami P, et al. Cytomegalovirus infection and the risk of mortality and frailty in older women: a prospective observational cohort study. Am J Epidemiol. 2010;171(10): 1144–52.

55. Yao X, Hamilton RG, Weng NP, et al. Frailty is associated with impairment of vaccine-induced antibody response and increase in post-vaccination influenza infection in community-dwelling older adults. Vaccine. 2011;29(31):5015–21.

56. Varadhan R, Chaves PH, Lipsitz LA, et al. Frailty and impaired cardiac autonomic control: new insights from principal components aggregation of traditional heart rate variability indices. J Gerontol A Biol Sci Med Sci. 2009;64(6):682–7.

57. Burks TN, Andres-Mateos E, Marx R, et al. Losartan restores skeletal muscle remodeling and protects against disuse atrophy in sarcopenia. Sci Transl Med. 2011;3(82):82ra37.

58. Morley JE, Vellas B, van Kan GA, et al. Frailty consensus: a call to action. J Am Med Dir Assoc. 2013;14(6):392–7.

59. Robinson TN, Wu DS, Sauaia A, et al. Slower walking speed forecasts increased postoperative morbidity and 1-year mortality across surgical specialties. Ann Surg. 2013;258(4):582–8.

60. Abellan van KG, Rolland Y, Bergman H, Morley JE, Kritchevsky SB, Vellas B. The I.A.N.A task force on frailty assessment of older people in clinical practice. J Nutr Health Aging. 2008;12(1):29–37.

61. Afilalo J, Eisenberg MJ, Morin JF, et al. Gait speed as an incremental predictor of mortality and major morbidity in elderly patients undergoing cardiac surgery. J Am Coll Cardiol. 2010;56(20): 1668–76.

62. Morley JE, Malmstrom TK, Miller DK. A simple frailty questionnaire (FRAIL) predicts outcomes in middle aged African Americans. J Nutr Health Aging. 2012;16(7):601–8.

63. Woo J, Yu R, Wong M, Yeung F, Wong M, Lum C. Frailty screening in the community using the FRAIL scale. J Am Med Dir Assoc. 2015;16(5):412–9.

64. van Abellan KG, Rolland YM, Morley JE, Vellas B. Frailty: toward a clinical definition. J Am Med Dir Assoc. 2008;9(2):71–2.

65. Ng TP, Feng L, Nyunt MS, et al. Nutritional, physical, cognitive, and combination interventions and frailty reversal among older adults: a randomized controlled trial. Am J Med. 2015;128(11):1225–36.

66. Cameron ID, Fairhall N, Langron C, et al. A multifactorial interdisciplinary intervention reduces frailty in older people: randomized trial. BMC Med. 2013;11:65.

67. Chow WB, Rosenthal RA, Merkow RP, Ko CY, Esnaola NF. Optimal preoperative assessment of the geriatric surgical patient: a best practices guideline from the American College of Surgeons National Surgical Quality Improvement Program and the American Geriatrics Society. J Am Coll Surg. 2012;215(4):453–66.

68. Rockwood K, Song X, MacKnight C, et al. A global clinical measure of fitness and frailty in elderly people. CMAJ. 2005;173(5):489–95.

69. Mitnitski AB, Mogilner AJ, Rockwood K. Accumulation of deficits as a proxy measure of aging. ScientificWorldJournal. 2001;1:323–36.

70. Rockwood K, Mitnitski A. Frailty defined by deficit accumulation and geriatric medicine defined by frailty. Clin Geriatr Med. 2011;27(1):17–26.

71. Theou O, Walston J, Rockwood K. Operationalizing frailty using the frailty phenotype and deficit accumulation approaches. Interdiscip Top Gerontol Geriatr. 2015;41:66–73.

72. Joseph B, Pandit V, Zangbar B, et al. Validating trauma-specific frailty index for geriatric trauma patients: a prospective analysis. J Am Coll Surg. 2014;219(1):10–7.

73. Guaraldi G, Brothers TD, Zona S, et al. A frailty index predicts survival and incident multimorbidity independent of markers of HIV disease severity. AIDS. 2015;29(13):1633–41.

74. Varadhan R, Yao W, Matteini A, et al. Simple biologically informed inflammatory index of two serum cytokines predicts 10 year all-cause mortality in older adults. J Gerontol A Biol Sci Med Sci. 2014;69(2):165–73.

75. Goldberg TH, Chavin SI. Preventive medicine and screening in older adults. J Am Geriatr Soc. 1997;45(3):344–54.

76. Walter LC, Covinsky KE. Cancer screening in elderly patients: a framework for individualized decision making. JAMA. 2001;285(21):2750–6.

77. Turner G, Clegg A. Best practice guidelines for the management of frailty: a British Geriatrics Society, Age UK and Royal College of General Practitioners report. Age Ageing. 2014;43(6):744–7.

78. Fiatarone MA, O'Neill EF, Ryan ND, et al. Exercise training and nutritional supplementation for physical frailty in very elderly people [see comments]. N Engl J Med. 1994;330(25):1769–75.

79. Hunter GR, McCarthy JP, Bamman MM. Effects of resistance training on older adults. Sports Med. 2004;34(5):329–48.

80. Miller ME, Rejeski WJ, Reboussin BA, Ten Have TR, Ettinger WH. Physical activity, functional limitations, and disability in older adults. J Am Geriatr Soc. 2000;48(10):1264–72.

81. McAuley E, Konopack JF, Morris KS, et al. Physical activity and functional limitations in older women: influence of self-efficacy. J Gerontol B Psychol Sci Soc Sci. 2006;61(5):270–7.

82. Milne AC, Potter J, Vivanti A, Avenell A. Protein and energy supplementation in elderly people at risk from malnutrition. Cochrane Database Syst Rev. 2009;2, CD003288.

83. Montero-Odasso M, Duque G. Vitamin D in the aging musculoskeletal system: an authentic strength preserving hormone. Mol Aspects Med. 2005;26(3):203–19.

84. Ensrud KE, Blackwell TL, Cauley JA, et al. Circulating 25-hydroxyvitamin D levels and frailty in older men: the osteoporotic fractures in men study. J Am Geriatr Soc. 2011;59(1):101–6.

85. Bauer JM, Verlaan S, Bautmans I, et al. Effects of a vitamin D and leucine-enriched whey protein nutritional supplement on measures of sarcopenia in older adults, the PROVIDE study: a randomized, double-blind, placebo-controlled trial. J Am Med Dir Assoc. 2015;16(9):740–7.

Delirium

2

Nicole T. Townsend and Thomas N. Robinson

2.1 Introduction

Delirium is a common medical condition that healthcare providers will encounter while caring for older adults, especially in the hospitalized patient. On a general medical service, rates of delirium range from 10 to 40 % [1–3]. Further, up to a quarter of hospitalized patients over age 65 will present with delirium [4]. An additional 30 % of hospitalized patients in this age group will develop delirium acutely during their hospitalization [5]. Familiarity with the clinical syndrome of delirium, identification of which patients are at risk, and knowledge on how to prevent, diagnose, and treat delirium are critical to healthcare professional's ability to provide high quality care of hospitalized older adults.

Delirium is critical to prevent and, should it occur, to recognize early because of its close association with increased morbidity and mortality in the hospitalized patient. Patients who experience delirium have long-term loss of cognitive function, higher complication rates, increased hospital length of stay, and higher mortality. Delirium has recently been recognized as a complex phenotype in older patients that shifts the prevalence focus from chronologic age and medical comorbidities to the functional impact of comorbidities especially frailty (discussed fully in a separate chapter) and disability. While the frail older adult is at higher risk for delirium in the hospitalized setting, any hospitalized patient can develop delirium.

2.2 Delirium Definition

Delirium is defined as a disturbance in attention and awareness, with a change in cognition that occurs over a short period of time (hours to days) and fluctuates during the course of the day. Differentiating preexisting dementia from delirium is critically important. Clinically, delirium presents with inattention, disordered thinking, and loss of orientation, with a component of both agitation and hyperactivity, or, especially in the elderly, with depressed affect and hypoactivity. Patients can appear confused, have hallucinations, be somnolent, or present with all of these symptoms during the course of delirium. Unlike dementia, delirium waxes and wanes over the course of the day, so patients may have normal behavior during one assessment, and be agitated or somnolent the next. Thus, a high level of clinical suspicion is necessary in order to recognize and diagnose a patient with delirium. The hypoactive delirium subtype is widely recognized as the most under-diagnosed presentation of delirium.

2.3 Delirium Risk Factors

The risk of developing delirium following surgery is best described as a relationship between a physiologic stressor, predisposing patient risk factors, and iatrogenic conditions (see Fig. 2.1) [6]. A multitude of risk factors have been identified that increase the chances of the development of delirium; this multiplicity includes both intrinsic patient factors and external precipitating factors during a hospital stay. Risk factors for delirium are multifactorial, and there is a dose-response to the number of risk factors and the odds of developing delirium [7]. Dementia is the most closely associated intrinsic patient vulnerability that increases risk of delirium [8, 9]. The greater the severity of dementia, the greater the risk of developing delirium [10]. Patients with underlying medical conditions associated with frailty such as poor mobility, fatigue, a high level of co-morbid medical conditions [11], and malnutrition [12] also place patients at

N.T. Townsend, MD, MS
Department of Surgery, School of Medicine, University of Colorado, 12631 E 17th Ave, C-305, Aurora, CO 80045, USA

T.N. Robinson, MD, MS (✉)
Department of Surgery, Denver VA Medical Center, 1055 Clermont St (MS 112), Denver, CO 80220, USA
e-mail: thomas.robinson@ucdenver.edu

© Springer International Publishing Switzerland 2017
J.R. Burton et al. (eds.), *Geriatrics for Specialists*, DOI 10.1007/978-3-319-31831-8_2

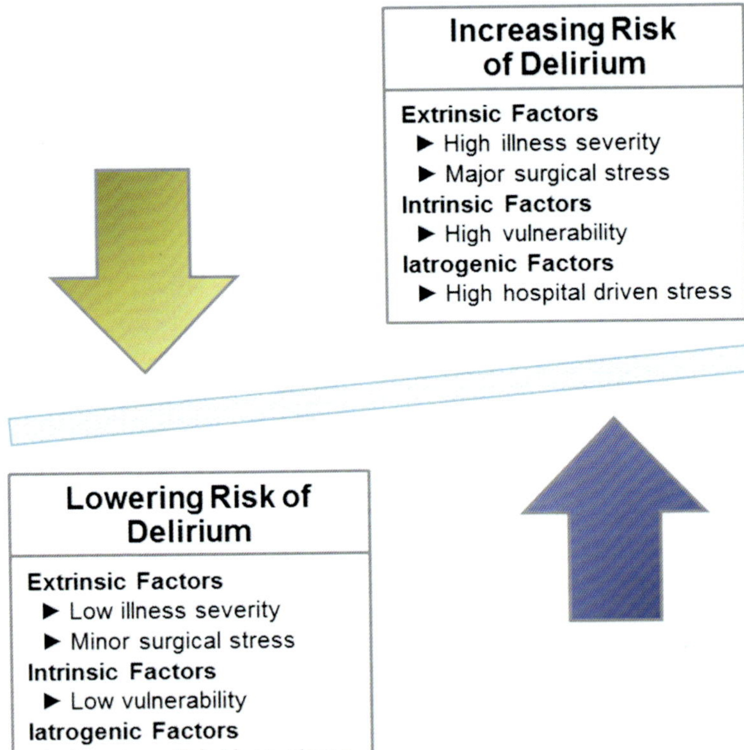

Fig. 2.1 Multifactorial model of delirium. The risk of a delirium is a combination of extrinsic factors to the patient (e.g., severity of medical illness, stress of surgical intervention), intrinsic factors to the patient (e.g., cognitive impairment, advanced age), and iatrogenic factors (e.g., sleep disruption, pain control)

risk for development of delirium [13]. Frail patients can have rates of delirium of up to 60 % [4]. Other intrinsic risk factors include increased age and sensory impairment (visual or hearing) [7].

Routine hospital care introduces external iatrogenic risk factors, including polypharmacy (discussed fully in a separate chapter), disruption of sleep–wake cycles, infection, psychoactive medication prescription (specifically benzodiazepines and anti-cholinergic drugs), physical restraints, use of bladder catheters, and iatrogenic adverse events have all been identified as risk factors for delirium [14]. See Table 2.1 for a summary of delirium risk factors.

Various specialty-specific rates of delirium have been reported that further identify groups of hospitalized patients who are more at risk for the development of delirium. Patients who present to the emergency department or are in the intensive care unit, oncology patients, and patients for multiple surgical specialties (e.g., vascular or orthopedic surgery) can have higher rates of delirium than the average hospitalized adult. Ten percent of patients present to the emergency department with delirium, although this number may under-represent the true incidence [13, 15]. Orthopedic injuries and operations also carry high risk, with 40 % of patients developing delirium after bilateral knee replacement [16] and up to 60 % following hip fracture [17]. Patients undergoing coronary artery bypass grafting have rates of postoperative delirium of 33–50 % [18, 19].

Table 2.1 Risk factors for delirium

Advancing age
Impaired cognition (e.g., dementia)
Severe illness or comorbidity burden
Functional dependence
Infection or sepsis
Hearing or vision impairment
Sleep disturbance
Depression
Poor nutrition
Anemia
Alcohol use
Hypoxia or hypercarbia
Dehydration
Electrolyte abnormalities
Inappropriate medication prescription • >5 new medications • benzodiazepines • anticholinergics • antihistamines • antipsychotics

Intensive care unit (ICU) patients, both medical and surgical, are at extremely high risk of delirium. The prevalence of delirium has been reported to be as high as 80 % [20]. There is, however, dramatic variability in the incidence of delirium in the ICU. Recently, because of the recognition of the risk of delirium, many ICUs have specific pathways for delirium prevention, which can significantly reduce the occurrence of delirium [21, 22]. ICU care is associated with disruption of sleep–wake cycling, high severity of illness, and use of many drugs that are associated with increased risk of delirium, so it is unsurprising these patients are more vulnerable to developing delirium.

2.4 Presentation of Delirium

Delirium is exceptionally heterogeneous in its presentation. The fact that the course of delirium waxes and wanes makes the diagnosis of delirium clinically challenging. This has led to a wide variety of diagnostic tools which can be used to diagnose delirium (see "Diagnostic Tools" section below and Chap. 8, Screening Tools for Geriatric Assessment by Specialists).

While there are several ways to define subtypes of delirium, one of the most commonly used strata is by motor activity, known as hyperactive, hypoactive, and mixed subtypes of delirium (see Fig. 2.2) [23]. The primary distinction between these motor subtypes is the presence of agitation versus lethargy in the patient's clinical presentation. Patients with evidence of both hyperactive and hypoactive delirium are described as having mixed delirium.

There are several checklists (see section below) that identify psychomotor symptoms that are associated with delirium, and when present in combination, increase the specificity of these symptoms to delirium [24]. Hyperactivity in delirium may be associated with increased involuntary movements, restlessness, wandering, increased speed, amount, or volume of speech, inability to sleep, distractibility, combativeness, hallucinations, or tangential thoughts (among others). Hypoactive delirium may present as apathy, decreased activity, decreased speed, amount, or volume of speech, somnolence, or decreased alertness. A mixed subtype presentation occurs when patient symptoms fluctuate between these two categories of agitation and lethargy.

Hypoactive delirium may be under-represented in the epidemiology of delirium because it is difficult to diagnose [25, 26]. A high level of clinical vigilance and suspicion of the diagnosis of delirium is especially necessary to diagnose hypoactive delirium. Hypoactive symptoms may be easy to attribute to other patient health conditions without a high clinical suspicion to monitor for delirium. Further, some studies have demonstrated that postoperative patients with hypoactive delirium have worse prognosis when monitoring 6-month mortality rate [27], although other studies have demonstrated improved outcomes for patients with hypoactive delirium [28].

2.5 Diagnostic Tools for Delirium

There are many diagnostic tools to identify delirium. They can be specifically designed for the ICU patient or other clinical settings, and may focus on certain diagnostic criteria, such as motor subtype. Below are brief descriptions of some commonly used diagnostic tools and comments about specific indications or limitations.

The confusion assessment method (CAM) is the most widely recognized tool to assess delirium and can be completed in under 5 min. [29] It uses four criteria: (1) acute onset of symptoms with fluctuating course, (2) inattention, (3) disorganized thinking, and (4) altered level of consciousness. The first 2 criteria must be present with either the 3rd or the 4th criteria. It has high inter-rater reliability with high accuracy compared to psychiatrist assessment for delirium.

The Delirium Rating Scale-Revised-98 (DRS-R98) is a 16-item scale, of which 13 items score for severity of symptoms. It has high inter-rater reliability, sensitivity, and specificity, including use in patients who have concomitant neurologic disease, such as dementia [30]. It is designed for use by any healthcare professional.

The cognitive test for delirium (CTD) is a diagnostic test specifically designed to assess critically ill hospitalized patients, including patients unable to communicate, such as those who are intubated and sedated [31]. It particularly emphasizes nonverbal domains, specifically visual and auditory symptoms. It is also able to reliably distinguish the difference between delirium and other psychiatric disorders.

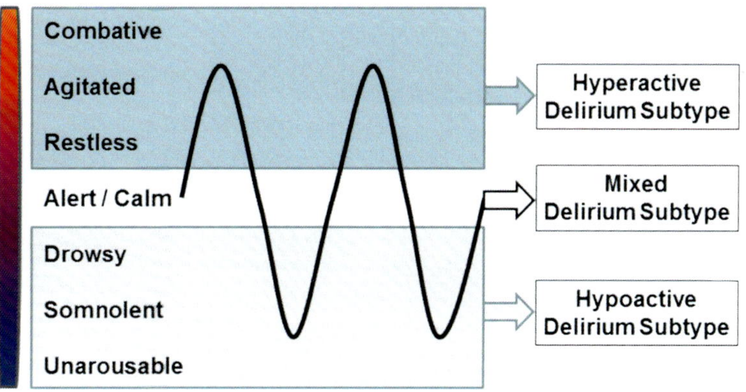

Fig. 2.2 The motor subtypes of delirium. The motor subtypes of delirium include hyperactive (pure overactive state represented in *blue*), hypoactive (pure underactive state represented in *gray*), and mixed (fluctuation between over- and underactive represented by *black line*)

The Delirium Motor Subtype Scale (DMSS) is used specifically to identify features of hyperactive and hypoactive delirium [24]. It is an 11-point scale any healthcare provider can use to assess patient behaviors, and includes 7 hypoactive features and 4 hyperactive features. Two symptoms must be present in order to classify delirium in a specific subtype.

The CAM for the Intensive Care Unit (CAM-ICU) was developed from the CAM assessment to better diagnose patients who are mechanically ventilated [32]. It uses nonverbal assessments to identify the same criteria of acute onset of symptoms with fluctuating course, inattention, and disorganized thinking or altered level of consciousness. It has high levels of sensitivity and specificity for delirium in ventilated patients, although the traditional CAM is more effective in patients able to fully participate in the assessment [20].

The intensive care delirium screening checklist is another test for patients in the ICU setting. It is a brief checklist of eight items based off of DSM criteria of delirium [33]. While it also has high sensitivity for delirium in the ICU, it is less specific than the CAM-ICU method. It is designed for use for all healthcare professionals.

The Memorial Delirium Assessment Scale was specifically developed to monitor development of delirium in ill patients enrolled in clinical trials [34]. It involves a 10-item checklist which was validated in patients with AIDS and metastatic cancer. It is well suited for use in repeated assessments over time for patients being seen longitudinally in trials.

The important issue is that a clinician should be very familiar with one or two of these screening tools and use them in daily practice.

2.6 Medical Evaluation of Delirium

Given the heterogeneous presentation of the clinical syndrome of delirium in combination with the complex intrinsic and iatrogenic precipitating factors, a structured, thorough, and routine approach to evaluation of the patient with delirium is necessary. A hospitalized patient may have presented at admission with delirium or develop it during their hospital course. While it is not only important to recognize the clinical syndrome, it is also important to identify correctable conditions which contributed to the state of delirium. Acute onset of delirium may have developed secondary to a single provocative factor (such as a symptomatic urinary tract infection (UTI), myocardial infarction (MI)), multiple medications (polypharmacy), admission to ICU, and others).

The appropriate workup of delirium involves methodical evaluation of the patient to identify treatable causes as well as initiate behavioral interventions. Table 2.2 outlines a comprehensive workup for patients with acute delirium which should supplement bedside examination. While many of these tests should be considered to be routine in an acute clinical change, others should only be considered if clinically indicated.

2.7 Prevention of Delirium

Although recognition and treatment of delirium once the patient develops the syndrome is essential, interventions to prevent delirium occurrence are essential for all patients at risk for delirium. Identification of individuals with multiple

Table 2.2 Medical evaluation of delirium

	Routinely ordered	Ordered if indicated
Laboratory tests	Complete blood count (infection, anemia) Basic metabolic panel (electrolyte disturbances, acid base status, renal function) Glucose (hypo- or hyper-glycemia) Arterial blood gas (hypoxia or hypercarbia) Urine analysis (infection but asymptomatic bacteriuria is not thought to cause delirium and is very common in older patients, especially women	Troponin (myocardial infarction) Thyroid levels (hypo- or hyper-thyroidism) ESR (inflammation) Viral titers or bacterial cultures (infection) Urine or blood drug screen (intoxication) Thiamine and Vitamin B12 (vitamin deficiency) HIV (infection) Sputum culture Blood culture
Imaging	Chest X-ray (infection)	Head CT (dementia, stroke) Brain MRI (dementia, stroke)
Clinical evaluation	Physical examination Medication review (BEERs list) [52] Social history (alcohol or benzo use)	Remove un-needed catheters
Ancillary tests	EKG (myocardial infarction) Pulse oximetry (hypoxia)	EEG (seizures, metabolic disturbance) Lumbar puncture (meningitis)

risk factors (e.g., frail, elderly, multiple comorbidities) allows the clinician to target preventive interventions to the at-risk population. Interventions such as making sure the patient has full use of their sensory aids, orientation protocols, early mobilization measures, minimization of sleep disturbance, and avoidance or discontinuation of high risk medications can all create an environment that will lower the risk of delirium for the at-risk patient [35]. Daily rounds that address these non-pharmacologic interventions utilize a multidisciplinary care team and plan that creates consistent assessment of these issues. Up to 40 % of hospitalized patients may have preventable delirium [14, 28]. Both of the current clinical practice guideline statements strongly recommend the implementation of multi-component delirium prevention protocols for patients at risk for delirium [35, 36].

Educational programs concerning delirium in every medical center are essential. These programs should be considered a system-level prevention tool. Education of healthcare providers about recognition, prevention, and treatment of delirium consistently reduces episodes of and duration of delirium, regardless of the specific intervention or protocol. [37–39] Further, educational interventions are cost-effective and associated with no patient harm [40–42].

2.8 Treatment of Delirium

When a patient does develop acute delirium, management of a potential underlying reversible cause of the delirium is essential. Appropriate treatment of identifiable causes will improve the patient's clinical condition. However, risks and benefits of aggressive or interventional therapies should be considered when treating a delirious patient, and weighed in the context of their clinical condition and goals of care. See Table 2.3 for modifiable causes of delirium with a proposed intervention. Behavioral modifications have been described above in the section regarding prevention of delirium. Interventions such as encouraging use of sensory aids, establishing day–night cycling, and the other interventions described in the previous section are effective in treating delirium in addition to their role in prevention.

Multiple pharmacologic interventions have been explored both as prophylaxis of delirium and as treatment. At this time, pharmacologic prophylaxis of delirium is not recommended. There are very few randomized, controlled trials exploring pharmacologic prophylaxis. Prophylactic use of epidural anesthesia, donepezil, and tryptophan administration has not been associated with a significant change in incidence or duration of delirium [43–45]. Prophylactic haloperidol is associated with no difference in the incidence of delirium, but has been associated with shorter duration of delirium and hospital length of stay in patients who were identified as being high risk for delirium [46]. Prophylactic haloperidol, however, is not recommended as this drug has its own serious side effects. Melatonin has been found to reduce delirium in both medical and surgical hospitalized patients but these data are not robust enough to recommend its routine use [47, 48].

Pharmacologic treatment of delirium should be reserved only for patients who have failed behavioral interventions and are at significant harm to themselves or others. Pharmacologic treatment typically is an antipsychotic, such

Table 2.3 Factors that cause delirium which can be clinically addressed

Modifiable delirium trigger	Clinical intervention
Immobility	• Ambulate in hallway three times daily • Early physical therapy consultation
Sensory impairments	• Glasses accessible at beside • Hearing aids accessible at beside
Impaired cognition	• Orientation three times daily • Family/friends at bedside
Medications	• Avoid high risk medications/polypharmacy • Daily medication review
Dehydration	• Assess and manage volume status • Adequate hydration
Pain	• Proactively assess and manage pain • Use non-opioid meds if possible
Nutrition	• Proactively encourage nutrition • May require swallowing evaluation
Sleep enhancement	• Allow overnight sleep without interruption • Reduce nighttime noise
Respiratory status	• Assess and manage hypoxia • Assess and manage hypercarbia
Infection	• Recognize delirium as presentation of infection • Work-up infection in delirium evaluation
Iatrogenic causes	• Remove unnecessary catheters/lines • Avoid dark daytime room

as haloperidol, but this treatment should not be universal and is not without risk. There is significant heterogeneity in the study designs and interventions observed in studies on the pharmacologic treatment of delirium. Antipsychotics are associated with adverse outcomes such as an increase in mortality and motor side effects, including the neuro-malignant syndrome. Nonetheless, haloperidol or other anti-psychotics have been used for severe agitated delirium only when behavioral interventions have failed and there is con-cern for patient safety or that of others [35]. Antipsychotic use in the treatment of delirium may improve the symptoms of agitation but does nothing for underlying delirium patho-physiology. If ever prescribed, the clinician should have a plan for tapering and discontinuing antipsychotics as soon as possible and typically within a few days. Benzodiazepines are contraindicated in treatment of the delirious patient and can actually exacerbate and prolong an acute episode of delirium [49].

2.9   Outcomes of Delirium

Delirium is not only a common condition in the hospitalized and elderly patient, it is associated with significantly worse long-term clinical outcomes for patients. Delirium has been associated as an independent predictor of increased morbi-dity and mortality across multiple patient groups, including postoperative patients (gastrointestinal, cardiac, and ortho-pedic), ICU patients, and cancer patients.

In a broad variety of surgical patients, delirium is associ-ated with significant increases in 30-day mortality [50, 51]. It has also been associated with increased 6-month mortality in general surgery and thoracic surgery patients [27]. ICU patients similarly have worsened 6-month survival if they suffered from delirium, independent of other conditions [20].

Delirium is also associated with increased morbidity in addition to increased mortality. Delirium is independently associated with increased ICU length of stay, hospital length of stay, and rate of discharge to an institutional facility [27, 50, 51]. These outcomes, especially the loss of independence with institutional discharge, may be of critical importance to patients and families when discussing prognosis and goals of care in the hospitalized patient with delirium.

2.10   Conclusion

Delirium is a common clinical syndrome in the hospitalized patient, with increasing rates in vulnerable populations, such as the frail, patients with multiple comorbidities, and those in the ICU. Delirium is a clinically heterogeneous condition, with psychomotor changes that can range from extreme agitation that endangers patient and provider safety, to subtle

lethargy that can be difficult to clinically detect. The most effective prevention and treatment of delirium involves mul-tifactorial and multidisciplinary behavioral modifications and medical optimization of underlying conditions. There is no consensus about uniformly effective pharmacologic pro-phylaxis or treatment. Delirium is a high risk condition, which is associated with increased morbidity and mortality, and is a critical syndrome for all healthcare providers to recognize.

References

1. Levkoff S, Cleary P, Liptzin B, Evans DA. Epidemiology of delir-ium: an overview of research issues and findings. Int Psychogeriatr. 1991;3(2):149–67. http://www.ncbi.nlm.nih.gov/pubmed/1811770. Accessed 22 Oct 2015.
2. Trzepacz PT. Delirium. Advances in diagnosis, pathophysiology, and treatment. Psychiatr Clin North Am. 1996;19(3):429–48. http://www.ncbi.nlm.nih.gov/pubmed/8856810. Accessed 22 Oct 2015.
3. Siddiqi N, House AO, Holmes JD. Occurrence and outcome of delirium in medical in-patients: a systematic literature review. Age Ageing. 2006;35(4):350–64. doi:10.1093/ageing/afl005.
4. Francis J, Martin D, Kapoor WN. A prospective study of delirium in hospitalized elderly. JAMA. 1990;263(8):1097–101. http://www.ncbi.nlm.nih.gov/pubmed/2299782. Accessed 22 Oct 2015.
5. Rudberg MA, Pompei P, Foreman MD, Ross RE, Cassel CK. The natural history of delirium in older hospitalized patients: a syndrome of heterogeneity. Age Ageing. 1997;26(3):169–74. http://www.ncbi.nlm.nih.gov/pubmed/9223710. Accessed 22 Oct 2015.
6. Inouye SK, Charpentier PA. Precipitating factors for delirium in hospitalized elderly persons. Predictive model and interrelationship with baseline vulnerability. JAMA. 1996;275(11):852–7. http://www.ncbi.nlm.nih.gov/pubmed/8596223. Accessed 1 Oct 2015.
7. Inouye SK. Delirium in hospitalized older patients: recognition and risk factors. J Geriatr Psychiatry Neurol. 1998;11(3):118–25. dis-cussion 157–158 http://www.ncbi.nlm.nih.gov/pubmed/9894730. Accessed 22 Oct 2015.
8. Elie M, Cole MG, Primeau FJ, Bellavance F. Delirium risk factors in elderly hospitalized patients. J Gen Intern Med. 1998;13(3):204–12. http://www.pubmedcentral.nih.gov/articlerender.fcgi?artid=14 96920&tool=pmcentrez&rendertype=abstract. Accessed 22 Oct 2015.
9. Schor JD, Levkoff SE, Lipsitz LA, et al. Risk factors for delirium in hospitalized elderly. JAMA. 1992;267(6):827–31. http://www.ncbi.nlm.nih.gov/pubmed/1732655. Accessed 22 Oct 2015.
10. Voyer P, Cole MG, McCusker J, Belzile E. Prevalence and symp-toms of delirium superimposed on dementia. Clin Nurs Res. 2006;15(1):46–66. doi:10.1177/1054773805282299.
11. Pompei P, Foreman M, Rudberg MA, Inouye SK, Braund V, Cassel CK. Delirium in hospitalized older persons: outcomes and predic-tors. J Am Geriatr Soc. 1994;42(8):809–15. http://www.ncbi.nlm.nih.gov/pubmed/8046190. Accessed 22 Oct 2015.
12. Inouye SK, Studenski S, Tinetti ME, Kuchel GA. Geriatric syn-dromes: clinical, research, and policy implications of a core geriat-ric concept. J Am Geriatr Soc. 2007;55(5):780–91. doi:10.1111/j.1532-5415.2007.01156.x.
13. Vasilevskis EE, Han JH, Hughes CG, Ely EW. Epidemiology and risk factors for delirium across hospital settings. Best Pract Res Clin Anaesthesiol. 2012;26(3):277–87. doi:10.1016/j.bpa.2012.07.003.

14. Inouye SK, Bogardus ST, Charpentier PA, et al. A multicomponent intervention to prevent delirium in hospitalized older patients. N Engl J Med. 1999;340(9):669–76. doi:10.1056/NEJM 199903043400901.

15. Hustey FM, Meldon SW, Smith MD, Lex CK. The effect of mental status screening on the care of elderly emergency department patients. Ann Emerg Med. 2003;41(5):678–84. doi:10.1067/mem.2003.152.

16. Williams-Russo P, Urquhart BL, Sharrock NE, Charlson ME. Post-operative delirium: predictors and prognosis in elderly orthopedic patients. J Am Geriatr Soc. 1992;40(8):759–67. http://www.ncbi.nlm.nih.gov/pubmed/1634718. Accessed 22 Oct 2015.

17. Holmes J, House A. Psychiatric illness predicts poor outcome after surgery for hip fracture: a prospective cohort study. Psychol Med. 2000;30(4):921–9. http://www.ncbi.nlm.nih.gov/pubmed/11037100. Accessed 22 Oct 2015.

18. Santos FS, Velasco IT, Fráguas R. Risk factors for delirium in the elderly after coronary artery bypass graft surgery. Int Psychogeriatr. 2004;16(2):175–93. http://www.ncbi.nlm.nih.gov/pubmed/15318763. Accessed 22 Oct 2015.

19. Mu D-L, Wang D-X, Li L-H, et al. High serum cortisol level is associated with increased risk of delirium after coronary artery bypass graft surgery: a prospective cohort study. Crit Care. 2010;14(6):R238. doi:10.1186/cc9393.

20. McNicoll L, Pisani MA, Zhang Y, Ely EW, Siegel MD, Inouye SK. Delirium in the intensive care unit: occurrence and clinical course in older patients. J Am Geriatr Soc. 2003;51(5):591–8. http://www.ncbi.nlm.nih.gov/pubmed/12752832. Accessed 22 Oct 2015.

21. Salluh JI, Soares M, Teles JM, et al. Delirium epidemiology in critical care (DECCA): an international study. Crit Care. 2010;14(6):R210. doi:10.1186/cc9333.

22. Pandharipande P, Cotton BA, Shintani A, et al. Prevalence and risk factors for development of delirium in surgical and trauma intensive care unit patients. J Trauma. 2008;65(1):34–41. doi:10.1097/TA.0b013e31814b2c4d.

23. Lipowski ZJ. Delirium in the elderly patient. N Engl J Med. 1989;320(9):578–82. doi:10.1056/NEJM198903023200907.

24. Meagher D, Moran M, Raju B, et al. A new data-based motor subtype schema for delirium. J Neuropsychiatry Clin Neurosci. 2008;20(2):185–93. doi:10.1176/jnp.2008.20.2.185.

25. Liptzin B, Levkoff SE. An empirical study of delirium subtypes. Br J Psychiatry. 1992;161:843–5. http://www.ncbi.nlm.nih.gov/pubmed/1483173. Accessed 22 Oct 2015.

26. Spronk PE, Riekerk B, Hofhuis J, Rommes JH. Occurrence of delirium is severely underestimated in the ICU during daily care. Intensive Care Med. 2009;35(7):1276–80. doi:10.1007/s00134-009-1466-8.

27. Robinson TN, Wallace JI, Wu DS, et al. Accumulated frailty characteristics predict postoperative discharge institutionalization in the geriatric patient. J Am Coll Surg. 2011;213(1):34–7. doi:10.1016/j.jamcollsurg.2011.01.056.

28. Marcantonio E, Ta T, Duthie E, Resnick NM. Delirium severity and psychomotor types: their relationship with outcomes after hip fracture repair. J Am Geriatr Soc. 2002;50(5):850–7. http://www.ncbi.nlm.nih.gov/pubmed/12028171. Accessed 22 Oct 2015.

29. Inouye SK, van Dyck CH, Alessi CA, Balkin S, Siegal AP, Horwitz RI. Clarifying confusion: the confusion assessment method. A new method for detection of delirium. Ann Intern Med. 1990;113(12):941–8. http://www.ncbi.nlm.nih.gov/pubmed/2240918. Accessed 22 Oct 2015.

30. Trzepacz PT, Mittal D, Torres R, Kanary K, Norton J, Jimerson N. Validation of the delirium rating scale-revised-98: comparison with the delirium rating scale and the cognitive test for delirium. J Neuropsychiatry Clin Neurosci. 2001;13(2):229–42. http://www.ncbi.nlm.nih.gov/pubmed/11449030. Accessed 22 Oct 2015.

31. Hart RP, Levenson JL, Sessler CN, Best AM, Schwartz SM, Rutherford LE. Validation of a cognitive test for delirium in medical ICU patients. Psychosomatics. 1996;37(6):533–46. doi:10.1016/S0033-3182(96)71517-7.

32. Ely EW, Margolin R, Francis J, et al. Evaluation of delirium in critically ill patients: validation of the confusion assessment method for the intensive care unit (CAM-ICU). Crit Care Med. 2001;29(7):1370–9. http://www.ncbi.nlm.nih.gov/pubmed/11445689. Accessed 20 July 2015.

33. Bergeron N, Dubois MJ, Dumont M, Dial S, Skrobik Y. Intensive care delirium screening checklist: evaluation of a new screening tool. Intensive Care Med. 2001;27(5):859–64. http://www.ncbi.nlm.nih.gov/pubmed/11430542. Accessed 16 Sep 2015.

34. Breitbart W, Rosenfeld B, Roth A, Smith MJ, Cohen K, Passik S. The memorial delirium assessment scale. J Pain Symptom Manage. 1997;13(3):128–37. http://www.ncbi.nlm.nih.gov/pubmed/9114631. Accessed 12 Oct 2015.

35. Postoperative delirium in older adults: best practice statement from the American geriatrics society. J Am Coll Surg. 2014;220(2):136–148.e1. doi:10.1016/j.jamcollsurg.2014.10.019.

36. Tahir TA, Morgan E, Eeles E. NICE guideline: evidence for pharmacological treatment of delirium. J Psychosom Res. 2011;70(2):197–8. doi:10.1016/j.jpsychores.2010.10.011.

37. Lundström M, Edlund A, Karlsson S, Brännström B, Bucht G, Gustafson Y. A multifactorial intervention program reduces the duration of delirium, length of hospitalization, and mortality in delirious patients. J Am Geriatr Soc. 2005;53(4):622–8. doi:10.1111/j.1532-5415.2005.53210.x.

38. Tabet N, Hudson S, Sweeney V, et al. An educational intervention can prevent delirium on acute medical wards. Age Ageing. 2005;34(2):152–6. doi:10.1093/ageing/afi031.

39. Robinson TN, Eiseman B, Wallace JI, et al. Redefining geriatric preoperative assessment using frailty, disability and co-morbidity. Ann Surg. 2009;250(3):449–55. doi:10.1097/SLA.0b013e3181b45598. pii: 00000658-200909000-00013.

40. Caplan GA, Harper EL. Recruitment of volunteers to improve vitality in the elderly: the REVIVE study. Intern Med J. 2007;37(2):95–100. doi:10.1111/j.1445-5994.2007.01265.x.

41. Rubin FH, Neal K, Fenlon K, Hassan S, Inouye SK. Sustainability and scalability of the hospital elder life program at a community hospital. J Am Geriatr Soc. 2011;59(2):359–65. doi:10.1111/j.1532-5415.2010.03243.x.

42. Rizzo JA, Bogardus ST, Leo-Summers L, Williams CS, Acampora D, Inouye SK. Multicomponent targeted intervention to prevent delirium in hospitalized older patients: what is the economic value? Med Care. 2001;39(7):740–52. http://www.ncbi.nlm.nih.gov/pubmed/11458138. Accessed 22 Oct 2015.

43. Díaz V, Rodríguez J, Barrientos P, et al. [Use of procholinergics in the prevention of postoperative delirium in hip fracture surgery in the elderly. A randomized controlled trial]. Rev Neurol. 33(8):716–9. http://www.ncbi.nlm.nih.gov/pubmed/11784964. Accessed 22 Oct 2015.

44. Liptzin B, Laki A, Garb JL, Fingeroth R, Krushell R. Donepezil in the prevention and treatment of post-surgical delirium. Am J Geriatr Psychiatry. 2005;13(12):1100–6. doi:10.1176/appi.ajgp.13.12.1100.

45. Robinson TN, Dunn CL, Adams JC, et al. Tryptophan supplementation and postoperative delirium – a randomized controlled trial. J Am Geriatr Soc. 2014;62(9):1764–71. doi:10.1111/jgs.12972.

46. Kalisvaart KJ, de Jonghe JFM, Bogaards MJ, et al. Haloperidol prophylaxis for elderly hip-surgery patients at risk for delirium: a randomized placebo-controlled study. J Am Geriatr Soc. 2005;53(10):1658–66. doi:10.1111/j.1532-5415.2005.53503.x.

47. Al-Aama T, Brymer C, Gutmanis I, Woolmore-Goodwin SM, Esbaugh J, Dasgupta M. Melatonin decreases delirium in elderly patients: a randomized, placebo-controlled trial. Int J Geriatr Psychiatry. 2011;26(7):687–94. doi:10.1002/gps.2582.

48. Chen S, Shi L, Liang F, et al. Exogenous melatonin for delirium prevention: a meta-analysis of randomized controlled trials. Mol Neurobiol. 2015. doi:10.1007/s12035-015-9350-8.

49. Marcantonio ER, Juarez G, Goldman L, et al. The relationship of postoperative delirium with psychoactive medications. JAMA. 1994;272(19):1518–22. http://www.ncbi.nlm.nih.gov/pubmed/7966844. Accessed 22 Oct 2015.

50. Gleason LJ, Schmitt EM, Kosar CM, et al. Effect of delirium and other major complications on outcomes after elective surgery in older adults. JAMA Surg. 2015:1. doi:10.1001/jamasurg.2015.2606.

51. Raats JW, van Eijsden WA, Crolla RMPH, Steyerberg EW, van der Laan L. Risk factors and outcomes for postoperative delirium after major surgery in elderly patients. PLoS One. 2015;10(8):e0136071. doi:10.1371/journal.pone.0136071.

52. American Geriatrics Society 2015 updated beers criteria for potentially inappropriate medication use in older adults. J Am Geriatr Soc. 2015;63(11):2227–46. doi:10.1111/jgs.13702.

Preoperative Evaluation

Susan E. Wozniak, JoAnn Coleman, and Mark R. Katlic

3.1 Introduction

As the population continues to age, the spectrum of health care practice is changing. The growth in population is especially evident in the growth of numbers of the "oldest old" (i.e., those over 85 years). It is rare for a surgeon not to encounter the "oldest old" as part of their practice spectrum. This is paralleled by an increase in conditions commonly found in older patients (e.g., atherosclerosis, diabetes, hypertension, degenerative joint disease, age related macular degeneration and cataracts, and cancer).

Some health care facilities have shown impressive outcomes for surgery in the geriatric population, outcomes similar to those in the general population. Remarkably, these similar outcomes have even been seen in complex surgical procedures such as aortic arch replacement [1], pancreaticoduodenectomy [2], gastrectomy [3], hepatectomy [4], and esophagectomy [5]. But even more importantly, there is overwhelming evidence that quality of life can be maintained or improved following surgery [6–9].

However, despite the encouraging nature of these results, age remains an independent risk factor for postoperative morbidity [10, 11] and mortality [12, 13]. Finlayson [13] found increased operative mortality in 70- and 80-year-olds undergoing high-risk cancer operations. This result is emulated in a study of 30,900 colorectal resections in the National Surgery Quality Improvement Program (NSQIP) database

[14]. Postoperative complications are sometimes higher and postoperative length of stay is often longer than that in younger patients [15, 16]. These results remind us there is continued room for quality improvement, a large part of which entails preoperative care uniquely fitted to the needs of geriatric surgical patients.

Perioperative evaluation entails multiple components for a detailed comprehensive preoperative evaluation; permits more informed decision making in recommending a certain surgery; encourages modification of a procedure to an individual patient's needs; and provides critical information regarding a patient's preoperative baseline to the team caring for a patient postoperatively. Thus, it is important to view the patient as an individual, with decisions based on functional rather than chronologic age alone.

Much literature has been published regarding "best" preoperative care for the older patient. Unfortunately no single, validated assessment has been found. The Holy Grail of Geriatric Surgery [17] is a simple, reliable test to assess perioperative risk in a geriatric patient. As the number of surgeries performed on older adults increases, a greater understanding of the unique needs of individual older surgical candidates will develop. Further, this allows expansion and improvement of well vetted best practice guidelines to optimize preoperative geriatric care.

3.2 The ACS/AGS Best Practice Guidelines

Recognizing the unique needs of the aging surgical populace, the American College of Surgeons National Surgical Quality Improvement Program (ACS NSQIP) and the American Geriatrics Society (AGS) partnered to construct best practices guidelines focused on perioperative care of the geriatric surgical patient. A 21-member, multidisciplinary included the ACS Geriatric Surgery Task Force, 14 medical centers, and experts from multiple surgical sub-specialties such as: urology, colorectal surgery, endocrine surgery,

S.E. Wozniak, MD, MBA • J. Coleman, DNP, ACNP, ANP, AOCN, GCN
Center for Geriatric Surgery, Department of Surgery, Sinai Hospital, 2401 West Belvedere Avenue, Hoffberger Building, Suite 42, Baltimore, MD 21215, USA

M.R. Katlic, MD, MMM (✉)
Center for Geriatric Surgery, Department of Surgery, Sinai Hospital, 2401 West Belvedere Avenue, Baltimore, MD 21215, USA
e-mail: mkatlic@lifebridgehealth.org

© Springer International Publishing Switzerland 2017
J.R. Burton et al. (eds.), *Geriatrics for Specialists*, DOI 10.1007/978-3-319-31831-8_3

advanced laparoscopic surgery, surgical oncology, anesthesiology, and geriatric medicine.

A focused, structured literature review (using PubMed) identified clinical trials, practice guidelines, systemic reviews, and meta-analyses published over the last decade. The expert panel reviewed the publications based on strength of evidence, relevance to geriatric patients, endorsement by professional associations, and most recent publications. With the initial search yielding 25,978 citations, a total of 5879 abstracts were screened and ultimately 309 publications chosen as appropriate for the study purposes. The final guidelines summarize evidence-based recommendations for improving preoperative assessment of geriatric patients [18].

Understanding the highlights of a comprehensive perioperative geriatric assessment is essential in providing quality care to the older surgical patient.

3.2.1 Assessing Cognitive Ability and Capacity to Understand

It is important that a patient understand the risks, benefits, and alternatives to surgery before any procedure. A physician must confirm that a patient is able to delineate in their own words basic understanding of a proposed surgical intervention. Legally based criteria to demonstrate decision-making capacity include: (1) the patient can clearly indicate his or her treatment choice; (2) the patient understands the relevant information communicated by the physician; (3) the patient acknowledges his or her medical condition, treatment options, and the likely outcomes, and (4) the patient can engage in a rational discussion about the treatment options [19].

Screening for mild cognitive impairment preoperatively in a patient without known cognitive impairment may identify patients at risk for postoperative complications. For a patient without a known history of mental decline it is recommended to obtain a detailed history and perform a cognitive assessment, such as the Mini-Cog [20]. If cognitive impairment is suspected, referral to a geriatrician or primary care provider should be considered for further workup [21]. It is critical to document a patient's preoperative zcognitive exam as it is often difficult to assess postoperative cognitive impairment without an accurate preoperative baseline.

As Americans are living longer, the proportion showing signs of cognitive impairment and dementia has dramatically increased, especially in those over age 60 [22, 23]. Preexisting cognitive impairment is associated with not only postoperative delirium [24], but also perioperative mortality risk [25], longer hospital stays, and functional decline [26].

Chapters 4 and 6—Psychiatry and Palliative Care have in-depth discussions of competency and decision capacity.

3.2.2 Screening for Depression

Depression in the elderly is not uncommon with major depression found in approximately 1–3 % with 8–16 % showing clinically significant depressive symptoms. [27] Patients with depression have been shown to have a greater level of pain and, in turn, require more postoperative analgesia [28]. Risk factors for depression among geriatric patients include bereavement, female sex, disability, sleep disturbance, and a history of depression. Poor health, living alone, and cognitive impairment have been associated with a higher likelihood of depression [29].

A simple screening test for depression is the Patient Health Questionnaire-225 [30]. Asking: 1. "In the last year, have you ever felt sad, blue, depressed or down for most of the time for at least 2 weeks?" 2. "In the last year, have you ever had a time, lasting at least 2 weeks, when you didn't care or enjoy the things you usually do?" If "yes" is answered to either question, then further evaluation is recommended. It is important to note that the PHQ-2 has not been validated in unique circumstances such as patients with severe medical illnesses, impaired communications skills, or frail elderly patients [30].

Chapters 4 and 8, Psychiatry and Tools of Assessment offer additional information on screening for depression.

3.2.3 Screening for Postoperative Delirium Risk Factors

Delirium is one of the most common postoperative complications in the older surgical population. The incidence of postoperative delirium cited in literature ranges widely, studies citing from 5.1 to 52.2 % [31]. The two strongest predisposing factors for delirium are preexisting cognitive impairment and dementia [32]. Further risk factors that should be considered preoperatively include substance abuse, depression, impaired hearing or vision, polypharmacy, and poor overall functional status.

Postoperative delirium is associated with many complications including greater mortality, decreased functional recovery, longer hospital stay, and higher chance of post-hospitalization institutionalization [24, 31]. Some studies cite up to 40 % incidence of delirium in older, hospitalized adults is preventable [33]. Hence, it is critical to understand a patient's risk factors for delirium and institute evidence-based interventions [34].

Chapter 2—Delirium provides an in-depth discussion of delirium.

3.2.4 Screening for Alcohol or Substance Abuse

Alcohol abuse is fairly common in the elderly population. Blazer et al. found 15.4 % of community-dwelling individuals aged >65 years to show signs of alcohol abuse [25, 35]. Preoperative alcohol abuse and dependence are associated with increased rates of postoperative complications such as wound infection, pneumonia, and sepsis [36, 37].

All patients should be screened for alcohol and substance abuse and if a patient answers "yes" to any of the CAGE questions, perioperative prophylaxis for withdrawal syndromes should be considered. In non-emergent surgeries one should highly consider sending motivated patients to substance abuse specialists [38–39]. Patients with alcohol use disorder may benefit from receiving perioperative vitamin B12, folic acid, thiamine, and other vitamin supplementation [18].

3.2.5 Cardiac and Pulmonary Evaluation

Adverse cardiac outcomes have a higher probability of occurring in older patients [40, 41]. In non-cardiac surgery patients Lee et al. found a 2 % risk of perioperative cardiac complications [42]. For patients with or at risk of cardiac disease, Devereaux et al. found a 3.9 % risk for cardiac complications [43], a rate almost double for high-risk cardiac patients [42, 43]. It is important to risk stratify patients to identify those with an increased chance of cardiac complications to provide appropriate perioperative management by anesthesia and surgeons as well to clearly delineate operative risk to the patient and their family.

The American College of Cardiology and the American Heart Association (ACC/AHA) recommend completing a perioperative cardiac risk assessment on everyone using the ACC/AHA algorithm for non-cardiac surgery to help establish perioperative cardiac risk in non-cardiac surgery patients (complete version is available at ACC/AHA and ESC websites) http://my.americanheart.org/professional/StatementsGuidelines/ByTopic/TopicsA-C/ACCAHA-Joint-Guidelines_UCM_321694_Article.jsp#.Vng5eZoQWJA (accessed 12/21/2015) [44, 45].

Postoperative pulmonary complications are not uncommon and affect postoperative morbidity and mortality in the older patient [46]. In non-cardiac surgery patients, postoperative pulmonary complications average 6.8 % increasing to 15 % in those over age 70 [47]. The *ACS NSQIP Best Practices Guidelines: Prevention of Postoperative Pulmonary Complications* delineates postoperative pulmonary complication risk factors as patient-related and surgery-related factors [48]. Of note, obesity, well-controlled asthma, and diabetes were not considered risk factors [48].

Strategies to prevent postoperative pulmonary complications include perioperative pulmonary function testing in patients with uncontrolled COPD and asthma, smoking cessation, and perioperative incentive spirometer instruction and usage [49–51]. In select patients, chest radiography and pulmonary function tests may also be helpful [48, 51]. Chapter 27 — Pulmonary and Critical Care Medicine provides details of assessing the pulmonary status.

3.2.6 Functional Status, Mobility, and Fall Risk

Consideration of functional status, mobility, and fall risk in a geriatric patient is critical. Functional dependence was the strongest predictor of postoperative 6-month mortality in a prospective review of older patients who underwent major surgery [52]. Impaired mobility in elderly surgical patients has also been associated with increased postoperative delirium [31, 53].

Patients should have their functional status evaluated by assessing their capability to carry out activities of daily living (ADL). A simple screening test includes four questions: 1. "Can you get out of bed or chair by yourself?" 2. "Can you dress and bathe yourself?" 3. "Can you make your own meals?" and 4. "Can you do your own shopping (e.g., for food or at the mall)?" [54, 55]. If a patient answers "no" to any of these questions, then further evaluation should be contemplated. An assessment of formal ADLs and instrumental ADLs can also be performed [56, 57]. It is important to document any identified functional limitations and referral to occupational and/or physical therapy [58, 59]. Particular attention should be paid to possible deficits in hearing, vision, or swallowing as these can impact postoperative recovery. Hearing deficits can affect postoperative delirium, falls, and communication. Gait and mobility can easily be tested using the timed-up-and-go test (TUGT) [60, 61]. Patients having a difficult time rising from a chair or necessitating more than 15 s to finish the test are at a greater risk of falling. Communication with all members of the team caring for the patient is critical along with instituting preventive measures whenever any of these deficits are identified. Chapter 8 — Tools of Assessment has a discussion of tools available to assess functional status.

3.2.7 Frailty

Frailty is a condition characterized by decreased physiologic reserve and vulnerability to stressors, leaving patients with a higher likelihood of experiencing unfortunate outcomes such as a decrease in mobility. In the worst case scenario it may be coupled with frequent hospitalizations, need for higher level of care, and often untimely death. This was validated by Makary and associates specifically in older surgical patients. Makary et al. demonstrated frailty to independently predict increased postoperative adverse events and an increased chance of discharge to an assisted living facility [63]. We are still learning about how to optimally assess frailty and its clinical impact [64, 65]. Chapter 1—Frailty provides a thorough discussion of this condition.

3.2.8 Nutrition Assessment

Rates of malnutrition in elderly communities are surprisingly high. Estimates rate malnutrition for elderly in the community at 5.8 %, nursing homes at 13.8 %, hospitals at 38.7 %, and rehabilitation at 50.5 % [66]. Poor nutrition is associated with infectious complications such as surgical site infections, wound dehiscence, and anastomotic leaks [67].

A nutritional status screen should include documentation of height and weight and calculation of body mass index. A patient should be asked about any unintentional weight loss in the last year. Obtaining a baseline serum albumin and pre-albumin level may also be considered [54, 68].

Nutritional risk should be considered if a patient has a serum albumin <3.0 g/dL (without hepatic or renal involvement), BMI <18.5 kg/m²b, or any inadvertent weight loss of 10–15 % over the past 6 months [69]. Referral to a dietician should be considered for individuals identified at risk for poor nutrition to develop a plan for "preoperative nutritional support." If this is not feasible, it may be helpful to prescribe nutritional supplements when preparing for surgery. The European Society for Clinical Nutrition and Metabolism (ESPEN) summarizes recommendations regarding nutritional support [69–71].

Chapter 8—Tools of Assessment provides more details on assessing nutrition status.

3.2.9 Medication Assessment

Elderly patients are at a high risk for incurring side effects from drugs. Older patients are sensitive to psychoactive effects of medications, especially those often used in the perioperative time period. Narcotics and benzodiazepines may be the cause of postoperative delirium. Chronic kidney disease and impaired renal function are also common in the older population. Ensuring renal dosing of medications is essential to prevent adverse drug side effects. Medication doses should be adjusted for renal function based on glomerular filtration rate (GFR) and not on serum creatinine alone.

Polypharmacy is common in the geriatric population as they have a greater burden of illnesses and disease. Polypharmacy is associated with not only adverse drug reactions but also greater risk of cognitive impairment and mortality [72, 73]. When possible, non-essential medications should be discontinued preoperatively and the addition of new medications should be kept to a minimum [74, 75].

It is essential for medication lists to be reviewed, reconciled, and documented including nonprescription pharmaceuticals such as vitamins, topical agents, herbal supplements, or non-steroidal anti-inflammatory agents [76]. This review can identify medications that should be discontinued or dose-altered prior to surgery. The American Geriatric Society (AGS) Updated Beers Criteria for Potentially Inappropriate Medication Use in Older Adults provides peer-reviewed guidelines regarding medications that should be avoided in the older population [75].

Conversely, it is necessary to continue those medications that are shown to reduce perioperative adverse events such as heart attack and stroke. Following the most current ACC/AHA guidelines for perioperative beta blockers and statins is also essential [44, 58, 77, 78].

Chapter 5—Medication Management provides a detailed discussion of this subject.

3.2.10 Patient and Family Counseling

Over the last decade many more people, including the elderly, are completing advance directives. Without advance directives, physicians rely on health care proxies to make end-of-life decisions for patients. Unfortunately, many never discuss their preferences with their next of kin [79]. Studies also show family members, surrogates, and physicians often fail to accurately predict patients' treatment preferences [80, 81].

It is strongly recommended that as part of preoperative planning a surgeon review if the patient has an advanced directive such as a living will or a durable power of attorney for health care. It is also imperative that a surgeon clearly communicate treatment goals, the expected postoperative course, and any potential complications in words that a patient understands.

Incorporating the appropriate health, language, and educational literacy (along with any written or audiovisual aids for explanation) is paramount in helping the patient and their family/social support system understand the risk and benefits of the proposed surgery. Having the patient along with his family at the same discussions can often be helpful as it allows everyone to hear the same information [82, 83].

Taking the time to understand a patient's family/caregiver and support network can also be beneficial when considering the patient's discharge disposition. Referral to a social worker or case manager should be made if there is concern for inadequate family or social support [84].

3.2.11 Preoperative Testing and Imaging

Preoperative screening tests indicated in the geriatric surgical population include hemoglobin, albumin, and renal function tests [54]. Hemoglobin assessment is important in suspected or known cases of anemia and in surgeries anticipating a large amount of blood loss [85, 86]. Renal function tests are necessary to assess for clearance of any medications (anesthetics, antibiotics, etc.) and as a baseline in patients taking medications that affect renal function such as angiotensin-converting enzyme inhibitors or NSAIDS [87, 88]. Measurement of serum albumin is particularly helpful in patients with multiple chronic conditions, like liver disease and those with malnutrition [89].

In specific geriatric surgical patients other preoperative laboratory tests that are helpful include white blood cell count, electrolytes, and coagulation tests. White blood cell count is helpful in cases of suspected infection or patients at high risk for leukopenia secondary to illness or drugs [51]. Electrolyte studies (e.g., Na, K, Cl, CO_2) are important not only in patients with renal insufficiency but also in patients taking diuretics, ACE inhibitors, and digoxin [51, 54]. Coagulation studies (e.g., PT/INR/PTT) are needed in patients with history of bleeding disorders or anticoagulants.

Preoperative diagnostic tests should be based on each patient's clinical history and physical exam, type of surgery, and comorbidities. Chest X-rays are important in patients >70 years of age with acute or chronic cardiopulmonary disease (e.g., asthma, COPD, and smoking). Electrocardiograms may be indicated in patients with a cardiac history (e.g., previous myocardial infarct, ischemic heart disease, heart failure, and cardiac arrhythmias), renal insufficiency, respiratory disease, or diabetes. In patients scheduled for lung resection or a clinical history of obstructive lung disease, pulmonary function tests can help quantify pulmonary function [47, 90]. Noninvasive stress testing is indicated in patients with increased risk factors who are undergoing intermediate risk or vascular surgeries [91, 92].

3.3 The Complete Meal: Best Practices

The Sinai Center for Geriatric Surgery in Baltimore, MD incorporated all of the ACS NSQIP/AGS Best Practices and have added several others: Charlson Comorbidity Index Score, Adult Fall Risk Assessment, Eastern Cooperative Oncology Group (ECOG) Performance Status, living situation, number of stairs a person can climb, hearing screen, oral/dental screen, tobacco use, pinch grip assessment, Core Healthy Days measures, Zarit Caregiver Burden Interview, and a pre-assessment and post-assessment eyeball score. This evaluation, performed by an experienced nurse practitioner on patients aged ≥75 years prior to any elective surgery, requires 20–30 min beyond a routine history and physical examination. It is performed in the preoperative assessment area. All information is entered into a database within our Cerner® electronic health record, accessible to all who care for the patient.

Problems identified preoperatively lead to more compulsive perioperative care. Alerts are placed in the chart for decreased hearing, fall risk, and potential for postoperative delirium. Patients who fail the mini-Cog are targeted for measures to prevent postoperative delirium. The Care Management Department is notified if a patient's caregiver is found to feel severely burdened preoperatively, as that patient may present a discharge disposition problem and is less likely to return directly home. Surgeons are called if their patient is frail—procedures are rarely cancelled but operations may be modified—or if the patient does not demonstrate understanding of the planned procedure.

The financial commitment for this comprehensive program includes the salary and benefits of the nurse practitioner (who also contributes to the academic and educational mission of the Center), a hand grip strength dynamometer (Jamar®, Sammons Preston Rolyan, Bolingbrook, IL), a screening audiometer (Audioscope®, Welch Allyn, Skaneateles Falls, NY), a pinch gauge dynamometer (Jamar®, Sammons Preston Rolyan, Bolingbrook, IL), information technology support to build the electronic database, and printed material to educate referring physicians. Patients potentially could be billed for a low-level evaluation in order to offset some of the expense.

3.4 The A La Carte Menu: More Practical Considerations

Options exist in a number of areas: the person who performs the evaluation, the location of the evaluation, a more limited dataset of tests, the location of the data, and prospective versus retrospective study.

3.4.1 Who Performs the Evaluation

The Clinical Coordinator of the Center for Geriatric Surgery at Sinai Hospital of Baltimore is a veteran of the Department of Surgery at a major university center, with a Doctorate of Nursing Practice and a Masters in Adulthood and Aging.

Table 3.1 Comprehensive versus limited dataset of tests

Comprehensive	Limited (one from each domain)
CAGE screen for alcohol abuse	*Cognition:*
Cardiac and pulmonary risk factors	Mini-Cog
Frailty, 5-point phenotype assessment	MMSE
ADL	*Frailty:*
IADL	5-point
TUG	Climbing
Nutrition screen	*Function:*
Hearing screen	ECOG
Medication review	ADL
Charlson comorbidity index score	IADL
Advanced directive counseling	
Fall risk assessment	
Performance status, ECOG	
Stair-climbing question	
Living situation	
Quality of life/health rating	
Estimated creatinine clearance/GFR	
Postoperative delirium risk factors	
Caregiver burden interview	
Provider "Gestalt" assessment	
Oral/dental screen	
Pincher strength assessment	

ADL activities of daily living, *CAGE* cut-down, annoyed, guilty, eye-opener, *ECOG* eastern cooperative oncology group performance scale, *GFR* glomerular filtration rate, *IADL* instrumental activities of daily living, *MMSE* Mini mental status examination, *TUG* timed-up-and-go test

However, she has taught others to do our complete evaluation, including residents and other nurse practitioners in the preoperative testing area. The total assessment could readily be performed by a nurse, resident, medical student, physician assistant, or the patient's surgeon.

3.4.2 Location of the Evaluation

The preoperative assessment area is ideal for the geriatric evaluation: many patients are there already for laboratory testing or a routine history and physical examination. However, any clinic or surgeon's office is suitable. The hand grip dynamometer, pinch gauge dynamometer, and screening audiometer are portable (and potentially expendable, see below). The timed-up-and-go, gait speed, mini-Cog, and other tests can be completed anywhere. A hospital or Department of Surgery might decide to pilot the program in one specialty, one division, or one large surgery group.

3.4.3 Dataset for Screening

Screening that assesses general domains of frailty, cognition, and function/performance status gives important details beyond a basic history and physical exam (Table 3.1). The ACS/NSQIP AGS Best Practices guidelines recommend a 5-point test of frailty popularized by Fried and proven valuable in a surgical population [62, 63]. Others, however, have employed simple gait speed or the timed-up-and-go test. A basic screen of cognition is the mini-Cog, which involves a 3-item recall and clock-drawing; this simple test has been correlated with risk of worse postoperative results [20]. Activities of Daily Living (ADL), Instrumental Activities of Daily Living (IADL), and performance status (e.g., Eastern Cooperative Oncology Group score) involve simple questions and assessment. Medication reconciliation and falls risk assessment have become routine in many institutions.

3.4.4 Location of the Data

An electronic health record is optimal for the location of testing results, as it is accessible by all throughout the patient's perioperative course. If the database is constructed with discrete fields, it may be queried subsequently for research or quality improvement purposes. A paper form which follows the patient is also possible, as is a simple addendum to the dictated history and physical examination.

Allowing access to the geriatric preoperative assessment allows not only the surgical management team but also physical therapy, occupational therapy, nursing and social workers to understand more clearly the patient's baseline. Physical and occupational therapy are able to better gauge a patient's preoperative activity status as physician admission notes often do not contain important information regarding details covered in a geriatric preoperative assessment. Social workers can often anticipate in advance what additional services may need to be obtained for the patient prior to discharge.

3.5 Best Practice Versus Reality

Recognizing that this comprehensive evaluation would require significant time and resources, the authors nevertheless believe that those burdens would be offset by the benefits of identifying high-risk individuals, improving communication between surgeon and patient, and potentially preventing adverse events.

The Sinai Center for Geriatric Surgery is a new initiative. Currently data about its impact and improvement of surgical outcomes is accumulating, is being entered into national databases, and ultimately will be submitted for publication. However, early impressions about the benefit of this program can be shared. Selected observations follow:

1. Preliminary data from the program revealed 20 % of elective geriatric patients, without a known history of cognitive impairment, displayed mild cognitive impairment

and, therefore, were more prone to have postoperative delirium. This led to brochure now being developed for patients and family to educate them about postoperative delirium.

2. A documented mental status baseline has helped postoperative care providers like anesthesiologists, intensivists, and consultants appreciate postoperative changes more reliably.

3. A few patients were found to not understand the information that was given to them by the surgeon and/or his/her team due to either not hearing the information correctly from an unknown hearing deficit or needing more basic explanation of the procedure. Surgeons were informed and typically they have more information about the proposed surgery.

4. Identifying a hearing deficit has alerted postoperative caregivers to know from which side to speak to a patient or ensure a patient's hearing aids are available postoperatively. Nurses have been particularly responsive to this extensive preoperative assessment as they have had an easier time communicating with patients postoperatively knowing in advance of hearing deficits and to take measures to optimize communication.

5. Case management has been called for a number of patients without identified caregivers to help plan more effectively for discharge by helping to establish a caregiver such as an unaware relative, neighbor, a friend, or church member. This on occasion has prevented postsurgical transfer to a nursing home or rehabilitation center.

6. Surgeons including faculty and trainees at Sinai Hospital of Baltimore generally have been responsive to the preoperative evaluation of the Geriatric Surgical Center and report a positive impact in their patient's postsurgical course.

3.6 Conclusion

The older preoperative patient benefits from an assessment that includes more than a routine physical examination and electrocardiogram. Such an assessment includes domains likely to affect the elderly: cognition, functionality, frailty, polypharmacy, nutrition, and social support. This fosters decisions based on functional age rather than chronologic age and on each patient as a unique individual.

One such assessment is that promulgated by the ACS NSQIP/AGS Best Practices Guideline. If this comprehensive evaluation is considered impractical for an institution or surgeon's office, a limited dataset of tests will still be valuable. Any opportunity to improve results in the growing population of older surgical patients should not be missed.

References

1. Shah PJ, Estrera AL, Miller 3rd CC, et al. Analysis of ascending and transverse aortic arch repair in octogenarians. Ann Thorac Surg. 2008;86(3):774–9.
2. Hatzaras I, Schmidt C, Klemanski D, et al. Pancreatic resection in the octogenarian: a safe option for pancreatic malignancy. J Am Coll Surg. 2011;212(3):373–7.
3. Kunisaki C, Akiyama H, Nomura M, et al. Comparison of surgical outcomes of gastric cancer in elderly and middle-aged patients. Am J Surg. 2006;191(2):216–24.
4. Menon KV, Al-Mukhtar A, Aldouri A, Prasad RK, Lodge PA, Toogood GJ. Outcomes after major hepatectomy in elderly patients. J Am Coll Surg. 2006;203(5):677–83.
5. Ruol A, Portale G, Zaninotto G, et al. Results of esophagectomy for esophageal cancer in elderly patients: age has little influence on outcome and survival. J Thorac Cardiovasc Surg. 2007;133(5):1186–92.
6. Amemiya T, Oda K, Ando M, et al. Activities of daily living and quality of life of elderly patients after elective surgery for gastric and colorectal cancers. Ann Surg. 2007;246(2):222–8.
7. Zierer A, Melby SJ, Lubahn JG, Sicard GA, Damiano Jr RJ, Moon MR. Elective surgery for thoracic aortic aneurysms: late functional status and quality of life. Ann Thorac Surg. 2006;82(2):573–8.
8. Huber CH, Goeber V, Berdat P, Carrel T, Eckstein F. Benefits of cardiac surgery in octogenarians—a postoperative quality of life assessment. Eur J Cardiothorac Surg. 2007;31(6):1099–105.
9. Moller A, Sartipy U. Changes in quality of life after lung surgery in old and young patients: are they similar? World J Surg. 2010;34(4):684–91.
10. Ngaage DL, Cowen ME, Griffin S, Guvendik L, Cale AR. Early neurological complications after coronary artery bypass grafting and valve surgery in octogenarians. Eur J Cardiothorac Surg. 2008;33(4):653–9.
11. Leo F, Scanagatta P, Baglio P, et al. The risk of pneumonectomy over the age of 70. A case-control study. Eur J Cardiothorac Surg. 2007;31(5):780–2.
12. Turrentine FE, Wang H, Simpson VB, Jones RS. Surgical risk factors, morbidity, and mortality in elderly patients. J Am Coll Surg. 2006;203(6):865–77.
13. Finlayson E, Fan Z, Birkmeyer JD. Outcomes in octogenarians undergoing high-risk cancer operation: a national study. J Am Coll Surg. 2007;205(6):729–34.
14. Kiran RP, Attaluri V, Hammel J, Church J. A novel nomogram accurately quantifies the risk of mortality in elderly patients undergoing colorectal surgery. Ann Surg. 2013;257(5):905–8.
15. Barnett SD, Halpin LS, Speir AM, et al. Postoperative complications among octogenarians after cardiovascular surgery. Ann Thorac Surg. 2003;76(3):726–31.
16. Jarvinen O, Huhtala H, Laurikka J, Tarkka MR. Higher age predicts adverse outcome and readmission after coronary artery bypass grafting. World J Surg. 2003;27(12):1317–22.
17. Katlic MR. The holy grail of geriatric surgery. Ann Surg. 2013;257(6):1005–6.
18. Chow WB, Rosenthal RA, Merkow RP, Ko CY, Esnaola NF. Optimal preoperative assessment of the geriatric surgical patient: a best practices guideline from the American College of Surgeons National Surgical Quality Improvement Program and the American Geriatrics Society. J Am Coll Surg. 2012;215(4):453–66.
19. Appelbaum PS. Clinical practice. Assessment of patients' competence to consent to treatment. N Engl J Med. 2007;357:1834–40.
20. Borson S, Scanlan J, Brush M, et al. The Mini-Cog: a cognitive 'vital signs' measure for dementia screening in multi-lingual elderly. Int J Geriatr Psychiatry. 2000;15:1021–7.

21. Knopman DS, Boeve BF, Petersen RC. Essentials of the proper diagnoses of mild cognitive impairment, dementia, and major subtypes of dementia. Mayo Clin Proc. 2003;78:1290–308.

22. Brookmeyer R, Evans DA, Hebert L, et al. National estimates of the prevalence of Alzheimer's disease in the United States. Alzheimers Dement. 2011;7:61–73.

23. Plassman BL, Langa KM, Fisher GG, et al. Prevalence of cognitive impairment without dementia in the United States. Ann Intern Med. 2008;148:427–34.

24. Ansaloni L, Catena F, Chattat R, et al. Risk factors and incidence of postoperative delirium in elderly patients after elective and emergency surgery. Br J Surg. 2010;97:273–80.

25. Robinson TN, Raeburn CD, Tran ZV, et al. Postoperative delirium in the elderly: risk factors and outcomes. Ann Surg. 2009;249:173–8.

26. Rudolph JL, Inouye SK, Jones RN, et al. Delirium: an independent predictor of functional decline after cardiac surgery. J Am Geriatr Soc. 2010;58:643–9.

27. Steffens DC, Fisher GG, Langa KM, et al. Prevalence of depression among older Americans: the aging, demographics and memory study. Int Psychogeriatr. 2009;21:879–88.

28. Taenzer P, Melzack R, Jeans ME. Influence of psychological factors on postoperative pain, mood and analgesic requirements. Pain. 1986;24:331–42.

29. Cole MG, Dendukuri N. Risk factors for depression among elderly community subjects: a systematic review and metaanalysis. Am J Psychiatry. 2003;160:1147–56.

30. Li C, Friedman B, Conwell Y, Fiscella K. Validity of the Patient Health Questionnaire 2 (PHQ-2) in identifying major depression in older people. J Am Geriatr Soc. 2007;55:596–602.

31. Dasgupta M, Dumbrell AC. Preoperative risk assessment for delirium after noncardiac surgery: a systematic review. J Am Geriatr Soc. 2006;54:1578–89.

32. Marcantonio ER, Juarez G, Goldman L, et al. The relationship of postoperative delirium with psychoactive medications. JAMA. 1994;272:1518–22.

33. Inouye SK, Bogardus ST Jr, Charpentier PA, et al. A multicomponent intervention to prevent delirium in hospitalized older patients. N Engl J Med. 1999;340:669–76.

34. American geriatrics society abstracted clinical practice guideline for postoperative delirium in older adults. J Am Geriatr Soc. 2015;63:142–50.

35. Blazer DG, Wu LT. The epidemiology of alcohol use disorders and sub-threshold dependence in a middle-aged and elderly community sample. Am J Geriatr Psychiatry. 2011;19(8):685–94.

36. Nath B, Li Y, Carroll JE, et al. Alcohol exposure as a risk factor for adverse outcomes in elective surgery. J Gastrointest Surg. 2010;14:1732–41.

37. Tonnesen H, Kehlet H. Preoperative alcoholism and postoperative morbidity. Br J Surg. 1999;86:869–74.

38. Hinkin CH, Castellon SA, Dickson-Fuhrman E, et al. Screening for drug and alcohol abuse among older adults using a modified version of the CAGE. Am J Addict. 2001;10:319–26.

39. Berks J, McCormick R. Screening for alcohol misuse in elderly primary care patients: a systematic literature review. Int Psychogeriatr. 2008;20:1090–103.

40. Gal J, Bogar L, Acsady G, et al. Cardiac risk reduction in noncardiac surgery: the role of anaesthesia and monitoring techniques. Eur J Anaesthesiol. 2006;23:641–8.

41. Davenport DL, Ferraris VA, Hosokawa P, et al. Multivariable predictors of postoperative cardiac adverse events after general and vascular surgery: results from the patient safety in surgery study. J Am Coll Surg. 2007;204:1199–210.

42. Lee TH, Marcantonio ER, Mangione CM, et al. Derivation and prospective validation of a simple index for prediction of cardiac risk of major noncardiac surgery. Circulation. 1999;100:1043–9.

43. Devereaux PJ, Goldman L, Cook DJ, et al. Perioperative cardiac events in patients undergoing noncardiac surgery: a review of the magnitude of the problem, the pathophysiology of the events and methods to estimate and communicate risk. CMAJ. 2005;173(6):627–34.

44. Fleischmann KE, Beckman JA, Buller CE, et al. ACCF/AHA focused update on perioperative beta blockade. J Am Coll Cardiol. 2009;54:2102–28.

45. Wijeysundera DN, Duncan D, Nkonde-Price C, Virani SS, Washam JB, Fleischmann KE, et al. ACC/AHA Task Force Members. Perioperative beta blockade in noncardiac surgery: a systematic review for the 2014 ACC/AHA guideline on perioperative cardiovascular evaluation and management of patients undergoing noncardiac surgery: a report of the American College of Cardiology/American Heart Association Task Force on Practice Guidelines. Circulation. 2014;130(24):2246–64.

46. Johnson RG, Arozullah AM, Neumayer L, et al. Multivariable predictors of postoperative respiratory failure after general and vascular surgery: results from the patient safety in surgery study. J Am Coll Surg. 2007;204:1188–98.

47. Smetana GW, Lawrence VA, Cornell JE. Preoperative pulmonary risk stratification for noncardiothoracic surgery: systematic review for the American College of Physicians. Ann Intern Med. 2006;144:581–95.

48. Roberts J, Lawrence VA, Esnaola NF. ACS NSQIP best practices guidelines: prevention of postoperative pulmonary complications. Chicago: American College of Surgeons; 2010.

49. Smetana GW. Postoperative pulmonary complications: an update on risk assessment and reduction. Cleve Clin J Med. 2009;76:S60–5.

50. Doyle RL. Assessing and modifying the risk of postoperative pulmonary complications. Chest. 1999;115:77S–81.

51. Smetana GW, Macpherson DS. The case against routine preoperative laboratory testing. Med Clin North Am. 2003;87:7–40.

52. Robinson TN, Eiseman B, Wallace JI, et al. Redefining geriatric preoperative assessment using frailty, disability and comorbidity. Ann Surg. 2009;250:449–55.

53. Brouquet A1, Cudennec T, Benoist S. Impaired mobility, ASA status and administration of tramadol are risk factors for postoperative delirium in patients aged 75 years or more after major abdominal surgery. Ann Surg. 2010;251(4):759–65.

54. Woolger JM. Preoperative testing and medication management. Clin Geriatr Med. 2008;24:573–83. vii.

55. Lachs MS, Feinstein AR, Cooney Jr LM, et al. A simple procedure for general screening for functional disability in elderly patients. Ann Intern Med. 1990;112:699–706.

56. Katz S, Downs TD, Cash HR, Grotz RC. Progress in development of the index of ADL. Gerontologist. 1970;10:20–30.

57. Lawton MP, Brody EM. Assessment of older people: selfmaintaining and instrumental activities of daily living. Gerontologist. 1969;9:179–86.

58. Carli F, Scheede-Bergdahl C. Prehabilitation to enhance perioperative care. Anesthesiol Clin. 2015;33(1):17–33.

59. Santa Mina D, Clarke H, Ritvo P, Leung YW, Matthew AG, Katz J, Trachtenberg J, Alibhai SM. Effect of total-body prehabilitation on postoperative outcomes: a systematic review and meta-analysis. Physiotherapy. 2014;100(3):196–207.

60. Gunter KB, White KN, Hayes WC, Snow CM. Functional mobility discriminates nonfallers from one-time and frequent fallers. J Gerontol A Biol Sci Med Sci. 2000;55:672–6.

61. Podsiadlo D, Richardson S. The timed "Up & Go": a test of basic functional mobility for frail elderly persons. J Am Geriatr Soc. 1991;39:142–8.

62. Fried LP, Ferrucci L, Darer J, et al. Untangling the concepts of disability, frailty, and comorbidity: implications for improved targeting and care. J Gerontol A Biol Sci Med Sci. 2004;59:255–63.

63. Makary MA, Segev DL, Pronovost PJ, et al. Frailty as a predictor of surgical outcomes in older patients. J Am Coll Surg. 2010; 210:901–8.

64. Clegg A, Rogers L, Young J. Diagnostic test accuracy of simple instruments for identifying frailty in community-dwelling older people: a systematic review. Age Ageing. 2015;44(1):148–52.

65. Sternberg SA, Wershof Schwartz A, Karunananthan S, Bergman H, Mark CA. The identification of frailty: a systematic literature review. J Am Geriatr Soc. 2011;59(11):2129–38.

66. Kaiser MJ, Bauer JM, Ramsch C, et al. Frequency of malnutrition in older adults: a multinational perspective using the mini nutritional assessment. J Am Geriatr Soc. 2010;58:1734–8.

67. Schiesser M, Kirchhoff P, Muller MK, et al. The correlation of nutrition risk index, nutrition risk score, and bioimpedance analysis with postoperative complications in patients undergoing gastrointestinal surgery. Surgery. 2009;145:519–26.

68. McGory ML, Kao KK, Shekelle PG, et al. Developing quality indicators for elderly surgical patients. Ann Surg. 2009;250:338–47.

69. Weimann A, Braga M, Harsanyi L, et al. ESPEN guidelines on enteral nutrition: surgery including organ transplantation. Clin Nutr. 2006;25:224–44.

70. Braga M, Ljungqvist O, Soeters P, et al. ESPEN guidelines on parenteral nutrition: surgery. Clin Nutr. 2009;28:378–86.

71. Deutz NE, Bauer JM, Barazzoni R, et al. Protein intake and exercise for optimal muscle function with aging: recommendations from the ESPEN expert group. Clin Nutr. 2014;33(6):929–36.

72. Barnett SR. Polypharmacy and perioperative medications in the elderly. Anesthesiol Clin. 2009;27:377–89.

73. Silveira MJ, Kim SY, Langa KM. Advance directives and outcomes of surrogate decision making before death. N Engl J Med. 2010;362:1211–8.

74. Charlesworth CJ, Smit E, Lee DS, Akramadhan F, Odden MC. Polypharmacy among adults aged 65 years and older in the United States: 1998–2010. J Gerontol A Biol Sci Med Sci. 2015; 70(8):989–95.

75. Steinman MA, Beizer JL, DuBeau CE, Laird RD, Lundebjerg NE, Mulhausen P. How to use the American Geriatrics Society 2015 beers criteria—a guide for patients, clinicians, health systems, and payors. J Am Geriatr Soc. 2015 – Beers criteria in AGS.

76. Whinney C. Perioperative medication management: general principles and practical applications. Cleve Clin J Med. 2009;76: S126–32.

77. Biccard BM, Sear JW, Foex P. Statin therapy: a potentially useful peri-operative intervention in patients with cardiovascular disease. Anaesthesia. 2005;60:1106–14.

78. Wijeysundera DN, Duncan D, Nkonde-Price C, Virani SS, Washam JB, Fleischmann KE, Fleisher LA. Perioperative beta blockade in noncardiac surgery: a systematic review for the 2014 ACC/AHA guideline on perioperative cardiovascular evaluation and management of patients undergoing noncardiac surgery: a report of the American College of Cardiology/American Heart Association Task Force on practice guidelines. J Am Coll Cardiol. 2014;64(22): 2406–25.

79. Seckler AB, Meier DE, Mulvihill M, Paris BE. Substituted judgment: how accurate are proxy predictions? Ann Intern Med. 1991;115:92–8.

80. Kossman DA. Prevalence, views, and impact of advance directives among older adults. J Gerontol Nurs. 2014;40(7):44–50.

81. Goede M, Wheeler M. Advance directives, living wills, and futility in perioperative care. Surg Clin North Am. 2015;95(2):443–51.

82. Pugliese OT, Solari JL, Ferreres AR. The extent of surgical patients' understanding. World J Surg. 2014;38(7):1605–9.

83. Sherlock A, Browne S. Patients' recollection and understanding of informed consent: a literature review. ANZ J Surg. 2014;84(4): 207–10.

84. Al-Zahrani R, Bashihab R, Ahmed AE, Alkhodair R, Al-Khateeb S. The prevalence of psychological impact on caregivers of hospitalized patients: the forgotten part of the equation. Qatar Med J. 2015;1:3.

85. Smilowitz NR, Oberweis BS, Nukala S, et al. Association between Anemia, bleeding and transfusion with long-term mortality following non-cardiac surgery. Am J Med. 2015;15 [Epub ahead of print].

86. Douglas WG, Uffort E, Denning D. Transfusion and management of surgical patients with hematologic disorders. Surg Clin North Am. 2015;95(2):367–77.

87. Levey AS, Becker C, Inker LA. Glomerular filtration rate and albuminuria for detection and staging of acute and chronic kidney disease in adults: a systematic review. JAMA. 2015;313(8):837–46.

88. Wasung ME, Chawla LS, Madero M. Biomarkers of renal function, which and when? Clin Chim Acta. 2015;438:350–7.

89. Rocha NP, Fortes RC. Total lymphocyte count and serum albumin as predictors of nutritional risk in surgical patients. Arq Bras Cir Dig. 2015;28(3):193–6.

90. Qaseem T. Risk assessment for and strategies to reduce perioperative pulmonary complications. Ann Intern Med. 2006;145:553. author reply 553.

91. Holt NF. Perioperative cardiac risk reduction. Am Fam Physician. 2012;85(3):239–46.

92. Fleisher LA, Fleischmann KE, Auerbach AD, et al. 2014 ACC/AHA guideline on perioperative cardiovascular evaluation and management of patients undergoing noncardiac surgery: executive summary: a report of the American College of Cardiology/American Heart Association Task Force on practice guidelines. J Nucl Cardiol. 2015;22(1):162–215.

Psychiatric Disorders in Older Adults

Kelly L. Dunn and Robert Roca

4.1 Introduction

The older patient with neuropsychiatric syndromes poses special challenges to specialists asked to provide consultation services or ongoing treatment. These syndromes complicate obtaining a clear and accurate history, may make it more difficult to perform a physical examination, contribute to noncompliance with treatment recommendations, and may directly compromise treatment outcomes. Many of these illnesses are chronic and have remitting and relapsing courses throughout the life span. Others tend to emerge as patients grow older (e.g., Alzheimer's disease) and may complicate pre-existing psychiatric illnesses. In this chapter, the presentation and treatment of five common syndromes (depression, anxiety, delirium, dementia, and psychosis) are discussed. Also, an approach to determining whether a patient has the capacity to make medical decisions—a question that arises frequently in the care of the mentally ill elderly—is presented.

4.2 Depressive Syndromes

4.2.1 Vignette

An 82-year-old widow was brought to her endocrinologist, the only physician she sees regularly, by her daughter because of a change in behavior. Mrs. S's husband of 52 years had recently died at home after a 10-year battle with prostate cancer. Since his death she had been withdrawn,

stopped attending weekly religious services, and abandoned her daily walking routine. She seemed less attentive to household chores and was frequently found "just sitting around" when her daughter stopped by for a visit. She wasn't eating adequately and had lost about 20 pounds. Prior to her decline, the patient had been in good health and took only levothyroxine and aspirin regularly. On examination, the patient was thin, neatly dressed, and subdued. She was slow in her movements and responses. She answered questions softly and simply and frequently returned to the subject of her husband's death. In response to questions about weight loss, she stated that she had no appetite, found it difficult to prepare meals for just herself, and was experiencing early satiety and some difficulties swallowing. She revealed a belief that she had developed cancer and that this was the source of her decline. She insisted on being referred to a gastroenterologist. The physician agreed to make the referral but also expressed concern to the patient and her daughter that she seemed to be struggling with a significant depressive disorder as well as grief related to the loss of her husband. While waiting for an appointment with the gastroenterologist, she agreed to start an antidepressant, mirtazapine 15 mg at bedtime. After 2 weeks the mirtazapine was increased to 30 mg. By the time she was evaluated by the endocrinologists, many of her symptoms had begun to resolve and she had regained 10 pounds. No further work up was suggested. She did begin to attend a grief support group offered by Hospice and returned to her other routine activities.

Depressive syndromes in the elderly are heterogeneous and can be difficult to identify and treat. According to the DSM-5, a major depressive episode is diagnosed when either lack of interest or pleasure or depressed mood is present along with four or more of the following symptoms: insomnia or hypersomnia, psychomotor agitation or retardation, fatigue or loss of energy, significant weight loss, diminished ability to concentrate or make decisions, recurrent thoughts of death or suicidal ideation, and feelings of worthlessness or excessive or inappropriate guilt. These symptoms must be present for at least 2 weeks [1]. It is common for older

K.L. Dunn, MD
1601 Airport Blvd., Suite 3, Melbourne, FL 32901, USA

R. Roca, MD, MPH, MBA (✉)
Sheppard Pratt Health System, Inc.,
6501 N. Charles Street, Baltimore, MD 21204, USA
e-mail: rroca@sheppardpratt.org

© Springer International Publishing Switzerland 2017
J.R. Burton et al. (eds.), *Geriatrics for Specialists*, DOI 10.1007/978-3-319-31831-8_4

patients to express their distress using somatic terms such as "sick" or "blah" rather than psychological terms such as "depressed." Compared to younger patients, older patients are more likely have psychomotor agitation or retardation [2] and to present with depression complicated by delusions [3]. When present delusions tend to be nihilistic, somatic, or revolve around themes of persecution or betrayal.

Because the older patient may be referred to another specialist for evaluation of a related somatic complaint or difficulty, it is important to be alert to the possibility of an underlying mood disorder. Formal screening with a standardized instrument such as the Patient Health Questionnaire (PHQ-9) [4] or the Geriatric Depression Scale (GDS) [5] may be helpful. It is also vital to supplement the history provided by the patient with information from family members or care providers. Chapter 8—Tools for Geriatric Assessment also provides information on simple screening instruments.

When depression symptoms are present in elderly patients, it is important to proceed with a thoughtful medical evaluation, even if there is a high index of suspicion of a mood disorder. Standard laboratory assessments should include a thyroid panel, a basic chemistry panel, and CBC with differential. Because symptoms of vitamin deficiency can mimic or co-occur with depression, levels of vitamin B12, vitamin D, and folate should be measured. Finally, an EKG should be obtained to rule out any contributing arrhythmia and to identify conduction system abnormalities that might affect drug selection.

Treatment of depression in the elderly should be multifaceted and comprehensive. Antidepressant medications are often indicated. The "start low, go slow" principle applies in initial dosing decisions, but older adults often require dosages comparable to those needed by younger patients. Antidepressant medications include selective serotonin reuptake inhibitors, serotonin-norepinephrine reuptake inhibitors, tricyclic compounds, monoamine oxidase inhibitors, and other agents (e.g., bupropion and trazodone); these agents differ in side effects but none has been shown to be superior to any other. Patients may require a mood stabilizer (e.g., lithium, valproate) if there has been a diagnosis of bipolar disorder or an antipsychotic (e.g., olanzapine, quetiapine, aripiprazole) if delusions or hallucinations are present. In general these medications should not be discontinued abruptly as this may precipitate withdrawal symptoms or the re-emergence of the symptoms for which the medications were being prescribed. A psychiatrist should be consulted if the clinician is unfamiliar with the use of psychoactive drugs, especially, because of their side effect profile, when prescribing monoamine oxidase inhibitors, mood stabilizers, and antipsychotics.

Psychotherapy is nearly always of benefit for patients willing to engage in it. In some instances, it may be the only acceptable treatment option available for patients who are unwilling to take or unable to tolerate medications. There are many kinds of psychotherapy (e.g., family therapy, cognitive behavioral therapy (CBT), individual and group dynamic therapy), and there is growing knowledge documenting the effectiveness of different kinds of psychotherapy for different conditions.

Faith-based interventions may be effective for religious patients [6]. Finally, electroconvulsive therapy (ECT) and transcranial magnetic stimulation may be appropriate treatment options, but are not always available and in any case require consultation with a mental health specialist. ECT is a very effective treatment for refractory depressive conditions.

The differential diagnosis of depression includes a number of psychiatric disorders. Depression tends to be a recurrent, relapsing, and remitting condition. Some individuals never achieve complete remission of symptoms and struggle with chronic depression; formerly called "dysthymia," this is termed "persistent depressive disorder" in DSM-5. Individuals with a history of cyclic mood swings marked by depression, irritability, and/or mania may have bipolar disorder; distinguishing recurrent major depression from bipolar depression is important because treatment is different. Finally, grief reactions are common in older adults in response to losses that grow more common with aging, e.g., bereavement, loss of independence, loss of roles and productivity, loss of health. These reactions frequently include such symptoms as sadness, anxiety, social withdrawal, difficulty making decisions, sleep disturbance, and loss of appetite. While the presence of such symptoms for a period of time after loss can be normal, the persistence of these symptoms, particularly if associated with suicidal ideation or irrational self-reproach, may signal an emerging major depressive disorder for which specific treatment will be necessary.

Major depression may accompany any medical disorder and may complicate the clinical presentation as well as treatment of the medical disorder. Cardiovascular disease [7], endocrinopathies, [8] neurologic disorders (e.g., Parkinson's disease [9]), cerebrovascular disease [10], and the degenerative major neurocognitive disorders (e.g., Alzheimer's disease) are commonly accompanied by depressive syndromes. In some instances, a depressive syndrome may herald a new onset neurologic disorder [11]. Regardless of the co-morbidity, a depressive syndrome should always be identified and treated and should never be dismissed as simply symptomatic of the underlying systemic process.

4.3 Anxiety Disorders

4.3.1 Vignette

A 78-year-old widow was brought to her cardiologist by her son because of complaints of chest pain and shortness of breath. She had been a resident of a local assisted living facility for the past 4 years. The assisted living facility staff was concerned about her increasingly frequent calls for assistance because of chest pain and shortness of breath, and her son indicated that he was receiving the same kinds of calls several times per day. She had been sent to a local hospital emergency department three times in the last 30 days, and the work-ups had revealed no acute cardiac or pulmonary findings. She had a long history of tobacco use and continued to smoke one pack of cigarettes daily. She had previously been diagnosed with congestive heart failure and COPD. Twelve months ago the patient developed atrial fibrillation and suffered an embolic stroke. She was subsequently hospitalized and then transferred to a rehabilitation facility. Review of her records indicated that she had been prescribed diazepam 5 mg twice daily for many years and that this was not prescribed during her hospitalization or subsequently. On examination, she was neatly dressed and had a slow and tentative gait with a walker. She was irritable, argumentative, and somatically focused. Her respirations were 22/min and she had an irregular pulse of 100/min. She abruptly terminated the examination, insisting that she needed to urinate. The cardiologist decreased the dose of her diuretic and rescheduled it to morning administration. Concern was expressed about a possible life-long anxiety disorder that should be treated, but preferably not with a benzodiazepine, given her advanced age and unsteady gait. The patient agreed to a trial of citalopram 5 mg daily. After 1 month, the dose was increased to 10 mg daily. After 3 months, the patient was much less irritable and demanding, the frequency of her calls to the staff for assistance had dropped to 3 times a week, and she had had no further trips to the emergency department. Her use of tobacco persisted, but dropped to four cigarettes a day, primarily because she was now engaged in structured activities at the assisted living facility.

Anxiety disorders are common among elderly patients, both as primary and as co-morbid conditions. As with depressive disorders, older patients may have difficulty identifying their symptoms as anxiety and may instead use somatic or non-specific terms. Anxiety disorders tend to be chronic conditions, waxing and waning in severity in response to life circumstances and stressors. They may not be diagnosed until late life as new stresses and losses ensue.

Anxiety disorders should be suspected when a patient presents with difficult to diagnosis and treat symptoms. DSM-5 distinguishes several specific types of anxiety disorders. Generalized anxiety disorder is characterized by excessive worry, often accompanied by tension, irritability, sleep disruption, vague gastrointestinal symptoms, fatigue, and impaired concentration. It is frequently the somatic symptoms—not complaints of anxiety—that precipitate the visit to the doctor or other health professional. Consequently, patients with generalized anxiety disorder are frequently prescribed muscle relaxants, benzodiazepines, or other hypnotics, all of which may be poorly tolerated, increasing

the risk of falls, confusion, and sedation. It is common for patients with anxiety disorders to have been prescribed benzodiazepines for decades without interruption until some medical crisis results in their discontinuation, precipitating an increase in anxiety symptoms as well as symptoms of benzodiazepine withdrawal. A careful history with corroboration by family may be needed to uncover the cause of worsening anxiety symptoms in scenarios such as this.

Other anxiety disorders are less common, and most begin earlier in life. Panic disorder typically is less severe—and panic attacks less frequent—as people age, but older patients may present with episodes of severe anxiety accompanied by multiple somatic complaints, including autonomic, cardiac, pulmonary, and gastrointestinal symptoms. A senior with obsessive compulsive disorder (OCD) may present to the physician because of physical symptoms associated with specific compulsions (e.g., dermatitis due to excessive hand washing). OCD usually becomes manifest in young adulthood but may have its onset in late life, sometimes secondary to a primary neurological disorder (e.g., basal ganglia lesion) [12]. Hoarding tends to be grouped with OCD, although persons who hoard differ from those with typical OCD in that they are not distressed by their behaviors; it is usually families or neighbors who are concerned and intervene. New onset hoarding behavior late in life may signal the onset of a progressive dementing syndrome [13]. Posttraumatic stress disorder (PTSD) is a chronic condition precipitated by one or several identifiable traumatic events. While it generally begins earlier in life and tends to grow less intense with age, PTSD may produce psychosocial disability that persists into late life. Also PTSD may develop in a senior after a profoundly traumatic event such as a severe physical trauma, including major surgery, or criminal violation such as a robbery. Specific phobias (e.g., fear of heights, animals, closed-in spaces, etc.) generally begin earlier in life and may persist into late life. One particular fear—fear of falling—tends to begin in late life [14]. It typically presents after medical events, such as a stroke or a series of falls. It may cause patients to become functionally homebound and interfere with their ability to comply with advice from their physician to pursue physical therapy, exercise, or undergo recommended evaluation.

In considering the diagnosis of an anxiety disorder in an elderly patient, it is vital to ask about prior anxiety symptoms to establish whether there is, in fact, a long-standing anxiety disorder. Anxiety symptoms truly appearing for the first time in late life should prompt a thorough medical evaluation given the possibility that a primary medical condition may be a contributing factor. New onset anxiety with shortness of breath or chest pain may be due to pulmonary emboli or coronary artery disease. New onset anxiety with insomnia, weight loss, and diarrhea may be secondary to thyroid disease. Acute onset of obsessive thinking or compulsive behavior may be symptomatic of acute basal ganglia disease or a new onset progressive neurologic disease.

Treatment should be multifaceted and comprehensive. Psychotherapy, particularly cognitive behavioral therapy, is effective in older adults [15]. Simple cognitive interventions (e.g., reassuring a patient with panic attacks that the panic symptoms will remit on their own after a few minutes) can be very powerful. Pharmacotherapy is often initiated, although the use of medications to treat anxiety disorders in the elderly has not been studied extensively. Benzodiazepines are frequently prescribed and in fact many patients have taken them for many years without apparent harm. However, benzodiazepines have serious side effects, including cognitive impairment and falls, and should be used infrequently and then with the help of a mental health professional, if possible. SSRIs are the first-line pharmacological intervention, although they are not immediately effective and are not without risk. It is best to begin with small doses and increase the dosage slowly to minimize the risk of an early paradoxical exacerbation of anxiety symptoms.

Anxiety disorders often co-exist with other psychiatric disorders. Nearly one half of older patients with a major depressive disorder have a concurrent anxiety disorder [16–18]. One quarter of those patients with anxiety disorders also have a co-morbid major depressive disorder [16]. This phenomenon has clinical implications as patients with co-morbid depression and anxiety are more impaired, have a higher risk of suicide [19], take longer to get better [20, 21], and have higher rates of relapse [22]. It is also important to note the relationship between anxiety and dementia. Late onset anxiety may herald the onset of a major neurocognitive disorder, particularly among persons who are aware of their declining cognitive function [23].

4.4 Delirium

4.4.1 Vignette

A 72-year-old businessman suffered a myocardial infarction while at work and underwent an uneventful emergency 4-vessel bypass procedure. Seventy-two hours postoperatively, he suddenly became confused, agitated, and uncooperative. He removed his IV access. Nursing staff placed wrist restraints to prevent him from removing his urinary catheter. He refused all oral medications, including prn haloperidol. Laboratory studies were ordered and were normal except for a thyroid stimulating hormone (TSH) of 10 ulU/ml, hematocrit level of 30%, a white blood cell count of 12,000 K/ cumm, and a urinalysis with 3+ bacteria, moderate leukocyte esterase and some red blood cells. There was no history of a pre-existing cognitive disorder according to the medical records. His wife confirmed this, insisting that he had no symptoms of memory impairment prior to surgery and suc-

cessfully managed his own marketing company. Although he denied regular alcohol use upon hospital admission, his wife acknowledged that he enjoyed his daily "cocktails" and consumed as many as four mixed drinks each evening. A presumptive diagnosis of alcohol withdrawal delirium was made. Treatment with lorazepam was ordered, and the agitation, restlessness, and combativeness began to respond almost immediately. Over the next few days, lorazepam was tapered and discontinued uneventfully. He was able to participate in physical therapy, and his cognition returned to baseline. The TSH remained elevated at 10 ulU/ml so thyroid replacement therapy was initiated. He was discharged home to his family, with referrals to AA and a strong recommendation that he refrain from drinking alcohol in any quantity.

Delirium is a very important syndrome that every clinician caring for older patients must master. It is discussed briefly here for convenience and is also discussed at length in the Delirium chapter. Delirium is a syndrome characterized by the sudden onset of disturbances in attention, awareness, and cognition usually caused by an acute medical condition, substance intoxication or withdrawal, exposure to toxins, some medications including over the counter agents or topical ophthalmologic agents or combinations of these factors. Psychotic symptoms (e.g., hallucinations, delusions, misperception of actual stimuli) and psychomotor abnormalities (e.g., agitation/hyperactivity or slowing/hypoactivity) are common. Disruptions of the sleep–wake cycle and emotional disturbances (e.g., apathy, emotional labiality, irritability, rumination, fear, and euphoria) may also occur.

Risk factors for delirium include advanced age (>75 years of age), baseline cognitive impairment, prior history of delirium, vision and hearing impairment, history of cerebrovascular disease, severe co-morbid illness, and substance abuse [24]. The rate of identification of delirium is only 30% [24]. Having a high index of suspicion is necessary in high risk populations, particularly the elderly, in whom delirium is often of the easily overlooked hypoactive type [24]. Delirium is a clinical diagnosis based on history and examination. Given the difficulty in detecting delirium, the incidence in various care settings is underestimated. Delirium is present in at least 8–17% of older patients presenting to hospital emergency departments and 40% of nursing home residents transferred to an emergency department for evaluation [25]. Studies have documented prevalence rates of 18–35% in general medical settings, 25% on geriatric inpatient units, 50% in intensive care units (ICUs), and up to 50% in the surgical, cardiac, and orthopedic care settings [25].

The complications of delirium are significant and potentially life threatening. Delirium in the ICU is associated with an extended length of stay, the extended use of mechanical ventilation, and a two to fourfold increase in mortality [25]. The risk of death in the first 6 months following a diagnosis of delirium in the emergency room increases by 70% [25, 26]. Patients who develop a delirium on a general medical floor or a geriatric unit have a 1.5 fold [25] increased risk of death in the year following the index hospitalization. Delirium present at the time of admission to a post-acute care setting is associated with a fivefold increase in mortality at 6 months [27]. Postoperative delirium and delirium in the ICU are also associated with persistent cognitive impairment 12 months after hospital discharge [25, 28].

It is common for the older patient to present with delirium as the only sign of an undiagnosed underlying medical or acute surgical condition. This is particularly true for patients who are unable to give a reliable history or articulate specific complaints, such as persons with a pre-existing cognitive disorder. If caregivers report an acute mental status change, delirium should be presumed until proven otherwise. The medical workup of acute mental status changes should begin with a thorough medical history and physical examination. Basic blood work (e.g., complete blood count, comprehensive chemistry panel), urinalysis, and an electrocardiogram should be obtained. In addition, thyroid function tests, vitamin B12 and vitamin D levels, ammonia level, and screens for alcohol and drugs of abuse should be considered. Without a history of falls or a change in the neurologic exam, neuroimaging is not recommended as part of the routine diagnostic workup; neuroimaging produces new findings in fewer than 2% of patients with previously diagnosed dementia or another determined medical cause of the delirium [29], and neuroimaging findings alter treatment interventions in fewer than 10% of patients [30]. An electroencephalogram typically demonstrates generalizing slowing in delirium but could have diagnostic findings suggestive of seizure activity [31, 32], including non-convulsive status epilepticus, and thus may be of value when non-convulsive seizure activity is a diagnostic consideration.

The etiology of delirium is typically multifactorial, and the standard treatment approach is to begin with identifying the underlying cause(s). Infections (symptomatic urinary tract infection (caution here is needed as asymptomatic bacteria is very common among seniors, especially women, and not a cause of delirium), pneumonia or sepsis) commonly present as or with an associated delirium. Metabolic abnormalities such as alterations in sodium, calcium, and magnesium can produce acute mental status changes. Respiratory conditions resulting in alterations in oxygenation can affect cognition acutely. Thyroid disease can also produce acute cognitive changes. Medications are estimated to be implicated in 40% of cases of delirium [33, 34], presumably through disruption of cholinergic neurotransmission resulting from the anticholinergic effects of many drugs. The Beers Criteria [35] identifies medications most frequently associated with delirium. (See also the Chap. 5.) Also not to be overlooked is the possibility of intoxication and/or withdrawal from such substances as alcohol, narcotic analgesics, and benzodiazepines.

Treatment of the acute delirium is multifaceted. In addition to treating the underlying medical cause(s) (including painful conditions) and removing any exacerbating medications, nonpharmacologic interventions are essential and include strategies of re-orientation, limiting overstimulation, and ameliorating sensory deficits by providing eyeglasses and hearing aids. The presence of reassuring family and staff is essential. Although commonly used, psychotropic medications such as antipsychotics should only be considered after nonpharmacologic interventions have been implemented. Finally, the use of physical restraints should be avoided as they intensify delirium. Most importantly, several controlled studies have demonstrated that the proactive intervention by the treatment team can both decrease the incidence of delirium [36–40] and improve the rate of recognition of a delirium when it occurs [41–43]. These interdisciplinary and environmental strategies are discussed in Chap. 2.

4.5 Dementia

4.5.1 Vignette

A 75-year-old married man was hospitalized emergently following a fall at home resulting in a fracture of the right femur. He and his wife agreed to surgical repair, which proceeded without complication. Thirty-six hours postoperatively, the orthopedic surgeon received phone calls from hospital nursing staff reporting that the patient was very lethargic. Laboratory studies were ordered and were unremarkable except for slightly decreased hemoglobin and hematocrit levels. He was receiving only acetaminophen for pain control. When examined by the surgeon, he was awake but confused, restless, agitated, and reaching for objects that were not present. A small dose of oral haloperidol was administered, and a neurology consultation was ordered. The neurologist found the patient awake and alert, but oriented only to his name and the name of hospital. He had mild cogwheel rigidity of the upper extremities but no tremor or psychomotor slowing. The patient denied distress and had no recollection of confusion or hallucinations. In speaking with his wife, the neurologist obtained a history of subtle but progressive memory loss over the past 3 years. Over that time he had begun awakening his wife at night, reporting nightmares as well as anxiety about "seeing people" who were not present; he eventually would accept redirection and reassurance and return to sleep. His wife also recounted a history of kicking and punching behaviors during sleep that had recently become so violent that she frequently slept in the guest room for her own safety. The neurologist made a diagnosis of acute delirium but also suspected an underlying dementia syndrome due to Lewy Body disease. He discontinued haloperidol and replaced it with quetiapine 12.5 mg QHS.

The patient continued to have occasional episodes of increased confusion and brief visual hallucinations, but the episodes of profound lethargy ceased. He was able to participate in physical therapy and was discharged home. Over the course of the next year he experienced the recurrence of distressing visual hallucinations each time quetiapine was discontinued, so the decision was made to continue quetiapine at a low dose. Over the next several years, he showed progressive short-term memory loss and increasingly prominent Parkinsonian signs (shuffling gait, resting tremor, cogwheel rigidity). Lewy Body disease was confirmed at autopsy 6 years after his initial hospitalization.

Dementia is a clinical syndrome caused by a diverse array of diseases and marked by declining cognitive ability of sufficient severity to produce significant functional impairment. The most common underlying pathologic entities are Alzheimer's disease (AD), Lewy Body disease (LBD), cerebrovascular disease, and frontotemporal lobar degeneration, but a wide range of other diseases may be implicated. Because this syndrome is present in as many as 30 % of persons over age 85, its prevalence is growing rapidly as the population ages [1].

In the most recent version of the Diagnostic Manual of Mental Disorders (DSM-5) [1], the term dementia has been supplanted by the term "Major Neurocognitive Disorder (MND)." For most purposes, these terms can be regarded as synonymous, although there are subtle differences; e.g., MND can be diagnosed in a person with significant impairment in only one cognitive domain, whereas the term dementia has been reserved for persons with impairments in several domains. One of the main purposes of this change was to facilitate the distinction between MND and "Mild Neurocognitive Disorder," a long-recognized condition in which the impairments in cognitive functioning are measurably less severe than in MND and do not preclude independent functioning.

The cardinal sign of dementia is the development of functionally significant impairment in the ability to think, reason, and remember. Impairments in learning and short-term memory impairment are prominent in dementia syndromes due to AD and LBD but in conditions such as frontotemporal lobar degeneration the most conspicuous early signs may be changes in personality and social behavior (e.g., use of profanity; inappropriate sexual behavior). Other affected cognitive domains include executive functioning (e.g., planning, prioritizing), complex attention (e.g., attending to more than one task at a time), language (e.g., ability to find words), social cognition (e.g., ability to recognize emotional cues in social situations), and perceptual-motor functioning (e.g., difficulty with way-finding). In addition to cognitive impairment, most persons with dementia manifest behavioral and psychological signs and symptoms over the course of their illness, and it is often these clinical features of dementia that are most distressing to patients and to their caregivers. These include delusions, hallucinations, depression, apathy, and various kinds of agitation and aggression. While dementia symptoms often develop gradually and progress slowly, particularly in AD and LBD, they may also present or worsen suddenly as a result of an acute medical (e.g., pneumonia) or neurological (e.g., stroke) event or an adverse drug effect (e.g., dopaminergic agents for Parkinson disease; anticholinergic agents for urinary incontinence). In such cases, patients usually also have a superimposed delirium (see below).

Patients and their families often present to physicians with concerns about forgetfulness. In many cases cognitive impairment is readily apparent and there is unequivocal evidence of functional disability. In such instances the first task is to determine whether the observed syndrome is dementia alone, delirium alone, or delirium superimposed upon dementia (as in this vignette). While delirium and dementia share many clinical features in common, the core deficits in uncomplicated delirium are disturbances in attention and awareness evidenced by drowsiness (e.g., the delirium associated with renal failure) or by hypervigilance and distractibility (e.g., delirium associated with alcohol withdrawal). It develops suddenly as a result of an acute medical event or adverse drug effect, and it resolves gradually but variably in response to treatment of the underlying condition. In uncomplicated cases, recovery is complete. In the presence of delirium, it is impossible to make a new determination that a dementia syndrome is also present; this must await the resolution of the delirium-defining disturbance in attention. As a practical matter, delirium and dementia frequently co-exist, particularly in persons with acute medical illnesses, since dementing illnesses make patients more vulnerable to delirium in the presence of potentially deliriogenic conditions such as in this vignette; thus, a delirious episode may be the occasion on which an underlying dementia is first suspected.

Once is it clear that a dementia syndrome is present, the next task—if not previously done—is to identify the likely etiology. The most common causes are AD, LBD, and cerebrovascular disease, either alone or in combination with AD and LBD. AD or LBD is usually present in cases with gradual onset, slow progression, and prominent initial memory impairment. Genetic testing (e.g., subtyping APO-E gene) and brain amyloid scanning may help identify persons with AD but currently are not recommended for routine use. There is no specific laboratory test for LBD, although visual hallucinations and Parkinsonian motor symptoms are clinical features strongly suggestive of LBD. Cerebrovascular disease in the form of major stroke or microvascular changes is readily apparent on brain imaging. Hematology and blood chemistry studies are indicated to screen for evidence of other contributory general medical conditions (e.g., renal failure, thyroid disease, B-12 deficiency). Patients with dementia, without delirium, whose cognitive impairment is documented to have occurred over a year or so typically don't benefit from an evaluation looking for a reversible cause of their condition. Many persons presenting with complaints of memory loss do not have a major neurocognitive disorder. Some of these patients meet criteria for a condition termed "mild neurocognitive disorder" (mild NCD) [1]. This is characterized by subjective complaints about cognition (e.g., need to make lists; difficulty multi-tasking) accompanied by objective evidence of subpar performance (i.e., between 1 and 2 SD below the mean or between the 16th and 3rd percentiles with respect to age- and education-adjusted norms) in the absence of actual functional impairment. It may be difficult in routine practice to distinguish Mild NCD from worry about age-related changes in subjective performance exacerbated by depression or anxiety disorders, and it may be advisable to refer these patients for assessment by a neurologist, psychiatrist, geriatrician, or neuropsychologist for formal neuropsychological testing.

The treatment of a dementia syndrome depends on the underlying cause. Unfortunately, **there are no disease-altering treatments for the most common causes of dementia.** The only FDA-approved drug treatments for AD are drugs that slow the enzymatic degradation of the neurotransmitter acetylcholine (e.g., cholinesterase inhibitors such as donepezil) and memantine, a drug that is believed to mitigate glutamate-mediated cellular excitotoxicity. None of these is believed to treat the underlying pathophysiology or to halt disease progression, although they may temporarily reduce impairment and ameliorate caregiver burden. Use of these drugs, therefore, should occur only after a thoughtful discussion with the patient and family considering these issues and the drug side effects. If used, they should be continued if, and only if, improvement in 1–3 months is seen and side effects are tolerable. There are no FDA-approved drug treatments for the behavioral and psychiatric complications of dementia. There is a general consensus that the preferred first-line approach to these problems involves attention to medical (e.g., pain), environmental (e.g., excessive noise or crowding), and interpersonal (e.g., impatient caregivers) triggers to emotional and behavioral dyscontrol, but frequently these measures are not completely effective [44]. Antipsychotic medications (e.g., haloperidol) have often been used "off-label" to treat psychosis, agitation, and aggression in persons with dementia. In the last few years their use has diminished significantly as a result of studies showing increases in morbidity and mortality and only modest, short-term benefit associated with their use. Such results, especially the associated increase in mortality, have resulted in a "black box warning" on the package insert. However they continue to be required for the acute management of aggressive emergencies and for the longer term treatment of psychosis, agitation, and aggression unresponsive to environmental and behavioral interventions [44]. Many other drugs have been studied, and some (e.g., citalopram [45]) have shown promise, but none has been FDA-approved for this indication.

4.6 Psychosis

4.6.1 Vignette

An 88-year-old widowed woman saw a dermatologist because of a rash. She had a long history of cognitive decline and had been a resident of a skilled nursing facility for 5 years following a series of falls resulting in rib and pelvic fractures. She was no longer ambulatory. Over the last few months she had developed non-healing lesions on her left hand, forearm, cheek, and shoulder. She also had a flat erythematous contiguous rash on her cheeks and forehead. Treatment with oral antihistamines (a group of drugs to be avoided in older patients—see Chap. 5—Medication Management for details) and multiple topical preparations had been unsuccessful. On exam, she was neatly dressed and seated comfortably in her wheelchair. She was confused but calm and cooperative. She denied pruritus and pain. She was insistent that "bugs" were all over her, burrowing into her skin. She was frustrated that the "stuff in the tube in the bathroom" was not helping and that her only recourse was to pull and scratch at the bugs until she extracted them. According to the family, she had always been a loner and considered eccentric but had never before verbalized these kinds of beliefs. The dermatologist discontinued all of the oral antihistamines and topical treatments, with no change in her condition. Concerned about the delusional quality of the patient's complaints, he prescribed risperidone 0.25 mg twice daily. Within 1 month, her belief that "bugs" were burrowing into her skin had resolved. Within 2 months, there was a 50 % reduction in lesions, and the remaining lesions were all healing. After 3 months, there were very few lesions remaining, and the patient denied having any concerns about her skin. The nursing home staff commented that her "picking" behavior had ceased. In addition, they mentioned having recently discovered that she was smearing toothpaste on her face. They removed the toothpaste from her room, and the rash on her cheeks and forehead resolved promptly.

The term "psychosis" is not a diagnosis but a generic term used to describe a complex of mental symptoms including false perceptions (hallucinations) in any sensory modality (i.e., auditory, visual, tactile, olfactory, or gustatory), fixed false idiosyncratic beliefs (delusions) with a variety of themes (e.g., persecutory, grandiose, religious, nihilistic, irrationally self-blaming), and gross disturbances in motor behavior (catatonia) or in the organization of speech (formal thought disorder). These may be of sufficient severity to render the patient "out of touch with reality." The presence of these symptoms, particularly if severe and sudden in onset, calls for an immediate diagnostic assessment and often for emergency treatment.

The differential diagnosis is broad and includes some of the disorders already discussed in this chapter. Of course psychosis is the defining feature of schizophrenia. Schizophrenia occurs in about 1 % of the population and generally emerges in early adulthood but may also have its onset in late life. Principal symptoms are delusions (often persecutory) and auditory hallucinations, although olfactory, visual, and tactile hallucinations may be prominent in late onset cases. Formal thought disorder and catatonia may also occur. Isolated delusions, often persecutory or somatic, are the defining features of the so-called delusional disorders. In addition, delusions and hallucinations can complicate both severe depression (e.g., delusions of guilt; hallucinations urging suicide) and mania (e.g., grandiose delusions; hallucinations involving hearing the voice of God). Psychosis, particularly as manifested by visual hallucinations, may be the most conspicuous initial sign of a delirium complicating an acute medical condition, such as sepsis or alcohol withdrawal, requiring urgent diagnostic and therapeutic intervention. Psychosis may also be a prominent and very distressing feature of dementing illnesses such as AD and LBD.

Because the management of psychosis depends on the underlying cause(s), it is essential to perform an appropriate diagnostic evaluation. In a patient with new onset symptoms, the psychosis should be presumed to be a sign of delirium, and a thorough evaluation should be undertaken urgently looking for acute medical and neurological conditions as well as for evidence of drug toxicity or withdrawal. While treatment of the underlying condition(s) is the most important therapeutic intervention, it may be necessary to use antipsychotic medications to manage acute psychotic symptoms on a short-term basis. An exception might be delirium due to alcohol withdrawal, in which case benzodiazepines (one of the very few indications for these drugs in the elderly) would serve both to treat the underlying condition and to manage the acute behavioral and psychological symptoms. Psychosis complicating primary mood disorders generally responds to effective pharmacologic treatment of the primary mood disorder (e.g., antidepressant medications) supplemented by antipsychotic medications, although oftentimes electroconvulsive therapy is necessary and is in general the most rapidly effective treatment in these cases. Antipsychotic medications are usually necessary at some point—if not chronically—in the treatment of schizophrenia and related psychotic conditions (e.g., schizoaffective disorder) and are generally as effective in older adults as in younger patients. Psychotic symptoms complicating dementia syndromes may require antipsychotic medications periodically and in some cases chronically but more often—particularly when not resulting in distress or dangerous behavior—respond to tactful redirection and distraction by caregivers.

4.7 Determining Decisional Capacity (Competency)

In general, medical services cannot be provided to patients without their informed consent. For a health professional to accept consent as meaningful, one must believe that the patient is "competent" or has decisional capacity. It is not unusual for physicians to question the competence of their patients to provide or withhold consent for treatment, particularly when they are elderly, gravely ill, or facing a particularly complex treatment decision. Determinations of capacity are issue specific (e.g. hip surgery) and require careful consideration and communication with the patient and other informants.

Patients are capable of informed consent if they have the ability to (1) express a choice, (2) understand and state in their own words what they have been told; (3) appreciate the consequences of the choice, and (4) manipulate the information rationally to arrive at a decision in line with values and preferences (ability to reason) [46].

From a clinical standpoint, determining whether these conditions are met requires pursuit of two lines of inquiry: (1) Does the patient have a potentially competency-compromising condition; and (2) if so, is there evidence that the symptoms are interfering with decision making in this particular situation [47].

4.7.1 Vignette

An 85-year-old woman was admitted to the hospital because of a hip fracture and refused surgical treatment. At the time of evaluation she reported having fallen 3 days before admission and had elected to stay at home rather than go to the hospital because she didn't want treatment of any kind. She ultimately agreed to be taken to the hospital only because of unbearable pain. Once admitted she accepted pain relief measures but declined the offer of surgery even when informed of the risks associated with prolonged bed rest. She explained that she had had a long, good life but was now unhappy at home with her indifferent, alcoholic son and was ready to die. She appeared to understand her condition and the treatment options, clearly expressed a choice to forgo surgery, and appeared to understand the risks associated with her choice.

She had no appetite, slept fitfully, and had no interest in activities that had formerly brought her pleasure. Her mental status examination revealed depressed mood, sad affect, and hopelessness, but no formal thought disorder, delusions, hallucinations, or cognitive impairment. She was not contemplating self-harm but was accepting of possibly dying soon. She met formal criteria for major depressive disorder, a condition that can make patients irrationally pessimistic about their prospects and thus compromise decision-making capacity. In this case, the clinical team was concerned that depression-related hopelessness might be responsible for her negative appraisal of the desirability of treatment; therefore, the clinical team elected to treat her for depression and reassess her openness to surgical repair if her mood improved. In response to psychosocial interventions as well as pharmacotherapy with a low-dose stimulating antidepressant, her mood and affect improved markedly over the next few days (indeed, the response often occurs in just a short time). She began eating and socializing, and her sleep normalized. She continued to deny suicidality but also continued to refuse surgery and to express a readiness to die. At this point— given the resolution of the depressive syndrome—there was no evidence of a clinical condition that might be compromising her decision-making capacity, so the team regarded her as having the capacity to refuse surgery. She was discharged with a plan for home-based nursing care focused on pain management.

4.7.2 Vignette

A 75-year-old woman was admitted to the hospital because of a hip fracture and refused surgical repair. Upon evaluation she claimed to understand that the surgeons believed that surgery was essential but she was not convinced because she had known others who had recovered uneventfully from hip fractures without surgery. She also explained that she didn't want surgery because radio-transmitting equipment had been implanted in her abdomen many years before during a prior procedure and she had been monitored by the surgeons since that time; she didn't want to be vulnerable to such treatment again. Her mental status examination showed persecutory delusions and auditory hallucinations but no evidence of depression, mania, or significant impairment in memory, language, or other basic cognitive functions. Based on past history and her current mental status findings, she was determined to have schizophrenia.

She appeared to understand the nature of her condition and clearly expressed a choice. However, she did not appear to fully appreciate the risks associated with her choice, and the choice was clearly influenced heavily by her delusions regarding the implantation of radio-transmitting equipment. Thus she had a capacity-compromising condition and her choice appeared to be a symptom of that condition. She clearly was not competent to refuse surgery. The clinical team sought a surrogate decision-maker who could make a decision on her behalf, taking into account her values and historical preferences.

As these cases illustrate, there are two principal considerations in judgments about decisional capacity or competence. The first is a diagnostic question, i.e., is there a potentially capacity-compromising condition present? If there is not—as was the case in Case 1 after treatment—then there is no clinical reason to question capacity. If such a condition is present, then the question is the relevance of the diagnosis, i.e., can it be shown that the symptoms of the condition are compromising the patient's ability to choose rationally? If not, then there is no clinical reason to question capacity. If there is—as was the case in Case 2—then the patient can clearly be said to lack capacity, and a substitute decision-maker must be sought.

If a clinician is uncertain about a patient's capacity, he or she must consider the potential consequences of any decision. In general, the more grave the consequences, in a "sliding scale" fashion, the more certain the clinician must be that capacity is present to accept the patient's choice [46]. It is always wise to seek consultation and engage a surrogate decision-maker in situations requiring the determination of capacity .

4.8 Conclusion

The neuropsychiatric syndromes described in this chapter occur commonly among elderly patients and must be taken into account by all health care professionals when obtaining a history, performing a physical examination, ordering studies, arriving at a diagnosis, and suggesting treatment. These syndromes may mimic other medical conditions and may co-occur with *any* medical or surgical condition, complicating profoundly evaluation and treatment. Fortunately all of these syndromes can be treated and managed, if not cured. The first and most important step is recognizing their presence. Once a syndrome is detected, the specialist may proceed down the path of differential diagnosis using familiar tools (e.g., history, exam, and laboratory studies) and develop a diagnosis-specific plan of care. The implementation of the plan of care will often call for—and depend on—the active involvement of family and other caregivers. At any point in this process of care it may be helpful to obtain psychiatric consultation, particularly if there are complex differential diagnostic questions, if treatment would involve the use of unfamiliar medications, or if there is disagreement about a patient's decisional capacity. However, all practitioners can develop the skills necessary to recognize and treat neuropsychiatric syndromes that may compromise the care of their elderly patients. These treatments must always be discussed with and agreed upon by the patient and caregivers. Specialty expertise should be solicited whenever the clinician is not fully experienced or comfortable with the situation or treatment.

References

1. American Psychiatric Association. Diagnostic and statistical manual of mental disorders. 5th ed. Washington: American Psychiatric Association; 2013.
2. Parker G, Roy K, Hadzi-Pavlovic D, et al. The differential impact of age on the phenomenology of melancholia. Psychol Med. 2001;31(7):1231–6.
3. Meyers BS, Kalayam B, Mei-Tal V. Late-onset delusional depression: a distinct clinical entity? J Clin Psychiatry. 1984;45(8):347–9.
4. Kroenke K, Spitzer RL, Williams JB. The PHQ-9: validity of a brief depression severity measure. J Gen Intern Med. 2001;16(9):606–13.
5. Yesavage JA, Brink TL, Rose TL, et al. Development and validation of a geriatric depression screening scale: a preliminary report. J Psychiatr Res. 1982–1983; 17(1):37–49.
6. Koenig HG, George LK, Titus P. Religion, spirituality and health in medically ill hospitalized older adults. J Am Geriatr Soc. 2004;52(4):554–62.
7. Sullivan MD, LaCroix AZ, Baum C, et al. Functional status in coronary artery disease: a one year prospective study of the role of anxiety and depression. Am J Med. 1997;103(5):348–56.
8. Blazer DG, Moody-Ayers S, Craft-Morgan J, et al. Depression in diabetes and obesity: racial/ethnic/gender issues in older adults. J Psychosom Res. 2002;53(4):913–6.
9. Zesiewicz TA, Gold M, Chari G, et al. Current issues in depression in Parkinson's disease. Am J Geriatr Psychiatry. 1999;7(2):110–8.
10. Robinson RG, Price TR. Post-stroke depressive disorders: a follow-up study of 103 patients. Stroke. 1982;13(5):635–41.
11. Butters MA, Young JB, Lopez O, et al. Pathways linking late-life depression to persistent cognitive impairment and dementia. Dialogues Clin Neurosci. 2008;10(3):345–57.
12. Chacko RC, Corbin MA, Harper RG. Acquired obsessive-compulsive disorder associated with basal ganglia lesions. J Neuropsychiatry Clin Neurosci. 2000;12(2):269–72.
13. Chou KL, Mackenzie CS, Liang K, et al. Three-year incidence and predictors of first-onset DSM-IV mood, anxiety, and substance use disorders in older adults: results from wave 2 of the National Epidemiologic Survey on Alcohol and Related conditions. J Clin Psychiatry. 2011;72(2):144–55.
14. Arfken CL, Lack HW, Birge JT, et al. The prevalence and correlates of fear of falling in elderly persons living in the community. Am J Public Health. 1994;84(4):565–70.
15. Wetherell JL, Gatz M, Craske MG. Treatment of generalized anxiety disorder in older adults. J Consult Clin Psychol. 2003;71(1):31–40.
16. Beekman ATF, de Beurs E, van Balkom AJLM, et al. Anxiety and depression in later life; co-occurrence and communality of risk factors. Am J Psychiatry. 2000;157(1):89–95.
17. Lenze EF, Mulsant BH, Shear MK, et al. Co-morbid anxiety disorders in depressed elderly patients. Am J Psychiatry. 2000;157(5):722–8.
18. Mulsant BH, Reynolds 3rd CF, Shear MK, et al. Comorbid anxiety disorders in late-life depression. Anxiety. 1996;2(5):242–7.
19. Allguadner C, Lavori PW. Cause of death among 936 elderly patients with "pure" anxiety neurosis in Stockholm County, Sweden, and in patients with depressive neurosis or both diagnoses. Compr Psychiatry. 1993;34(5):299–302.
20. Alexopoulos GS, Katz IR, Bruice ML, et al. Remission in depressed geriatric primary care patients: a report from the PROSPECT study. Am J Psychiatry. 2005;162(4):718–24.
21. Lenze EJ, Mulsant BH, Dew MA, et al. Good treatment outcomes in late-life depression with comorbid anxiety. J Affect Disord. 2003;77(3):247–54.
22. Andreescu C, Lenze EJ, Dew MA, et al. Effect of comorbid anxiety on treatment response and relapse risk in late life depression: controlled study. Br J Psychiatry. 2007;190:344–9.
23. Seignourel PJ, Kunik ME, Snow L, et al. Anxiety in dementia: a critical review. Clin Psychol Rev. 2008;28(7):1071–82.
24. Inouye SK, Foreman MD, Mion LC, et al. Nurses recognition of delirium and its symptoms: comparison of nurse and researcher ratings. Arch Intern Med. 2001;161(20):2467–73.
25. Inouye SK, Westendorp RG, Saczynski JS, et al. Delirium in elderly people. Lancet. 2014;383(9920):911–22.
26. Pandharipande PP, Girard TD, Jackson JC, et al. BRAIN-ICU Study investigators: long term cognitive impairment after critical illness. N Engl J Med. 2013;369(14):1306–16.
27. Marcantonio ER, Kiely DK, Simons SE, et al. Outcomes of older people admitted to post-acute facilities with delirium. J Am Geriatr Soc. 2005;53(6):963–9.
28. Saczynski J, Marcantonio ER, Quack L, et al. Cognitive trajectories after post operative delirium. N Engl J Med. 2012;367(1):30–9.
29. Hufschmidt A, Shabarin V. Diagnostic yield of cerebral imaging in patients with acute confusion. Acta Neurol Scand. 2008;118(4):245–50.
30. Hirao K, Ohnishi T, Matsuda H, et al. Functional interactions between entorhinal cortex and posterior cingulated cortex at the very early stage of Alzheimer's disease using brain perfusion single photon emission computed tomography. Nucl Med Commun. 2006;27(2):151–6.
31. Jacobson S, Jerrier H. EEG in delirium. Semin Clin Neuropsychiatry. 2000;5(2):86–92.
32. Jenssen S. Electroencephalogram in the dementia work-up. Am J Alzheimers Dis Other Demen. 2005;20(3):159–66.
33. Inouye SK. The dilemma of delirium: clinical and research controversies regarding diagnosis and evaluation of delirium in hospitalized elderly medical patients. Am J Med. 1994;97(3):278–88.
34. Inouye SK, Charpentier PA. Precipitating factors for delirium in hospitalized elderly persons: predictive model and interrelationships with baseline vulnerability. JAMA. 1996;275(11):852–7.
35. American Geriatric Society. American Geriatrics Society updated Beers Criteria for potentially inappropriate medication use in older adults. J Am Geriatr Soc. 2012;60:616–31.
36. Bermann MA, Murphy KM, Kiely DK, et al. A model of management of delirious post-acute care patients. J Am Geriatr Soc. 2005;53(10):1817–25.
37. Deshodf M, Braes T, Flamaing J, et al. Preventing delirium in older adults with recent hip fracture through multidisciplinary geriatric consultation. J Am Geriatr Soc. 2012;60(4):733–9.
38. Lundstrom M, Edlund A, Karlsson S, et al. A multifactorial intervention program reduces the duration of delirium, length of hospitalization, and mortality in delirious patients. J Am Geriatr Soc. 2005;53(4):622–8.
39. Nayhton BJ, Saltzman S, Ramadan F, et al. A multifactorial intervention to reduce prevalence of delirium and shorten hospital length of stay. J Am Geriatr Soc. 2005;53(1):18–23.
40. Pitkala KH, Lairila JV, Strandberg TE, et al. Multicomponent geriatric intervention for elderly patients with delirium: a randomized, controlled trial. J Gerontol A Biol Sci Med Sci. 2006;61(2):176–81.
41. Marcantonio ER, Bergmann MA, Kiely DK, et al. Randomized trial of a delirium abatement program for post-acute skilled nursing facilities. J Am Geriatr Soc. 2010;58(6):1019–26.
42. Milisen K, Foreman MD, Abraham K, et al. A nurse-led interdisciplinary intervention program for delirium in elderly hip-fracture patients. J Am Geriatr Soc. 2001;49(5):523–32.
43. Tabet N, Hudson S, Sweeney V, et al. An educational intervention can prevent delirium on acute medical wards. Age Ageing. 2005;34(2):152–6.
44. Rabins PV, Rovner BW, Rummans T, Schneider LS, Tariot PN. Guideline watch (October 2014): practice guideline for the treatment of patients with Alzheimer's disease and other dementias. American Psychiatric Association. 2014. Accessed at http://psychiatryonline.org/guidelines.
45. Porsteinsson AP, Drye LT, Pollock BG, et al. Effect of citalopram on agitation in Alzheimer disease: the CITAD randomized clinical trial. JAMA. 2014;311:682–91.
46. Applebaum P. Assessment of patients' competence to consent to treatment. N Engl J Med. 2007;357:1834–40.
47. Roca R. Determining decisional capacity: a medical perspective. Fordham Law Rev. 1994;62:1177–96.

Medication Management

5

Nicole J. Brandt

5.1 Background

There are an estimated 44.7 million individuals over age 65 in 2013 (14.1% of the US population). This senior population is estimated to grow to 21.7% in 2040 [1]. And by 2060, demographers predict about 98 million seniors or twice their number in 2013. This senior population is characterized by medical complexity and disability. Nearly all seniors have at least one chronic condition, and about 75% have at least two [2]. Some level of disability was reported by 36% of adults aged 65 years or older. These reported disabilities increase each decade of life and include difficulty with hearing, vision, cognition, and ambulation [3]. Additionally this population dominates assisted living and skilled nursing facilities. Reports estimate that approximately 23% of new admissions to skilled nursing facilities are due to medication non-adherence [4]. Furthermore, it is estimated that 85% of residents within assisted living facilities need medication management administration and oversight [4].

With such a high percentage of the senior populations affected by multiple chronic medical conditions, the likelihood of increased medication use rises proportionally. A cross-sectional study on medication prevalence among adults showed that 28% of men and 33% of women aged 65–74 used five or more prescription medications, so-called polypharmacy. Polypharmacy is also defined by consensus as the "administration of more medications than medically necessary" [5]. The prevalence of drug use increases with age: nearly 40% of men and women 75–85 years had polypharmacy [6]. To complicate medication management further, older adults were found to be the largest consumer of over-the-counter (OTC) medications and dietary suppléments [6].

N.J. Brandt, PharmD, MBA, BCPP, CGP, FASCP (✉)
Department of Pharmacy Practice and Science,
University of Maryland, School of Pharmacy, Baltimore,
20 North Pine St N529, Baltimore, MD 21201, USA
e-mail: nbrandt@rx.umaryland.edu

This high use of medications and age related physiological losses among older adults results in disproportionately more medication related problems. This problem affects the well-being of many seniors and has enormous financial implications for health care insurers. According to a recent IMS Institute for HealthCare Informatics study, the misuse of medications contributes to \$500 billion in international healthcare spending. In order to address this preventable and expensive problem, the IMS Institute recommends "investing in medical audits that focus on elderly patients" [7]. In the USA, medication-related problems in the older adult population are associated with an annual expense of \$8 billion [8]. With the US aged population growing at a faster rate than ever before, the need to ensure safe medication management is increasingly urgent. This chapter will discuss selected age related physiological functions and syndromes that complicate medication management. Strategies to minimize common prescribing problems are discussed.

5.2 Factors Impacting Drug Response in Older Adults

5.2.1 Physiologic Alterations

Frailty has been defined as a "physiological syndrome characterized by decreased reserve and diminished resistance to stressors, resulting from cumulative decline across multiple physiological systems, causing vulnerability to adverse outcomes and high risk of death" [9]. Conceptualizing frailty through the four main underlying processes—changes in body composition, energetic imbalance, homeostatic dysregulation, and neurodegeneration—recognizes that the processes that underlie frailty start early in life and progress rapidly later in life but with a high degree of heterogeneity among individuals. Perhaps, even more important, this approach provides common criteria by which aging, disease, and environmental pressure contribute to the "aging pheno-

© Springer International Publishing Switzerland 2017
J.R. Burton et al. (eds.), *Geriatrics for Specialists*, DOI 10.1007/978-3-319-31831-8_5

type" and, in turn, to frailty [10]. The syndrome of frailty is discussed in more depth in Chap. 1.

This section will highlight selected organ system changes that result in alterations in pharmacokinetic and pharmacodynamic responses in older adults. Pharmacokinetic (i.e., absorption, distribution, metabolism, elimination) processes affect disposition of a medication and determine the concentration at the site(s) of action. Pharmacodynamic processes involve the interaction between a medication and the receptors and the effector organ, which results in the pharmacological response of a medication [11].

5.2.2 Nervous System

Some central nervous system (CNS) active biogenic amines decline with age, notably norepinephrine and dopamine. For this reason the clinician must be vigilant when prescribing medications that are associated with inducing Parkinson symptoms. Table 5.1 provides a summary of such drugs. Should Parkinson symptoms develop in association with drugs, every effort is needed to discontinue the medication and use a less offensive agent. Drug induced Parkinson (DIP) is generally reversible once the medication is stopped but it may persist for 4 to even 18 months [12].

In addition to DIP other agents adversely affect the central and peripheral nervous system. Especially important are the numerous medications with anticholinergic properties (Table 5.2). These agents commonly cause delirium, urinary retention, constipation, dry mouth, and blurry vision which can impact quality of life as well as functional capabilities of older adults. That is why it is important to minimize the cumulative anticholinergic burden on older adults.

5.2.3 Cardiovascular System

One age related change in the heart is a decline of the ability to respond to stress with an increasing heart rate and coronary blood flow. In part this is due to the decreased response to catecholamines (i.e., epinephrine), which is related to the diminished number or decreased sensitivity of beta-receptors in older adults [14]. This is why it is imperative to be aware of medications that reduce cardiac output (e.g., calcium blockers) or cause sodium retention (e.g., glucocorticosteroids, nonsteroidal anti-inflammatory drugs) as these could stress the myocardium causing heart failure exacerbation.

5.2.4 Gastrointestinal Tract

There are numerous age related physiological changes in the GI tract including:

- Increase in gastric pH secondary to reduction in gastric acid secretion;
- Decrease in splanchnic blood flow (estimated about 30–40 %);
- Increase in gastric emptying time; and a decrease in gastric motility

However, there appears to be no effect of these changes on drug absorption.

5.2.5 Hepatic System

The liver is involved in the catabolism and elimination of many medications. Age related changes impacting this hepatic function include:

- Decrease in the liver mass as well as blood flow impacting medications such as propranolol
- Decline in metabolic reactions such as:

- Hydroxylation (e.g., phenytoin)
- Dealkylation (e.g., diazepam)
- Sulfide oxidation (e.g., chlorpromazine)
- Hydrolysis (e.g., aspirin)

While there is great variability in age related changes in hepatic metabolism among older adults, clinicians must be vigilant that age related hepatic functional decline could

Table 5.1 Medications and drug-induced parkinsonism

Drugs commonly implicated	Drugs less commonly or rarely implicated
Typical antipsychotic agents (e.g., chlorpromazine, promazine, haloperidol, trifluoperazine, sulpiride, flupentixol, pimozide, fluphenazine)	Atypical antipsychotic agents (e.g., quetiapine, clozapine)
	Calcium channel agents (e.g., diltiazem, verapamil)
Calcium channel agents (e.g., flunarizine, cinnarizine)	Antiarrhythmic agents (e.g., amiodarone)
	Antidepressants (MAOI, SSRI, TCA)
	Anticonvulsants (e.g. sodium valproate)
Antiemetic agents (e.g., prochlorperazine, metoclopramide)	Lithium
Atypical antipsychotic agents, particularly at higher doses (e.g., risperidone, olanzapine) Antihypertensive agents (e.g., reserpine, a-methyldopa)	Miscellaneous: anticancer drugs (tamoxifen, thalidomide), hormones (levothyroxine, medroxyprogesterone), some of the antibiotics, antiviral and antifungal agents

Table 5.2 Medications with strong anticholinergic activity and alternative approaches [13]

Therapeutic class	High anticholinergic activity medications	Alternative approaches
Antihistamines	Brompheniramine Carbinoxamine Chlorpheniramine Clemastine Cyproheptadine Dexchlorpheniramine Dimenhydrinate Diphenhydramine (oral) Doxylamine Hydroxyzine Meclizine Triprolidine	Intranasal normal saline Second generation antihistamine (e.g., loratadine) Intranasal steroid (e.g., beclomethasone, fluticasone)
Antidepressants	Amitriptyline Amoxapine Clomipramine Desipramine Doxepin (>6 mg) Imipramine Nortriptyline Paroxetine Protriptyline Trimipramine	For depression: selective serotonin reuptake inhibitors (SSRI) (except paroxetine); selective norepinephrine reuptake inhibitor (SNRI), bupropion For Neuropathic Pain: SNRI, gabapentin, capasaicin topical, pregabalin, lidocaine patch
Antimuscarinics (urinary incontinence)	Darifenacin Fesoterodine Flavoxate Oxybutynin Solifenacin Tolterodine Trospium	Mirabegron
Antiparkinson agents	Benztropine Trihexyphenidyl	Carbidopa/levodopa
Antipsychotics	Chlorpromazine Clozapine Loxapine Olanzapine Perphenazine Thioridazine Trifluoperazine	Second generation antipsychotics except olanzapine if clinically warranted and benefit>risks especially in dementia patients
Antispasmodics	Atropine (excludes ophthalmic) Belladonna alkaloids Clidinium-chlordiazepoxide Dicyclomine Homatropine (excludes ophthalmic) Hyoscyamine Propantheline Scopolamine (excludes ophthalmic)	Loperamide Rifaximin
Skeletal muscle relaxants	Cyclobenzaprine Orphenadrine	For acute mild or moderate pain: acetaminophen, nonacetylated salicylate (e.g., salsalate), propionic acid derivatives (e.g., ibuprofen, naproxen)—yet consider co-morbidities and duration of use
Antiarrhythmic	Disopyramide	Atrial fibrillation: For rate control: nondihydropyridine CCB (e.g., diltiazem), beta blocker For rhythm control: dofetilide, flecainide, propafenone
Antiemetic	Prochlorperazine Promethazine	Ondansetron

Adapted from American Geriatrics Society 2015 Beers Criteria Update Expert Panel American Geriatrics Society 2015 Updated Beers Criteria for Potentially Inappropriate Medication Use in Older Adults. J Am Geriatr Soc 2015; 63:2227–2246, and Hanlon JT, Semla TP, Schmader KE. Alternative medications for medications in the use of high-risk medications in the elderly and potentially harmful drug-disease interactions in the elderly quality measures. J Am Geriatr Soc 2015; 63

result in greater concentrations of drugs resulting in increased risk for adverse drug events. Furthermore, it is important to note that other factors influence hepatic metabolism such as gender (e.g., women eliminate zolpidem (drug rarely indicated in seniors) slower than men), hepatic congestion from heart failure (e.g., reduces metabolism of warfarin and increases INR), and smoking (e.g., increases clearance of theophylline as it increases monooxygenase enzymes).

5.2.6 Renal System

Age related changes in renal function must be considered carefully. The following age related changes occur variably in the kidney [11]:

- Decrease in renal mass (due to number and size of intact nephrons) and blood flow;
- Decrease in glomerular filtration rate as well as tubular secretion and reabsorption.

The creatinine clearance is generally used as an index of renal function in order to make appropriate adjustments for dose when using drugs primarily or significantly eliminated by the kidney. The Cockcroft and Gault equation utilizes serum creatinine measurement, age, and weight. Despite limitations, this estimate is used widely within drug handbooks to dose adjust commonly used medications such as antibiotics and anticoagulants [15]. The clinical significance has been noted with the novel oral anticoagulant agents (e.g., dabigatran, rivaroxaban) with the increased risk of bleeding when not dosed appropriately [16]. Chapter 25—Nephrology provides a detailed discussion of the assessment of renal function and managing patients with various degrees of renal failure.

5.2.7 Body Composition

Body composition changes with aging and this can potentially influence the distribution of drugs. This could be clinically significant. One additional change that is important for practitioners is the impact of stress on the aged nervous system. Change in mental status is often a warning of a more insidious disease. Often times an acute infection, electrolyte abnormality or an addition or dose change of a medication may be the underlying etiology. Such changes include:

- Decrease in total body water influencing the serum and tissue concentration of medications such as digoxin;
- Decrease in lean body mass;
- Decrease in serum albumin which is known to bind medication such as phenytoin, valproic acid, and warfarin;

- Increase in total body fat leading to an increased volume of distribution of fat-soluble medications such as sedative-hypnotics and other CNS medications.

The magnitude of these changes is heterogeneous among seniors and is not predictable. Clinicians, therefore, must be hyper-vigilant for drug side effects or drug–drug interactions in supervising the care of all seniors. In summary, age related physiological changes in all seniors place them at a variable but marked increase in risk for an adverse drug event. The clinician must thoughtfully attempt to choose the correct dosage of the correct drug for the condition recognizing the heterogeneity in the population. The general prescribing dictum of starting medications at a low doses and then titrating up slowly while monitoring closely and regularly for adverse effects is prescient.

5.2.8 Adverse Drug Events

Adverse drug events (ADEs) in seniors are very common. Thirty-six percent of identified ADEs involved elderly individuals. Twenty-eight percent of all hospitalizations for seniors were medication related: 11 % due to non-adherence and 17 % due to adverse drug events [17]. Among ambulatory older adults, each ADE adds approximately $1300 in the cost of an individual's care [18]. The most common ADEs in seniors leading to urgent hospitalizations are gastrointestinal bleeding due to hematologic agents or gastrointestinal irritants, volume and electrolyte disturbances due to cardiovascular agents, altered mental status due to central nervous system agents, and hypoglycemia due to endocrine agents such as oral hypoglycemic agents or insulin [19].

Adverse drug events are very common but highly preventable. ADEs among older adults were serious, life threatening, or fatal in 38 %; and over 27 % of all ADEs were felt preventable. Over half of these ADEs were attributed to the lack of careful monitoring! [20, 21].

In addition to ADEs, medication non-adherence is a significant clinical problem. The average rate of poor or non-adherence is estimated to be between 30 and 50 %, irrespective of the burden of a patient's disease or prognosis [22]. Medication non-adherence contributed close to two-thirds of medication-associated hospitalizations in the USA [23]. In contrast, patients with high rates of medication adherence have significantly lower hospitalization rates [23]. The more complexity a patient's medication regimen the more likely is poor on non-adherence leading to a higher risk for medication errors [24]. There are high monetary costs to society from poor or non-adherence to drugs. For example, one study showed good adherence (compared to poor adherence) to medications decreased disease-associated costs [25]. In the USA, non-adherence is estimated to cost about $100 billion a year (including hospital costs), as well as contributing to about one-tenth of total hospitalizations [22].

Emerging models of health care incorporate an interdisciplinary approach to improve medication management for older adults. Currently Medicare Part D plans (prescription coverage) offer a covered benefit for eligible beneficiaries called Medication Therapy Management (MTM). MTM is a "patient-centric and comprehensive approach to improve medication use, reduce the risk of adverse events, and improve medication adherence." This program was developed to minimize ADEs and poor adherence among seniors who obtain Part D coverage [26]. The MTM program is available at no cost if a patient meets three conditions: more than one chronic condition; taking several medications; and combined annual cost of medications is more than $3507 (2016).

5.3 Polypharmacy (Polymedicine)

Medication adverse events are common in polypharmacy. Polypharmacy (using five or more drugs) often results when a clinician is prescribing for a patient with multiple conditions. In that scenario, a clinician may prescribe the medications suggested in several disease specific guidelines. However, such guidelines were typically designed by specialty experts for a patient with just a single disease.

Difficulty in sorting out problems from polypharmacy is especially profound because it is often uncertain what drugs are actually being taken and what symptoms are attributable to an ADE versus the symptoms from a patient's illnesses. There are many clinical tools and resources to combat polypharmacy and optimize prescribing. The following section highlights some of the most valuable of these.

5.3.1 Pharmacists' Care

Interprofessional teams including pharmacists have been shown to have overall positive impact on the care of older adults. A recent meta-analysis examining the effect of US pharmacists showed a positive effect on therapeutic safety, hospitalization, and adherence outcomes [27]. These findings support the expanding role of pharmacist in direct patient care services to improve the care of older adults with chronic co-morbidities.

5.3.2 American Geriatrics Society (AGS) Beer's Criteria

The initial Beers Criteria was published in 1991. It was a consensus panel's attempt to catalogue potentially inappropriate medications for nursing home residents. It was updated in 1997 to address older adults across all settings of care. This updated criteria was then adopted by the Health Care Finance Administration (now CMS), and used in the evaluation of nursing homes during the required survey process. A 2003 update occurred prior to the initiation of Medicare Part D. At that time some of the criteria were adopted into various quality prescribing metrics for Medicare Part D plans. The Beers Criteria were updated under the direction of the American Geriatrics Society (AGS) in 2012 and 2015 [28].

The criteria are intended for use in all ambulatory, acute, and long-term settings of care (except in hospice and palliative care) for populations aged 65 years and older in the USA. The intentions of the criteria are to: (1) improve medication selection; (2) educate clinicians and patients; (3) reduce adverse drug events; and (4) serve as a tool for evaluating quality of care, cost, and patterns of drug use in older adults. The Beer's Criteria are readily available on the American Geriatrics Society website.

5.3.3 STOPP & START Criteria

The Screening Tool for Older People's potentially inappropriate Prescriptions (or STOPP) criteria is another explicit criteria created in 2008 in Ireland in response to the limited applicability of Beers criteria for medications outside the USA, due to differences in medication approvals. The STOPP criteria list medications by drug class or by adverse drug event type. Furthermore, the STOPP/START criteria address inappropriate prescribing (IP) by discussing two issues related to prescribing: potentially inappropriate medications (PIMs)—so-called STOPP and potential prescribing omissions (PPOs)—START [27]. Information on this tool as well as international initiatives can be found at: http://www.senator-project.eu (December 2015).

The STOPP/START criteria when used upon admission to an acute hospital significantly improved medication appropriateness [29], which was maintained 6 months later. Furthermore, if applied within 72 h of hospital admission there was significant reduction in ADEs and average length of stay by 3 days in older patients [30]. The process of routinely reviewing an older adult's medications with the goal of minimizing those that are potentially inappropriate is beneficial [31].

5.3.4 AGS Managing Multi-Morbidity Guiding Principles

Clinicians caring for older adults with multiple medical chronic conditions can find guidance in prescribing using the AGS Managing Multi-Morbidity Guiding Principles.

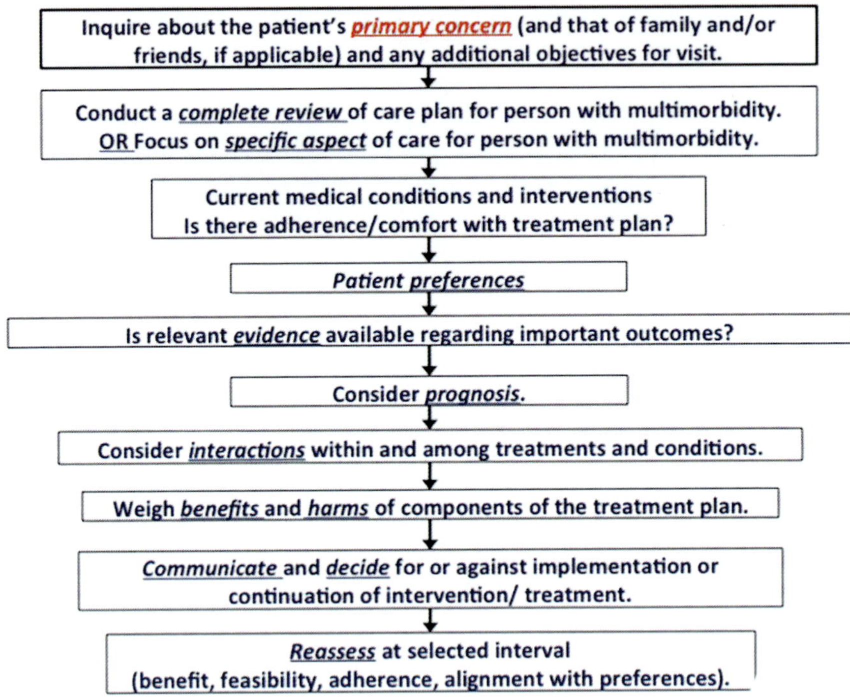

Fig. 5.1 AGS managing multi-morbidity guiding principles

This document was created by a panel of experts under the auspices of the American Geriatrics Society [32]. The goal of this effort was to develop an evidence base by which clinicians could better make sound clinical decisions. Figure 5.1 provides this decision template, which is available on the American Geriatrics Society website. While somewhat time consuming, using this template approach will optimize each patient's therapy consistent with their unique goals. Withdrawing medications, deprescribing, is a result of following these "Guiding Principles.".

Table 5.3 Levels of disease prevention [2]

Primary prevention	Avoids the development of a disease. Most population-based health promotion activities are primary preventive measures
Secondary prevention	Activities are aimed at early disease detection, thereby increasing opportunities for interventions to prevent progression of the disease and emergence of symptoms
Tertiary prevention	Reduces the negative impact of an already established disease by restoring function and reducing disease-related complications

5.4 Deprescribing

Deprescribing is "the systematic process of identifying and discontinuing drugs when existing or potential harms outweigh benefits within the context of an individual patient's care goals, current level of functioning, life expectancy, values, and preferences" [33]. This assessment needs to be frequently redone as patients health, goals, and values change. "You never step into the same river twice" is a useful expression of this concept. (Like a river, a patient's health situation, goals, and their assessment of benefit and burden from any intervention evolve with time.)

A patient's and his or her family's goals (prolong life, prevent morbidity, slow disease progression, or comfort care) must be repeatedly assessed. The results of these reassessments allow the clinician to identify proper patient goals and then logical therapeutic interventions in primary prevention, secondary prevention, control of chronic diseases, treatment of acute disease, and management of symptoms. This process is the foundation for deprescribing [34]. Table 5.3 outlines the theoretical levels of disease prevention.

An example of the application of these concepts is seen in the context of cardiovascular disease. Clinical trials and clinical guidelines encourage the initiation of long-term medication therapy for primary or secondary prevention of cardiovascular disease, as with statins. However these guidelines rarely define the timing, safety, or risks of discontinuing the agents. As a result of this, the number of medications used by a patient with cardiovascular (or other chronic illnesses) accumulates leading to multiple medications and an increase in ADEs. Not surprisingly, in the last year of life, the number of medicines prescribed increases by 50 % but this may not be consistent with a patient's goals [35]. This increase in medication use coupled with the effects of advanced disease at the end of life increases the risk of ADEs [36].

Fig. 5.2 Approach to deprescribing

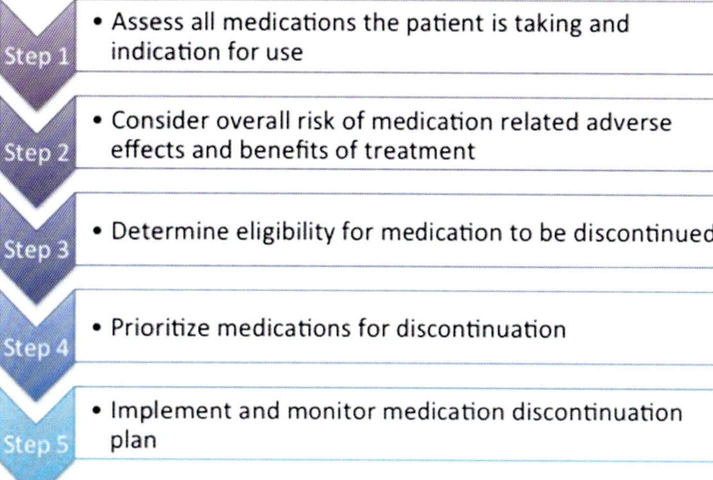

Accordingly, a focused effort by the clinician is imperative to identify the goals of care and deprescribe medications whenever possible. Clinicians in the setting of advanced life-limiting illness should always do this to reduce ADEs and potentially enhance quality of life (QOL) and sometimes survival [37, 38]. However, the choice of which medicines to discontinue, as well as estimating the time to benefit and safety, is not well studied. Therefore, thoughtful clinical judgment with sensitive patient and family communication is mandatory [37–40]. Figure 5.2 provides an approach when faced with these complex judgments [34]. Unfortunately this approach is not commonly used: one study reported that only one third of older adults did not have a conversation with their health care providers about priorities in health care decision-making [41].

A common example of this situation is statin therapy in older adults for primary and secondary prevention of cardiovascular disease. Although there is compelling evidence for prescribing statins for secondary prevention for people who are expected to live for many years, no evidence exists to guide decisions to discontinue statin therapy in patients with limited life expectancy. A randomized trial evaluated the safety and clinical impact of statin discontinuation in the palliative care setting. This issue was addressed in nearly 400 patients with an estimated life expectancy of less than 1 year and who were all taking statin for primary or secondary prevention for at least 3 months (69 % used >5 years). Remarkably, days until death after stopping statin was 229 with discontinuation versus 190 with continuation. Additionally to improving survival and reducing ADEs, studies of deprescribing, in appropriate situations, have financial benefit: $603 million in US healthcare expenditures with statins alone [42]. Similar results of deprescribing proton pump inhibitors have been published [43].

5.5 Summary

In order to optimize prescribing for older adults, reduce polypharmacy, decrease the number and burden of ADEs and reduce inappropriate health care costs, clinicians of every discipline must focus on medication management. Increasingly, interprofessional teams that include a pharmacist show great improvements in helping patients and their families meet their unique care goals while at once decreasing ADEs, improving outcomes and reducing costs.

References

1. Administration on Aging (AoA) Aging Statistics. Available at http://www.aoa.acl.gov/Aging_Statistics/index.aspx. Accessed 4 Dec 2015.
2. Centers for Disease Control and Prevention. Available at http://www.cdc.gov/aging/index.html. Accessed 4 Dec 2015.
3. National Council on Aging. Available at: https://www.ncoa.org. Accessed 4 Dec 2015.
4. Strandberg LR. Drugs as reasons for nursing home admissions. J Am Health Care Assoc. 1984;10:20–3.
5. Tjia J, Velten SJ, Parsons C, et al. Studies to reduce unnecessary medication use in frail older adults: a systematic review. Drugs Aging. 2013;30:285–307.
6. Qato D, Alexander GC, Conti R, Johnson M, Schumm P, Lindau S. Use of prescription and over-the-counter medications and dietary supplements among older adults in the United States. JAMA. 2008;300(24):2867–78.
7. IMS Institute. IMS Institute Study: $500B in global health spending can be avoided annually through more responsible use of medicines [Internet]. Oct. 2012; Available from: http://www.imshealth.com/portal/site/ims/menuitem.d248e29c86589c9c30e81c033208c22a/?vgnextoid=563637d68412a310VgnVCM10000076192ca2RCRD&vgnextchannel=437879d7f269e210VgnVCM10000071812ca2RCRD&vgnextfmt=default.
8. Burton MM, Hope C, Murray MD, et al. The cost of adverse drug events in ambulatory care. AMIA Annu Symp Proc. 2007:90–3.

9. Walston J, Hadley EC, Ferrucci L, et al. Research agenda for frailty in older adults: toward a better understanding of physiology and etiology: summary from the American Geriatrics Society/National Institute on Aging Research Conference on Frailty in Older Adults. J Am Geriatr Soc. 2006;54:991–1001.

10. Rowe JW, Kahn RL. Human aging: usual and successful. Science. 1987;237:143–9.

11. Higbee MD. The geriatric patient: general physiologic and pharmacologic considerations. J Pharm Pract. 2000;18(4):250–62.

12. Thanvi B, Treadwell S. Drug induced parkinsonism: a common cause of parkinsonism in older people. Postgrad Med J. 2009;85:322–6.

13. Hanlon JT, Semla TP, Schmader KE. Alternative medications for medications in the use of high-risk medications in the elderly and potentially harmful drug-disease interactions in the elderly quality measures. J Am Geriatr Soc. 2015;63:e8.

14. Klausner SC, Schwartz AB. The aging heart. Clin Geriatr Med. 1985;1(1):119–41.

15. Creatinine Clearance Calculator. Available at: http://reference.medscape.com/calculator/creatinine-clearance-cockcroft-gault. Accessed 4 Dec 2015.

16. Morill AM, Ge D, Willett KC. Dosing of target-specific oral anticoagulants in special populations. Ann Pharmacother. 2015;49(9):1031–45.

17. Rollason V, Vogt N. Reduction of polypharmacy in the elderly: a systematic review of the role of the pharmacist. Drugs Aging. 2003;20(11):817–32.

18. Field T, Gilman BH, Subramanian S, Fuller JC, Bates DW, Gurwitz JH. The costs associated with adverse drug events among older adults in the ambulatory setting. Med Care. 2005;43:1171–6.

19. Budnitz D, Lovegrove M, Shehab N, et al. Emergency hospitalizations for adverse drug events in older Americans. N Engl J Med. 2011;365(21):2002–12.

20. Gurwitz J, Field T, Harrold L, Rothschild J, Debellis K, Seger A, Cadoret C, Fish L, Garber L, Kelleher M, Bates D. Incidence and preventability of adverse drug events among older persons in the ambulatory setting. JAMA. 2003;289(9):1107–16.

21. Steinman MA, Handler SM, Gurwitz JH, et al. Beyond the prescription: medication monitoring and adverse drug events in older adults. J Am Geriatr Soc. 2011;59(8):1513–20.

22. Vermeire E, Hearnshaw H, Van Royen P, Denekens J. Patient adherence to treatment: three decades of research. A comprehensive review. J Clin Pharm Ther. 2001;26(5):331–42.

23. Osterberg L, Blaschke T. Adherence to medication. N Engl J Med. 2005;353(5):487–97.

24. Sokol MC, McGuigan KA, Verbrugge RR, Epstein RS. Impact of medication adherence on hospitalization risk and healthcare cost. Med Care. 2005;43(6):521–30.

25. Mansur N, Weiss A, Beloosesky Y. Looking beyond polypharmacy: quantification of medication regimen complexity in the elderly. Am J Geriatr Pharmacother. 2012;10(4):223–30.

26. Centers for Medicare & Medicaid Services. Medication therapy management. Available at: http://www.cms.gov/Medicare/Prescription-Drug-Coverage/PrescriptionDrugCovContra/MTM.html. Accessed 23 Nov 2015.

27. Lee JK, Slack MK, Martin J, et al. Geriatric patient care by U.S. pharmacists in healthcare teams: systematic review and meta-analyses. J Am Geriatr Soc. 2013;61(7):1119–27.

28. American Geriatrics Society. Beers Criteria Update Expert Panel American Geriatrics Society 2015 Updated Beers Criteria for potentially inappropriate medication use in older adults. J Am Geriatr Soc. 2015;2015(63):2227–46.

29. Hamilton H, Gallagher P, Ryan C, Byrne S, O'Mahony D. Potentially inappropriate medications defined by STOPP criteria and the risk of adverse drug events in older hospitalized patients. Arch Intern Med. 2011;171:1013–9.

30. O'Mahony D, O'Sullivan D, Byrne S, et al. STOPP/START criteria for potentially inappropriate prescribing in older people: version 2. Age Ageing. 2015;44:213–8.

31. Gallagher PF, O'Connor MN, O'Mahony D. Prevention of potentially inappropriate prescribing for elderly patients: a randomized controlled trial using STOPP/START criteria. Clin Pharmacol Ther. 2011;89:845–54.

32. Grace AR, Briggs R, Kieran RE, et al. A comparison of Beers and STOPP criteria in assessing potentially inappropriate medications in nursing home residents attending the emergency department. J Am Med Dir Assoc. 2014;15(11):830–4.

33. American Geriatrics Society (AGS). Guiding principles for the care of older adults with multimorbidity: an approach for clinicians: American Geriatrics Society Expert Panel on the Care of Older Adults with Multimorbidity. J Am Geriatr Soc. 2012;60(10):E1–25.

34. Scott IA, Hilmer SN, Reeve E, et al. Reducing inappropriate polypharmacy: the process of deprescribing. JAMA Intern Med. 2015;175(5):827–34.

35. Brandt N, Stefanacci R. Discontinuation of unnecessary medications in older adults. Consult Pharm. 2011;26:845–54.

36. Currow DC, Stevenson JP, Abernethy AP, et al. Prescribing in palliative care as death approaches. J Am Geriatr Soc. 2007;55(4):590–5.

37. Holmes HM, Hayley DC, Alexander GC, Sachs GA. Reconsidering medication appropriateness for patients late in life. Arch Intern Med. 2006;166(6):605–9.

38. Bain KT, Holmes HM, Beers MH, Maio V, et al. Discontinuing medications: a novel approach for revising the prescribing stage of the medication-use process. J Am Geriatr Soc. 2008;56(10):1946–52.

39. Sinclair C, Vollrath AM, Hallenbeck J. Discontinuing cardiovascular medications at the end of life: lipid-lowering agents. J Palliat Med. 2005;8(4):876–81.

40. Holmes HM, Min LC, Yee M, et al. Rationalizing prescribing for older patients with multimorbidity: considering time to benefit. Drugs Aging. 2013;30(9):655–66.

41. Case SM, O'Leary J, Kim N, Tinetti ME, Fried TR. Older adults' recognition of trade-offs in healthcare decision-making. J Am Geriatr Soc. 2015;63(8):1658–62.

42. Kutner JS, Blatchford PJ, Taylor Jr DH, et al. Safety and benefit of discontinuing statin therapy in the setting of advanced, life-limiting illness: a randomized clinical trial. JAMA Intern Med. 2015;175(5):691–700.

43. Reeve E, Andrews JM, Wiese MD, et al. Feasibility of a patient-centered deprescribing process to reduce inappropriate use of proton pump inhibitors. Ann Pharmacother. 2015;49(1):29–38.

Danielle J. Doberman and Elizabeth L. Cobbs

6.1 Introduction

Palliative care is an important dimension in the care of older adults, who account for a disproportionate percent of health-care use, with more than half of all older adults having three or more chronic diseases [1]. The person-centered focus of palliative care is especially relevant because multi-morbidity is associated with many negative consequences for older adults, including higher rates of adverse events from treatments, decreased quality of life (QOL), increased risk of disability, institutionalization and death, and greater health care expenditures [1].

Heterogeneity within the older population is multifactorial, and extends beyond variability in physical capabilities. Life experience, cultural and ethnic background, and religious or spiritual identification lead to individual differences in values and goals for health care. These values are likely to be especially meaningful when serious illness is present. In order to provide optimal, person-centered care, clinicians must communicate thoughtfully and compassionately with patients and families to develop goals and plans for care that are practical and reflect each patient's personal preferences [1].

D.J. Doberman, MD, MPH
Division of Geriatrics and Palliative Medicine, George Washington University, 2150 Pennsylvania Avenue N.W., Washington, DC 20037, USA

E.L. Cobbs, MD (✉)
Division of Geriatrics and Palliative Medicine, George Washington University, 2150 Pennsylvania Avenue N.W., Washington, DC 20037, USA

Geriatrics, Extended Care and Palliative Care,
Washington DC Veterans Affairs Medical Center,
50 Irving Street NW, Washington,
DC 20422, USA
e-mail: ecobbs@mfa.gwu.edu

6.2 The General Principles of Palliative Care

Three case examples of older adults of the same age and diagnoses but with differing health circumstances and preferences exemplify this point and will be referred to throughout the text:

(1) Anna: is a frail 85-year-old, with chronic obstructive pulmonary disease (COPD) from years of smoking, chronic kidney disease (CKD), peripheral-vascular disease (PVD), and atrial fibrillation. She ambulates with a rolling walker containing her oxygen canister. She recently moved in with her daughter after her last exacerbation of COPD when she became more forgetful and fearful of being by herself. Her need for 2 L of oxygen at all times makes it challenging to leave the apartment. Over the last 4 months, she was hospitalized three times: twice for respiratory ailments and once for Clostridium difficile colitis following a rehabilitation stay. She now presents to the Emergency Department (ED) with a dusky, cold, and painful right foot.

(2) Bob: is a robust 85-year-old with COPD from years of smoking, CKD, PVD, and atrial fibrillation. He plays golf twice a week and lives independently with his wife in a senior community. He volunteers at his church every Sunday to teach in the second grade class. He now presents to the ED with painless jaundice.

(3) Claire: is an 85-year-old nursing home resident with advanced dementia, COPD from years of smoking, CKD, PVD, and atrial fibrillation. Dependent on others for help with all activities of daily living, Claire often wanders aimlessly around the nursing facility looking for a lost kitten. She now presents to the ED with a hip fracture following a fall.

These cases illustrate three common scenarios of serious illness for older adults. Each person has nearly the same

© Springer International Publishing Switzerland 2017
J.R. Burton et al. (eds.), *Geriatrics for Specialists*, DOI 10.1007/978-3-319-31831-8_6

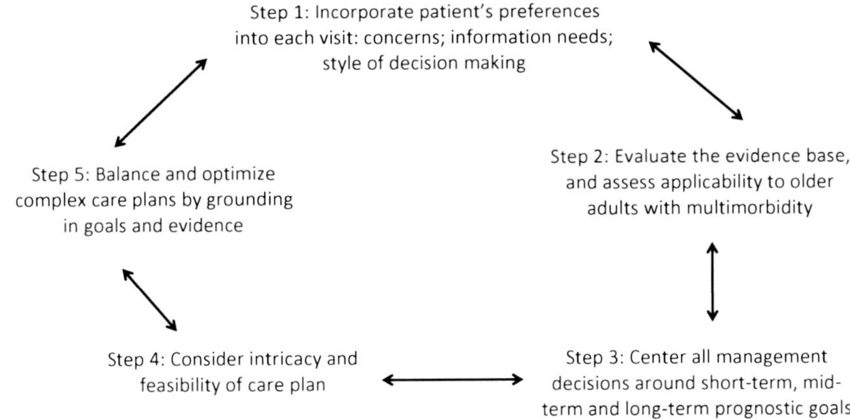

Fig. 6.1 Evaluation and management of those with multimorbidity [1]

past medical history. However, there is enormous heterogeneity in their multimorbidity, with varied implications for cognitive function, prognosis, and decision making. What questions should be asked by the emergency medicine physician, the hospitalist, the surgeon, the anesthesiologist, the cardiologist or pulmonologist? Who would ask about her advance directives? Which provider(s) would ponder the patient's prognosis at the outset of this new serious condition? How the patient's pre-existing life expectancy should be balanced with the prognosis resultant from the new problem? Would questions differ based on the patient's decision-making capacity or level of frailty? Do the answers to these questions alter the treatments offered? Given the heterogeneity of these patients, yet with a similar pattern of chronic disease burden, what advice would you provide to each?

If none of the physicians already involved with these patients are comfortable addressing all of these questions, a consultation with a palliative care provider would be helpful to develop the relevant information, options for treatment, risks and benefits and to assist the patient and family in defining goals and plans for care. Even with palliative care consultation, effective communication among providers, patients and families is critical to achieving optimal care. Good communication reduces physical and emotional distress, increases treatment adherence, and improves patient satisfaction [2]. One model for implementing a patient-centered care approach for older adults with multimorbidity has been advanced by the American Geriatrics Society (AGS). Items of value to the patient are integrated into outcomes [1, 3]. Models of shared decision are especially useful for older patients with multimorbidity [1, 4]. An overview of the AGS model can be viewed in Fig. 6.1 and in its totality at www.geriatricscareonline.org.

For older patients with multimorbidity and a new serious problem, as described above, short-, medium-, and long-term goals now may be achievable only over a few weeks or months.

6.2.1 Trajectories of Decline

Four prototypic healthcare trajectories for serious illness have been described in the literature: [5, 6] (1) sudden death; (2) death following a disease of progressive, linear decline (e.g., non-treatable cancer); (3) death following an illness with intermittent, acute exacerbations, or a "sawtoothed" functional decline (e.g., congestive heart failure or COPD); and (4) death from gradual progressive functional decline (e.g., neuromuscular disease or dementia). The three patterns of decline are shown in Fig. 6.2. In these patterns, the patient typically has been living in a state of variable, but limited, functional reserve often with dependence in activities of daily living (ADLs) for months or years prior to death. These situations, especially with a superimposed new illness or injury, require complex judgments by clinicians.

6.3 The Specialty of Palliative Care Medicine and Its Interface with Other Programs and Specialties

The World Health Organization (WHO) defines palliative care as healthcare that *"Improves the quality of life of patients and their families facing the problems associated with life-threatening illness, through the prevention and relief of suffering."* *"It affirms life, and regards dying as a normal process; it intends neither to hasten nor postpone death."* [7] Palliative care focuses not only on the patient, but also on his or her supporters, as all are profoundly impacted: physically, emotionally, socially, and spiritually. While the terms, "palliative care" and "palliative medicine" are often used inter-changeably, the broader term "palliative care" is preferred when referring to the multidisciplinary services including interdisciplinary teams and programs aimed at maintaining hope, preserving dignity and autonomy, and improving quality of life (QOL) for patients and families.

Fig. 6.2 Serious illness trajectories [5, 6]

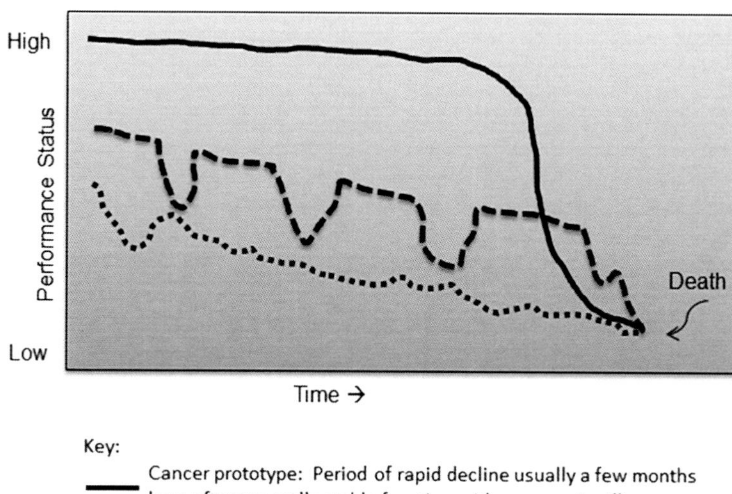

"Palliative medicine" is a phrase reserved for the portion of a team who are the medical providers only [8]. Palliative support is appropriate at any stage of illness—from diagnosis onward—and can be combined with treatments aimed at disease modification or cure. Team assistance and recommendations differ depending on the stage of illness and the preferences of the patient [9]. For example, while the hospitalized patient's goal is focused on disease cure or prolongation of life soon after learning of a new serious diagnosis, the palliative team may assist in building rapport with the patient and family and assisting with the practical burdens of illness.

As serious illness evolves, patient goals evolve, often shifting away from attempts at disease modification or cure as treatment options diminish or become more burdensome. During the evolution away from curative or disease-modifying treatment, the options for palliative treatments increase. Patients and families may focus on other goals such as being able to return home, improving physical comfort, alleviating spiritual distress, and other means of maximizing quality of life. Over time, the role of the palliative team will also change, likely assisting with increased symptom management. The palliative team may provide continuity of care and can assist in creating seamless transitions to home or other settings for post-acute care. Hospice services at home, or in an inpatient setting maybe a vital option to help the patient leave the hospital, or prevent admission.

6.4　Hospice Versus Palliative Care (Table 6.1)

While palliative care includes hospice care it is not limited to this. Hospice services are limited to those whose life expectancy is estimated to be less than 6 months, and focuses on end-of-life care. Palliative care providers care for patients at any point in the trajectory of a serious disease, regardless of prognosis [10].

In the USA, hospice is an integrated bundle of services that is covered by medical insurance. Hospice provides services, durable medical equipment and medications related to the terminal diagnosis (not to other co-morbidities). The care is provided by an interdisciplinary team. The Medicare Hospice Benefit requires each hospice to provide nurse case management services, access to physician services, chaplaincy, social work, and volunteer support. Bereavement counseling for 13 months after a patient's death is also offered. To enroll a patient in hospice, two physicians must certify they believe the patient has a life expectancy of 6 months or less. Patients are reassessed for hospice service eligibility at regular intervals, and services may extend beyond 6 months if a patient's condition is continuing to decline. However, if the patient's condition stabilizes, regulations dictate consideration of discharging the patient from hospice. Patients can revoke the hospice benefit at any time, such as if they are

Table 6.1 Palliative care vs. hospice

	Palliative care	Hospice
Primary goal	– Assist patient to achieve goals – Improve quality of life – Alleviate suffering	– Improve quality of life – Relieve suffering
Recipients	– Anyone with a serious illness	– Patients whose physicians certify a life limiting illness and a prognosis of 6 months (or less) if illness runs usual course and – Patients who elect their "hospice benefit" (e.g., insurance)
Providers	– Interdisciplinary Team may include MD, APN, SW, Chaplain, and other staff	– Interdisciplinary Team must include MD, RN, SW, Chaplain, volunteer, and a bereavement specialist.
Time frame	– Can be initiated at any time from diagnosis onward – Indefinite access	– Life expectancy of less than 6 months. – Services typically continue through death, but may be discontinued if patient's condition improves and life expectancy exceeds 6 months, or if patient elects to resume disease-modifying treatments.
Special benefits	– Treatments aimed at cure or disease-modification may be continued	– Provides and pays for medications, durable medical equipment related to the hospice diagnosis. – Volunteers provide some additional services.
Location	– Mostly hospitals, oncology practices, nursing homes, and group practices.	– Mostly at home. – Widely available.
Challenges	– Not widely available in the community setting.	– Typically, hospice benefit does not cover disease-modifying therapies such as chemotherapy, IV antibiotics, transfusions, etc. – New models of "concurrent care" (e.g., hospice and some chemotherapy) in some areas, especially if commercial insurance underwrites treatment. – Most hospices require caregiver in the home. – Personal care aide hours very limited.
Payment	– Professional fees are reimbursed by medical insurance, e.g., MD/NP fees covered by Medicare Part B. – Support from other programs (e.g., hospital, oncology practice) – No payment mechanism from Medicare for non-medical providers e.g., chaplain, personal care aides.	– Medicare Hospice Benefit or as defined by commercial payers.

APN advanced practice nurse, *IV* intravenous, *MD* physician, *NP* nurse practitioner, *RN* registered nurse, *SW* social worker

hospitalized. A re-evaluation for eligibility is required before enrolling in hospice again.

Hospice services are provided in the location the patient defines as "home" and, for example, may be engaged in a patient's private home, a nursing home, group home, or assisted living facility. The Medicare Hospice Benefit is commonly used and serves as the prototype for most other insurers.

6.5 Palliative Medicine vs. Geriatric Medicine

Palliative medicine and geriatric medicine share many common features. Both rely on interdisciplinary teams to provide care. Geriatric medicine emphasizes the importance of comprehensive assessment to optimize a patient's function. Palliative medicine focuses primarily on optimizing quality of life through alleviation of adverse symptoms, helping patients and families identify goals of care, and supporting effective emotional coping for patients and families. Both specialties encompass the care of older adults near the end of life and overlap in the care of frail elders. Both palliative and geriatric medicine teams have expertise in evaluating a patient's expected course, communication with patients and families to decide goals of care, develop advance care plans, and providing care throughout the course of the illness. Palliative providers have additional training and expertise in determining life expectancy, symptom control at end of life, and management of special populations of patients, such as those in the intensive care unit (ICU), patients with oncologic emergencies, nearing death with heart failure, human immunodeficiency virus (HIV), amyotrophic lateral sclerosis (ALS) and other degenerative neurological diseases, COPD, and chronic incapacitation from trauma. Geriatricians more typically have expertise caring for patients needing palliative care in nursing home, assisted living and home care venues. Both geriatric and palliative medicine specialists identify patient goals of care and address the comprehensive elements of function and well-being.

6.6   Evidence Base for Palliative Care

The Center to Advance Palliative Care (CAPC) (www.capc. org) has developed a venue for sharing expertise, tools, and resources in order to promote the integration of palliative care into every clinical setting serving those with serious illness. When palliative care is integrated into the care of patients in the ICU, research shows increased family satisfaction and comprehension; decreased family anxiety, depression and post-traumatic stress disorder; decreased conflict over goals of care; decreased time from recognition of poor prognosis to comfort-focused goals; increased symptom assessment; increased patient comfort; decreased use of non-beneficial treatments, and decreased ICU and hospital length of stay.

In the ED, there is evidence that proactive palliative care results in decreased hospitalizations, decreased in-hospital deaths, and increased use of hospice care. While the sites of care for palliative medicine consultation have historically been centered in the hospital setting, palliative services are moving to other places of need including outpatient clinics, assisted living environments, and nursing homes. Various models for outpatient palliative care services have been implemented. In one randomized trial, early palliative care for patients with non-small cell lung cancer in the outpatient setting resulted in improvements in both quality of life and mood. Participants also had less aggressive medical care at the end of life and longer survival [11].

The Institute of Medicine (IOM) report "Dying in America" described the state of end-of-life care in the USA [12]. This 2014 report concluded that improved medical and social supports to both patients and family could enhance quality of life while reducing costs. However, additional research suggested that many studies do not include adequate numbers of seniors [13]. "Geriatric Palliative Care" has been proposed as an "intersection subspecialty" for seniors. The cases presented early in the chapter exemplify this point and highlight the unique complexity present in each patient. Anna requires chronic management of COPD and other co-morbidities. Her acute problem is likely to worsen her other conditions and lead to more debility. Also, she is at high risk for a delirium, which if not prevented will worsen markedly her prognosis [14, 15]. Geriatric palliative care also must carefully address the needs of caregivers who are typically daughters or a senior partner often already overwhelmed with the care of supporting their children, grandchildren or meeting their own care needs. Such situations often preclude home hospice [16–18]. Palliative care planning, therefore, must consider all involved with helping the patient if an effective plan is to be developed [13].

6.7   Skilled Home Health vs. Home Hospice

Home health agencies offer many of the same services as home hospice: nurse case management, durable medical equipment, medication management, and social work assessment. Both skilled home health and hospice are provided by most insurers. The primary goal of hospice services is to improve quality of life through the end of life and this service continues through death (unless the patient is discharged from hospice). The goal of skilled home health services, however, is to resolve a medical or surgical problem (e.g., a wound) or functional loss from an illness or injury (e.g., therapy after a stroke). Services are short term and stop once the patient maximally improves. Hospice agencies provide 24-h telephone access to assist caregivers in managing urgent issues with the goal of caring for the patient effectively at home and avoiding hospital care. On the other hand, most skilled home health agencies do not have a 24 h on-call program and urgent needs must be provided by the primary care provider.

6.8   Palliative Care for all Clinicians

Basic palliative medicine attitudes and knowledge are appropriate for all clinicians caring for patients with serious illness [19, 20]. Such training and expertise in so-called primary palliative care has been endorsed by the 2014 IOM report [19, 21]. These proposed primary palliative skills needed by all clinicians include:

- Ability to elicit patient-centered goals of care
- Ability to develop and convey prognostic information and treatment options
- Assessment of pain and other physiologic and psychological symptoms
- Assessment of spiritual or social/practical burdens of illness
- Coordination of care for a safe transition to the next level of services

A study of over 1000 patients over age 80 years with serious illness showed the unique issues in this population compared to younger adults and children [22]. These older patients had a higher prevalence dementia, reduced prevalence of cancer, fewer recommendations for symptom management, and more questions concerning decision-making capacity, more issues related to withholding/withdrawing life-sustaining treatments and took more time to complete. These differences were substantiated in a slightly younger group, which showed that 70 % of patients older than 60 years lacked decision-making capacity at the time health care decisions were made [23]. In a third study, prior advance care planning conversations have been shown to reduce the emotional distress of surrogate decision makers of ICU patients [24]. These three studies point out the complexity of palliative care for seniors and the importance of advance care planning.

6.9 Communication and Shared Decision Making

Even today, many clinicians have received limited training in communication, estimating life expectancy, or breaking bad news [4, 25, 26]. As a result, many clinicians feel unprepared to help patients needing palliative and end-of-life care [4]. Patients with serious illnesses and their families or other caregivers desire and need clear and honest information [27, 28] from clinicians in order to wisely plan all aspects of their future: who will provide care, where will it be provided, what are the goals of care, what will become of their finances, what about their employment, and how do they think about dying. A stepwise approach of a compassionate explanation of the development of their current situation and the current options is best in hosting a family meeting and/or breaking bad news. Doing this thoughtfully and openly, with a wise sense of the course of the illness, and with sensitivity and empathy, decreases stress, confusion, false hopes, and anger for all. Such a conversation allows for the development of a satisfactory and shared decision that will help address all aspects of care including venue transitions and potential self-pay concerns [4, 27, 29].

A review of communication strategies with patients who have serious illness provides best practices and advocates for shared decision making using the patient-centered care model [27]. These strategies mirror the AGS [1] decision-making paradigm: (1) assess the patient's and family's understanding of the disease state and prognosis; (2) ascertain patient preference about information sharing and decision making; (3) involve family as guided by the patient; (4) discuss patient priorities, fears and thoughts about quality of life and function; (5) explore tradeoffs in quality of life, as patients often have goals more important than longevity, and (6) convey as accurate prognostic information as possible.

One approach to breaking bad news and negotiating a patient-centered care plan uses the mnemonic SPIKES, for **S**etting up the encounter, asking the patient their **P**erception of the medical situation, requesting an **I**nvitation to share prognostic information, provide **K**nowledge, **E**mpathize with emotion and **S**ummarize and **S**trategize for next steps [4]. An example of how this approach could be employed to assist in a conversation with Bob, a patient story early in the chapter, is shown in Table 6.2.

Contrary to the belief of some clinicians, patients are not harmed by discussions of end-of-life issues or goals of care planning [27]. Rather, patients and families wish to control the amount and timing of information they receive, especially when it relates to the prognosis of an illness(s) [28]. Commonly, patients and families need for information diverges as an illness progresses: family members typically want more detailed information and patients less.

The wise clinician must acknowledge and responding to patient and family emotions [30]. Unaddressed emotions can interfere with the ability to process and retain information, and may impair decision-making ability. Promptly responding to emotion—either verbally or non-verbally—legitimizes the feelings expressed and conveys openness on behalf of the clinician to discuss concerns fully and as they arise in the future [27, 30].

Finally, sensory and cognitive impairments are common in older adults, and may affect their ability to understand information presented verbally or visually (Table 6.3) [31, 32].

6.10 Symptom Relief in Serious Illness and EOL

Palliative assessment and treatment must incorporate considerations of the distinct pattern and severity of a patient's co-morbidities. Persons with dementia have unique needs in palliation. Cognitive impairment decreases a patient's ability to articulate complaints of distressing symptoms and to understand the disease process and develop and voice goals of care. Therefore, recognizing nonverbal cues are especially important to effective management. In situations of cognitive impairment, behavioral interventions (e.g., a compassionate and appropriate touch) are helpful. In the hospital, seniors are affected greatly by their environment. Noise, lighting, multiple visitors or providers at once, irritating interventions (e.g., IVs, oxygen, or catheters) can worsen agitation and discomfort, and these must be routinely assessed and modified. Seniors with chronic conditions and/or frailty often experience severe and distressing symptoms, such as limited activity, fatigue and physical discomfort or pain, which must be addressed [33, 34]. Because of co-morbidities and age-related physiological loses, drug management is complex in older patients needing palliative care. Chapter 5 provides an in-depth consideration of these issues. Of special consideration in palliative care two cardinal points should be made: use oral medications whenever possible, and when significant pain is present, avoid long-acting opioids, until the appropriate drug and formulation using short acting agents has been established.

Table 6.2 The SPIKES model employed in Bob's case

		Context	Words to consider:

S	Setup	• Find a private space, if in double room, draw curtain
		• Ensure patient comfort
		• Ensure uninterrupted time
		  o Turn off pager, phone
		  o Ensure presence of significant others
		  o Family/friends
		  o Medical team
			• Use non-verbal actions which show commitment to the patient and value to the dialogue:
			  o Sit down
			  o Ensure patient's physical comfort
			  o Attentive, open posture

P	Perception	• Assess patient/family's understanding of what is happening • Note vocabulary used by patient • Share decision making on meeting agenda	• "What is your understanding thus far about your jaundice, and what did you hope to learn today?" • "To make sure we are starting in same place, can you tell me what you understand about your yellow eyes, and what I can help you understand?"
I	Invitation	• Obtain patient's invitation to discuss details of illness; "ask" • Key with cross-cultural dialogues • Key with prognostic information	• "Are you the type of person who likes to know all the details about what is going on, or would you prefer I speak with your son?" • "How much information would you like to know about the future? About your diagnosis?" • "Would discussing prognosis be helpful to you?"
K	Knowledge	• Give a warning shot • Provide information info in small chunks and check for understanding • Avoid technical words and mirror patient's word choice o If patient says "growth," you say "growth"	• "I have your test results, and I have some bad news…" • E.g., "It appears as if we are unable to provide surgery due to the position of the cancer." • "What questions do you have? Is there anything I can help clarify?"
E	Empathize	• Empathize and explore the emotions expressed by the patient • Acknowledge emotion • Normalize feelings • Explore • Use "I wish" statements	• "I know these are not the results we wanted." • "Tell me what the hardest part of this is for you?" • "I am upset! Why did that surgeon examine my dad! I thought that meant he was going to have surgery!"
S	Summarize and Strategize	• Summarize what has been said • Clear plan for next steps and follow-up	• "Are there any last items I can help clarify?" • "Let's meet again at noon tomorrow to continue this discussion, after the medical oncologist has visited." • "I want to make sure I have clearly explained your dad's situation. Can you give me your understanding of what is ahead?"

Adapted from Baile et al. [4]

6.10.1 Symptom Assessment

A structured review of patients' goals and their current distressing symptoms needing attention is key to successful treatment. Such a review will need to be repeated frequently. For example, symptom management for a patient with only hours or days to live is likely to focus solely on comfort measures without concern of over sedation. When life expectancy is measured in weeks to months, concern for adverse effects of medications typically remains prominent. While cognitive impairment can make symptom assessment and management more challenging, nursing home residents with mild-to-moderate cognitive impairment have been shown to have self-reports of pain as valid as those without cognitive impairment [35]. Tools for symptom assessment include the easy to use Edmonton Symptom Assessment Scale [36]. This measures ten levels of distress for ten common symptoms including pain, fatigue, nausea, anorexia, dyspnea, and several affective features.

Patients with cognitive impairment have difficulty recalling previous symptoms making their comparison of interventions difficult. In this situation, the clinician must rely on changes in function, behavior or mood, as these may mirror improvement or deterioration of symptoms [37]. Several validated instruments are available to use in patients who are unable to communicate because of aphasia or intubation [38–40].

6.10.2 Approach to Management (Table 6.4)

With the goals of care established and assessment of symptoms complete, a comprehensive approach to symptom relief should be pursued. First, medications that do not

Table 6.3 Communication challenges and strategies with older adults

Potential challenges	Strategies
Low vision	– Ask and assess if low vision is present. – Adjust communication materials to avoid visual prompts. – Use "teach back" technique to assure understanding.
Hearing loss	– Ask and assess if able to hear adequately. – Establish optimal environment to promote communication, e.g., quiet, well lit room, seated directly in front of patient, minimize distractions. – Provide "pocket talker" or similar hearing augmentation tools. – Use "teach back" technique.
Low health literacy	– Reduce complexity of communication. – Avoid jargon and technical terms. – Try to use their words when possible. – Reduce the density of communication, no more than three concepts per encounter. – Use "teach back" technique.
Memory impairment	– Assess cognitive function by history-taking, chart review, or cognitive screen. – Identify family or health care proxies to participate.
Reduced concentration	– Optimize environmental factors to promote concentration. – Assess ability to concentrate and receive information. – Identify family or health care proxies to participate.
Cultural influences	– Recognize language and cultural barriers to communication. – Ask about communication preferences. – Ask about individual values and cultural backgrounds and seek to understand and integrate into care. – Use "teach back" technique for patient and family/health care proxies.
Role expectations	– Ask what and to whom information should be disclosed. – Ask about preferences for decision-making strategies.

further the patient's goals should be discontinued. Medications traditionally avoided in the older adult could now be considered if consistent with the goals of care. The mantra of "Start Low, Go Slow" guides prescribing. A second step is to optimize the "environment of care," a term that refers to practices related to the patient's experience. The goal is to promote quality of life, such as liberalizing diet, and visiting hours, reducing or eliminating vital signs, and allowing family, pets, and children to visit and even to sleep over.

6.10.2.1 Persistent Somatic Pain

Many older adults suffer from chronic non-malignant pain associated with musculoskeletal and other disorders. In some seniors, pain sensation may diminish; inherently reflecting age associated physiological deterioration in the nociceptive pathways, typically occurring after age 80 [41]. However, patients with cancer seem not to benefit from nervous system aging and are likely to experience significant pain from the cancer [42] and as a consequence of treatment [43].

Expert groups recommend beginning pharmacologic therapy with non-opioids such as acetaminophen at or less than 3 g per day (or lower in the presence of liver disease or alcohol excess) and with caution (see below) non-steroidal anti-inflammatory drugs (NSAIDs), then adding opioids of the necessary strength for worsening moderate pain, and stronger opioid plus non-opioid plus adjuvant therapy for more severe pain [39].

NSAIDs are particularly risky in older adults. Chronic NSAID use is associated with an increased risk of peptic ulcer disease, acute renal failure, fluid retention, stroke, and myocardial infarction. In addition, NSAIDs interfere with a number of commonly used medications such as warfarin and corticosteroids. Older adults are at higher risk for adverse effects due to age-related loss of physiologic reserve, polypharmacy, and multi-morbidities. It is advised to avoid chronic NSAID use if possible. Even the so-called safer NSAID celecoxib in higher doses has a greater incidence of gastrointestinal and cardiovascular adverse events. While naproxen, a longer acting NSAID, may have less cardiovascular toxicity than other NSAIDs, this and other long-acting NSAID preparations (e.g., piroxicam and oxaprozin) are best avoided, if possible [44].

Opioids are recommended for moderate to severe cancer pain but are generally under-prescribed in older patients with cancer pain [45, 46]. Key to effective pain relief is dosing the medicine at regular intervals, decided by its duration of relief of the patient's pain. Morphine sulfate is the standard in the treatment of pain at end of life, but oxycodone may be preferred for those with severely compromised renal or hepatic function (see Table 6.5).

6.10.2.2 Neuropathic Pain

Neuropathic pain is caused by damage to the somatosensory nervous system. Seniors are at increased risk because many diseases that cause neuropathic pain increase in incidence with age, including diabetes mellitus (painful diabetic neuropathy), herpes zoster (post-herpetic neuralgia), low back pain (lumbar spinal stenosis), cancers, limb amputation, and stroke. Treatment options are influenced by heterogeneity, multimorbidity, changes in pharmacodynamics and pharmacokinetics, polypharmacy, and limited evidence base for treatment decisions in older adults. Older adults are underrepresented in clinical trials and this reduces the generalizability of results to older populations [47]. Gabapentin and pregabalin are anticonvulsants that may be effective for neuropathic pain. Tricyclic antidepressants also may help, but are less desirable in older adults because of

Table 6.4 Palliative treatments for symptoms

Symptom	Special features	Treatments	Special considerations
Somatic pain	• Opioids first line for cancer pain.	• Morphine oral/IV/SQ • Oxycodone oral • Hydromorphone oral/IV/SQ • Fentanyl transdermal/IV	• Always start bowel medications at the same time as opioids to prevent constipation. • Start with half the opioid dose recommended for younger adults • Fentanyl and oxycodone are safer than morphine in those with renal impairment.
Neuropathic pain	• Adjuvants or co-analgesics helpful in addition to opioids.	• Gabapentin— may cause dizziness. • Pregabalin—25–50 bid in debilitated patients • Tricyclic antidepressants (TCA) • Carbamazepine • Selective serotonin reuptake inhibitors (SSRI) • Mixed reuptake inhibitors (SNRI) • Topical lidocaine patches. • Ketamine IV/PO (limited data in older adult) • Methadone	• Start with gabapentin 100 mg at bedtime. Increase weekly, as tolerated. • If stopping gabapentin or pregabalin, taper over a week to avoid seizures. • Gabapentin and pregabalin both require renal adjustment • Methadone is dangerous due to unpredictable metabolism and interaction with many other medications. May prolong QTc. For use by experienced prescribers only.
Dyspnea	• If bronchospasm present, give bronchodilators. • If volume overloaded, give furosemide 40 mg PO/IV one dose. • If oxygen sats <90, give oxygen 2 l/min. • Low dose opioids relieve dyspnea	• Albuterol 2 inhalations every 4 h prn or 3 ml nebulizations every 2 h prn. • Morphine 5 mg PO every 2 h prn or 2 mg SQ/IV every hour prn.	• Monitor respirations. • Consider non-pharmacologic options including fans, relaxation, CPAP, BiPAP, physical comfort measures.
Anxiety	• Investigate causes.	• Non-pharmacologic treatments first (empathic listening, psychotherapy, integrative therapies such as music, relaxation mindfulness, Reiki, massage) • SSRI—may take weeks for full effect. • Gabapentin or Trazodone. • Short acting benzodiazepine e.g., lorazepam. • Long-acting benzodiazepine if chronic (e.g., clonazepam).	
Delirium	• Common in older adults, especially those with low vision and hearing and cognitive impairment. Seek underlying cause. Anticholinergic medications likely to precipitate or worsen (e.g., diphenhydramine).	• Haloperidol 0.5 mg PO/IV/SQ every 4 h as needed. Increase by 1 mg every hour until desired effect. Maximum daily dose 20 mg.	• Consider QTc monitoring at higher doses.
Constipation	• Fecal impaction more common in older adults. Can lead to urinary retention.	• Senna • Docusate • Add milk of magnesia concentrate if supported by renal function 10 mg PO daily or bisacodyl 10 mg PO/PR every day. • Methylnaltrexone SQ every other day until BM.	• Start prophylactic senna daily or twice daily with start of opioid treatment. • Rectal exam to rule out fecal impaction. • Consider KUB to rule out obstruction.

(continued)

Table 6.4 (continued)

Symptom	Special features	Treatments	Special considerations
Fatigue	• Most common EOL symptom across all disease states	• Methylphenidate 2.5 in morning and at noon. Avoid taking near evening hours.	• Evidence for effective treatment is lacking.
Nausea/Vomiting	• Common in advanced cancer. Symptoms derive from disease or its treatment. Multiple neurotransmitters may be targeted simultaneously for symptom relief.	• See separate table.	
Anorexia	• Almost universal in seriously ill persons. • May be more distressing to family than patient. • Evaluate and treat reversible causes, such as constipation, nausea, or oral thrush	• Lift dietary restrictions and encourage patients to eat whatever is most appealing. • Avoid enteral feedings in patients with advanced dementia. Instead offer oral assisted feeding and "comfort feeding" by hand. • Enteral feedings might be considered in patients with proximal GI obstruction and high level of function, or patients with ALS, or patients receiving chemotherapy or radiation involving proximal GI tract.	• Megestrol acetate may improve appetite, weight, and quality of life in some patients but has not been shown to prolong life or improve tolerance of cancer therapies. • Corticosteroids may increase appetite, weight, and quality of life in some patients, but has not been shown to prolong life or improve other outcomes.
Depression	• Commonly under-recognized and under-treated in older adults and those near the end of life. • Mistaken belief that depression is normal in older adults and seriously ill persons.	• Standard treatments (SSRIs) are effective but take 2–6 weeks before therapeutic. • Psychostimulants are generally safe and can be given concurrently with standard antidepressants, e.g., methylphenidate 2.5 mg PO q am and lunch time. • Electroconvulsive therapy (ECT) is safe and may be used when a rapid response is needed. Presence of space-occupying CNS lesions precludes ECT. • Cognitive behavioral therapy and active listening are helpful.	
Bladder spasms	• Obtain urinalysis and culture/sensitivity. Treat UTI if believed to be present (asymptomatic bacteriuria is common). • If Foley present, can it be removed?	• Oxybutinin 5 mg PO TID for 48 h. Maximum daily dose is 20 mg. • Tolterodine 1–2 mg PO BID. • Scopolamine patch every 72 h. • Phenazopyridine 200 mg PO TID x48 h	• Anticholinergic therapy may worsen delirium

their anticholinergic effects. Topical lidocaine in patch or gel may be useful for some. Please see Table 6.5 for additional agents which may be helpful.

6.10.2.3 Dyspnea

Dyspnea is multifactorial in etiology, and results from the interplay of pathophysiologic stimuli from hypoxemia, bronchospasm, airway obstruction, pneumonia, and anxiety. Self-reported dyspnea occurs in more than 75 % with advanced heart failure [48] and is a more reliable measure than the respiratory rate, presence of pulmonary congestion, hypercarbia or hypoxemia. Managing a patient with dyspnea should be a blend of disease-targeted treatments and symptom-relief interventions. Opioids are especially effective in the treatment of dyspnea. They act both cen-trally to reduce the perception of dyspnea and peripherally on lung opioid receptors that influence respiratory drive and through capillary vasodilation. Opioids are considered safe in the treatment of dyspnea and remote concerns about them causing respiratory depression and CO2 retention are unfounded. Oxygen is an important treatment, especially for those who are hypoxemic. One large randomized and double-blind study of palliative oxygen versus canister room air for non-hypoxemic patients suggested that patients may benefit from moving air alone. Simple maneuvers such as a handheld fan directed at the face may also provide benefit. Non-pharmacologic interventions such as acupuncture and pulmonary rehabilitation have potential benefit but have not yet been carefully studied [49].

Table 6.5 Commonly used opioids

Name	Preparations	Dosing	Precautions
Morphine	• Versatile as available in oral or parenteral formulations. May be used IV, SQ, IM, PO, although IM avoided in comfort-focused care. • Short acting oral-form also called *"Morphine Immediate Release."* • Morphine elixir *concentrate* 20 mg/ml may be used with patients no longer taking oral sustenance. Place in buccal fold. • Morphine, sustained release (MS Contin©). Typically used every 12 h but may be used every 8 h with increasing up-titration.	• Start with 2.5–5 mg PO every 4 h PRN, or 1–2 mg IV every 3 h PRN based on renal function and opioid naïve status.	• Start with low dose short acting form PRN. • Titrate up as needed after 1–2 doses. • No ceiling. • Avoid in renal failure. • Prevent constipation. • Use opioid conversion chart to guide change of one opioid or form of opioid to another.
Oxycodone	• Oral preparations only. • Oxycodone: short acting opioid (approximately 3–4 h) • Oxycodone sustained release (Oxycontin©): longer acting (approximately 12 h)	• Start with 2.5–5 mg PO every 4 h PRN	• Start with low dose short acting. • Avoid using fixed combinations (e.g., Acetaminophen 325 mg-oxycodone 5 mg) when escalating doses. • Prevent constipation. • Use opioid conversion chart to change from one opioid to another.
Hydromorphone (Dilaudid)	• Available for oral, IV, SQ delivery. • More potent than morphine: 1 mg IV hydromorphone ~ 6.5 mg IV morphine	Oral elixir option may be ideal for some older adults	• A preferred opioid in renal failure. • Start with low dose and titrate up as needed. • Prevent constipation. • Use opioid conversion chart to guide change of one opioid to another.
Fentanyl	• Available for IV, SQ or transdermal application. • Parenteral forms have short half life	Fentanyl transdermal patch doses 12, 25, 50, 75 and 100 mcg/h. Change q 72 h. Use opioid conversion chart to calculate dose if switching from short acting opioids.	• Not removed by dialysis, therefore a preferred option for patients undergoing hemodialysis • No analgesia from patch for 8–14 h. • Do not start patch on opioid naïve patient with cancer pain. • Use opioid conversion chart to guide change from one opioid to another. • Prevent constipation.

IV intravenous, *SQ* subcutaneous, *IM* intramuscular, *PO* oral

6.10.2.4   Anxiety

Anxiety is common in association with medical illnesses and depression. Medical illnesses (e.g., COPD) and the medications used to treat them may cause symptoms that mimic or exacerbate underlying primary anxiety disorders. Standard treatments for generalized anxiety disorders in late life include cognitive behavioral therapy and medications such as selective serotonin reuptake inhibitors (SSRIs) and selective serotonin and norepinephrine reuptake inhibitors (SNRIs). Benzodiazepines are usually avoided in older adults because of the risk of falls, cognitive impairment, depression, and the potential for abuse [50]. However, in the last days and weeks of life, as a patient's goals of care evolve, they may be appropriate for symptom relief.

6.10.2.5   Delirium

Delirium is common near the end of life and may be a manifestation of a modifiable clinical condition, especially a reaction to a drug, an infection, urinary retention, obstipation, or pain. Accordingly, an underlying etiology should always be sought to guide appropriate management. Patients with cognitive impairment are at an especially high risk for delirium, but delirium is a prominent feature of the end stage of many neurologic, oncologic, and organ failure conditions and it is not always reversible. Agitation, hallucinations, and confusion from delirium cause distress to both patients and families and these symptoms should be treated. Patients and families will need education and reassurance about the course of delirium and that it may last for weeks or months. Behavioral treatments such as avoidance of over stimulation, reassurance, reorientation, treasured photos or other items are helpful. The presence of trusted caregivers or pets typically helps greatly. Non-pharmacologic approaches such as favorite music may be particularly effective in all but especially in those with dementia. Haloperidol remains the neuroleptic of choice. Anticholinergics (such as diphenhydramine) and benzodiazepines often exacerbate delirium and should be avoided except at the very end of life [51]. Chapter 2 provides an in-depth review of delirium in all situations.

6.10.2.6 Constipation

Constipation is the most common distressing symptom in seriously ill persons. It is the only persistent adverse effect of chronic opioid use. There are no data to support one laxative over another. Most experienced clinicians begin with a bowel stimulant (e.g., Senna) and escalate doses as needed. Osmotic agents (e.g., polyethylene glycol) may be added if needed. Suppositories, enemas, or manual disimpaction may be required. Methylnaltrexone is an opioid receptor antagonist given subcutaneously and may be used in cases of refractory opioid-related constipation. While this is the best studied, there are still limited data to support using this agent, or other opioid receptor antagonists, in seniors. Newer agents for chronic constipation, such as the small intestinal secreta-gogues lubiprostone and linaclotide, have limited data supporting their use at the end of life.

6.10.2.7 Fatigue

Fatigue is experienced by up to 60–97 % of end stage renal disease (ESRD), COPD and heart failure patients and is associated with poor quality of life [33, 52]. Mechanisms likely include age-related changes in muscle strength and mass, as well as organ dysfunction and adverse medication effects. Fatigue is a subjective complaint with no ideal quantifying measure. It is a part of the important syndrome of frailty, discussed at length with guidance to its assessment in Chap. 1. There are limited data to guide treatment of this common symptom and stimulants, such as methylphenidate, are often used, but no evidence supports this. Finally, sleep disordered breathing, such as sleep apnea, may be an important contributor to a patient's symptom of fatigue. It is widely under-recognized and should be considered. Chapter 27 provides guidance to the evaluation and treatment of sleep disordered breathing.

6.10.2.8 Nausea and/or Vomiting

Nausea and/or vomiting occur under a variety of conditions in response to activation of one or more emetic triggers and are present in up to 70 % of those with advanced cancer. Nausea is mediated through the gastrointestinal lining, the chemoreceptor trigger zone in the medulla oblongata, the vestibular system, and the cerebral cortex. Vomiting is coordinated through the brainstem. Because of the multiple neurotransmitters involved in nausea, there are a number of treatment options (Table 6.6) and typically more than one scheduled agent is needed for control.

6.10.2.9 Anorexia

Anorexia is almost always seen near the end of life but may be distressing to family although not to the patient. Ice chips, popsicles, moist compresses, artificial saliva, and good

Table 6.6 Nausea relief

Medications	Class	Special comments
Haloperidol (Haldol)	Dopamine antagonist	Very effective. Commonly used by hospice. Avoid in patients with Parkinson's disease
Olanzapine (Zyprexa)	Dopamine antagonist	Very effective. May be more effective than haloperidol, but more costly.
Prochlorperazine (Compazine)	Dopamine antagonist	May precipitate sedation, delirium, and urinary retention in older persons.
Promethazine (Phenergan)	Dopamine antagonist	May precipitate sedation, delirium, and urinary retention in older persons.
Perphenazine (Trilafon)	Dopamine antagonist	May precipitate sedation, delirium, and urinary retention in older persons.
Diphenhydramine	Antihistamine	May precipitate sedation, delirium, and urinary retention in older persons.
Meclizine	Antihistamine	May precipitate sedation, delirium, and urinary retention in older persons. Helpful with vestibular nausea
Hydroxyzine	Antihistamine	May precipitate sedation, delirium, and urinary retention in older persons.
Scopolamine	Anticholinergic	Especially helpful in vestibular causes of nausea. May cause delirium and urinary retention in older adults
Ondansetron	Serotonin antagonist	Effective for chemotherapy induced nausea.
Granisetron	Serotonin antagonist	Effective for chemotherapy induced nausea.
Metoclopramide	Prokinetic agent	If dysmotility present. May cause dystonia in rare cases.
Cimetidine, famotidine, ranitidine	H2 receptor antagonists	If dyspepsia and/or gastritis present.
Omeprazole, lansoprazole	Proton-pump inhibitors	If dyspepsia and/or gastritis present. If gastritis present.
Lorazepam	Benzodiazepam	Helpful for anticipatory nausea, or nausea worsened by smell, sight, sound, or emotion
Hypnosis, biofeedback	Non-pharmacologic	Helpful for anticipatory nausea
Reiki (a Japanese alternative medicine approach), ceiling fan, small meals	Non-pharmacologic	Useful for all types of nausea

mouth care are helpful. Lemon glycerin swabs irritate dry mucous membranes and should be avoided. While corticosteroids and megestrol acetate are associated with appetite enhancement and some weight gain, and may improve quality of life in some, they have not been associated with prolongation of life or improved treatment outcomes. With the exception of amyotrophic lateral sclerosis or proximal gastrointestinal obstruction associated with a good functional status and active treatment, there is no evidence that enteral feedings at the end of life improve survival or quality of life and are not routinely recommended. All experts recommend that dietary restrictions be liberalized and patients be encouraged to eat whatever they wish: so-called comfort feeding.

6.10.2.10 Depression

Depression is common in older adults with and without serious illness. Prevalence may be as high as 42 % in palliative care settings. Mood disorders also include anxiety and anticipatory grief, commonly seen in older adults with advanced illness. These symptoms are correlated with poor quality of life and increased mortality. Anticipatory grief is defined as a feeling of loss associated with current and anticipated changes related to illness. Grief should be distinguished from depression as the treatment and course often differ. Vegetative symptoms such as insomnia, weight change, and anorexia are not reliable markers of depression, and may stem from the underlying disease. Change in mood, suicidal ideation, and anhedonia are more reliable indicators. Treatment of depression in older adults with advanced illness is similar to treatment in other adult populations and can improve both depressive symptoms and mortality [53]. However, patients with advanced dementia are less likely to benefit from treatment with antidepressants. Cognitive behavioral therapy may offer substantial benefit. If prognosis is long enough, SSRIs are the pharmacologic treatment of choice. When life expectancy is short, psychostimulants such as methylphenidate are generally safe in older adults and may be effective. Electroconvulsive therapy may also be considered when a rapid response is needed (and CNS lesions are absent). Chapter 4 provides an in-depth discussion of depression in seniors.

6.10.2.11 Loud Respirations

Loud respirations (tracheal congestion or the "death rattle") often occur near the very end of life. This phenomena occurs because the patient is unable to clear secretions from the oropharynx, typically in the last few hours or days of life, and reflects the oscillation of secretions during inspiration and expiration. Although there is no evidence this is distressing to patients near the end of life, families and caregivers themselves often find the noisy respirations alarming. Optimal management includes preparing and educating the family about this occurrence. Sometimes gentle oral suction with a soft catheter helps, but deep suction is generally discouraged, as stimulation of the mucosa can trigger greater production of secretions. If pharmacological intervention is needed, anticholinergic medications can dry the secretions (Table 6.7).

6.11 Determining the Prognosis

Prognosis is a variable of enormous importance in palliative care and it must be assessed and thoughtfully communicated to the patient and caregivers [54]. Using age alone to estimate life expectancy without considering the clinical situation and disease burden leads to over treatment of frail and fragile patients or under treatment of highly active functional patients [55]. While "prognosis" is often assumed to refer to "remaining life expectancy," a prognosis can also forecast other outcomes, e.g., referring to the earlier cases, the likelihood that Anna will need an amputation, or Bob's ability to tolerate chemotherapy. Estimating mortality can be performed reliably for a population but poorly for an individual. Prognosis is a point estimate and will evolve in any patient over time as new issues and data emerge. Life tables are one means of deriving broad estimates of survival, but do not necessarily apply to individual patients. Mortality estimates can also be derived by applying disease-specific prognostic indices, such as such as the BODE Index for COPD [56] or the MELD score [57] for advanced liver disease. However, the applicability of a single disease-specific prognostic index to an individual with multiple severe illnesses is unknown.

A recent systematic review [54] identified 16 validated, non-disease specific prognostic tools in adults over age 60 and assessed each for quality and utility as an index for mortality. The review evaluated indices for older adults who reside in the community, nursing facilities, and eight tools which were validated for use in hospitalized patients: five for patients in the emergency department or at hospital admission, and three at hospital discharge. In sum, the most common predictors of mortality were functional status and comorbidities [54]. None of the studies reported a C statistic greater than 0.90: showing a lack of precision in mortality forecasting. Typically, mortality indices do not include positive factors such as social support or family history, which could be pertinent in families with exceptional longevity [58, 59].

Not all patients with a serious illness want a clinician's prediction of prognosis. It is important, therefore, to ascertain if the patient wishes to receive such information [28]. In the majority of patients, prognostic estimates are desired and the clinician must then use his or her judgment in presenting as accurate an estimate as possible, while acknowl-

Table 6.7 Management of active dying

Signs and symptoms	Management
Neurologic changes: Decreasing level of consciousness • Increasing drowsiness • Absence of eyelash reflexes	• Prepare families on what to expect • Assume continued "awareness" of patient and encourage family members to talk to patient • Promote familiar and comfortable environment of care (e.g., loved ones, pets, music) • Encourage family to show affection with touch
Terminal delirium • Confusion • Restlessness or agitation • Day/night reversal • Visions/hallucinations	• Education and support for family and caregivers • Consider treatment of underlying causes if death not imminent • Trial of opioids as first line (assess for worsening agitation, myoclonic jerks) • Benzodiazepines • Haloperidol (avoid in Parkinson's disease)
Respiratory changes: Diminished breathing • Shallow breathing • Periods of apnea or Cheyne–Stokes respirations • Use of accessory muscles • Appearance of breathlessness	• Educate and support family • Opioids or benzodiazepines in low doses for breathlessness
Circulatory changes create: • Cool, clammy skin • Increased perspiration • Mottled extremities • Decreased urinary output • Decreasing blood pressure • Increasing heart rate	• Educate and support family • Encourage gentle bathing • Blankets will not warm patient's periphery
Gastrointestinal changes: Ileus as peristalsis ceases Loss of sphincter control Incontinence of urine and/or stool	• Prepare and educate family • Maintain cleansing and skin care • Typically can manage with absorbent pads • Consider urinary catheter or rectal tube if cleansing care is distressing to patient, increasing caregiver burden, or threatening skin breakdown

Loss of ability to swallow
"Death rattle"
• Reflects accumulation of saliva or oropharyngeal secretions
• May sound like gargling
	• Educate and support family; often alarming, despite patient's comfort
	• Discontinue all unnecessary IV fluids; consider IV diuretic if BP favorable
	• Reposition patient to help clear secretions, e.g., turning side to side, lowering head of bed briefly, or raising head
	• Avoid suctioning
	• Reduce production of saliva and secretions with scopolamine or glycopyrrolate
	  o Glycopyrrolate 1 mg PO/IV/SQ BID/TID prn (Glycopyrrolate does not cross the blood brain barrier, thus lower risk for delirium with use.)
	  o Scopolamine transdermal 1.5 mg q 3 days; takes 12 h for full effect
	  o Hyoscyamine 0.125–0.25 mg PO/SL q 4 h prn
	  o Atropine ophthalmic drops may be used orally or sublingually, 1–2 gtt TID

edging significant uncertainty. For example, consider saying to Bob: "Patients with your condition often live several months, and by that I mean three to six, but this estimate could be more or less."

6.12 Ethical and Legal Considerations

One of the key steps in health care decision making is determining if the patient has decision-making capacity. Determination of decision-making capacity should be decision– or issue-specific, e.g., focused on a specific question, such as the capacity for Claire to consent to surgery, or for Anna to participate in discharge planning decisions. The need to consider a patient's decision-making capacity is especially challenging in patients with delirium or progressive cognitive decline.

If a patient is found to lack decision-making capacity, the patient's surrogate decision maker should be asked to provide informed consent about the goals of care including for diagnostic procedures, treatments or placement. In the absence of a previously designated proxy, each state has specific legal statutes detailing the order of surrogacy for patients unable to speak on their own behalf.

It is suggested that surrogates make decisions using the ethical principle of *"substituted judgment,"* or in effect, speaking on behalf of the patient: "What would the patient say if he were here with us and speaking for himself?" If a living will or other advanced directive document exists—including informal communications, such as social media postings or email writings—the health care team and the surrogate can use these to guide the understanding of the patient's wishes. Ideally a proxy has an in-depth understanding of the values by which the person leads their

Table 6.8 Key distinctions in major EOL ethical concerns

	Withhold life-sustaining technology	Withdraw life-sustaining technology	Palliative care and use of opioid analgesics	Physician-assisted suicide	Euthanasia
Intent of treatment	Avoid unwanted treatments	Discontinue unwanted or ineffective treatments	Relieve suffering	Terminate life	Terminate life
Cause of death	Underlying disease	Underlying disease	Underlying disease	Intervention prescribed by physician and administered by patient	Intervention administered by physician

Adapted from Swetz and Kamal [10]

life, and will be equipped to make choices using substituted judgment. Alternatively, if it is unclear what the patient would choose, or if the surrogate does not know the patient well, a *"best interests standard"* can be used to inform decision making. This standard is used when the patient's values are unknown, and the care team and surrogate choose what a "reasonable person" or "what most people choose in this situation." [60] States vary in what is used for the legal term for a health care proxy, but two common terms are Durable Power of Attorney (DPOA) and Health Care Power of Attorney (HCPA).

A growing body of literature exists that surrogate decision makers may develop post-traumatic stress disorder following the extreme emotional duress of serving as a health care proxy [24, 61]. Clinicians can lessen this burden if they facilitate conversations with surrogates using phrases such as "What would your Mother say if she were able to talk to us now?" rather than "Do you want us to resuscitate your Mother?"

A common and difficult decision for a proxy is to consider not using a medical intervention (e.g., do-not-resuscitate, or do-not-intubate), or, especially, to discontinue medical treatments that are not helpful or becoming more of a burden, such as cessation of dialysis, artificial nutrition, or ventilator support. Families may equate the withdrawal of non-beneficial medical treatments as equal to euthanasia or a deliberate action undertaken to end life. However, this is not the case and the courts have found it ethical and legal for patients or their surrogates to elect to withhold or withdraw medical treatments that are burdensome or have become ineffective [10]. Decisions to avoid burden also apply to less dramatic choices such as hospital transfer, imaging or phlebotomy as these all may feel assaultive, especially in cognitively compromised individuals [62].

The Alzheimer's Association advocates that patients with dementia document their end-of-life preferences early in the course of their disease, while they have capacity, and can fully and freely participate in the advance directive process. They further state those with dementia *"have a moral and legal right to limit or forgo medical or life sustaining treatment including the use of artificial feeding, mechanical ventilators, cardiopulmonary resuscitation, antibiotics, dialysis and other invasive technologies."* [63]

Further consider our case of Claire, whose situation was described at the beginning of the chapter. She developed a sudden change in consciousness with tachypnea and tachycardia on post-operative Day 3. Chest X-ray findings were consistent with aspiration pneumonitis. Her son was urgently telephoned to re-address the goals of care and whether Claire would want to be treated with endotracheal intubation. When the benefits and burdens of mechanical ventilation are described the clinician must present the immediate and long-term impact of the procedure. Informed consent must include this full spectrum of information, as well as a full range of treatment options including those that provide comfort and dignity focused care. It is important to inform all that the goal of palliative care is to provide dignity and comfort, and it is not euthanasia. The cause of death is the underlying disease, and not the medications used to provide comfort (Table 6.8). Chapter 4 also provides information on determining capacity.

6.13 Culture

Culture and ethnicity are often significant determinants of a senior's perspective on serious illness and health-care decision making. Cultural background includes religion and spiritual beliefs, ethnicity, educational background and any identification with a particular community. Cultural heritage also influences communication with health care providers. Clinicians should recognize the influence of personal cultural context on communications and goals of care.

Older adults as a group often display minimal assertiveness with providers and are more reluctant to express their opinions when they disagree with recommended treatments [64, 65]. Older adults are often accompanied by family members or others whose presence may affect their own autonomy [66].

Culture may affect the values of and preferences for care. For example, African Americans select hospice care at a lower rate than Caucasians, especially for non-cancer diagnoses [67, 68]. African Americans are more likely than other groups to discontinue hospice services in order to seek life-prolonging treatments [69]. In addition, older African

Americans from the southeastern USA are more likely than older Caucasians from the same region to hold spiritual beliefs that conflict with choosing palliative goals, distrust the health care system, experience discomfort when discussing death and want more aggressive medical care at the end of life. These elements influence decisions near the end of life [70].

Cultural background inevitably shapes patient and family expectations regarding the roles to be played by the patient, family, provider, and other members of the community. While US culture values autonomy and truth-telling with respect to health care, some subcultures are wary of truth-telling with respect to their elderly loved ones with serious illness. Traditional Navajo beliefs, for example, hold that talking about potential negative outcomes causes them to occur [71]. Some cultures outside the US value withholding information from the patient and allowing the family or provider to make health care decisions [72]. The clinician must identify these variable cultural beliefs and acknowledge them, if patient appropriate care is to be provided.

6.14 Health Literacy

Older adults have among the lowest health literacy rates, increasing the risk of misunderstanding issues concerning medical decision making and they experiencing higher rates of poor health outcomes [73]. Health literacy is a concern for all patient–provider communications, but especially when language barriers and cultural differences are present. In some cultures, family decision making is valued over individual decision making. Bias or insensitivity to cultural differences leads to negative interactions of patients with health care providers and the health care system in general. Clinicians must avoid making assumptions about decision-making style and ask patients and families directly about their preferences for communication. Often the differences within cultural groups are greater than those between different groups.

References

1. American Geriatrics Society Expert Panel on the Care of Older Adults with Multimorbidity. Guiding principles for the care of older adults with multimorbidity: an approach for clinicians. J Am Geriatr Soc. 2012;60(10):E1–25.
2. Griffin SJ, Kinmonth AL, Veltman MW, Gillard S, Grant J, Stewart M. Effect on health-related outcomes of interventions to alter the interaction between patients and practitioners: a systematic review of trials. Ann Fam Med. 2004;2(6):595–608.
3. American Geriatrics Society Expert Panel on the Care of Older Adults with Multimorbidity. Patient-centered care for older adults with multiple chronic conditions: a stepwise approach from the American Geriatrics Society. J Am Geriatr Soc. 2012;60(10):1957–68.
4. Baile WF, Buckman R, Lenzi R, Glober G, Beale EA, Kudelka AP. SPIKES-A six-step protocol for delivering bad news: application to the patient with cancer. Oncologist. 2000;5(4):302–11.
5. Lunney JR, Lynn J, Foley DJ, Lipson S, Guralnik JM. Patterns of functional decline at the end of life. JAMA. 2003;289(18):2387–92.
6. Murray SA, Kendall M, Boyd K, Sheikh A. Illness trajectories and palliative care. BMJ. 2005;330(7498):1007–11.
7. Sepúlveda C, Marlin A, Yoshida T, Ullrich A. Palliative care and end-of-life issues: the World Health Organization's global perspective. J Pain Symptom Manage. 2002;24(2):91–6.
8. Campion EW, Kelley AS, Morrison RS. Palliative care for the seriously ill. N Engl J Med. 2015;373(8):747–55.
9. Morrison RS, Meier DE. Palliative care. N Engl J Med. 2004;350(25):2582–90.
10. Swetz KM, Kamal AH. Palliative care. Ann Intern Med. 2012;156(3):ITC2-1.
11. Temel JS, Greer JA, Muzikansky A, Gallagher ER, Admane S, Jackson VA, et al. Early palliative care for patients with metastatic non-small-cell lung cancer. N Engl J Med. 2010;363(8):733–42.
12. Committee on Approaching Death, Institute of Medicine (U.S.). Dying in America: improving quality and honoring individual preferences near the end of life. 2014.
13. Goldstein NE, Morrison RS. The intersection between geriatrics and Palliative care and end-of-life issues: a call for a new research agenda. J Am Geriatr Soc. 2005;53(9):1593–8.
14. Bellelli G, Mazzola P, Morandi A, Bruni A, Carnevali L, Corsi M, et al. Duration of postoperative delirium is an independent predictor of 6-month mortality in older adults after hip fracture. J Am Geriatr Soc. 2014;62(7):1335–40.
15. Girard T, Pandharipande P, Ely EW. Delirium in the intensive care unit. Crit Care. 2008;12:S3.
16. Arbaje AI, Wolff JL, Yu Q, Powe NR, Anderson GF, Boult C. Postdischarge environmental and socioeconomic factors and the likelihood of early hospital readmission among community-dwelling Medicare beneficiaries. Gerontologist. 2008;48(4):495–504.
17. Coleman EA, Min S, Chomiak A, Kramer AM. Posthospital care transitions: patterns, complications, and risk identification. Health Serv Res. 2004;39(5):1449–66.
18. Adelman RD, Tmanova LL, Delgado D, Dion S, Lachs MS. Caregiver burden: a clinical review. JAMA. 2014;311(10):1052–60.
19. Weissman DE, Meier DE. Identifying patients in need of a palliative care assessment in the hospital setting a consensus report from the center to advance palliative care. J Palliat Med. 2011;14(1):17–23.
20. von Gunten CF. Secondary and tertiary palliative care in US hospitals. JAMA. 2002;287(7):875–81.
21. Weissman DE. Consultation in palliative medicine. Arch Intern Med. 1997;157(7):733–7.
22. Evers MM, Meier DE, Morrison RS. Assessing differences in care needs and service utilization in geriatric palliative care patients. J Pain Symptom Manage. 2002;23(5):424–32.
23. Silveira MJ, Kim SYH, Langa KM. Advance directives and outcomes of surrogate decision making before death. N Engl J Med. 2010 04/01; 2015/09;362(13):1211–18.
24. Wendler D, Rid A. Systematic review: the effect on surrogates of making treatment decisions for others. Ann Intern Med. 2011;154(5):336–46.
25. Glare PA, Sinclair CT. Palliative medicine review: prognostication. J Palliat Med. 2008;11(1):84–103.
26. Lloyd-Williams M, MacLeod RD. A systematic review of teaching and learning in palliative care within the medical undergraduate curriculum. Med Teach. 2004;26(8):683–90.
27. Bernacki RE, Block SD. Communication about serious illness care goals: a review and synthesis of best practices. JAMA Intern Med. 2014;174(12):1994–2003.
28. Parker SM, Clayton JM, Hancock K, Walder S, Butow PN, Carrick S, et al. A systematic review of prognostic/end-of-life

communication with adults in the advanced stages of a life-limiting illness: patient/caregiver preferences for the content, style, and timing of information. J Pain Symptom Manage. 2007;34(1):81–93.

29. Wilson DM, Hewitt JA, Thomas R, Mohankumar D, Kovacs Burns K. Age-based differences in care setting transitions over the last year of life. Curr Gerontol Geriatr Res. 2011;2011:101276.

30. Back AL, Arnold RM, Baile WF, Tulsky JA, Fryer-Edwards K. Approaching difficult communication tasks in oncology1. CA Cancer J Clin. 2005;55(3):164–77.

31. Caban AJ, Lee DJ, Gomez-Marin O, Lam BL, Zheng DD. Prevalence of concurrent hearing and visual impairment in US adults: The National Health Interview Survey, 1997–2002. Am J Public Health. 2005;95(11):1940–2.

32. Bernstein AB, Remsburg RE. Estimated prevalence of people with cognitive impairment: results from nationally representative community and institutional surveys. Gerontologist. 2007;47(3):350–4.

33. Walke LM, Gallo WT, Tinetti ME, Fried TR. The burden of symptoms among community-dwelling older persons with advanced chronic disease. Arch Intern Med. 2004;164(21):2321–4.

34. Shega JW, Dale W, Andrew M, Paice J, Rockwood K, Weiner DK. Persistent pain and frailty: a case for homeostenosis. J Am Geriatr Soc. 2012;60(1):113–7.

35. Ferrell BA, Ferrell BR, Rivera L. Pain in cognitively impaired nursing home patients. J Pain Symptom Manage. 1995;10(8):591–8.

36. Watanabe SM, Nekolaichuk C, Beaumont C, Johnson L, Myers J, Strasser F. A multicenter study comparing two numerical versions of the Edmonton Symptom Assessment System in palliative care patients. J Pain Symptom Manage. 2011;41(2):456–68.

37. Ferrell BA. Pain evaluation and management in the nursing home. Ann Intern Med. 1995;123(9):681–7.

38. Herr K, Coyne PJ, Key T, Manworren R, McCaffery M, Merkel S, et al. Pain assessment in the nonverbal patient: position statement with clinical practice recommendations. Pain Manag Nurs. 2006;7(2):44–52.

39. AGS Panel on Persistent Pain in Older Persons. The management of persistent pain in older persons. J Am Geriatr Soc. 2002;50(6 Suppl):S205–24.

40. Kapo J, Morrison LJ, Liao S. Palliative care for the older adult. J Palliat Med. 2007;10(1):185–209.

41. Helme RD, Gibson SJ. The epidemiology of pain in elderly people. Clin Geriatr Med. 2001;17(3):417–31.

42. Rao A, Cohen HJ. Symptom management in the elderly cancer patient: fatigue, pain, and depression. J Natl Cancer Inst Monogr. 2004;(32):150–7.

43. Potter J, Higginson IJ. Pain experienced by lung cancer patients: a review of prevalence, causes and pathophysiology. Lung Cancer. 2004;43(3):247–57.

44. Marcum ZA, Hanlon JT. Recognizing the risks of chronic nonsteroidal anti-inflammatory drug use in older adults. Ann Longterm Care. 2010;18(9):24–7.

45. Higginson IJ, Gao W. Opioid prescribing for cancer pain during the last 3 months of life: associated factors and 9-year trends in a nationwide United Kingdom cohort study. J Clin Oncol. 2012;30(35):4373–9.

46. Barbera L, Seow H, Husain A, Howell D, Atzema C, Sutradhar R, et al. Opioid prescription after pain assessment: a population-based cohort of elderly patients with cancer. J Clin Oncol. 2012;30(10):1095–9.

47. Treatment considerations for elderly and frail patients with neuropathic pain. Mayo Clinic Proceedings: Elsevier; 2010.

48. Martin-Pfitzenmeyer I, Gauthier S, Bailly M, Loi N, Popitean L, d'Athis P, et al. Prognostic factors in stage D heart failure in the very elderly. Gerontology. 2009;55(6):719–26.

49. Kamal AH, Maguire JM, Wheeler JL, Currow DC, Abernethy AP. Dyspnea review for the palliative care professional: treatment goals and therapeutic options. J Palliat Med. 2012;15(1):106–14.

50. Wolitzky-Taylor KB, Castriotta N, Lenze EJ, Stanley MA, Craske MG. Anxiety disorders in older adults: a comprehensive review. Depress Anxiety. 2010;27(2):190–211.

51. LeGrand SB. Delirium in palliative medicine: a review. J Pain Symptom Manage. 2012;44(4):583–94.

52. Horigan AE. Fatigue in hemodialysis patients: a review of current knowledge. J Pain Symptom Manage. 2012;44(5):715–24.

53. Gallo JJ, Bogner HR, Morales KH, Post EP, Lin JY, Bruce ML. The effect of a primary care practice-based depression intervention on mortality in older adults: a randomized trial. Ann Intern Med. 2007;146(10):689–98.

54. Yourman LC, Lee SJ, Schonberg MA, Widera EW, Smith AK. Prognostic indices for older adults: a systematic review. JAMA. 2012;307(2):182–92.

55. Walter LC, Covinsky KE. Cancer screening in elderly patients: a framework for individualized decision making. JAMA. 2001;285(21):2750–6.

56. Celli BR, Cote CG, Marin JM, Casanova C, Montes de Oca M, Mendez RA, et al. The body-mass index, airflow obstruction, dyspnea, and exercise capacity index in chronic obstructive pulmonary disease. N Engl J Med. 2004;350(10):1005–12.

57. Botta F, Giannini E, Romagnoli P, Fasoli A, Malfatti F, Chiarbonello B, et al. MELD scoring system is useful for predicting prognosis in patients with liver cirrhosis and is correlated with residual liver function: a European study. Gut. 2003;52(1):134–9.

58. Gill TM. The central role of prognosis in clinical decision making. JAMA. 2012;307(2):199–200.

59. Barzilai N. Discovering the secrets of successful longevity. J Geront Series A: Biol Sci Med Sci. 2003;58(3):M225–6.

60. American Medical Association. Surrogate decision making. Code of medical ethics, opinion E-8.081. Chicago, IL: AMA; 2006.

61. Detering KM, Hancock AD, Reade MC, Silvester W. The impact of advance care planning on end of life care in elderly patients: randomised controlled trial. BMJ. 2010;340:c1345.

62. Gabow P. The fall: aligning the best care with standards of care at the end of life. Health Aff. 2015;34(5):871–4.

63. The Alzheimer's Association. Ethical considerations: issues in death and dying. Available at: http://www.alz.org/alzwa/documents/alzwa_Resource_EOL_FS_Death_and_Dying_ethical_issues.pdf. Accessed November, 19, 2015.

64. Greene M, Adelman R, Rizzo C. Problems in communication between physicians and older patients. J Geriatr Psychiatry. 1996;29(1):13–32.

65. Elkin EB, Kim SH, Casper ES, Kissane DW, Schrag D. Desire for information and involvement in treatment decisions: elderly cancer patients' preferences and their physicians' perceptions. J Clin Oncol. 2007;25(33):5275–80.

66. Clayman ML, Roter D, Wissow LS, Bandeen-Roche K. Autonomy-related behaviors of patient companions and their effect on decision-making activity in geriatric primary care visits. Soc Sci Med. 2005;60(7):1583–91.

67. Colon M, Lyke J. Comparison of hospice use and demographics among European Americans, African Americans, and Latinos. Am J Hosp Palliat Care. 2003;20(3):182–90.

68. Johnson KS, Kuchibhatla M, Tanis D, Tulsky JA. Racial differences in the growth of noncancer diagnoses among hospice enrollees. J Pain Symptom Manage. 2007;34(3):286–93.

69. Johnson KS, Kuchibhatla M, Tanis D, Tulsky JA. Racial differences in hospice revocation to pursue aggressive care. Arch Intern Med. 2008;168(2):218–24.

70. Johnson KS, Kuchibhatla M, Tulsky JA. What explains racial differences in the use of advance directives and attitudes toward hospice care? J Am Geriatr Soc. 2008;56(10):1953–8.

71. Carrese JA, Rhodes LA. Western bioethics on the Navajo reservation: benefit or harm? JAMA. 1995;274(10):826–9.

72. Hancock K, Clayton JM, Parker SM, der Wal S, Butow PN, Carrick S, et al. Truth-telling in discussing prognosis in advanced life-limiting illnesses: a systematic review. Palliat Med. 2007;21(6):507–17.

73. Paasche-Orlow MK, Parker RM, Gazmararian JA, Nielsen-Bohlman LT, Rudd RR. The prevalence of limited health literacy. J Gen Intern Med. 2005;20(2):175–84.

Anna Stepczynski, Tejo K. Vemulapalli, and Mindy J. Fain

7.1 Demographics

The marked rise in the number of older adults is reflected in US hospital data. Although adults age 65 and older currently represent approximately 13 % of the US population, they account for a disproportionate amount of healthcare utilization and 40 % of hospitalizations. In 2030, adults age 65 and older will represent nearly 20 % of the population. Adults age 85 years and older constitute the most rapidly growing segment, and although they currently only account for approximately two percent of the population, by 2030 their numbers will increase by 20 % [1]. Those 80 and over as a group are the heaviest users of health care and hospitalizations. The most common reasons for admission to the hospital for older adults include heart failure, cardiac arrhythmias, acute coronary syndromes, and pneumonia. Although these diagnoses are similar to those of a younger adult population, older patients have a longer average length of stay (5.5 days vs 5.0 days for adults 45–64 years old) [2]. For adults over age 80, the most common causes of hospitalization are heart failure, pneumonia, urinary tract infection, septicemia, stroke, and hip fracture [3]. Patients over 80 have been found to receive fewer invasive procedures and less costly care than a younger cohort. This difference has not been shown to

A. Stepczynski, MD, BSc
Division of Geriatrics, General Internal Medicine and Palliative Medicine, Department of Medicine, University of Arizona College of Medicine, 1501 N Campbell Ave, Tucson, AZ 85719, USA

T.K. Vemulapalli, MD
Division of Inpatient Medicine, Department of Medicine, University of Arizona College of Medicine, 1501 N Campbell Avenue, Tucson, AZ 85719, USA

M.J. Fain, MD (✉)
Department of Medicine, Arizona Center in Aging, University of Arizona College of Medicine, 1821 E. Elm Street, Tucson, AZ 85719, USA
e-mail: mfain@aging.arizona.edu

be due to the patient's preferences regarding life-sustaining care or their severity of illness [4]. They are also more likely to be transferred to long-term care: approximately 40 % of patients over the age of 85 are transferred to a skilled nursing facility [3].

- Older adults account for nearly 40 % of all hospital admissions and nearly 50 % of all costs related to hospitalization [3]. They also suffer more adverse events in the hospital, including delirium, hospital-acquired infections, and adverse drug reactions.

7.2 The Vulnerable Older Adult

Aging results in significant, progressive reduction in physiologic reserves across multiple organ systems. Despite this, older adults sustain themselves in homeostasis in spite of declining reserves called "homeostenosis"—a delicate state invisible to the clinician's eye. These physiological losses make a senior vulnerable to any significant perturbation or stress. Older adults have muted physiologic responses to acute stressors such as an infection, an adverse medication effect, dehydration, or surgery. These stressors expose the elders' underlying vulnerability due to their lack of compensatory reserve.

- Aging-related physiologic vulnerability combined with the increased prevalence of chronic disease with aging is manifested as unexpected clinical failure of the heart, lungs, kidney, brain, or other organ systems that were not the primary reason for admission to the hospital [5] (Table 7.1).

7.3 Marked Heterogeneity Among Older Adults

Descriptions of age-related physiologic declines and comorbidities give the impression that the older population is clinically homogenous, but this is not true. Older adults

© Springer International Publishing Switzerland 2017
J.R. Burton et al. (eds.), *Geriatrics for Specialists*, DOI 10.1007/978-3-319-31831-8_7

Table 7.1 Physiologic changes of aging

Organ/system	Age-related physiologic change	Consequences of aging, not disease
General	↑ Body fat	Altered drug distribution
	↓ Total body water	
Endocrine	Impaired glucose homeostasis	↑ glucose during stress
	↑ ADH, ↓ renin, and ↓ aldosterone	Disrupted volume homeostasis
Respiratory	↓ Lung elasticity and ↑ chest wall stiffness	Increased effort, atelectasis when bed or chair bound
	Decreased recoil	↓ Exercise tolerance
	Decreased DL_{CO}	
	Decreased cough reflex	Micro-aspiration
		Ventilation/perfusion mismatch
	Increased A-a gradient	Decreased resting PO_2
Hematologic/immune system	↓ T cell function	↓ Response to pathogens
	↑ Autoantibodies	
Musculoskeletal	↓ Lean body mass, muscle	↓ Strength
	↓ Bone density	Osteopenia
Cardiovascular	↑ LVH, arterial stiffness	Impaired orthostatic responses; HFpEF (e.g., diastolic dysfunction)
	↓ B-adrenergic responsiveness	↓ baroreceptor sensitivity
		↓ cardiac output and HR response to stress
		Hypotensive response to ↑ HR or dehydration
Renal	↓ GFR	Impaired drug excretion
	↓ urine concentration/dilution	Delayed response to salt/fluid restriction or overload

Adapted with permission from Fedarko NS, McNabney MK. Biology. In: Durso SC, Sullivan GM, eds. Geriatrics Review Syllabus: A Core Curriculum in Geriatric Medicine, 8th ed. New York, NY: American Geriatrics Society; 2013, and Kasper et al., Harrison's Principles of Internal Medicine, 16th Edition, McGraw-Hill, adapted with permission of McGraw Hill Education

experience physiologic aging at very different rates, and even in the same person, different organ systems age at varying rates; and as a result, older adults are more different from one another than are younger patients. Older adults also suffer from age-related chronic conditions such as heart disease, diabetes, and geriatric syndromes such as dementia, frailty, and incontinence, in unpredictable ways. More than 50 % of older adults have more than three chronic conditions, called multi-morbidity [6]. As a result, there is marked clinical heterogeneity and the overriding lesson is that age itself does not predict a person's state of health or wellness, which may range from resilient to frail.

- An individualized geriatric assessment is a major step in the management of the older hospitalized adult. It provides the essential framework to deliver personalized, high quality and safe care for this high-risk and diverse group of patients.

7.4 Assessment of the Hospitalized Older Adult: Key Themes and Common Pitfalls

Although the hospital is often lifesaving, for an older adult, it also presents serious challenges with potentially devastating consequences. Approximately one-third of patients older than age 70 develop a potentially preventable hospitalization-associated disability despite successful treatment of the acute illness. This often results in impairment of activities of daily living (ADLs) and an inability to continue to live independently [7, 8]. A systematic approach is required to identify and manage these challenges, which include cognitive and functional decline, adverse effects from medications [9], and other components. Several risk-prediction scoring tools are available to identify hospitalized older adults at risk for new-onset disability, adverse medication effects, and other hospital-associated complications. These tools can assist in targeting the high risk patients and inform clinical care [10]. Identification of frailty provides important prognostic information regarding morbidity and mortality [11–13].

7.4.1 Geriatric Assessment in the Hospital

Geriatric assessment (GA) has evolved to meet diverse clinical needs in a variety of settings. Core GA components involve the identification of medical, physical, functional, social, and psychological issues that then link to a coordinated team-based plan of care. GA focuses on a senior's unique presentation of acute illness, and plans for the prevention of common adverse events during hospitalization. A recent review reported that hospitalized patients who received GA with a subsequent individualized care plan compared to those without GA were more likely to be alive and in their own homes after a year (and not be institutionalized) and more likely to have maintained their baseline cognitive function [14].

- A geriatric assessment on admission to hospital identifies the patient's baseline status, targets common geriatric problems and hazards that would otherwise have been unsuspected or disregarded, expands upon usual medical assessment to reduce hospital-associated risks and improve outcomes, and initiates planning for transition of care (Table 7.2).

The following is a list of recommended steps, recognizing that there is significant overlap and that the order and timing of each may be modified based on the patient's acuity and clinical scenario.

7.4.1.1 Step 1: Assess Capacity for Medical Decision Making

The patient must have the capacity for medical decision-making in order to fully engage in a discussion about goals, values, and preferences. Since approximately 1/4 of hospitalized elders lack decision-making capacity, all hospitalists must be skilled in assessing decision-making capacity and must routinely determine this capacity in older patients—not just when prompted by a patient's unusual behavior or denial of a recommended treatment [15]. Importantly, a patient with dementia may still maintain decisional capacity. The assessment of a patient's medical decisional capacity involves his or her ability to understand the consequences of a decision. Four elements of a decision-making capacity assessment include: (1) communicating a choice, (2) understanding the

Table 7.2 Routine assessment for hospitalized older adults

History and physical	Geriatric area	Specific geriatric assessment	Why assess?
Care preferences	Advance care planning	• Review DMPOAHC and/or Living Will (if available)	• Guides care
		• Assess capability of medical decision making	
		• Assess goals of care, values, and preferences	
Past history	Healthcare utilization	• Review ED or hospital admission within 30 days	• Targets risk and informs transitions
	Vaccination	• Review pneumococcal and influenza immunization status	• Hospital is good site for updating vaccinations
Functional status	Functional status	• Assess ADLs, IADLs	• Targets risk and informs transitions
		• Ask: Have you recently had a decline in your functioning?	
		• Ask: Do you have help at home? What do they help you with? (e.g., shopping, meals, taking a bath or shower, transportation, managing finances)	
Medication review	Over-and-under treatment	• Review each medication for indication, dose, and adverse effects	• Mitigates adverse medication effects and errors
	Adverse effects	• Review high risk medications (e.g., psychotropics, anticholinergics)	• Informs transitions
		• Ask: Are there any medications that have been recently started?	
	Adherence	• Ask: About how many doses do you miss a week?	
		• Ask: What do you do to make sure you get your mediations? (e.g., caregiver help, pill boxes)	
Social history	Social support	• Ask: Where do you live? (e.g., home, assisted living, nursing home).	• Informs transitions
		• Ask: Who lives with you?	• Assists with prevention strategies (ETOH withdrawal)
		• Ask: Are you a caregiver for someone else?	• Informs transition; may need to report
	Alcohol use	• Ask: How many drinks (alcohol) do you have a week?	
		• Administer: CAGE	
	Elder mistreatment	• Ask: Do you feel safe at home?	

(continued)

Table 7.2 (continued)

History and physical	Geriatric area	Specific geriatric assessment	Why assess?
Review of systems	Cognition	• Ask: Have you had problems with your memory or confusion?	• Informs hospital course and transition (don't make diagnosis of dementia in hospital setting)
	Mood	• Ask: (PHQ-2): Over the past month, have you often had little interest or pleasure in doing things? Have you been bothered by feeling down, depressed, or hopeless?	
	Incontinence	• Ask: Do you have trouble holding your urine? Do you wear a pad?	
	Falls	• Ask: Have you fallen in the past 6 months?	
	Nutrition	• Ask: Have you lost weight in the past 6 months? How much?	
	Vision/hearing	• Ask: Do you have problems seeing or hearing?	
	Skin	• Ask: Do you have any skin sores or ulcers?	
	Pain	• Ask: Are you having pain?	
Physical assessment	General/VS	• Assess temperature	• Informs hospital course and transition
		• Check orthostatic BP and heart rate	
		• Calculate BMI	
		• Consider frailty assessment	
		Perform daily skin exam	
		• Assess for delirium	
	Cognition	• Perform Mini-Cog (3-item recall and clock or other cognitive screen	
	Gait	• Observe patient getting up and walking	
Labs	Renal function	• Estimate CrCl (Cockcroft–Gault formula)	• Mitigates errors in dosing

Modified with permission from: Pierluissi E, Sotelo M. Hospital Care. In: Durso SC, Sullivan GM, eds. Geriatrics Review Syllabus: A Core Curriculum in Geriatric Medicine, 8th ed. New York, NY: American Geriatrics Society; 2013

question asked, (3) appreciating the situation, and (4) demonstrating reasoning. Capacity is determined in relation to a specific question or situation and must be reassessed as the clinical picture changes [16]. Several tools are available to help structure the assessment including the Aid to Capacity Evaluation tool [17]. Specialty consultants, including psychiatrists, may be brought in when there is evidence for depression or psychosis complicating the discussion. Chapters 4 and 6 also provide information on determining decision-making capacity.

- Assessing a patient's medical decision-making capacity is within the hospitalist's scope of practice.

7.4.1.2 Step 2: Establish Goals, Values, and Preferences

Establishing the patient's goals, values, and preferences is a very early step in GA. Specific treatment decisions follow this understanding and it should drive the hospital management plan. Determine if the patient has any advance care planning in place (e.g., durable medical power of attorney for health care, living will, etc.) and follow the patient's desired wishes as best as possible. A helpful framework in discussion with patients with multi-morbidity includes attention to treatment-related risks, burdens, and benefits, including their anticipated life expectancy, functional impairments, and quality of life [6, 18].

To develop a plan of care in alignment with patient/family goals, preferences, and values, engage in a discussion following these guidelines. Before beginning the discussion, be as prepared as you can be with the facts of the case and share this information with the patient and family to ensure understanding. Ask open-ended questions and be prepared to listen and respond to the patient's questions and concerns. Examples of how to start the conversation include: "What would you like to see happen?", "What would you like to avoid?", "What fears or worries do you have about your illness or medical care?", and "What are you hoping for now?", and "What is important to you?" Specific issues to discuss (in addition to resuscitation orders and code status) may include (as appropriate) ICU care, dialysis, nutritional support, future hospitalizations, and the role of comfort measures. Confirm understanding of the patient's wishes at the end of discussion.

With a structured approach and practice, the discussion can be completed within a short time. The benefit to patient, family, consultants, and all involved hospital personnel is invaluable in focusing on the goals of care. In many cases, managing patient and family expectations is a key part of the initial and follow-up discussions.

At times, these expectations may be overly optimistic, failing to appreciate an extremely poor prognosis. Other times, the expectations may be based on age-related stereotypes that unreasonably deny the opportunity for an elder to recover from their acute illness. For example, a family may misunderstand the clinical picture of delirium and acute onset of urinary incontinence (two common adverse effects in the hospital setting) and come to the conclusion that their loved one suffers from dementia and chronic urinary incontinence. They may then believe that they can no longer care for the patient at home. These inappropriate diagnoses, if unchallenged by the hospital team, impact further care. The family may decide that a transfer to a more supervised setting is in their loved one's best interests, and the family's lowered expectations for recovery often solidify cognitive and functional losses.

- Directly discuss the patient's goals, values, and preferences. Develop and implement a care plan based on achieving these goals, as best as possible. Strongly consider consulting the palliative care team (discussed in depth in Chap. 6) or the ethics committee if patient and/or family expectations appear to be unrealistic or if there is conflict.

7.4.1.3 Step 3: Conduct an Effective and Efficient History and Physical

The traditional history and physical includes past medical history, medication review, social history, review of systems, and physical exam. Within these domains, several assessments should be systematically incorporated to elicit important geriatric issues. For example, in addition to gathering the list of medications, directly ask the patient and/or caregiver to describe the strategies they use to ensure medication adherence and carefully consider whether the medications (or lack thereof) could be contributing to the patient's acute illness. In addition to usual social history questions, ask the patient about any help they require from others to meet their Activities of Daily Living (ADLs) or Instrumental Activities of Daily Living (IADL) needs, or if they feel safe at home. In the review of systems, ask about vision and hearing problems or weight loss in the prior 6 months. For the physical examination, checks of orthostatic blood pressure and gait are very informative. Utilize the hospital team (e.g., nurses, social workers, pharmacists, dietitians, and therapists) to broaden and deepen the assessment in a time-efficient manner (Table 7.2).

- Incorporate key geriatric domains into the standard history and physical (rather than an "add-on"). With practice, this will allow for more focused and efficient care in the fast-paced hospital setting.

7.4.1.4 Step 4: Avoid Misdiagnosis: Know About Unique Presentations of Common Conditions

It is essential to maintain a high degree of skepticism and carefully re-evaluate the initial diagnosis of older patients admitted through the emergency department. Signs and symptoms due to adverse medication effects are often incorrectly ascribed to a medical or psychiatric problem. Up to 30 % of hospitalizations in the older population involve an adverse medication effect [19]. Although chest pain is the most common presenting symptom of acute coronary syndrome (ACS) in all ages, elderly patients often present with non-typical symptoms, including dyspnea, delirium, GERD, or fatigue [20]. In addition, ACS can be precipitated by other stresses, such as infection or dehydration, further delaying clinical recognition when the symptoms are non-classical. Older adults often have severe infection without fever or other typical signs and symptoms. Even in the setting of pneumonia or sepsis, fever is absent in 30–50 % of elderly patients [21]. Clinically, these infections present as non-specific symptoms of functional decline (abrupt change in self-care ability), a new geriatric syndrome (falls or delirium) — or exacerbation of an underlying chronic condition. There is often a recognized pattern to this common "atypical" presentation of acute illness, whereby the elder's symptoms are reflective of the system with the least physiologic reserve (termed the "weakest-link principle") [22].

In addition, the presence of clinically significant chronic kidney disease is often missed (and medications incorrectly dosed) because of pseudo-normalization of the serum creatinine in older adults with low muscle mass and diminished renal function. To avoid this, renal function must be assessed by estimated glomerular filtration rate or creatinine clearance, rather than the MDRD that often appears in lab reports. Dementia or the new onset of acute confusion (delirium) interferes with obtaining a history and assessing symptoms. See Chap. 2 for a discussion of diagnosis and prevention of delirium. Lastly, the negative impact of ageism, combined with the absence of a reliable history, results in the inaccurate assumption of a terminal illness or advanced dementia in a malnourished, confused elderly patient who is suffering from an acute illness.

Finally, a common conundrum for hospitalists: is the excessive information from imaging and laboratory assessments typically developed in a patient admitted through the emergency department. Seniors have many comorbidities and incidental findings. Therefore, often there are data that are irrelevant to the patient's acute problem. Reviewing these data carefully and deciding what is important or irrelevant requires judgment and thoughtful communication with the patient and family but is important in developing a wise care plan and avoiding iatrogenic complications.

- The interplay of normal age related physiological change, comorbidities, and geriatric syndromes results in heterogeneous, clinical presentations of common conditions. Overall, it's essential to maintain a high index of suspicion for mis-diagnosis or under-diagnosis in the older adult.

7.4.1.5 Step 5: Continuous Transition Planning: Begin on Admission

Care transitions (often termed "handoffs," "discharges," or "transfers") can be complicated and costly for older adults with complex needs, and planning for a safe and effective transition of care should begin on the day of admission. Care transitions occur between providers, between levels of care (e.g., from intensive care unit to the floor), or across healthcare settings (e.g., from hospital to a skilled-nursing facility, or hospital to home) and require several, well-orchestrated steps that address patient and family/caregiver, physician/healthcare provider, and health system factors [23]. While making every attempt to respect the patient's autonomy and privacy, an important first step involves including caregivers and family members in the process.

Elements of transition include care coordination, discharge planning, and disease management and hospitalists are responsible for the patient's care from admission until the transition of care is complete. Hospitalists are encouraged by the National Transition of Care Coalition to adopt the concept of "transfer with continuous management" [24]. Unless a team-based, structured approach is utilized, key elements can get lost in the transition, resulting in highly fragmented and poor quality care. The transition plan should include a complete and clear medication list (reconciled with preadmission medication list), assessment of cognitive and functional level, lists of diagnoses, pending tests and appointments (and attention to logistical needs), assessment of caregiver needs and resources, and advance care directives. It should also include specific education regarding self-management, warning symptoms or signs ("red flags") of their disease condition and who to call and what to do when these arise, instructions as to what to expect (including other clinical disciplines that may be involved in care, such as nursing or physical therapy), and how to navigate the next site of care (Table 7.3). At the time of any transition, a brief

Table 7.3 Improving care transitions for older adults

Discharge/transition barriers	Recommended approaches
Physician to provider communication	• Collaborate with primary care provider (PCP) in discharge and follow-up planning • Promptly and accurately transfer information to the provider at the next level of care • Utilize a standardized template to ensure comprehensive communication • Communicate specifically about diagnoses, advance care plans, medications, allergies, adverse events, follow-up needs/pending tests and studies, red flags and possible next steps
Medication management	• Partner with clinical pharmacists to manage medication information and reconciliation, including over-the-counter products, and work to eliminate high risk medications for older adults (Chap. 5, Medication Management for Beers list) • Reconcile medications at all care transitions, and communicate list to PCP, including allergies and adverse medication events, and medications discontinued and added • Educate patients about changes to their medications, and develop a plan to ensure medication adherence for complex regimens
Patient and family factors	• Involve patient and family members early in the process of hospitalization • Work with interprofessional transfer/discharge teams to assess needs, and ensure available resources to optimize patient's medical condition, functioning and safety, and to support the caregiver • Ensure that the patient and caregiver understand and agree with the goals and purpose of the transfer, and what to expect at next level of care • Assess the health literacy of patient and family, and provide access to patient care navigators to help negotiate the health system • Schedule and prepare for specific follow-up appointments prior to discharge • Utilize home health and/or hospice services when indicated, and consider home visits for high risk or frail elderly patients. Use established community networks and ensure coordination
Physician–patient communication	• Provide discharge counselling regarding diagnoses, medication changes, self-care instructions, appointments for follow-up, red flag symptoms, what to do if problems arise, and plans for durable medical equipment (if home) • Reaffirm patient's goals of care, values, and preferences, and confirm advance care plans • Provide simply written materials with illustrations to reinforce verbal instructions and promote patient self-management • Utilize teach-back techniques to assess the gaps in patient and family's understanding • Give opportunity to ask questions and spend time answering them • Encourage use of personal health record to manage information

Adapted with permission from Sunil Kripalani, Amy T. Jackson, Jeffrey L. Schnipper, and Eric A. Coleman, Recommendations for improving care Transitions at Hospital Discharge, Journal of Hospital Medicine, Vol 2 No 5 Sept/Oct 2007 Page 316 phone call between the current and receiving provider is very helpful.

Suboptimal care transitions are hazardous to older adults and it impacts safety, costs, functional outcomes, morbidity, and mortality. Current high hospital readmission rates in part are a sobering reflection of our failures in transitional care, and a focus of national scrutiny. Nearly 20 % of Medicare beneficiaries are re-admitted within 30 days, and 30 % are readmitted within 90 days [25]. Risk for poor transitions in older adults include: living alone, limited self-care abilities, poor health literacy, low income, prior hospitalization, five or more comorbidities, functional impairments and limited resources or caregiver support, or transition to home with home-care services (because of the challenges involved in coordinating care at home for patients with complex needs). Specific diagnoses, including depression, heart disease, diabetes, and cancer, also predict poor transitions [26].

Many problems occur if the hospitalists are not familiar with the capabilities of various settings, which include: home with family support, home with home-health care, custodial care (e.g., assisted living), skilled nursing facilities (SNF), acute rehabilitation hospital, long-term acute care (LTAC), and hospice care (home support or inpatient). Unless the hospitalist is familiar with resources at care settings, such as the availability of on-site medical care, specific medications, imaging or lab tests at SNF, the discharge plan may be unrealistic and unsustainable. It would be wise for hospitalists to briefly visit the most common community institutions used in his or her discharges to gain firsthand knowledge of their unique resources and limitations. Table 7.4 provides a synopsis of post-acute care services and institutions. For a planned discharge to home, access to ongoing medical care, cognitive or functional capabilities of the patient, availability of a caregiver, financial resources to pay for care, and the availability of community resources are especially important to consider. Ultimately, the choice of the discharge site of care should be the best match between the patient's needs and the resources and services available at the location.

There are many well-recognized barriers to achieving a safe transition and the process is further challenged in the

Table 7.4 Synopsis of post-acute care settings

Post-acute care setting[a]	Services	Type of therapy available	Care requirements	Specialty services	Limitations
Long-term Acute Care (LTAC) Hospitals	Respiratory care, Wound care, IV Antibiotic therapy	Short-term rehabilitation	Trach and vent patients Complex wound care	Dialysis Pain management	Only for patients whose LOS is predicted to be close to 25 days
In-hospital Sub-acute Unit	Pulmonary, cardiac care, wound care	Intensive short-term rehabilitation	Reconditioning	Orthopedic Rehab	Not many hospitals have these units
Inpatient Rehab Centers	Wound Care, Pulmonary Therapy, Complex physical and neurological therapy	Intensive short-term rehabilitation	Patient is expected to be able to return to independent living after the rehab stay	Pulmonary rehabilitation Dialysis Stroke and other Neurological rehabilitation	Patients should be able to participate in at least 3 h of daily rehabilitation
Skilled Nursing Facilities (SNFs)	Cardiac, pulmonary, wound care, and antibiotic administration	Orthopedic, neurological, and speech-language rehabilitation	Patients should have skilled care needs otherwise will be downgraded to Long-term care facilities	Dialysis	Care provided may vary at different SNFs Patients must have a preceding hospital stay
Home Health Services	Wound care, IV antibiotic administration, skilled nursing and physical therapy	Physical therapy, occupational therapy, and speech therapy	Patient has to be homebound[b] No need for preceding hospital stay	Medical social work and aide services	Physician has to certify patient is homebound and is in need of services
Home Hospice Care	Medical and support services for terminal illness	Pain management	Patient has to be certified by a physician to have less than 6 months of life expectancy	Palliative care	Patient has the choice to elect or revoke hospice services

[a]Some variations may exist based on state regulations and services available in a particular institution
[b]Per Medicare (https://www.medicare.gov/Pubs/pdf/10969.pdf accessed on 12/8/2015), to be homebound means the following:
    Leaving your home isn't recommended because of your condition
    Your condition keeps you from leaving home without help (such as using a wheelchair or walker, needing special transportation, or getting help from another person)
    Leaving home takes a considerable and taxing effort

often chaotic acute care environment. The recent trend of institution-based physicians providing care in one specific setting (i.e., hospitalists, SNFists), the lack of knowledge about other sites of care, and the lack of communication between these providers are the primary factors in failure of transitions of care. Adding to the insult are various electronic health record systems that lack interoperability, leading to poor handoffs. Different care settings have their own formulary restrictions and different medication reconciliation requirements. New roles have emerged, such as patient care navigators, transition nurses/coaches, and home visiting nurses, to facilitate safe care transitions and decrease fragmentation of the care provided [23].

In addition to preparing the patient and family for a safe and effective transition, it is clear that communications between physicians taking care of patients in acute and post-acute setting needs to improve [27]. The Transitions of Care Consensus policy statement released by a multi-stakeholder consensus group in coalition with the Stepping Up to the Plate alliance of the American Board of Internal Medicine (ABIM) outlined the standards of transitions of care between inpatient and outpatient setting [28]. Several models such as the Nurses Improving Care for Healthsystem Elders (NICHE) [29], Project BOOST [30], and the Care Transition Program [31] can be of great help in improving the transition process, and hospitalists are positioned to play a key role in their health system in selecting and implementing care transition policies to improve health outcomes [32, 33].

- Several tools are available to identify geriatric patients at risk during transitions, and to provide a team-based framework with protocols to address the complexities of care. Championing evidence-based hospital and health system transition programs, and utilizing tools such as the 'discharge checklist' proposed by the Society of Hospital Medicine's Hospital Quality and Patient Safety committee [34], can prevent fragmentation of the care provided during the critical time of transition (Table 7.3).

7.4.2 Management of the Hospitalized Older Adult: Key Themes and Common Pitfalls

7.4.2.1 Step 6: Mitigate Hospitalization-Associated Disability

Despite successful treatment of the admitting condition, approximately 1/3 of older hospitalized adults develop new functional (cognitive and physical) impairments that affect their ability for self-care and limit their ability to continue to live independently. These patients are at high risk for readmission within 30 days, most often for an acute medical condition other than the initial admission diagnosis. The cause of this post-hospital syndrome—an acquired, transient condition of generalized risk—is believed to be due to the impact of bed rest and the usual processes of care that result in significant and global physiological stress, and a period of vulnerability [7]. The elderly hospitalized patient experiences substantial stress, including poor nutrition, sleep deprivation, pain, adverse medication effects, sensory deprivation, delirium, cognitive challenges, and physical deconditioning. These hospitalization related events contribute to a cycle of decline, resulting in recurrent hospitalizations, institutionalization, morbidity, and mortality. Patients remain disabled long after even a brief, seemingly minor hospitalization. One year following discharge, fewer than 50 % of adults recovered to previous level of function [35].

- An acute medical illness resulting in hospitalization is a sentinel event for an older adult. Be aware of hospital-associated disability and in addition to addressing the urgent needs of the patient's acute illness, look beyond the admitting diagnosis and prevent these predictable and devastating events. (See Managing Common Risks and Adverse Events below) [7, 8].

7.4.2.2 Step 7: Manage Multiple Consultants

Beyond the role of calling and coordinating the efforts of several consultants and working with the interprofessional team, the hospitalist must take primary responsibility for developing and implementing a plan of care that is aligned with the patient's and family's goals, values, and preferences. This includes engaging in difficult conversations, guiding the patient and family through medical and/or surgical disease management options, managing patient and family expectations, and appropriately integrating palliative symptom management and end-of-life care.

- In complex patients with multiple consultants, assume a leadership role and navigate the course of the hospitalized older adult with a keen eye on the patient's goals of care, preferences, and values.

7.4.2.3 Step 8: Identify Patients in Need of Palliative Care Assessment

Many older hospitalized patients with serious, complex, and potentially life-threatening or life-limiting medical conditions benefit from a palliative care assessment. In most hospitals, this is accomplished through a palliative care consult. Expert consensus checklists are available to identify patients at high risk for unmet palliative care needs, both on admission and during daily rounds. Checklist components include: advancing chronic conditions, failure-to-thrive, worsening physical symptoms, or disagreements regarding treatment options. A "no" answer to the "surprise question" asked of yourself: "Would you be surprised if the patient died within 12 months?" is a very helpful criteria [36]. Chapter 6 provides detailed information in this area including what expertise in palliative care a hospitalist should have.

- The palliative care consultation service is designed to provide specialty-level care to help manage challenging symptoms, navigate complex family dynamics, and guide the patient and family in achieving difficult care decisions regarding potentially life-sustaining therapies.

7.4.2.4 Step 9: Manage Common Risks and Adverse Events

Acute hospitalization of older adults places them at risk for specific adverse events that result from vulnerability to "usual" processes of care—from bed rest, to standing orders for pain, anxiety, and sleep that are not targeted to the special needs of older adults, to complications from interventions intended to be therapeutic. The following is a brief review of common and/or high-risk events that predispose hospitalized elders to poor clinical outcomes, and includes recommended approaches to improve outcomes. Chapters 1–8 provide important information on these issues, especially frailty, delirium, psychiatry, medication management, palliative care, and tools for assessment (Table 7.5).

- Many of the poor outcomes from hospitalization are due to predictable risks and many are preventable. The hospitalist should have strategies to prevent or mitigate these adverse events, although some decline may be unavoidable due to the impact of the acute illness or injury.

Table 7.5 Common risks and hazards of hospitalization

Malnutrition
Poor skin integrity/pressure ulcers
Polypharmacy and adverse med effects
Atypical presentation/misdiagnoses
Nosocomial infections
Depression
Delirium
Frailty
Cognitive impairment
Sensory impairments
Functional impairments
Falls and immobility
Constipation
Urinary incontinence
Volume shifts
Uncontrolled pain
Sleep disturbances
Managing multiple specialty consultants
Lack of identified goals, values, and preferences
Lack of medical decision-making capacity
Complex care transitions

7.5 Common High Risk Events and Recommendations

7.5.1 Falls and Immobility

Hospitalized older adults are at high risk of falling due to many factors: underlying co-morbidities and functional impairments; the impact of acute illness; hospital-associated deconditioning due to bed rest; adverse treatment effects targeting the acute illness (e.g., diuretics for heart failure), hospital-induced symptom management (e.g., inappropriate use of anticholinergics or sedative-hypnotics), and challenges navigating unfamiliar surroundings. A history of prior falls, or abnormalities in gait, balance, leg strength, ability to get up from the bed, or cognition identify older adults at risk for falls. Immobility during hospitalization leads rapidly to decreased strength, impaired ambulation, and increased risk for falls. Falls increase hospital costs and lengths of stay. In the hospital setting, attention to several components have been shown to reduce falls: (1) avoid medications with psychotropic and anticholinergic effects, (2) monitor regularly at the bed-side volume status, including orthostatic blood pressure measurements, especially for those patients on diuretic or anti-hypertensive medications, and manage adverse effects, (3) provide ambulatory supervision for high risk older adults (by nursing, or physical therapy if needed) and appropriate adaptive equipment (e.g., walkers), (4) avoid bed rest only orders, and ensure that patients have time throughout the day to sit in the chair and ambulate, (5) encourage independent ambulation for those who are able to walk independently, directly countering some elder's and health care professionals' belief that bed rest is restorative, (6) attend to patient's toileting needs, and (7) minimize the use of tethers (e.g., urinary catheters, cardiac telemetry, and IVs) and avoid mechanical restraints that limit movement in the bed. Promptly discontinue tethers no longer needed as they contribute to immobility and increase the rate of delirium, infections, and falls.

7.5.2 Orthostatic Hypotension

Orthostatic hypotension (OH) is a common, serious, and often unrecognized issue, estimated to occur in approximately 30 % of older adults in the community and twice as common in those admitted to hospital [37]. It is defined as a drop of at least 20 mmHg in systolic pressure or a 10 mmHg drop in diastolic pressure within 3 min of standing. Aging-related changes in plasma volume, baroreflexes and venomotor tone, exacerbated by comorbid conditions (e.g., diabetes, hypertension, and Parkinson's disease) contribute to OH. Since most older adults are asymptomatic (e.g., they don't complain of lightheadedness) and orthostatic pressures are usually not routinely measured unless there is clinical suspicion, it is frequently missed. OH is exacerbated by bed rest, dehydration, medications, and other interventions. Hospitalized patients with OH are at increased risk for falls and injury, and it often persists after discharge, where it is associated with falls, syncope, cardiovascular complications, and all-cause mortality. It is an easily diagnosed and remediable condition and OH should be routinely assessed on admission and at intervals throughout the hospital stay. Contributing factors should be systematically addressed to reduce falls and other complications. Patients with OH should be taught behavioral modification techniques like standing and waiting a few minutes before attempting to walk in order to minimize falls.

7.5.3 Sleep Disturbances

Sleep disturbances occur in approximately 30 % of hospitalized older adults and contribute to significant adverse effects, including delirium. Sleeplessness is due to multiple factors, including the illness itself (e.g., pain, dyspnea), high noise and light levels, medication effects or withdrawal, and frequent disruptions from usual processes of care (e.g., phlebotomy, vital signs, medication administration). Hospitalists should enter orders and work with nurses and others to minimize these disruptions. Despite the known risks associated with sedative-hypnotics, including falls, hip fractures, and delirium, approximately 30 % of hospitalized patients receive these medications, often because it is included in routine standing orders. This is inappropriate and sleep deprivation is best managed by including bundling care processes at night (e.g., ordering that vital signs, blood draws, and daily weights be obtained during the same hour rather than intermittently throughout the night), optimizing the sleeping environment, utilizing non-pharmacological sleep aids such as warm drinks and soothing music, and avoiding generic order sets for sleep, anxiety, and pain.

7.5.4 Malnutrition

Nutritional deficiencies are a common occurrence in acutely ill hospitalized older adults, and are associated with increased risk of complications, institutionalization, and death [37]. Approximately 35 % of hospitalized adults age 70 and older suffer from moderate or severe protein-calorie malnutrition, and vitamin and electrolyte deficiencies further complicate the clinical course. A standardized approach to assessing nutritional risk is recommended, such as the brief Mini Nutritional Assessment (MNA) [37]. At-risk patients should receive a dietitian-led individualized nutri-

tional treatment plan. In addition to considering supplements, important remedial factors include difficulty in self-feeding or chewing, need for dentures, dysphagia, anorexic side effects from medications, or a too restrictive diet. Constipation also contributes to poor oral intake. Easily implemented interventions include sitting the patient up to eat, relaxing dietary restrictions, and providing assistance as needed to promote oral feedings whenever possible. The decision to consider a feeding tube is complex, and demands a careful discussion with the patient and family with an honest and full appraisal of the immediate and long-term burdens and benefits of this intervention. In certain circumstances, such as advanced dementia, feeding tubes have not been shown to prolong survival or improve comfort [38].

7.5.5 Nosocomial (Hospital-Acquired) Infections

Nosocomial infections are common in older adults with severe illness, comorbid conditions, functional impairment, and malnutrition. The lack of fever and the presence of atypical symptoms in many elders contribute to misdiagnosis. Common infections include pneumonia, intravascular catheter-related infections, Clostridium difficile associated diarrhea, and urinary tract infections (UTIs). The strongest risk factor for hospital-acquired pneumonia is mechanical ventilation. Patients with dementia and Parkinson's disease, as well as those on antipsychotics, are at higher risk. Strategies to prevent aspiration pneumonia include attention to oral hygiene and safe feeding techniques. Clostridium difficile associated diarrhea is a serious and often persistent nosocomial infection and causes significant morbidity and mortality. Risk factors include exposure to antibiotics, advanced age, duration of hospitalization, and use of a proton pump inhibitor (PPI). Key strategies include using antibiotics with the narrowest spectrum possible, avoiding PPIs when possible, early recognition and treatment, and implementation of contact precautions. UTIs associated with indwelling urinary catheters are the leading cause of nosocomial bacteremia and carry high morbidity and mortality. As seen with other serious infections in older adults, these patients often present only with unexplained confusion, hypotension, or acidosis. It is strongly recommended to limit catheter use, routinely monitor the need for the catheter, and remove it as soon as possible. Overall, adherence to infection control programs in the hospital can prevent and reduce the rates of nosocomial infections. Bacteriuria is very common and often leads to erroneously asymptomatic prescribing antibiotic (see discussion in Sec. 7.5.9). Chapter 24 provides in-depth information.

7.5.6 Pressure Ulcer

A hospital acquired pressure ulcer (HAPU) is a CMS designated "never event" and as such, Medicare does not reimburse hospitals for the costs of treating an acquired Stage III or IV ulcer. The incidence of HAPU ranges from 7 to 9%, and it is associated with significant morbidity and mortality, high costs, and directly impacts transition planning [39]. Several hospital factors increase the risk of acquiring a pressure ulcer: immobility, malnutrition, incontinence, and cognitive/neurologic impairment. The Braden and Norton scales are commonly used in hospitals to assess risk, and target patients for preventive interventions, including: **daily skin assessment**, proper repositioning for bed-bound or mobility-limited patients, use of moisturizing creams, optimizing nutritional status, use of pressure-reducing products as indicated, and encourage ambulation. It is important to learn how to safely move and position a patient in bed (e.g., from lying to sitting up at 45°) without increasing pressure, shear, or friction forces on the skin, as an incorrect technique inadvertently causes pressure ulcers. The hospitalist should review daily with nursing the status of a patient's skin or do the evaluation her- or himself.

7.5.7 Volume Shifts, Impaired Response

Usual aging is the result of a complex interplay among the normal physiologic aging changes in the renal, endocrine, cardiovascular, and other systems, along with the additional impact of age-associated diseases such as hypertension, heart disease, and diabetes. The aging kidney is less able to concentrate urine or excrete free water, and is less able to mount an effective and efficient response to dehydration, salt restriction, or volume excess. The left ventricle is hypertrophied, and the vasculature is stiffer and less responsive to β-adrenergic stimulation. With increased heart rate, volume depletion, loss of atrial contraction or other stresses, the aged heart is less able to maintain hemodynamic stability. In the hospital, the volume status of older patients is frequently challenged by interventions such as intravenous hydration, diuretics, salt/fluid restriction, and keeping patients NPO for procedures. Because of an impaired ability to appropriately respond to volume shifts, older patients often become dehydrated, experience fluctuations in blood pressure and pulse, develop signs and symptoms of volume overload, or rapidly develop serum chemical abnormalities, such as hypo- or hypernatremia. It is important to monitor weight and physical signs of dehydration (increased skin turgor, dry oral mucosa (if not mouth breathing), lack of axillary moisture) and volume overload (jugular venous pressure, edema) to detect and treat these problems early.

7.5.8 Constipation

Constipation is common in older people, and complicates the hospital course of many older adults if not anticipated and prevented. It is estimated that 50% of community-dwelling elders suffer from constipation, and climbs to almost 70% in nursing home residents. Risk factors include diseases like Parkinson's disease, dementia, post-stroke syndromes and endocrinopathies as well as medications such as opiates, diuretics, and antacids. The hospital environment puts elders at further risk of constipation due to bed rest and immobility, use of constipating medications, uremia, and electrolyte abnormalities (hypokalemia, hypercalcemia, hyponatremia).

Elders may show the typical symptoms and signs of constipation, but they often present instead with delirium, urinary retention, and overflow diarrhea or fecal incontinence/seepage in the setting of impaction. Prevention and treatment of constipation involves encouraging mobility, treating electrolyte disturbances, ensuring adequate hydration and dietary fiber along with regular screening to reduce constipating medications. If those cannot be discontinued, instituting a bowel regimen is essential. Once constipation develops, the use of stool softeners such as docusate has little to no benefit. Preferred agents include osmotic laxatives such as polyethylene glycol, along with stimulants such as bisacodyl and senna. Caution should be used when considering phosphate and magnesium containing products as these can lead to worsening kidney function and electrolyte disturbances in those with reduced GFR. If enemas are needed, tap water is safer in seniors. In addition, using lactulose in patients with significant colonic dilation or pseudo-obstruction can lead to further gas production from sugar fermentation, causing worsening abdominal pain, bloating, and even perforation [40]. Chapter 24, Geriatric Gastroenterology has a detailed review on managing constipation.

7.5.9 Urinary Incontinence

Acute urinary incontinence occurs in approximately 35% of hospitalized older adults [41], and is a high-risk condition for several reasons, including: (1) moisture contributes to the development of sacral pressure ulcers, (2) indwelling urinary catheters are used to keep track of output (and to keep the area dry), leading to serious urinary tract infections, (3) patients may fall and suffer serious injury while urgently attempting to reach the bathroom, and (4) patients feel overwhelmed and isolated to now have developed another age related infirmity especially when this problem is not often even recognized or acknowledged by nurses or physicians. Hospitalists should communicate daily with nursing staff to recognize acute urinary incontinence and initiate an investigation for retention or diuresis. Too often acute urinary incontinence is ignored or assumed to be chronic or functional. However, it is important to remember that asymptomatic bacteriuria is very common among older adults and should not be treated with antibiotics as is too often the case. Delirium is not a result of bacturia without fever otherwise unexplained or urinary tract symptoms. Following the assessment, potential interventions include medication review to discontinue potentially offending medications, such as diuretics or anticholinergics, avoidance of tethers or restraints, cued or scheduled voiding, use of a bedside commode, limiting continuous intravenous fluids during the night, and encouraging mobility [42].

7.6 Bring It All Together: Engineer Geriatric Issues into Daily Rounds

As has been detailed above, the elderly are at an increased risk relative to other hospitalized patients due to a greater susceptibility to delirium and functional decline. Many of these risks are modifiable if careful protocol driven precautions are initiated. Table 7.6 proposes a checklist to use as an adjunct to daily rounds, in an effort to screen for and potentially prevent the common hospital related complications specific to the geriatric population.

Table 7.6 Tips for daily rounds

Area of concern	Check/ask
Goals of care/transition plan	• Daily update on care transition plan • Is plan still consistent with patient goals, preferences, and values?
Cognition/mood	• Use delirium screen • Ask orientation re: person, place, time • Test for inattention (count from 1 to 10 and back from 10 to 1) • 3-item recall; consider mini-Cog • Assess interaction and mood
Environment	• Wake patient, help sit them up • Ensure they have glasses, hearing aids, teeth • Open blinds, turn on TV, hand them newspaper • Encourage family to come visit, stay the night
Mobility	• Don't use "Bed rest" or "Out of Bed prn" orders • Be specific: Sit in chair for meals; walk with assist 3 times daily • Physical Therapy or Occupational Therapy evaluation as needed • Consider briefly watching patient stand/walk during rounds
Tethers	• Check need for all tethers every day • Is telemetry still required? • Is the IV needed (for medication, for fluids) continuously? • Is continuous pulse oximetry required? Can a different option such as the ear be used? • Is there an indwelling urinary catheter in place? Is it required? • Are SCDs really needed? • Any restraints? REMOVE and consider a sitter, if possible
Fluid balance	• Check for adequate hydration (PE, weight, access to water, within reach?) • Actively encourage patients to drink (as appropriate) • Check for volume overload • Check for orthostatic hypotension • Trend daily weights
Nutrition	• Consider nutrition consult • Assess appetite
Continence (urine/bowel)	• Check for last bowel movement, screen for constipation • Assess urine incontinence/retention • Use cueing and bedside commode
Skin	• Check skin daily, especially pressure points; check with nursing for skin status daily • Use skin-safe techniques to move patient in bed for general exam (e.g., don't pull or drag across sheets; support when sitting up) • Check IV sites
Sleep	• Ask about sleep • Use environmental/nonpharmacologic options
Medications (scheduled and prn)	• Review medication list daily; check for new and prn medications; check against Beers Criteria (Chap. 5) • Avoid anticholinergics, antihistamines, and benzodiazepines (but be aware of chronic use and do not stop abruptly) • Assess for withdrawal symptoms (alcohol, other medications) • Address adequate pain control

7.6.1 Alternatives to Hospital Care

It is important to recognize that hospitalizations and care transitions present significant challenges for older, frail patients. In response to this, it has been demonstrated that many older adults with selected medical conditions may safely be offered alternatives to hospitalization depending upon their clinical setting, available resources, and their goals and preferences. The alternatives to hospitalization may include bringing in home health services, or continuing medical care in the elder's facility without transfer. Although hospital-level care can be provided safely in the home for several conditions, including pneumonia and urinary tract infection, current reimbursement rules in non-capitated systems limit its feasibility [43]. The hospitalist will likely have a central role in helping to define alternatives to hospital care, an emerging field that is driven by advancements in technology, quality and safety outcomes, and reimbursement strategies [44, 45].

7.6.2 Bring High Value to the Hospital and Healthcare System

Hospitalists are ideally and uniquely positioned to play a major role in improving quality and safety for older hospitalized adults and in championing and supporting hospital-wide interventions [34]. Some of these interventions are targeted to prevent specific adverse events, such as hospital-wide fall prevention programs that use information technology, patient education, and plans of care to communicate patient-specific alerts to the team [46]. Other targeted interventions identify older patients at risk for adverse drug reactions [47] or employ protocols for medication appropriateness, including computerized decision support and alerts [48–50]. Hospital-based mobilization programs are an effective method to promote older adults to get out of bed and maintain function [51, 52]. The Hospital Elder Life Program targets delirium prevention and management through practical, hospital-wide interventions that address sleep, orientation, and cognition, successfully decreasing rates of delirium, thus reducing hospital length of stay and costs [53]. The use of checklists and admission order sets can improve quality of care for older adults by ensuring that evidence-based principles of geriatric care are integrated into daily care, such as orders for daily mobilization, assessing the presence of delirium, or restricting the use of high-risk medications.

Many hospitals have developed designated inpatient geriatric units to provide interprofessional care for high risk elders through a combination of structural modifications, order sets and protocols, and dedicated and skilled geriatric staffing. Often called Acute Care of Elders (ACE) units, they have been demonstrated to improve function and reduce discharge of patients to long-term care facilities. In place of geographic units, some hospitals utilize mobile geriatric interprofessional teams to provide consults for high-risk older patients throughout the hospital. The results of such programs show benefit but have more variable results than ACE units [14, 54].

References

1. Living. AfC. Census Data & population Estimates. 2015.
2. http://www.cdc.gov/nchs/fastats/hospital.htm. National Hospital Discharge Survey: 2010 table. Number and rate of hospital discharges.
3. Levant S, Chari K, DeFrances CJ. Hospitalizations for patients aged 85 and over in the United States, 2000–2010. NCHS Data Brief. 2015(182):1–8.
4. Hamel MB, Lynn J, Teno JM, et al. Age-related differences in care preferences, treatment decisions, and clinical outcomes of seriously ill hospitalized adults: lessons from SUPPORT. J Am Geriatr Soc. 2000;48(5 Suppl):S176–82.
5. Halter J, Ouslander J, Tinetti M, Studenski S, High K, Asthana S. Hazzard's geriatric medicine and gerontology. McGraw-Hill Prof Med/Tech; 2009.
6. Guiding principles for the care of older adults with multimorbidity: an approach for c. Guiding principles for the care of older adults with multimorbidity: an approach for clinicians: American Geriatrics Society Expert Panel on the Care of Older Adults with Multimorbidity. J Am Geriatr Soc. 2012;60(10):E1–25.
7. Krumholz HM. Post-hospital syndrome—an acquired, transient condition of generalized risk. N Engl J Med. 2013;368(2):100–2.
8. Covinsky KE, Pierluissi E, Johnston CB. Hospitalization-associated disability: "She was probably able to ambulate, but I'm not sure". JAMA. 2011;306(16):1782–93.
9. Zwart SR, Pierson D, Mehta S, Gonda S, Smith SM. Capacity of omega-3 fatty acids or eicosapentaenoic acid to counteract weightlessness-induced bone loss by inhibiting NF-kappaB activation: from cells to bed rest to astronauts. J Bone Miner Res. 2010;25(5):1049–57.
10. Mehta KM, Pierluissi E, Boscardin WJ, et al. A clinical index to stratify hospitalized older adults according to risk for new-onset disability. J Am Geriatr Soc. 2011;59(7):1206–16.
11. Wyrko Z. Frailty at the front door. Clin Med. 2015;15(4):377–81.
12. Fried LP, Tangen CM, Walston J, et al. Frailty in older adults: evidence for a phenotype. J Gerontol A Biol Sci Med Sci. 2001;56(3): M146–56.
13. Rodriguez-Manas L, Fried LP. Frailty in the clinical scenario. Lancet. 2015;385(9968):e7–9.
14. Ellis G, Whitehead MA, Robinson D, O'Neill D, Langhorne P. Comprehensive geriatric assessment for older adults admitted to hospital: meta-analysis of randomised controlled trials. BMJ. 2011;343:d6553.
15. Sessums LL, Zembrzuska H, Jackson JL. Does this patient have medical decision-making capacity? JAMA. 2011;306(4):420–7.
16. Appelbaum PS. Clinical practice. Assessment of patients' competence to consent to treatment. N Engl J Med. 2007;357(18):1834–40.
17. Toronto. Aid to Capacity Evaluation tool. 2015.
18. Ritchie CS, Zulman DM. Research priorities in geriatric palliative care: multimorbidity. J Palliat Med. 2013;16(8):843–7.
19. Chan M, Nicklason F, Vial JH. Adverse drug events as a cause of hospital admission in the elderly. Intern Med J. 2001;31(4):199–205.
20. Jokhadar M, Wenger NK. Review of the treatment of acute coronary syndrome in elderly patients. Clin Interv Aging. 2009;4:435–44.

21. Norman DC. Fever in the elderly. Clin Infect Dis. 2000;31(1): 148–51.
22. Lyons W. Principles of geriatric care. In: al MSe, editor. Principles and practice of hospital medicine. New York, NY: McGraw-Hill; 2012.
23. Arbaje AI, Kansagara DL, Salanitro AH, et al. Regardless of age: incorporating principles from geriatric medicine to improve care transitions for patients with complex needs. J Gen Intern Med. 2014;29(6):932–9.
24. Coalition NToC. 2015.
25. Takahashi PY, Haas LR, Quigg SM, et al. 30-day hospital readmission of older adults using care transitions after hospitalization: a pilot prospective cohort study. Clin Interv Aging. 2013;8:729–36.
26. Arbaje AI, Wolff JL, Yu Q, Powe NR, Anderson GF, Boult C. Postdischarge environmental and socioeconomic factors and the likelihood of early hospital readmission among community-dwelling Medicare beneficiaries. Gerontologist. 2008;48(4):495–504.
27. Halasyamani L, Kripalani S, Coleman E, et al. Transition of care for hospitalized elderly patients—development of a discharge checklist for hospitalists. J Hosp Med. 2006;1(6):354–60.
28. Snow V, Beck D, Budnitz T, et al. Transitions of Care Consensus Policy Statement American College of Physicians-Society of General Internal Medicine-Society of Hospital Medicine-American Geriatrics Society-American College of Emergency Physicians-Society of Academic Emergency Medicine. J Gen Intern Med. 2009;24(8):971–6.
29. Fulmer T, Mezey M, Bottrell M, et al. Nurses Improving Care for Healthsystem Elders (NICHE): using outcomes and benchmarks for evidenced-based practice. Geriatr Nurs. 2002;23(3):121–7.
30. BOOST P. Project BOOST. http://www.hospitalmedicine.org/ BOOST/. Accessed 2015.
31. Program CT. Care Transitions Program. 2015; http://caretransitions.org/.
32. Naylor MD, Aiken LH, Kurtzman ET, Olds DM, Hirschman KB. The care span: the importance of transitional care in achieving health reform. Health Aff. 2011;30(4):746–54.
33. Hansen LO, Young RS, Hinami K, Leung A, Williams MV. Interventions to reduce 30-day rehospitalization: a systematic review. Ann Intern Med. 2011;155(8):520–8.
34. Medicine SoH. Hospitalist/Hospitalist Job/Leadership/Education. 2015; http://www.hospitalmedicine.org/. Accessed November 18, 2015.
35. Covinsky KE, Palmer RM, Fortinsky RH, et al. Loss of independence in activities of daily living in older adults hospitalized with medical illnesses: increased vulnerability with age. J Am Geriatr Soc. 2003;51(4):451–8.
36. Weissman DE, Meier DE. Identifying patients in need of a palliative care assessment in the hospital setting: a consensus report from the Center to Advance Palliative Care. J Palliat Med. 2011;14(1):17–23.
37. Feldblum I, German L, Castel H, Harman-Boehm I, Shahar DR. Individualized nutritional intervention during and after hospitalization: the nutrition intervention study clinical trial. J Am Geriatr Soc. 2011;59(1):10–7.
38. Medicine ABoI. Choosing Wisely. 2015.
39. Lyder CH, Wang Y, Metersky M, et al. Hospital-acquired pressure ulcers: results from the national Medicare Patient Safety Monitoring System study. J Am Geriatr Soc. 2012;60(9):1603–8.
40. Rao SS, Go JT. Update on the management of constipation in the elderly: new treatment options. Clin Interv Aging. 2010;5: 163–71.
41. Zurcher S, Saxer S, Schwendimann R. Urinary incontinence in hospitalised elderly patients: do nurses recognise and manage the problem? Nurs Res Pract. 2011;2011:671302.
42. Dowling-Castronovo A. Urinary incontinence assessment in older adults Part I–transient urinary incontinence. Obstet Gynecol. 1985;109(2):277–80.
43. Leff B, Burton L, Mader SL, et al. Hospital at home: feasibility and outcomes of a program to provide hospital-level care at home for acutely ill older patients. Ann Intern Med. 2005;143(11): 798–808.
44. Cheng J, Montalto M, Leff B. Hospital at home. Clin Geriatr Med. 2009;25(1):79–91. vi.
45. Leff B, Burton L, Mader SL, et al. Comparison of functional outcomes associated with hospital at home care and traditional acute hospital care. J Am Geriatr Soc. 2009;57(2):273–8.
46. Dykes PC, Carroll DL, Hurley A, et al. Fall prevention in acute care hospitals: a randomized trial. JAMA. 2010;304(17):1912–8.
47. Onder G, Petrovic M, Tangiisuran B, et al. Development and validation of a score to assess risk of adverse drug reactions among in-hospital patients 65 years or older: the GerontoNet ADR risk score. Arch Intern Med. 2010;170(13):1142–8.
48. By the American Geriatrics Society Beers Criteria Update Expert P. American Geriatrics Society 2015 Updated Beers Criteria for potentially inappropriate medication use in older adults. J Am Geriatr Soc. 2015.
49. Hamilton H, Gallagher P, Ryan C, Byrne S, O'Mahony D. Potentially inappropriate medications defined by STOPP criteria and the risk of adverse drug events in older hospitalized patients. Arch Intern Med. 2011;171(11):1013–9.
50. Mattison ML, Afonso KA, Ngo LH, Mukamal KJ. Preventing potentially inappropriate medication use in hospitalized older patients with a computerized provider order entry warning system. Arch Intern Med. 2010;170(15):1331–6.
51. Zisberg A, Shadmi E, Sinoff G, Gur-Yaish N, Srulovici E, Admi H. Low mobility during hospitalization and functional decline in older adults. J Am Geriatr Soc. 2011;59(2):266–73.
52. Fisher SR, Kuo YF, Graham JE, Ottenbacher KJ, Ostir GV. Early ambulation and length of stay in older adults hospitalized for acute illness. Arch Intern Med. 2010;170(21):1942–3.
53. Inouye SK, Bogardus Jr ST, Baker DI, Leo-Summers L, Cooney Jr LM. The Hospital Elder Life Program: a model of care to prevent cognitive and functional decline in older hospitalized patients. Hospital Elder Life Program. J Am Geriatr Soc. 2000;48(12):1697–706.
54. Landefeld CS, Palmer RM, Kresevic DM, Fortinsky RH, Kowal J. A randomized trial of care in a hospital medical unit especially designed to improve the functional outcomes of acutely ill older patients. N Engl J Med. 1995;332(20):1338–44.

Screening Tools for Geriatric Assessment by Specialists

8

John R. Burton and Jane F. Potter

A specialist clinician can and should use easily performed assessment tools to help in the evaluation of older patients. Such assessment instruments help any clinician screen for underlying problems that could put a patient at high risk for an adverse outcome from a new medication or procedure a specialist is considering. Such underlying clinical problems often are subtle and may not be listed on the patient list of chronic problems or in the referral letter.

The senior population roughly over the age of 80 years is characterized by increasing vulnerability. This vulnerability has many causes but to simplify it relates to three cardinal differences in this population compared to those that are younger:

1. *The presence of multiple chronic health problems in an individual.* Typically an octo- or nona-genarian has 10–15 chronic health problems. One health problem may mask the symptoms of another and treating one problem may have an adverse impact on another. Such a situation typically leads to polypharmacy and the high risk of an adverse drug effect including a drug–drug interaction.
2. *The continuous loss of physiological reserve.* Such losses demonstrated consistently by several longitudinal studies begin around the age of 30 years. The physiological losses are subtle and deterioration occurs slowly. Most typically these progressing changes are appreciated earliest among athletes who notice they have lost their competitive edge. Competition times in running and swimming, for example, gradually get slower over the years even with continued vigorous training and without injury. These physiological changes are quite variable among organs and individuals. However, by age 80 or so an individual has lost so much physiological reserve that they are at increased risk of a significant clinical problem developing after a perturbation such as an operation, a diagnostic procedure, a fall, or a new medication.
3. *Heterogeneity among individuals,* therefore, is remarkable. This heterogeneity makes the care of an older person unique and often precludes the clinician from applying published clinical trials (which rarely include very old individuals) and, especially, clinical guidelines to a patient over age 80 or so. This heterogeneity requires the clinician to apply considerable judgment when advising a diagnostic test, surgical intervention, or medical treatment for such a patient. Always a careful clinical risk–benefit judgment must be made and the patient needs to be a part of such discussions if complications and unexpected outcomes are to be minimized and patient understanding and satisfaction are to be maximized. While this heterogeneity is frustrating to many clinicians, it is remarkably rewarding to others as it demands maximum clinical knowledge, ideal communication skills, and knowing each patient and their goals extremely well.

Therefore, for a specialist trying to guide a senior, screening for subtle associated problems is important. Simple tools may be of value in this regard. Many of these tools are discussed in detail in other chapters, but here are discussed practical and common assessment tools that have been well studied and disseminated. They are discussed in a single chapter to make access easier when a clinician is seeing a patient and time is limited. These assessment tools are most often done by various members of an interdisciplinary team (a group of clinicians of different professions and/or training working regularly and collaboratively to achieve a unified approach). In the office setting these assessment tools are often performed by a nurse working in close partnership with a physician, nurse practitioner, or physician assistant.

J.R. Burton, MD (✉)
Professor of Medicine, Johns Hopkins University School of Medicine, The Johns Hopkins Bayview Medical Center, 5505 Hopkins Bayview Circle, Baltimore, MD 21224, USA
e-mail: jburton4@jhmi.edu

J.F. Potter, MD
Harris Professor of Geriatric Medicine, Chief, Division of Geriatrics and Gerontology, Director, Home Instead Center for Successful Aging, Department of Internal Medicine, University of Nebraska Medical Center, 986155 Nebraska Medical Center, Omaha, NE 68198-6155, USA

© Springer International Publishing Switzerland 2017
J.R. Burton et al. (eds.), *Geriatrics for Specialists*, DOI 10.1007/978-3-319-31831-8_8

8.1   Fall Risk

Falls by older patients are common after the initiation of certain new medications, procedures, or hospitalization. Estimation of the risk may help the clinician avoid a fall by alerting all to the increased fall risk and can lead to developing preemptive preventive strategies. *The Timed Up and Go Test* is the most popular for a quick assessment of fall risk. This evaluation can be done in a few seconds. It is easy and provides some sense of a patient's mobility and risk of falling [1, 2]. Some experienced clinicians simply observe the patient coming into the office or getting on to the examination table. While valuable, this simple observation strategy seems to be less accurate than The Timed Up and Go Test.

To perform the Timed Up and Go Test, the clinician gives the following instructions to the patient and informs the patient he or she is being timed. The patient is instructed to:

1. Rise quickly from the arm chair;
2. Walk 10 feet using a cane or walker if they normally do so;
3. Turn around;
4. Walk back to the chair and sit down.

The clinician or an assistant starts the patient by indicating that they will be timed and then giving a precise start command. Accomplishing this is recorded in seconds and the fall risk is related to the elapsed time from the Go command until the patient sits back down: 10 or less—low risk for fall; 11–19—moderate; 20–29—high risk; and 30 or greater is impaired mobility and a very high risk of falling. A clinician knowing the risk for a fall will want to talk with the patient and ideally with the primary care provider to weigh the risk and benefit of any considered intervention. If the potential for a fall is significant and the benefit of a new therapeutic or diagnostic perturbation is consider to outweigh the risk, preventive strategies such as precautionary guidance to the patient or physical therapy consultation may be appropriate. The Timed Up and Go test is not completely predictive of the fall risk in community dwelling elders but it is simple and the most popular and it when markedly abnormal gives the clinician some sense of the likelihood of a fall.

Other gait assessment tools have been validated and are of considerable value. The simplest of these is Gait Speed. Gait speed in one study was assessed by timing a patient's walk (at their normal or usual pace) over a measured 5 m. If six or more seconds is required (0.833 m/s or slower), there is an incremental higher risk of mortality and major morbidity in a study of older patients undergoing cardiac surgery [3]. The same cut off appears in numerous studies supporting that gait speed 0.8 m/s or better is necessary for independent community ambulation [4]. A simple approach is to measure a 5 or 4 (see frailty below) m or longer distance in an office hallway, time the patient, and calculate his or her speed.

8.2   Dementia

Cognitive impairment of any level is a significant risk factor for complications from any clinical perturbation such as hospitalization, a diagnostic or therapeutic procedure, or medication. Such impairment may effect up to 20 % of seniors over the age of 80. Further cognitive impairment is not always obvious to even a trained clinician and for specialists it may not be in the referral note of a patient especially when this problem is only mild or modest. Accordingly, if cognitive impairment has not earlier been evaluated, it is in the best interest of the patient if the specialist or his or her staff screens an older patient for cognitive impairment. The *Mini Cog*™ [5] is the simplest and most popular such assessment tool:

1. Instruct the patient to listen carefully and remember three unrelated but simple words and then repeat the words. Pen, watch, and tie are examples.
2. Instruct the patient to draw the numbers of the face of a clock after handing the individual a paper with only a blank circle representing the outline of the clock.
3. Instruct the patient to draw the hands of a clock to represent a specific time such as 9:15 or 1:25. The patient may take as much time as needed to complete this task.
4. Then instruct the patient to repeat the three words given before the clock drawing distraction.

Scoring is simple: one point is given for each correctly recalled word after completing the clock drawing.

Zero is a positive screen for dementia; one-two with an abnormal clock drawing is a positive screen; one-two with a normal clock drawing is a negative screen; a score of three is a negative screen.

A clock drawing is normal only if the numbers are placed in appropriate sequence and the hands are displayed properly. A positive screen for dementia should alert the specialist to the risk of potentially underlying cognitive impairment.

The Mini-Cog test is copyrighted and cannot be modified, reproduced or disseminated without the permission of its primary developer, Soo Borson, MD, of the University of Washington. Other cognitive assessment tools are available [6] but the Mini-Cog [7] seems to be the simplest and most popular.

There are several other more elaborate assessment tools to evaluate and monitor over time cognitive impairment. Perhaps one of the most popular is the Mini-Mental State Examination (MMSE). The MMSE was developed decades ago [8] and has been well validated and widely disseminated. It is a 30-point evaluation that takes about 7–10 min to complete. It is influenced by age and education but remains popular. Currently its copyright is held by Psychology Assessment Services (PAS) who offer copies of it and a training manual for sale on line. One can enter MMSE in web search engine to find examples. Another is the Montreal

Cognitive Assessment (MoCA). This test is especially valuable in early dementia and in those with vascular dementia. Information on performing and interpreting this test is readily available on the following web site: www.mocatest.org. On this site one can access detailed information, in many languages, about the instrument. There are no copyrights or restrictions on its use.

8.3 Delirium

Delirium is in older people often of the hypoactive type (as opposed to the hyperactive, typical more common in younger individuals). Because of this, the diagnosis of delirium is easily missed by even experienced clinicians. Recognizing delirium is of critical importance as its presence in a patient portends a serious situation that often will markedly worsened with a new insult such as a procedure or new medication. Delirium in all forms is a serious risk factor for rapid mental deterioration, prolonged hospitalization, complications, and death. Risk factors for delirium are advanced age, multiple co-morbidities, and underlying brain disease, even if mild. Many medications including those not requiring a prescription are associated with the development of delirium.

The well-validated *Confusion Assessment Method (CAM)* is the most widely used screening tool [9]. Delirium is diagnosed classically by evaluating nine features: acute onset, inattention, disorganized thinking, altered level of consciousness, disorientation, memory impairment, perceptual disturbances, psychomotor agitation or retardation, and altered sleep–wake cycle.

These nine criteria are well described in the Diagnostic and Statistical Manual for Mental Disorders. Classically studies on delirium used an expert psychiatrist's evaluation as the gold standard for the diagnosis of delirium. To make the evaluation of delirium more accessible to all clinicians a simplified assessment tool was created and validated [10, 11]. The Confusion Assessment Method (CAM) is based on evaluating the patient for a change in cognition and has four cardinal features:

1. A rapid onset with a fluctuating course with changes over minutes to hours;
2. Inattention;
3. Disorganized thinking; and/or
4. Altered level of consciousness.

The diagnosis of delirium requires the presence 1, 2 and either 3 or 4.

The timing of the onset and the nature of the course of the symptoms are self-evident. However, hypoactive delirium is often mistaken for dementia in a clinical setting and it is imperative to establish the onset of symptoms especially by asking other observers such as family members. Delirium is different from dementia. Dementia is only properly evaluated in a patient with a clear consciousness and is manifest by a slowly progressive course and without fluctuation from 1 min, hour, or day to the next as occurs in delirium. Delirium frequently occurs in cognitively impaired individuals making the evaluation of the level of dementia difficult to assess.

Inattention can be assessed by observing that the patient is not tuned into the conversation or is not fully aware of the surroundings. A patient with delirium will often drift off in midsentence or just stare at something other than the clinician. A quick test is to have patients say the months of the year backward.

Disorganized thinking is detected by illogical or disconnected responses to questions. Responses are often irrelevant, rambling, or incoherent or the patient may have hallucinations or delusions.

Consciousness can be assessed by evaluating the mental status for hypo or hyperactivity (agitation). A common clinical trap is to assume that the patient is sleepy or just waking up when, in fact, this is hypoactive delirium.

The optimal use of the CAM is based on observations during cognitive testing such as performing the mini-mental state examination (see above). Some experience and training is suggested for the best results. A CAM training manual is available from the scholars who first introduced it by entering into a web search engine Hospital Elder Life Program or www.elderlifeprogram.med.yale.edu. The menu bar can direct one to the Assessment Instruments.

A valuable guideline for post-operative delirium is available. It was published in late 2014 by an expert panel sponsored by the American College of Surgeons and the American Geriatrics Society with support from the John A. Hartford Foundation. This guideline may be found on the following AGS website: www. geriatricscareonline.org. The guideline can be downloaded for no charge to AGS members and for a small fee for non-members. A more detailed discussion of delirium can be found in the Delirium chapter.

8.4 Frailty

Frailty is a clinical phenotype that is a marker for increased vulnerability to adverse health outcomes and increased mortality after surgical or medical interventions or other perturbation. The diagnosis of 'frailty' to date has mostly been utilized in research settings to identify those at increased risk of adverse outcomes and for biological studies. For example, in a study of over 1000 older adults receiving general surgery, those who were frail were up to 20 times more likely to need care in a post-acute facility as compared to those who were robust or not frail [12]. Subspecialists are increasingly interested in the identification of the frail subset of older adults in order to help predict and potentially prevent adverse outcomes related to procedures and treatments. Dozens of frailty assessment methods have evolved over the past several years that may be useful to clinicians as they attempt to determine which older adults may be at most risk for adverse outcomes. Most of the tools perform well at identifying vulnerable older adults. A recent consensus conference on frailty suggested that those over age 70 should be screened for physical frailty, in part because physical frailty can be potentially treated or prevented with specific modalities, and the adverse outcomes associated with frailty ameliorated [13]. Use of any of these tools by clinicians has been delayed because of confusion about which tool to choose, and because of lack of research on how to manage a patient differently once frailty status is determined.

In general, there have been two approaches to the identification of frailty, which in turn has driven the development of multiple frailty assessment tools. The physical frailty or phenotype approach suggests that frailty emerges from an age-related biological process that results in weakness, fatigue, low levels of activity. The frailty index approach suggests that frailty is driven by an accumulation of illnesses as well as cognitive and social decline that can be ultimately additive. Few guidelines exist on how to best choose a tool for the purpose at hand. Most tools have not been extensively validated or utilized across populations, and few comparison studies have been done that show clear benefit of using one tool over the other. In addition, different tools may or may not be good matches for the intended use. For example, a brief screening tool may be appropriate for risk stratification while a more formal frailty assessment could be required to define preoperative interventions meant to modify surgical outcomes.

8.4.1 Frailty Measures

Given the wide array of tools and the wide variety of populations in which the tools may need to be implemented, the choice of which to use must be tailored to a clinical situation and clinical need. In addition, choosing tools that have been previously used in a variety of populations and have demonstrated predictive validity in several settings should also influence the choice of tools. Time to complete a frailty assessment also matters in a clinical setting. The development of discipline specific clinical guidelines of how best to manage frail older adults in a variety of clinical settings is needed to more fully utilize assessment tools.

8.4.1.1 Single-Item Surrogate Frailty Assessments (2–3 min)

For feasibility, single-item measurement tools have been proposed to stand in for a more formal frailty measurement. Gait speed measured over a 4 m distance is recognized as a highly reliable single measurement tool that predicts adverse outcomes [14, 15]. A timed up-and-go score (the time it takes to rise from a chair, walk 10 feet, turn around, and return to sitting in the chair) $\geq$15 s is closely related to both postoperative complications and 1-year mortality [16]. Some of these single measures are components of both the frailty index and frailty phenotype approaches, and although they can be easy to use and predictive of certain outcomes, they can lack sensitivity and specificity of the full frailty assessment tools.

8.4.1.2 Frail Scale (<5 min)

The Frail Scale was developed as a quick screening tool [17]. The Geriatric Advisory Panel of the International Academy of Nutrition and Aging developed this approach to define frailty as a case-finding tool [14]. This brief tool simply requires asking 5 questions and scoring a 1 for each yes. Those who are frail score 3, 4, and 5, and those who are robust score 0 [18].

> **F**atigue (Are you fatigued?)
> **R**esistance (Can you climb 1 flight of stairs?)
> **A**mbulation (Can you walk 1 block?)
> **I**llnesses (greater than 5)
> **L**oss of weight (greater than 5 %)

8.4.1.3 Physical or Phenotypic Frailty (10 min)

Phenotypic or physical frailty is the most widely used measurement tool used by frailty researchers, and especially those interested in learning about the biology that may underlie frailty. This frailty evaluation was 1 of 2 strategies recognized by the American College of Surgeons/American Geriatric Society's optimal preoperative assessment of the older adult [19]. The tool requires a questionnaire, a hand-held dynamometer, and a stopwatch for implication. The recent development of a web-based calculator has further accelerated the ease of use for this tool. Access to needed measurement equipment, training guides, and web-based calculator is available at https://jhpeppercenter.jhmi.edu/a1b1/login.aspx. This clinical phenotype has five components that can be assessed using readily available measurement equipment and a web-based frailty calculator as described below. The score is determined on a 0–5 scale with 0 being not frail; 1–2 pre frail; and 3–5 frail. The severity of the risk is linear.

The major measurement domains include:

1. Shrinking (greater than 5 % loss of body weight in the last year).
2. Weakness (grip strength of the dominate hand in the lowest 20 % of the age and body mass index (BMI).
3. Poor endurance (self-reported exhaustion).
4. Slowness (lower 25 % of population average measures 4 m walking time).
5. Low activity (assessed by activity questions that identify weekly energy expenditure of less than 383/270 kcals for males and females, respectively).

Although this tool is commonly utilized in research settings, it takes more effort than other methods in that it requires specialized equipment (i.e., dynamometer and a stop watch) to measure it. Hence, it may not be a practical method for a busy clinician to assess frailty.

8.4.1.4 Deficit Accumulation Index

The most widely recognized deficit accumulation method to measure frailty was developed from the Canadian Health and Aging Study [20]. Between 21 and 70 deficits are suggested to be measured. Although considerable time may be needed to gather information in the initial developmental stages of individualized frailty indices, data may be quickly accessible if they are already available in the electronic medical record. The frailty index score is calculated as the number of characteristics that are abnormal (or "deficits") divided by the total number of characteristics measured. Scoring has mostly been done by summing the total deficits and comparing to a published cut off score, or by calculating a ratio between deficits and total number of characteristics. This tool can be accessed in a series of references [21–23]. Recent adaptations of this tool for risk assessment in a variety of clinical settings including trauma surgery outcomes have demonstrated the tool's predictive ability for adverse outcomes [24]. However, beyond risk assessment, the wide variety of unrelated variables included in the tool and its conceptual basis as a tool with cumulative unrelated deficits make it less useful for designing targeted interventions or biological studies in vulnerable frail patients.

8.4.1.5 Additional Tools

There are many additional published measures of frailty but to date are not as well studied or as broadly validated [25]. One of these was popularized by The Journal of the American College of Cardiology. They have created an on-line frailty calculator for patients with cardiac disease such as aortic stenosis: http://tools.cardiosource.org/Tools/ccpFrailty.html. This tool derives a frailty score based on a patient's BMI, gait speed, calf circumference, ADL and cognitive assessments, and the answers to several questions about function and activities. This tool is now being studied for use in other conditions and as a general indicator of recovery after surgery. The authors of this chapter are grateful to Dr. Jeremy Walston (Chap. 1—Frailty) for his review and embellishment of this section.

8.5 Depression

Depression is a common problem in seniors and one that is often under recognized. The presence of a significant clinical depression is important to recognize as it can be associated with poor outcomes in the treatment of associated illnesses and in recovery from major interventions such as a surgical procedure.

The simplest screen is the *PHQ 2 Question Tool* [26, 27]. Ask the patient if, in the last 2 weeks, they have:

1. Felt down, depressed, or hopeless and
2. Little interest or pleasure in doing things.

A positive screen may indicate a significant depression and this should be followed up. For the non-psychiatric specialists the most appropriate action would be to raise the question of depression with the referring or primary care provider before initiating any major intervention or starting medications with known adverse effect on mood.

8.6 Physical Self-Maintenance

A chronic loss of any physical independence by an older person is a harbinger for adverse outcomes after any significant perturbation such as an acute injury or surgical procedure. Physical independence can be measured by several tools.

The Katz Index of Activities of Daily Living (ADLs) [28] may be the best known, most studied, and simplest to use. The ADL index has been simplified since originally introduced and assesses an individual's ability to perform six functions:

1. Bathing
2. Dressing
3. Toileting
4. Transferring
5. Continence
6. Feeding

These ADLs are activities necessary for daily living and are typically readily performed by a 7 year old. Each is scored on a 1 or 0 basis for each of the 6 items: a score of 1 if the patient is fully independent and a score of 0 if partially dependent (needing some help) or totally dependent. A score of 6 indicates fully independent function and a low risk for complications or poor outcome. A good source for this and other valuable geriatric assessment information can be found at The Hartford Institute for Geriatric Nursing at the New York University College of Nursing (www.hartfordign.org). The lower the ADL score, the worse the prognosis for the patient and the more likelihood that complications will result from a clinical perturbation. Patients with the lowest scores have a higher mortality rate and are at risk for long-term care placement. Identified impairments are also important for the specialist to consider in planning a diagnostic or therapeutic intervention as the strategies to achieve an ideal outcome may need to be modified from those used in a patient with normal ADLs.

A parallel tool, The Lawton Instrumental Activities of Daily Living (IADLS) is also available and measures more complex skills required to live in the community [29]. The IADL scale measures 8 functions also on a 1-0 scale and the lower the score the less independent the patient. This scale measures the following activities:

1. The use of a telephone;
2. Shopping;
3. Food preparation;
4. Housekeeping;
5. Laundry;
6. Transportation;
7. Responsibility for medications; and
8. Finances.

One can download from The Hartford Institute for Geriatric Nursing web site (see above) a useful two-page guide and scale of this instrument.

8.7 Nutritional Assessment and Screening for Malnutrition

In a variety of populations of surgical (orthopedic, gastrointestinal, etc.) and medical (older acute care, oncology, etc.) patients, malnutrition is associated with longer length of hospital stay, complications, and mortality. The American Society for Enteral and Parenteral Nutrition (ASPEN) defines malnutrition as "an acute, sub-acute, or chronic state of nutrition in which varying degrees of over nutrition or under nutrition with or without inflammatory activity have led to a change in body composition and diminished function." In a clinical practice guideline [30], ASPEN recommends the following with respect to adult nutrition screening and assessment:

1. Screening for nutrition risk is recommended for hospitalized patients.
2. Nutrition assessment is suggested for all patients who are at risk as identified by nutrition screening.
3. Nutrition support intervention is recommended for patients identified by screening and assessment as at risk for malnutrition or malnourished.

Also in that practice guideline is a brief review of 11 different screening instruments and two nutrition assessment tools: the Mini Nutritional Assessment [31] and the Subjective Global Assessment of nutrition status [32]. While no single screening or assessment tool is specifically recommended, disciplines whose interventions (e.g., surgery and oncology) or patient populations (orthopedic hip fracture, pulmonary disease) that are associated with significant nutritional risk will want to implement a screening and assessment tool. Reference [33] provides a general review of this topic.

8.8 Social Assessment

While a complete social assessment is not feasible in an office practice, any clinician caring for older patients should be aware of the factors involved in social assessment and when assistance from a social worker will be important to achieving the desired outcomes. Key elements of social assessment include [34]:

1. Patient characteristics: culture, ethnicity, education, economic situation
2. Family care system: identifying the primary and other caregivers and their level of burden
3. Environment: home safety, formal services
4. Advanced care planning: living will, powers of attorney for health and finance, advance directives.

A single question often used to explore an older individuals access to family care is: "In case of illness or emergency, who is available to assist you." When an individual is identified, that information needs to be in the patient's health record as should the items listed in item 4 above. When the patient answers that there is no one identified to provide care, a full social assessment is needed.

8.9 Potential for Urinary Retention in Men

Urinary retention is a common problem among older men. This problem is often precipitated by a new medication, hospitalization, or surgical procedure. The specialists planning one of these interventions should be aware of an increased risk for urinary retention. This can be easily screened for by the *International Prostrate Symptom Score (I-PSS)*. This tool can be administered by a member of an interdisciplinary team in an office practice or completed independently by a patient. Knowing that a patient is at increased risk of urinary retention will alert the specialist to caution the patient. The answers to the I-PSS are weighted on a 0–5 scale. The seven questions asked concern the following symptoms noticed in the last month:

1. Incomplete emptying;
2. Frequency;
3. Intermittency (how often have you stopped and started again during urination);
4. Urgency;
5. Weak stream;
6. Straining;
7. Nocturia.

The sum of these seven questions is the final score. The higher the score (35 is the highest), the greater the severity of prostatic hypertrophy and therefor the more concern for the possibility of retention with an intervention. The I-PPS asks an eighth question concerning the quality of life due to urinary symptoms. The I-PPS in a usable format can be downloaded from the web by putting BPH Score Sheet in a search engine or going to the following web site: www.urospec.com/uro/forms/ipps.pdf.

8.10 Polypharmacy

Polypharmacy is very common among seniors and is considered a geriatric syndrome leading to poor health outcomes and increased mortality. The most common definition of polypharmacy is the use of four or more drugs regularly by a single patient. Often seniors with multiple health problems are taking eight or more drugs daily and continuously. The increased vulnerability from multiple chronic illnesses and loss of physiological reserve of the octogenarian predisposes to drug toxicities, adverse effects, and drug–drug interactions. This predisposition increases with each drug. Treating an older patient by guideline protocols is especially precarious because of their inherent increased vulnerability [35]. The specialist will need to use caution in prescribing new medications for these reasons. New and just released drugs are a special hazard when prescribed to seniors. Studies of new drugs almost never include individuals over age 80. So prescribing such a drug is like entering the older patient in an uncontrolled clinical trial in an individual at increased risk of adverse events. Except in urgent situations and without an alternative, most geriatricians wait at least 2 years after a new drug has been released before prescribing it outside of a clinical trial. Often by that time a more accurate drug profile is emerging. The vulnerability to drugs is not just to those taken systemically but occurs in topical agents, especially those administered in the conjunctiva. There is no simple tool available that can guide a clinician in prescribing medications to the very old patient. The wise clinician will make a thoughtful risk–benefit judgment and include the patient and primary care provider in the decisions about initiating drugs.

The Beers Criteria [36] are commonly used by clinicians as a guide to prescribing medications to seniors. This list of drugs that are best avoided, if at all possible, in seniors includes 53 classes of drugs or specific medications. These drugs are presented in three categories:

1. Potentially inappropriate medications in all seniors;
2. Potentially inappropriate medications in seniors with certain conditions; and
3. Drugs that should be used with caution.

Knowledge of this Beers Criteria can provide a clinician with guidance to which individual judgment must then be applied. The Beers Criteria have become widely disseminated. Increasingly they have been used, arguably sometimes perhaps too aggressively [37], by insurance companies to deny payment for a drug. In fact, the American Geriatrics Society (AGS) has received numerous calls and letters concerning drug payment denials based solely on the Beers Criteria. In response they have generated a letter used to send to insurers when complaints about payment for drugs on the Beers list [38]. That letter re-emphasizes that the Beers Criteria should never be used as the sole criteria for formula decisions but rather they are intended to inform clinical decision-making, research, training, and policy. The Beers Criteria have been used in evaluating health care quality. The Beers Criteria have been available for over 20 years but have been periodically updated by a panel of experts and is sponsored by the AGS. Information concerning the Beers Criteria and a list of the drugs is available on line. It is easiest to obtain this information from the AGS by putting geriatricscareonline.org in your web electronic search engine. The Beers Criteria pocket cards can be downloaded for free to AGS members and for $5.00 for non-members. Chapter 5—Medication Management develops the issue of polypharmacy more fully.

8.11 Tools Available from the National Institutes of Health

The NIH created a valuable resource for tools in assessing issues related to the neurosciences. The NIH Toolkit covers the domains of cognitive, sensory, motor, and emotional functions. While it is designed a resource for research and covers all ages, many of the tools are applicable to clinical practice. Tools have been carefully vetted and are applicable up to age 85. The tools are available on line and are free. One can get general information about these many evaluation tools from the following website: http://www.nihtoolbox.org/WhatAndWhy/Assessments/NIH%20Toolbox%20Brochure-2012.pdf.

One can find a list of the tools and information on registering to access them at www.NIHtoolbox.org.

References

1. Shumway-Cook A, Brauer S, Woollacott M. Predicting the probability for falls in community-dwelling older adults using the timed up & go test. Phys Ther. 2000;80:896–903.
2. Barry E, Galvin R, Keogh C, Horgan F, Fahey T. Is the timed up and go test a useful predictor of risk of falls in community dwelling older adults: a systemic review and meta-analysis. BMC Geriatr. 2014;14:1–14.
3. Afilalo J, Eisenberg MJ, Morin J-F, et al. Gait speed as an incremental predictor of mortality and major morbidity in elderly patients undergoing cardiac surgery. J Am Coll Cardiol. 2010;56:1668–76.

4. Artuad F, Singh-Manoux A, Dugravot A, et al. Decline in gait speed as a predictor of disability in older adults. J Am Geriatr Soc. 2015;63:1129–36.

5. Borson S, Scanlan J, Brush M, Vitalliano P, Dokmak A. The Mini-Cog: a cognitive "vital signs' measurement for dementia screening in multi-lingual elderly. Int J Geriatr Psychiatry. 2000;15:1021–7.

6. Lin JS, O'Connor E, Rossom RC, Purdue LA, Eckstrom E. Screening for cognitive impairment in older adults: a systemic review for the U.S. Preventive Services Task Force. Ann Intern Med. 2013;159:601–12.

7. Borson S, Scalan JM, Chen P, Ganguli M. The mini-cog as a screen for dementia: validation in a population-based sample. J Am Geriatr Soc. 2003;51:1451–4.

8. Folstein MF, Folstein SE, McHugh PR. Mini-mental state: a practical method for grading cognitive state of patients for the clinician. J Psychiatr Res. 1975;12:189–98.

9. Wei LA, Fearing MA, Sternberg EJ, Inouye SK. The confusion assessment method: a systemic if current usage. J Am Geriatr Soc. 2008;56:823–30.

10. Inouye SK, van Dyck CH, Alessi CA, Balkin S, Siegal AP, Horowitz RI. Clarifying confusion: the confusion assessment method. Ann Intern Med. 1990;113:941–8.

11. The American Geriatrics Society expert panel on postoperative delirium in older adults. J Am Geriatr Soc. 2015;63:142–50.

12. Varadhan R, Yao W, Matteini A, Beamer BA, Xue QL, Yang H, Manwani B, Reiner A, Jenny N, Parekh N, Fallin MD, Newman A, Bandeen-Roche K, Tracy R, Ferrucci L, Walston J. Simple biologically informed inflammatory index of two serum cytokines predicts 10 year all-cause mortality in older adults. J Gerontol A Biol Sci Med Sci. 2014;69:165.

13. Makary MA, Segev DL, Pronovost PJ, Syin D, Bandeen-Roche K, Patel P, Takenaga R, Devgan L, Holzmueller CG, Tian J, Fried LP. Frailty as a predictor of surgical outcomes in older patients. J Am Coll Surg. 2010;210:901–8.

14. Morley JE, Vellas B, van Kan GA, Anker SD, Bauer JM, Bernabei R, Cesari M, Chumlea WC, Doehner W, Evans J, Fried LP, Guralnik JM, Katz PR, Malmstrom TK, McCarter RJ, Gutierrez Robledo LM, Rockwood K, von HS, Vandewoude MF, Walston J. Frailty consensus: a call to action. J Am Med Dir Assoc. 2013;14:392–7.

15. van Abellan KG, Rolland Y, Bergman H, Morley JE, Kritchevsky SB, Vellas B. The I.A.N.A task force on frailty assessment of older people in clinical practice. J Nutr Health Aging. 2008;12:29–37.

16. Afilalo J, Eisenberg MJ, Morin JF, Bergman H, Monette J, Noiseux N, Perrault LP, Alexander KP, Langlois Y, Dendukuri N, Chamoun P, Kasparian G, Robichaud S, Gharacholou SM, Boivin JF. Gait speed as an incremental predictor of mortality and major morbidity in elderly patients undergoing cardiac surgery. J Am Coll Cardiol. 2010;56:1668–76.

17. Robinson TN, Wu DS, Sauaia A, Dunn CL, Stevens-Lapsley JE, Moss M, Stiegmann GV, Gajdos C, Cleveland Jr JC, Inouye SK. Slower walking speed forecasts increased postoperative morbidity and 1-year mortality across surgical specialties. Ann Surg. 2013;258:582–8.

18. van Abellan KG, Rolland YM, Morley JE, Vellas B. Frailty: toward a clinical definition. J Am Med Dir Assoc. 2008;9:71–2.

19. Woo J, Yu R, Wong M, Yeung F, Wong M, Lum C. Frailty screening in the community using the FRAIL scale. J Am Med Dir Assoc. 2015;16:412–9.

20. Chow WB, Rosenthal RA, Merkow RP, Ko CY, Esnaola NF. Optimal preoperative assessment of the geriatric surgical patient: a best practices guideline from the American College of Surgeons National Surgical Quality Improvement Program and the American Geriatrics Society. J Am Coll Surg. 2012;215:453–66.

21. Rockwood K, Song X, MacKnight C, Bergman H, Hogan DB, McDowell I, Mitnitski A. A global clinical measure of fitness and frailty in elderly people. CMAJ. 2005;173:489–95.

22. Mitnitski AB, Mogilner AJ, Rockwood K. Accumulation of deficits as a proxy measure of aging. ScientificWorldJournal. 2001;1:323–36.

23. Rockwood K, Mitnitski A. Frailty defined by deficit accumulation and geriatric medicine defined by frailty. Clin Geriatr Med. 2011;27:17–26.

24. Theou O, Walston J, Rockwood K. Operationalizing frailty using the frailty phenotype and deficit accumulation approaches. Interdisc Top Gerontol Geriatr. 2015;41:66–73.

25. Joseph B, Pandit V, Zangbar B, Kulvatunyou N, Tang A, O'Keeffe T, Green DJ, Vercruysse G, Fain MJ, Friese RS, Rhee P. Validating trauma-specific frailty index for geriatric trauma patients: a prospective analysis. J Am Coll Surg. 2014;219:10–7.

26. Kroenke K, Spitzer RL, Williams JBW. The patient health questionnaire-2: validity of a two-item depression screener. Med Care. 2003;41:1284–92.

27. Gillbody S, Richards D, Brealey S, Hewitt C. Screening for depression in medical settings with the patient health questionnaire (PHQ): a diagnostic meta-analysis. J Gen Intern Med. 2007;22:1596–602.

28. Katz S, Downs TD, Cash HR, Grotz RC. Progress in development of the index of ADL. Gerontologist. 1970;10:20–30.

29. Lawton MP, Brody EM. Assessment of older people: self-maintaining and instrumental activities of daily living. Gerontologist. 1969;9:179–86.

30. Mueller C, Compher C, Ellen DM, et al. A.S.P.E.N. clinical guidelines: nutrition screening, assessment, and intervention in adults. JPEN J Parenter Enteral Nutr. 2011;35(1):16–24.

31. Guigoz Y. The mini-nutritional assessment review of the literature-what does it tell us? J Nutr Health Aging. 2006;10:466–85.

32. Detsky AS, McLaughlin JR, Baker JP, et al. What is subjective global assessment of nutritional assessment? JPEN J Parenter Enteral Nutr. 1987;11:8–13.

33. Carlson C, Merel SE, Yukawa M. Geriatric syndromes and geriatric assessment for the generalist. Med Clin North Am. 2015;99:263–79.

34. Roth DL, Haley WE, Wadley VG, et al. Race and gender differences in perceived caregiver availability for community-dwelling middle-aged and older adults. Gerontologist. 2007;47(6):721–9.

35. Boyd CM, Darer J, Boult C, Fried LP, Boult L, Wu AW. Clinical practice guidelines and quality of care for older patients with multiple comorbid diseases. JAMA. 2005;294:716–24.

36. The American Geriatrics Society 2012 Beers Criteria Update Expert Panel. American Geriatrics Society updated Beers criteria for potentially inappropriate medication use in older adults. J Am Geriatr Soc. 2012;60:616–31.

37. Barger MS. Misuse of Beers Criteria, let to ed. J Am Geriatr Soc. 2014;62:1411.

38. McCormick WC. American Geriatrics Society response to letter to the editor from Marc S. Berger "misuse of Beers criteria". J Am Geriatr Soc. 2014;62:2466.

## Part II

Surgical and Related Specialties

Stacie Deiner and Deborah J. Culley

9.1 Introduction

Advances in both surgery and anesthesia allow older patients to be candidates for surgical procedures and have increased the number and type of surgical procedures performed in patients aged 65 and older. In 2009 alone, 17.8 million surgical procedures were performed on older patients in the USA [1] While older age is a risk factor for postoperative complications, there is significant heterogeneity between elders such that chronologic age alone does not predict whether an individual will experience a complicated perioperative course (2002, 2011). Despite the size of this demographic, guidance for the anesthetic management of older patients is still in its infancy. In this chapter we present data from recent studies and national expert panels that should be considered when planning the anesthetic management of an older surgical patient.

9.2 Preoperative Assessment: The ACS/AGS Preoperative Guidelines in Your Practice

A number of studies have suggested that a comprehensive geriatric assessment prior to surgery in older patients can decrease hospital length of stay and postoperative complications [2]. However, in practice it is often difficult to obtain a geriatric consult for every older patient and the preoperative preparation of the older patient is often left to the anesthesiologist and surgeon. To aid in providing geriatric centered

care the Geriatrics for Specialists Initiative (GSI), sponsored by the American Geriatrics Society (AGS), developed core competencies for surgical subspecialists involved in the care of older surgical patients[3] and the American College of Surgeons (ACS) National Surgical Quality Improvement Program (NSQIP) in collaboration with the AGS released "Best Practice" Guidelines in 2012 [4]. Both the competencies and the Best Practices Guidelines are resources for nurses, surgeons, proceduralists, and anesthesiologists and highlight the special needs of this aging population. The AGS Guidelines help highlight geriatric specific concerns including frailty, cognitive impairment, decision making, depression, and potentially inappropriate medications in the perioperative period (Table 9.1). While the integration of functional and cognitive assessments into routine preoperative care is in its infancy, studies suggest that baseline physical and cognition performance are highly predictive of physical and cognitive recovery [5–8] (Table 9.2). See Chap. 3, Preoperative Evaluation.

9.3 Frailty and Postsurgical Outcomes

Frailty is a syndrome which transcends comorbidity and is characterized by fatigue, weight loss, and low functional activity levels[9]. The frailty phenotype is associated with significant perioperative morbidity and mortality[10, 11]. Frailty is more common in older surgical patients when compared to community dwelling older people. Recent studies in both cardiac and noncardiac surgical populations suggest that preoperative frailty is a predictor of complications such as infection, reintubation, pneumonia, hospital length of stay, institutionalization, and mortality (Table 9.3) [6, 12–15]. Frailty may be amenable to treatment with nutritional support, prehabilitation, rehabilitation, and vitamin supplementation [16, 17]. Therefore, preoperative identification of frailty is useful for risk stratification, discharge planning and may identify patients whose condition could be optimized prior to surgery [18].

S. Deiner, MS, MD (✉)
Department of Anesthesiology, The Icahn School of Medicine at Mount Sinai, One Gustave Levy Place, New York, NY 10029, USA
e-mail: Stacie.deiner@mssm.edu

D.J. Culley, MD
Department of Anesthesiology, Perioperative and Pain Medicine, Brigham and Women's Hospital, 75 Francis Street, Boston, MA 02115, USA

© Springer International Publishing Switzerland 2017
J.R. Burton et al. (eds.), *Geriatrics for Specialists*, DOI 10.1007/978-3-319-31831-8_9

Table 9.1 Selected medications potentially inappropriate for the elderly, modified from American Geriatrics 2015 Beer's Criterion

Drug	Rationale	Recommendation	Quality of evidence	Strength of recommendation
Diphenhydramine, meclizine	Clearance reduced, risk of confusion	Avoid, except in for the use of diphenhydramine for allergic reaction	Moderate	Strong
Atropine, scopolamine	Uncertain effectiveness	Avoid	Moderate	Strong
Clonidine	High risk of CNS effects, bradycardia, orthostasis	Avoid as first line antihypertensive	Low	Strong
First and second generation antipsychotics	Increased risk of stroke and greater rate of cognitive decline, avoid for behavioral problems (including delirium) unless nonpharmacologic interventions have failed and patient is a harm to self or others	Avoid	Moderate	Strong
Lorazepam, Diazepam	Elderly have increased sensitivity to benzodiazepines and decreased metabolism of longer acting agents	Avoid	Moderate	Strong
Zolpidem	Minimal improvement in sleep latency and duration	Avoid	Moderate	Strong
Insulin Sliding Scale	Higher risk of hypoglycemia without improvement of hyperglycemia management regardless of care setting	Avoid	Moderate	Strong
Metoclopramide	Can cause extrapyramidal effects including tardive dyskinesia, risk may be greater in frail elderly	Avoid, unless for gastroparesis	Moderate	Strong
Meperidine	Higher risk of delirium than other opioids, safer alternatives available	Avoid	Moderate	Strong
Ketorolac	Increased risk of GI bleeding, acute kidney injury	Avoid	Moderate	Strong

From The American Geriatrics Society 2015 Beers Criteria Update Expert Panel, American Geriatrics Society 2015 Updated Beers Criteria for Potentially Inappropriate Medication Use in Older Adults, J Am Geriatr Soc 63:2227–2246, 2015

Table 9.2 Frailty tools and associated outcomes

Frailty measure	Description	Clinical outcome
Frailty phenotype	Weight loss, grip strength, exhaustion, low physical activity and 15 feet walking speed[a]	30-day complications, institutionalization, length of stay
Frailty Index/deficit accumulation	30–70 measures of comorbidity, ADL, physical and neurological exam	Mortality and institutionalization
Modified frailty index	History of diabetes; COPD, or pneumonia; congestive heart failure; myocardial infarction; angina/PCI; hypertension requiring medication; peripheral vascular disease; dementia; TIA or CVA; CVA with neurological deficit; ADL	30 days, 1-year, and 2-year mortality, 30 days major postoperative complications
Gait speed	5-m Gait >6 s[a]	Mortality, major postoperative complications, institutionalization, and length of stay
Timed up and go (TUG)	TUG <10s, 11–14 s, >15 s[a]	1-year mortality
Robinson	Katz Score, Mini cognition, Charlson Index, anemia <35%, albumin <3.4, hx of falls	30 days major postoperative complications, length of stay, 30 days readmission, 6 months postoperative mortality

Used with permission from Amrock LG, Deiner S., The implication of frailty on preoperative risk assessment. Curr Opin Anaesthesiol. 2014 Jun;27(3):330–5

[a]See Chap. 8, Screening Tools for Geriatric Assessment by Specialists, for details on employing these measures

Traditional frailty assessments are time consuming and require trained personnel [19] although short form screening tools have been developed and can be administered by a layperson making them more relevant to the preoperative evaluation when attempting to identify older frail patients [20]. While frailty screening is currently not the universal standard of care, such a holistic approach will likely become useful to identify patients at risk for adverse outcomes and allow not only for risk stratification, but to aid in patient and family counseling, and identify interventions to reduce postoperative complications. The reader is referred to Chap. 1 on Frailty for a full discussion.

Table 9.3 Summary of recommendations from the AGS expert panel on postoperative delirium clinical practice guideline

Strong Recommendations: (The evidence for each intervention where either the benefits clearly outweighed the risks or that the risks clearly outweighed the benefits.)

- Multicomponent nonpharmacologic interventions delivered by an interdisciplinary team should be administered to at-risk older adults to prevent delirium.
- Ongoing educational programs regarding delirium should be provided for healthcare professionals.
- A medical evaluation should be performed to identify and manage underlying contributors to delirium.
- Pain management (preferably with non-opioid medications) should be optimized to prevent postoperative delirium.
- Medications with high risk for precipitating delirium should be avoided.
- Cholinesterase inhibitors should not be newly prescribed to prevent or treat postoperative delirium.
- Benzodiazepines should not be used as first-line treatment of agitation associated with delirium.
- Antipsychotics and benzodiazepines should be avoided for treatment of hypoactive delirium.

Weak Recommendations: (The evidence favors these interventions, but the current level of evidence or potential risks did not support a strong recommendation.)

- Multicomponent nonpharmacologic interventions implemented by an interdisciplinary team may be considered when an older adult is diagnosed with postoperative delirium to improve clinical outcomes.
- The use of regional anesthetic at the time of surgery and postoperatively to improve pain control with the goal of preventing delirium may be considered.
- The use of antipsychotics (e.g., haloperidol, risperidone, olanzapine, quetiapine, or ziprasidone) at the lowest effective dose for the shortest possible duration may be considered to treat delirious patients who are severely agitated or distressed or who are threatening substantial harm to self and/or others.

Statements with Insufficient evidence: (The current level of evidence or potential risks of the treatment did not support either a strong or weak recommendation.)

- Use of processed electroencephalographic (EEG) monitors of anesthetic depth during intravenous sedation or general anesthesia may be used to prevent delirium.
- Prophylactic use of antipsychotic medications to prevent delirium

From The American Geriatrics Society Expert Panel on Postoperative Delirium in Older Adults. American Geriatrics Society Abstracted Clinical Practice Guideline for Postoperative Delirium in Older Adults. J Am Geriatr Soc 63:142–150, 2015

9.4 Perioperative Assessment and Management of Medications

Geriatric surgical patients are at high risk for polypharmacy and medication errors. This is compounded by frequent discrepancies between the surgical and anesthesiology medication records [21]. Polypharmacy is a strong predictor of such discrepancies [22]. Strategies to reduce discrepancies include encouraging patients to carry an updated medication list provided by their physician [22, 23] and medication reconciliation conducted by a clinical pharmacist at both hospital admission and discharge. Most chronic medications can be continued throughout the perioperative period while others may complicate intraoperative anesthetic management and affect postoperative outcomes. In this section we discuss the perioperative management of medications commonly used by older people.

Antihypertensive medications are commonly prescribed for older patients for blood pressure control. In most circumstances antihypertensive medications should be continued in the perioperative period, however, some antihypertensive medications require special consideration. Perioperative use of angiotensin converting enzyme (ACE) inhibitors/angiotensin receptor blockers (ARB) have been associated with protracted perioperative hypotension due to suppression of the renin-angiotensin-aldosterone-system (RAAS) preventing the normal hormonal and sympathetic response to surgical stress. However, the traditional practice of withholding ACE inhibitors and ARBs prior to elective surgery has recently been challenged because ACE/ARB related intraoperative hypotension has not been linked to adverse perioperative outcomes [24]. The 2014 ACC/AHA guidelines state that continuation of ACE inhibitors and ARBs is reasonable, and that if they are discontinued they should be restarted as soon as medically feasible [25, 26]. Generally, it seems reasonable to withhold ACE/ARB based on the patient's presenting blood pressure, likelihood of intraoperative fluid shifts, and risk of hypotension in the light of either surgical or medical conditions. Beta blockers are another commonly prescribed class of antihypertensive drugs that were thought to decrease risk of perioperative cardiac events. However, the PeriOperative ISchemic Evaluation (POISE) trial demonstrated that the benefit of beta blockers on the incidence of perioperative cardiac events was off-set by an increased incidence of perioperative stroke [27]. Current ACC/AHA guidelines recommend continuing beta blockers in the perioperative period for patients who take them chronically (Class 1 evidence) [25].

9.5 Antiplatelet Agents

Chronic use of antiplatelet drugs is common in older surgical patients to prevent thrombosis in patients with known history of atrial fibrillation, coronary artery disease, cardiac stents, or stroke. Prevention of thrombosis may be even more important in the perioperative period, which is characterized by a proinflammatory state which increases platelet activity and aggregation. However, the benefits of antiplatelet drugs must be balanced by the risk of intra and postoperative hemorrhage.

9.5.1 Aspirin

Aspirin is an irreversible cyclooxygenase-1 (COX-1) inhibitor which disables platelet aggregation. Aspirin has become ubiquitous in the treatment, primary and secondary prevention of myocardial infarction and stroke [28]. The benefits of aspirin for secondary prevention of cardiovascular disease are well established and according to ACC/AHA guidelines should be continued indefinitely in most patients with established coronary artery and other atherosclerotic disease. However, the risk-versus-benefit ratio for primary prevention is less clear. A meta-analysis of six primary prevention trials found that there was no reduction in vascular-related mortality attributed to aspirin use and that the rates of gastrointestinal bleeding and hemorrhagic stroke were increased [29]. Furthermore, administration of aspirin in the perioperative period has not been shown to affect perioperative death or nonfatal myocardial infarction but does increase the risk of major bleeding [30]. Whether to continue aspirin in patients who are at high risk of perioperative thrombosis should be discussed with the patient, surgeon, and cardiologist prior to surgery.

9.5.2 Thienopyridines

Thienopyridines prevent platelet aggregation by inhibiting the $P2Y_{12}$ receptor on platelet membranes and preventing adenosine diphosphate binding. Clopidogrel is the most commonly used antiplatelet medication in this class. These medications are used for primary and secondary prevention thromboembolic events in patients with cardiovascular and cerebrovascular disease and have gained widespread use as a component of dual antiplatelet therapy with aspirin in patients with cardiac stents to prevent thrombosis. Most centers discourage elective surgery in the immediate period following cardiac stent placement when it would require early cessation of clopidogrel due to risk of stent thrombosis and mortality. However, the definition of early discontinuation is evolving and many new generation stents require only 6 months of therapy [31]. Appropriate timing of antiplatelet therapy discontinuation after stent placement should be discussed with the cardiologist, surgeon, and patient. In particular it is important to discuss the balance between the location and type of stent, the time since the stent was placed, and the urgency of the surgical procedure.

9.6 Antidepressants

Depression affects 15–20 % of elders and is the most common psychiatric disorder in older people. Many older patients are prescribed antidepressant medications and consequences of their use in the perioperative period should be considered preoperatively [32]. Older generation antidepressants such as monoamine oxidase inhibitors (MAO-I) may interact with medications (e.g., meperidine and ephedrine) administered in the perioperative period leading to increasing anesthetic requirements, hypertensive crises, and potentially to life threatening hyperthermia and coma. It is unclear how long or whether patients should discontinue use of MAOIs prior to surgery. Although traditional recommendations have been to discontinue these agents for 2 weeks to 30 days before surgery, many of these recommendations were not based on high quality studies. There is some concern that doing so may result in significant morbidity or even mortality in patients who depend on these medications for the management of their depression. The newer generations of antidepressants such as serotonin reuptake inhibitors (SSRIs) tend to have fewer side effects and are generally continued throughout the perioperative period. However SSRIs are associated with platelet dysfunction and bleeding [33, 34] and this risk should be balanced with the risk of postoperative depression [35]. Accordingly, it is important to identify older patients taking antidepressants prior to surgery so that a treatment plan can be developed between the patient and primary care provider or psychiatrist.

9.7 Analgesics

9.7.1 Non-Opioid Analgesics

Many older people depend on NSAIDs and COX inhibitors for daily relief of mild to moderate chronic pain. However, NSAIDs have significant systemic side effects and are associated with up to a quarter of all adverse drug reactions in the older people [36]. Side effects of NSAIDS and COX inhibitors include: increases in mean arterial pressure, renal vasoconstriction, and sodium reabsorption leading to fluid retention and edema. Most surgeons advocate for cessation of NSAIDs 7–10 days prior to surgery due to concerns of perioperative hemorrhage; other studies suggest that the effects of NSAIDS and COX wane quickly and may be clinically irrelevant [37]. For patients that depend on NSAIDs, their continuation should be discussed with the surgeon to balance the risk of bleeding and with the need for pain control.

Non-opioid analgesics (e.g., acetaminophen and gabapentin) can usually be continued through the perioperative period and have been shown to decrease opioid requirements, improve functional outcome, and increase patient satisfaction postoperatively [38, 39]. Note that the dose of gabapentin and pregabalin is limited by side effects [40, 41]. Overall, multimodal analgesia may be beneficial but there is little data regarding the best regimen in elders [42].

9.7.2 Opioid Analgesics

Approximately 15–20 % of the community dwelling geriatric population and over 40 % of those living in nursing homes experience chronic pain that may require management with opioid medications [43]. Appropriate opioid dosing is complicated by age-related changes in total body water, lean muscle mass, and increased in body fat. These changes may lead to unpredictable drug responses due to changes in the volume of distribution, plasma concentration, and elimination profiles. Physiologic and pathophysiologic changes in renal function, hepatic metabolism, and central nervous system sensitivity may increase drug effects, duration of action, and incidence of side effects [44].

In most circumstances, opioid medications should be continued in the perioperative period. Withholding chronic pain medications results in patient discomfort and may cause symptoms of withdrawal. Chronic opioid use results in habituation which does not meet criteria for addiction. Opioid addiction occurs in older people, although at a lower rate compared to younger patients. The prevalence of drug abuse by Americans aged ≥65 years is tenfold lower than that of younger patients [45].

An important part of the preoperative assessment involves a plan for intraoperative and postoperative opioid administration. For example, calculating daily morphine equivalents based on home medications may be helpful in estimating baseline need. While baseline opioid dose may not be adequate in the perioperative period, calculation of daily opioid equivalents provides a starting point for therapy [46].

9.8 Intraoperative Anesthetic Management of an Older Patient

9.8.1 Physiology of Aging Organ Systems and Their Impact on Anesthetic Management

Cardiac changes that occur with advanced age include increased afterload due to arterial stiffening, elevated systolic blood pressure, left ventricular hypertrophy (LVH), valvular disease, and coronary artery disease. Notably, baroreceptor function is depressed, whereas cardiac output appears to be maintained in healthy individuals. LVH of normal aging causes some level of diastolic dysfunction which may only be symptomatic under stress as occurs with aggressive fluid therapy which may be necessary to support blood pressure during anesthesia. Increased vagal tone and decreased sensitivity of adrenergic receptors lead to a decline in heart rate by approximately one beat per minute per year of age after age 50 [47]. Fibrosis of the conduction system and loss of sinoatrial node cells increase the incidence of dysrhythmias, particularly atrial fibrillation and flutter. This physiology predisposes the older patient to exaggerated drops in blood pressure under anesthesia.

In the pulmonary system, decreased elasticity of lung tissue results in shallower alveoli and reduced size of small airway that in turn results in decreased alveolar surface area and an increase in the alveolar-arterial gradient with age and calculated by the following formula, $Pao_2 = 110 - (0.4 \times age)$. Respiratory mechanics are also altered in normal aging due to calcification of the costo-chondral margins and sarcopenia of the intercostal and diaphragmatic muscles. These changes increase closing volume so that it exceeds functional residual capacity by 45 years of age in the supine position and age 65 in the sitting position [48]. When this happens, some airways are closed during all or part of normal tidal breathing, resulting in a mismatch of ventilation and perfusion. Both anatomic and physiological dead space increase contribute to a higher risk of hypoxia with even mild hypoventilation or brief apnea. In the immediate postoperative period, protective laryngeal reflexes may be subdued and this may lead to a higher risk of pulmonary aspiration.

Renal blood flow and kidney mass decreases with age reducing glomerular filtration rate and creatinine clearance in most older people. Serum creatinine levels remain normal because of a proportional decrease in muscle mass [49]. Renal responsiveness to antidiuretic hormone is blunted resulting in free water wasting and dehydration during underhydration, while age-related cardiac-diastolic dysfunction reduces ability to excrete excess fluid volume during overhydration. Fluid management and choice of fluids has not been well studied in geriatric surgical patients. Most studies in this area are over 10 years old. One small study of older hip fracture patients showed that central venous pressure guided fluid administration with bolus challenges resulted in decreased time to discharge in comparison with standard care [50]. This is in line with meta-analyses that suggest patients at high risk of mortality benefit from goal directed fluid therapy [51]. Whether this is true for low to moderate risk older surgical patients is less clear when one considers the risk of central line placement. Similar to the overall population, there is no high quality evidence to guide the choice of crystalloid vs. colloid therapy in older people. With respect to blood transfusion, there is no evidence for liberal transfusion (10 g/dl) thresholds vs. restrictive (8 g/dl) ones even in patients with a history or risk factors for coronary artery disease [52]).

Normal age-related changes in physiology and pathophysiologic states predispose the older patient towards sensitivity to both the primary and side effects of anesthetic agents [53]. Liver mass, hepatic blood flow, and hepatic function decrease with age [54] leading to reductions in biotransformation of drugs, albumin production, and plasma cholinesterase levels. Minimum alveolar concentration required for general anesthesia with volatile anesthetics decreases 6–7 % per decade after age 40 [55] as does the dose of propofol needed for induction of anesthesia (1–1.5 mg/kg vs. 2–2.5 mg/kg in the general adult population) (Dundee et al. 1986). In general, the interaction between the physiology of aging and patient comorbidity suggests that dosing strategies should be based on the principle of "start low, go slow" [56].

Evidence that the particular medications or anesthetic techniques (general vs. regional anesthesia) prevent perioperative complications in older people is lacking. Studies comparing regional nerve blocks vs. general anesthesia, or comparing total intravenous anesthesia (TIVA) vs. gas are either small or have a high risk of bias. Evaluating whether anesthetic choice modifies patient outcomes is limited due to the requirements of the procedure, the patient's medical condition, and patient and practitioner preferences. Contrary to prior reports a recent retrospective study showed no mortality benefit for regional over general anesthesia in patients undergoing hip fracture repair (Neuman et al. 2014). While the results of this finding may not be generalizable to the overall geriatric population, it is the largest study to date on the subject. The definitive prospective trial is currently underway.

9.8.2 Depth of Anesthesia

Over the past decade, many anesthesiologists have used processed EEG in the operating room to judge anesthetic depth. While raw EEG requires interpretation of waveforms and often a dedicated EEG technician, the numerical output of processed EEG allows anesthesiologists to monitor brain activity. The Bispectral Index (BSI) monitor (BISTM Complete 4 Channel Monitor System, Covidien, Mansfield, MA) is the most widely used intraoperative measure of EEG. 2 or 4 channels of frontal lobe raw and processed EEG are recorded. In general, processed EEG involves an algorithm which transforms raw EEG data to a number which describes the state of how awake or deeply asleep a patient may be. The algorithms are generally based on studies which examine raw EEG parameters such as power spectral analysis and phase transitions in volunteers with very specific anesthetic regimens. The limitations of processed EEG is that the algorithms are only valid when the anesthetics being used have been studied for use with the monitor and evidence that older patients have different EEG responses when compared to younger patients [57].

Potential benefits of processed EEG include that they directly look at the brain compared to blood pressure and heart rate that indirectly judge anesthetic depth. This is particularly important in older patients due to the alterations in physiology known to occur with aging.

While processed EEG directly shows the anesthesiologist how a combination of drugs has affected the patient's consciousness, the best anesthetic depth for older patients is uncertain. While some studies suggest that greater depth of anesthesia is associated with adverse outcomes, other studies find that greater anesthetic depth is protective [58, 59]. In contrast, other studies suggest that processed EEG directed anesthesia care may decrease some adverse outcomes including delirium [60, 61]. Most recently, it has been recognized that EEG patterns under anesthesia are age dependent, which may not be accounted for in the processing algorithm [57]. This implies that reliance on processed EEG to judge depth could result in overly anesthetized older patients and will be an important area of investigation to determine whether depth of anesthesia as measured by processed EEG will be useful in optimizing outcomes for older people.

9.9 Intraoperative Care for Prevention of Postoperative Delirium

The AGS released best practice guidelines for prevention of postoperative delirium [62] and those recommendations are summarized in Table 9.3. Evidence for anesthetic selection to reduce delirium is also limited. Areas of interest for future research include manipulation of anesthetic depth to prevent postoperative delirium. Deeper plains of sedation in a hip fracture cohort are associated with greater incidence of delirium [61]. It is less clear whether depth of sedation is related to longer term cognitive outcomes such as postoperative cognitive dysfunction [60, 63]. Sessler et al suggest that patients who demonstrate greater depth of anesthesia and lower blood pressure combined with low concentration of anesthetic ("Triple Low Condition") may be predisposed to poor outcomes [59]. However, the risks of light anesthesia include awareness and sympathetic stimulation. Others have not found an association between a "triple low condition" and adverse patient outcomes [64].

In terms of pharmacologic prevention of delirium, there is no evidence to support the prophylactic use of antipsychotics or cholinesterase inhibitors (AGS Expert Panel on Postoperative Delirium in Older Adults. Electronic address: mjsamuel@americangeriatrics.org and AGS Society Expert Panel on Postoperative Delirium in Older Adults 2015). Use of antipsychotics is indicated only at the lowest dosage and the shortest duration to patients who pose harm to themselves or others. Benzodiazepines are not indicated for treatment or prevention of delirium and may be harmful.

The literature regarding the ability of anesthetic adjuncts such as ketamine and Dexmedetomidine to prevent delirium is still under development. A small prospective study showed that a single ketamine bolus decreased the odds of delirium in cardiac surgery patients [65]. The reader is referred to Chap. 2. Delirium for a full discussion of this topic.

9.10 Postoperative Care

9.10.1 Management of Postoperative Pain

While a full discussion of postoperative pain management in older people is beyond the scope of this chapter a range of techniques are available including opioid-sparing techniques with field blocks, and indwelling neuraxial and regional nerve catheters. Intravenous acetaminophen has shown some promise as a useful adjunct, although the advantage over pre-operative high dose oral acetaminophen has not been demonstrated [66]. There is low to moderate quality evidence that intravenous lidocaine infusion may decrease pain scores and has an impact on recovery of gastrointestinal recovery and opioid requirements [67].

Best practices for postoperative pain control in older patients remain underdeveloped and therefore pain management strategies are based on factors such as age, frailty, opioid tolerance, and practitioner familiarity. Both classic [68] and recent studies suggest that pain detection and pain tolerance thresholds are higher in older adults compared to younger adults irrespective of gender [69, 70]. However, the assumption that older patients have less pain could contribute to under medication in the postoperative period. Intravenous patient controlled analgesia (PCA) and patient controlled epidural analgesia (PCEA) have been used with good success in older patients. Both techniques involve a pump set to deliver a bolus dose when the patient presses a button; while continuous basal infusions are available these are best avoided in older patients. Older patients have similar attitude and readiness to use PCA pumps as younger adults [71] and PCA with frequent nursing assessments has been associated with improved pain scores [72]. Narcotics used in PCA pumps include fentanyl, hydromorphone, and morphine. Narcotic selection is crucial as older patients have a decrease in GFR and hepatic blood flow. Therefore, hydrophilic opioids such as morphine, which has an active metabolite, may accumulate and must be used with caution [73–75].

9.10.2 Strategies to Prevent Postoperative Complications in the Older Patients

The Department of Health and Human Services identified 10 hospital acquired conditions which were both high cost/volume and "reasonably preventable" using evidence based practices [76]. The term "never events" refers to things that should never occur in hospitals [77]. As an inducement to improve patient safety, the Center for Medicare and Medicaid Services no longer reimburses hospitals for the costs associated with these complications. However, some argue that this penalizes hospitals who care for frail older people who are at particularly high risk for these complications.

Older surgical patients are at high risk for "never events" including: catheter associated urinary tract infections, vascular catheter infections, pressure ulcers, and falls. Patients over 80 years old have a higher incidence of catheter related UTIs, associated with an increased length of stay leading, and an increase cost of care [78]. Prolonged use of indwelling Foley catheters increases the likelihood of UTI and 30-day mortality [79]. Hospitals that decrease their catheter days also decrease UTI [80]. Early mobilization, within 24 h of acute care admission, is associated with reduced length of stay, and maintenance or improvement of functional status [81].

9.10.3 Geriatric Specialized Units

Many of the problems in postoperative care for older patients can be minimized in specialized units and programs (e.g., the Hospital Elder Life Program) that incorporate strategies such as early mobilization, sensory enhancement (hearing aids, glasses), cognitive stimulation and orientation, nutritional support, and sleep enhancement [82]. These units and programs reduce cognitive and functional decline and achieve a higher level of patient and provider satisfaction and lower hospital costs. The reader is referred to Chap. 7. Hospital Medicine.

9.11 Conclusion

The evidence base for optimal geriatric care in the perioperative period remains under development. Support from the American Geriatrics Society, American College of Surgeons and the American Society of Anesthesiologist has provided research funding, resources, and guidelines to help identify geriatric specific conditions that need to be addressed to enhance patient outcomes. Training programs should at a minimum introduce resources to residents and fellows to increase awareness of special circumstances that are unique to this high risk patient population. In the future, perioperative care will be dictated by knowledge of geriatric physiology, pharmacology, comorbid conditions, and evolving evidence to enhance care to this vulnerable patient population. Postoperatively anesthesiologists should be at the forefront in preventing adverse peri-procedural adverse events in older patients.

References

1. CDC/National Center for Health Statistics. http://www.cdc.gov/nchs/fastats/insurg.htm (2013). Accessed 10 Dec 2013.

2. Partridge JS, Harari D, Martin FC, et al. The impact of pre-operative comprehensive geriatric assessment on postoperative outcomes in older patients undergoing scheduled surgery: a systematic review. Anaesthesia. 2014;69 Suppl 1:8–16. doi:10.1111/anae.12494.

3. Bell RH Jr, Drach GW, Rosenthal RA. Proposed competencies in geriatric patient care for use in assessment for initial and continued board certification of surgical specialists. J Am Coll Surg. 2011;213(5):683–90. doi:10.1016/j.jamcollsurg.2011.08.004.

4. Chow WB, Merkow RP, Cohen ME, et al. Association between postoperative complications and reoperation for patients undergoing geriatric surgery and the effect of reoperation on mortality. Am Surg. 2012;78(10):1137–42.

5. Amrock LG, Deiner S. The implication of frailty on preoperative risk assessment. Curr Opin Anaesthesiol. 2014;27(3):330–35. doi:10.1097/ACO.0000000000000065.

6. Makary MA, Segev DL, Pronovost PJ, et al. Frailty as a predictor of surgical outcomes in older patients. J Am Coll Surg. 2010;210(6):901–8. doi:10.1016/j.jamcollsurg.2010.01.028.

7. Moller JT, Cluitmans P, Rasmussen LS, et al. Long-term postoperative cognitive dysfunction in the elderly ISPOCD1 study. ISPOCD investigators. Lancet. 1998;351(9106):857–61.

8. Steinmetz J, Christensen KB, Lund T, et al. Long-term consequences of postoperative cognitive dysfunction. Anesthesiology. 2009;110(3):548–55. doi:10.1097/ALN.0b013e318195b569.

9. Fried LP, Tangen CM, Walston J, et al. Frailty in older adults: evidence for a phenotype. J Gerontol A Biol Sci Med Sci. 2001;56:M146–56.

10. Afilalo J, Alexander KP, Mack MJ, et al. Frailty assessment in the cardiovascular care of older adults. J Am Coll Cardiol. 2014;63(8):747–62. doi:10.1016/j.jacc.2013.09.070.

11. Hamaker ME, Jonker JM, de Rooij SE, et al. Frailty screening methods for predicting outcome of a comprehensive geriatric assessment in elderly patients with cancer: a systematic review. Lancet Oncol. 2012;13(10):e437–44. doi:10.1016/S1470-2045(12)70259-0.

12. Adams P, Ghanem T, Stachler R, et al. Frailty as a predictor of morbidity and mortality in inpatient head and neck surgery. JAMA Otolaryngol Head Neck Surg. 2013;139:783–9.

13. Bagnall NM, Faiz O, Darzi A, et al. What is the utility of preoperative frailty assessment for risk stratification in cardiac surgery? Interact Cardiovasc Thorac Surg. 2013;17:398–402.

14. McAdams-DeMarco MA, Law A, King E, et al. Frailty and mortality in kidney transplant recipients. Am J Transplant. 2015;15(1):149–54. doi:10.1111/ajt.12992.

15. Robinson TN, Wu DS, Pointer L, et al. Simple frailty score predicts postoperative complications across surgical specialties. Am J Surg. 2013;206:544–50.

16. Hirani V, Naganathan V, Cumming RG, et al. Associations between frailty and serum 25-hydroxyvitamin D and 1,25-dihydroxyvitamin D concentrations in older Australian men: the Concord Health and Ageing in Men Project. J Gerontol A Biol Sci Med Sci. 2013;68(9):1112–21. doi:10.1093/gerona/glt059; 10.1093/gerona/glt059.

17. Walston J, Hadley EC, Ferrucci L, et al. Research agenda for frailty in older adults: toward a better understanding of physiology and etiology: summary from the American Geriatrics Society/National Institute on Aging Research Conference on Frailty in Older Adults. J Am Geriatr Soc. 2006;54:991–1001.

18. Revenig LM, Canter DJ, Taylor MD, et al. Too frail for surgery? Initial results of a large multidisciplinary prospective study examining preoperative variables predictive of poor surgical outcomes. J Am Coll Surg. 2013;217:665.e1–70.

19. Theou O, Brothers TD, Mitnitski A, et al. Operationalization of frailty using eight commonly used scales and comparison of their ability to predict all-cause mortality. J Am Geriatr Soc. 2013;61:1537–51.

20. Morley JE, Malmstrom TK, Miller DK. A simple frailty questionnaire (FRAIL) predicts outcomes in middle aged African Americans. J Nutr Health Aging. 2012;16(7):601–8.

21. Burda SA, Hobson D, Pronovost PJ. What is the patient really taking? Discrepancies between surgery and anesthesiology preoperative medication histories. Qual Saf Health Care. 2005;14(6):414–6.

22. Cornu P, Steurbaut S, Leysen T, et al. Effect of medication reconciliation at hospital admission on medication discrepancies during hospitalization and at discharge for geriatric patients. Ann Pharmacother. 2012;46(4):484–94. doi:10.1345/aph.1Q594.

23. Frydenberg K, Brekke M. Poor communication on patients' medication across health care levels leads to potentially harmful medication errors. Scand J Prim Health Care. 2012;30(4):234–40. doi:10.3109/02813432.2012.712021.

24. Smith I, Jackson I. Beta-blockers, calcium channel blockers, angiotensin converting enzyme inhibitors and angiotensin receptor blockers: should they be stopped or not before ambulatory anaesthesia? Curr Opin Anaesthesiol. 2010;23(6):687–90. doi:10.1097/ACO.0b013e32833eeb19.

25. Fleisher LA, Fleischmann KE, Auerbach AD, et al. 2014 ACC/AHA guideline on perioperative cardiovascular evaluation and management of patients undergoing noncardiac surgery: executive summary: a report of the American College of Cardiology/American Heart Association Task Force on practice guidelines. Developed in collaboration with the American College of Surgeons, American Society of Anesthesiologists, American Society of Echocardiography, American Society of Nuclear Cardiology, Heart Rhythm Society, Society for Cardiovascular Angiography and Interventions, Society of Cardiovascular Anesthesiologists, and Society of Vascular Medicine Endorsed by the Society of Hospital Medicine. J Nucl Cardiol. 2015;22(1):162–215. doi:10.1007/s12350-014-0025-z.

26. Turan A, You J, Shiba A, et al. Angiotensin converting enzyme inhibitors are not associated with respiratory complications or mortality after noncardiac surgery. Anesth Analg. 2012;114(3):552–60. doi:10.1213/ANE.0b013e318241f6af.

27. POISE Study Group, Devereaux PJ, Yang H, et al. Effects of extended-release metoprolol succinate in patients undergoing noncardiac surgery (POISE trial): a randomised controlled trial. Lancet. 2008;371(9627):1839–47. doi:10.1016/S0140-6736(08)60601-7.

28. Antithrombotic Trialists' (ATT) Collaboration, Baigent C, Blackwell L, et al. Aspirin in the primary and secondary prevention of vascular disease: collaborative meta-analysis of individual participant data from randomised trials. Lancet. 2009;373(9678):1849–60. doi:10.1016/S0140-6736(09)60503-1.

29. Brotons C, Benamouzig R, Filipiak KJ, et al. A systematic review of aspirin in primary prevention: is it time for a new approach? Am J Cardiovasc Drugs. 2015;15(2):113–3. doi:10.1007/s40256-014-0100-5.

30. Devereaux PJ, Mrkobrada M, Sessler DI, et al. Aspirin in patients undergoing noncardiac surgery. N Engl J Med. 2014;370(16):1494–503. doi:10.1056/NEJMoa1401105.

31. Abualsaud AO, Eisenberg MJ. Perioperative management of patients with drug-eluting stents. JACC Cardiovasc Interv. 2010;3(2):131–42. doi:10.1016/j.jcin.2009.11.017.

32. Sutherland AM, Katznelson R, Clarke HA, et al. Use of preoperative antidepressants is not associated with postoperative hospital length of stay. Can J Anaesth. 2014;61(1):27–31. doi:10.1007/s12630-013-0062-0.

33. Movig KL, Janssen MW, de Waal Malefijt J, et al. Relationship of serotonergic antidepressants and need for blood transfusion in orthopedic surgical patients. Arch Intern Med. 2003;163(19): 2354–8. doi:10.1001/archinte.163.19.2354.

34. van Haelst IM, Egberts TC, Doodeman HJ, et al. Use of serotonergic antidepressants and bleeding risk in orthopedic patients. Anesthesiology. 2010;112(3):631–6. doi:10.1097/ALN.0b013e3181cf8fdf.

35. Kudoh A, Katagai H, Takazawa T. Antidepressant treatment for chronic depressed patients should not be discontinued prior to anesthesia. Can J Anaesth. 2002;49(2):132–6. doi:10.1007/BF03020484.

36. American Geriatrics Society Panel on the Pharmacological Management of Persistent Pain in Older Persons. Pharmacological management of persistent pain in older persons. Pain Med. 2009;10(6):1062–83. doi:10.1111/j.1526-4637.2009.00699.x.

37. Scott WW, Levy M, Rickert KL, et al. Assessment of common nonsteroidal anti-inflammatory medications by whole blood aggregometry: a clinical evaluation for the perioperative setting. World Neurosurg. 2014;82(5):e633–8. doi:10.1016/j.wneu.2014.03.043.

38. Clarke HA, Katz J, McCartney CJ, et al. Perioperative gabapentin reduces 24 h opioid consumption and improves in-hospital rehabilitation but not post-discharge outcomes after total knee arthroplasty with peripheral nerve block. Br J Anaesth. 2014;113(5):855–64. doi:10.1093/bja/aeu202.

39. Durmus M, Kadir But A, Saricicek V, et al. The post-operative analgesic effects of a combination of gabapentin and paracetamol in patients undergoing abdominal hysterectomy: a randomized clinical trial. Acta Anaesthesiol Scand. 2007;51(3):299–304.

40. Dahl JB, Nielsen RV, Wetterslev J, et al. Post-operative analgesic effects of paracetamol, NSAIDs, glucocorticoids, gabapentinoids and their combinations: a topical review. Acta Anaesthesiol Scand. 2014;58(10):1165–81. doi:10.1111/aas.12382.

41. Khan ZH, Rahimi M, Makarem J, et al. Optimal dose of pre-incision/post-incision gabapentin for pain relief following lumbar laminectomy: a randomized study. Acta Anaesthesiol Scand. 2011;55(3):306–12. doi:10.1111/j.1399-6576.2010.02377.x; 10.1111/j.1399-6576.2010.02377.x.

42. Makris UE, Abrams RC, Gurland B, et al. Management of persistent pain in the older patient: a clinical review. JAMA. 2014;312(8):825–36. doi:10.1001/jama.2014.9405.

43. Pergolizzi J, Boger RH, Budd K, et al. Opioids and the management of chronic severe pain in the elderly: consensus statement of an International Expert Panel with focus on the six clinically most often used World Health Organization Step III opioids (buprenorphine, fentanyl, hydromorphone, methadone, morphine, oxycodone). Pain Pract. 2008;8(4):287–313. doi:10.1111/j.1533-2500.2008.00204.x.

44. Abdulla A, Adams N, Bone M, et al. Guidance on the management of pain in older people. Age Ageing. 2013;42 Suppl 1:i1–57. doi:10.1093/ageing/afs200.

45. Tracy B, Sean Morrison R. Pain management in older adults. Clin Ther. 2013;35(11):1659–68. doi:10.1016/j.clinthera.2013.09.026.

46. Brallier JW, Deiner S. The elderly spine surgery patient: pre- and intraoperative management of drug therapy. Drugs Aging. 2015;32(8):601–9. doi:10.1007/s40266-015-0278-5.

47. Rooke GA. Autonomic and cardiovascular function in the geriatric patient. Anesthesiol Clin North Am. 2000;18(1):31–46. v-vi.

48. John AD, Sieber FE. Age associated issues: geriatrics. Anesthesiol Clin North Am. 2004;22(1):45–58. doi:10.1016/S0889-8537(03)00119-6.

49. Baldea AJ. Effect of aging on renal function plus monitoring and support. Surg Clin North Am. 2015;95(1):71–83. doi:10.1016/j.suc.2014.09.003.

50. Venn R, Steele A, Richardson P, et al. Randomized controlled trial to investigate influence of the fluid challenge on duration of hospital stay and perioperative morbidity in patients with hip fractures. Br J Anaesth. 2002;88(1):65–71.

51. Cecconi M, Corredor C, Arulkumaran N, et al. Clinical review: goal-directed therapy-what is the evidence in surgical patients? The effect on different risk groups. Crit Care. 2013;17(2):209. doi:10.1186/cc11823.

52. Carson JL, Terrin ML, Noveck H, et al. Liberal or restrictive transfusion in high-risk patients after hip surgery. N Engl J Med. 2011;365(26):2453–62. doi:10.1056/NEJMoa1012452.

53. Mangoni AA, Jackson SH. Age-related changes in pharmacokinetics and pharmacodynamics: basic principles and practical applications. Br J Clin Pharmacol. 2004;57(1):6–14.

54. Tajiri K, Shimizu Y. Liver physiology and liver diseases in the elderly. World J Gastroenterol. 2013;19(46):8459–67. doi:10.3748/wjg.v19.i46.8459.

55. Nickalls RW, Mapleson WW. Age-related iso-MAC charts for isoflurane, sevoflurane and desflurane in man. Br J Anaesth. 2003;91(2):170–4.

56. Shi S, Klotz U. Age-related changes in pharmacokinetics. Curr Drug Metab. 2011;12(7):601–10.

57. Purdon PL, Pavone KJ, Akeju O, et al. The ageing brain: age-dependent changes in the electroencephalogram during propofol and sevoflurane general anaesthesia. Br J Anaesth. 2015;115 Suppl 1:i46–57. doi:10.1093/bja/aev213.

58. Farag E, Chelune GJ, Schubert A, et al. Is depth of anesthesia, as assessed by the Bispectral Index, related to postoperative cognitive dysfunction and recovery? Anesth Analg. 2006;103(3):633–40.

59. Sessler DI, Sigl JC, Kelley SD, et al. Hospital stay and mortality are increased in patients having a "triple low" of low blood pressure, low bispectral index, and low minimum alveolar concentration of volatile anesthesia. Anesthesiology. 2012;116(6):1195–203. doi:10.1097/ALN.0b013e31825683dc.

60. Chan MT, Cheng BC, Lee TM, et al. BIS-guided anesthesia decreases postoperative delirium and cognitive decline. J Neurosurg Anesthesiol. 2013;25(1):33–42. doi:10.1097/ANA.0b013e3182712fba.

61. Sieber FE, Zakriya KJ, Gottschalk A, et al. Sedation depth during spinal anesthesia and the development of postoperative delirium in elderly patients undergoing hip fracture repair. Mayo Clin Proc. 2010;85(1):18–26. doi:10.4065/mcp.2009.0469.

62. American Geriatrics Society Expert Panel on Postoperative Delirium in Older Adults. Electronic address: mjsamuel@americangeriatrics.org, American Geriatrics Society Expert Panel on Postoperative Delirium in Older Adults. Postoperative delirium in older adults: best practice statement from the american geriatrics society. J Am Coll Surg. 2015;220(2):136–48.e1. doi:10.1016/j.jamcollsurg.2014.10.019.

63. Radtke FM, Franck M, Lendner J, et al. Monitoring depth of anaesthesia in a randomized trial decreases the rate of postoperative delirium but not postoperative cognitive dysfunction. Br J Anaesth. 2013;110 Suppl 1:i98–105. doi:10.1093/bja/aet055.

64. Kertai MD, White WD, Gan TJ. Cumulative duration of "triple low" state of low blood pressure, low bispectral index, and low minimum alveolar concentration of volatile anesthesia is not associated with increased mortality. Anesthesiology. 2014;121(1):18–28. doi:10.1097/ALN.0000000000000281.

65. Hudetz JA, Patterson KM, Iqbal Z, et al. Ketamine attenuates delirium after cardiac surgery with cardiopulmonary bypass. J Cardiothorac Vasc Anesth. 2009;23(5):651–7. doi:10.1053/j.jvca.2008.12.021.

66. Macario A, Royal MA. A literature review of randomized clinical trials of intravenous acetaminophen (paracetamol) for acute postoperative pain. Pain Pract. 2011;11(3):290–96. doi:10.1111/j.1533-2500.2010.00426.x.

67. Kranke P, Jokinen J, Pace NL, et al. Continuous intravenous perioperative lidocaine infusion for postoperative pain and recovery. Cochrane Database Syst Rev. 2015;7:CD009642. doi:10.1002/14651858.CD009642.pub2.

68. Sherman ED, Robillard E. Sensitivity to pain in the aged. Can Med Assoc J. 1960;83(18):944–7.

69. Petrini L, Matthiesen ST, Arendt-Nielsen L. The effect of age and gender on pressure pain thresholds and suprathreshold stimuli. Perception. 2015;44(5):587–96.

70. Racine M, Tousignant-Laflamme Y, Kloda LA, et al. A systematic literature review of 10 years of research on sex/gender and experimental pain perception - part 1: are there really differences between women and men? Pain. 2012;153(3):602–18. doi:10.1016/j.pain.2011.11.025.

71. Gagliese L, Jackson M, Ritvo P, et al. Age is not an impediment to effective use of patient-controlled analgesia by surgical patients. Anesthesiology. 2000;93(3):601–10.

72. Mann C, Pouzeratte Y, Boccara G, et al. Comparison of intravenous or epidural patient-controlled analgesia in the elderly after major abdominal surgery. Anesthesiology. 2000;92(2):433–41.

73. Epstein M. Aging and the kidney. J Am Soc Nephrol. 1996;7(8):1106–22.

74. Owen JA, Sitar DS, Berger L, et al. Age-related morphine kinetics. Clin Pharmacol Ther. 1983;34(3):364–8.

75. Zoli M, Magalotti D, Bianchi G, et al. Total and functional hepatic blood flow decrease in parallel with ageing. Age Ageing. 1999;28(1):29–33.

76. Kizer KW, Stegun MB. Serious reportable adverse events in health care. In: Henriksen K, Battles JB, Marks ES, et al., editors. Advances in patient safety: from research to implementation (volume 4: programs, tools, and products). The Agency for Healthcare Research and Quality (US) and the book is in the public domain Rockville (MD); 2005.

77. National Quality Forum. Serious Reportable Events. 2006. http://www.qualityforum.org/projects/sre2006.aspx. Accessed 12 Dec 2015.

78. Morse BC, Boland BN, Blackhurst DW, et al. Analysis of centers for medicaid and medicare services 'never events' in elderly patients undergoing bowel operations. Am Surg. 2010;76(8):841–5.

79. Wald HL, Ma A, Bratzler DW, et al. Indwelling urinary catheter use in the postoperative period: analysis of the national surgical infection prevention project data. Arch Surg. 2008;143(6):551–7. doi:10.1001/archsurg.143.6.551.

80. Barnes ZJ, Mahabir RC. Catheter use and infection reduction in plastic surgery. Can J Plast Surg. 2013;21(2):79–82.

81. Pashikanti L, Von Ah D. Impact of early mobilization protocol on the medical-surgical inpatient population: an integrated review of literature. Clin Nurse Spec. 2012;26(2):87–94. doi:10.1097/NUR.0b013e31824590e6.

82. Bjorkelund KB, Hommel A, Thorngren KG, et al. Reducing delirium in elderly patients with hip fracture: a multi-factorial intervention study. Acta Anaesthesiol Scand. 2010;54(6):678–88. doi:10.1111/j.1399-6576.2010.02232.x.

Cardiothoracic Surgery

10

Joseph C. Cleveland Jr.

Cardiovascular disease remains the leading cause of death and disability in the USA. Cardiovascular disease (CVD) is age-related with both the incidence and prevalence of cardiovascular disease increasing dramatically with increasing age. It is believed that the annual costs in 2015 in the USA for CVD and stroke will exceed $320 billion [1]. Further, the total number of inpatient cardiovascular operations and procedures increased 28 % from 2001 to 2010. Given the strong association of age and cardiovascular disease, the increasing population over age 65 is primarily responsible for this rise in cardiovascular surgery demand. The purpose of this chapter is to outline the considerations clinicians face when operating or intervening on the elderly patient with specific focus on the management of the two most common problems: coronary artery disease (CAD) and aortic stenosis.

The assessment of the geriatric patient who requires cardiovascular surgery is critical to providing optimal care. Frailty describes a biological syndrome whereby a patient is more vulnerable to stressors—i.e., acute or chronic changes in health status [2]. For the purpose of this chapter, frailty will mostly focus on an acute change in health that results from an intervention—either surgical or other catheter based procedure. With newer technological options being offered for patients, many new therapies can be offered to elderly patients. The overarching question is whether these newer procedures will provide more benefit than burden or, indeed, be futile.

Frailty and its assessment are discussed in depth in Chap. 1—Frailty. Several pertinent aspects of frailty related to cardiothoracic surgery are presented here for convenience and emphasis. The underlying mechanisms that promote frailty are multiple (Fig. 10.1). Inflammation [3], insulin resistance [4], and decreased levels of testosterone [5] are all

J.C. Cleveland Jr., MD (✉)
Division of CT Surgery, University of Colorado Anscutz Medical Center, 12631 East 17th Avenue, Academic Office 1, Room 6602, Aurora, CO 80045, USA
e-mail: joseph.cleveland@ucdenver.edu

thought to play a role in promoting frailty. The production of inflammatory cytokines in response to cardiac surgery is more pronounced in elderly patients [6]. This pathophysiological state results in catabolism of muscle, weakness, and malnutrition. In essence, there is little reserve present in the state of frailty and as such, major operations and procedures can exacerbate the frail phenotype.

10.1 Assessment of Frailty

There are several methods for assessing a patient to discover if frailty is present preoperatively. It is no longer acceptable to simply look at the patient and make this judgment, as was a method in the past. Rather, a protocol driven assessment is mandatory to identify the frail patient. If frailty is present, the patient is at a much increased risk for a poor outcome after a major perturbation such as surgery. At the University of Colorado Multidisciplinary Heart Valve Clinic consisting of surgeons, cardiologists, and others, three tools for the preoperative assessment to identify frailty seem effective: the 5-m walk test, grip strength as assessed by a dynamometer, and the Fried scale. The 5-m walk test is simple to conduct. One only needs a well-lighted hallway with 1-m lengths marked off to conduct this test. This test is perhaps the easiest to utilize and understand. Afilalo [7] and colleagues established that slow gait speed, defined as >6 s to walk 5 m, was an incremental risk factor for increased mortality and morbidity following cardiac surgery. These authors combined the robust risk-adjusted models of predicted mortality from the Society of Thoracic Surgeons (STS) Adult Cardiac Surgery Database and the 5-m walk test in 131 patients. Importantly, the combination of a high predicted STS risk with slow gait speed predicts a nearly 50 % chance of mortality or major morbidity (e.g., stroke, renal failure, prolonged ventilation, deep sternal wound infection, or need for reoperation) (Fig. 10.2). Finally, this study showed that slow gait speed will increase the STS predicted risk 2–3 fold. This finding is of great value in directing contemporary therapy

© Springer International Publishing Switzerland 2017
J.R. Burton et al. (eds.), *Geriatrics for Specialists*, DOI 10.1007/978-3-319-31831-8_10

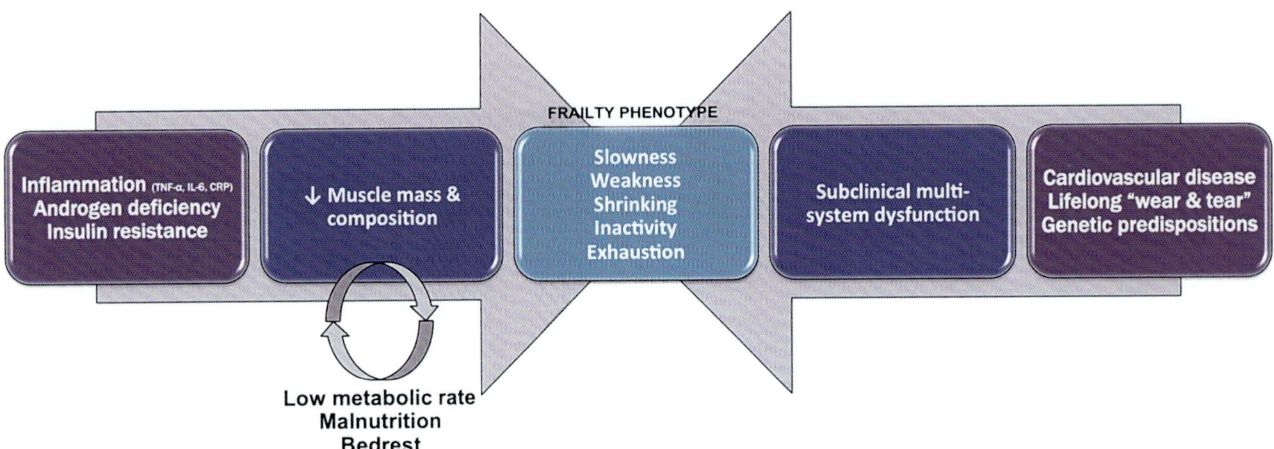

Fig. 10.1 (*Left*) The age-associated activation of inflammatory cells and decline in androgen hormones upset the balance between catabolic and anabolic stimuli, respectively, leading to a decline in muscle mass and composition known as sarcopenia. This detrimental response is aggravated in patients with insulin resistance and metabolic syndrome. Addition of bed rest and malnutrition initiates a vicious cycle of further decline in muscle mass, limiting the necessary mobilization of amino acids in times of stress. (*Right*) The accumulation of subclinical impairments in multiple organ systems resulting from cardiovascular disease, lifelong "wear and tear," and/or genetic predisposition lead to decreased homeostatic reserve and resiliency to stressors. Other pathophysiological pathways have been proposed. Biological pathways may manifest clinically as slow walking speed, weakness, weight loss, physical inactivity, and exhaustion—termed the phenotype of frailty. *CRP* C-reactive protein, *IL* Interleukin, *TNF* tumor necrosis factor. Reproduced with permission from Afilalo, J, et al. Frailty assessment in the cardiovascular care of older adults. JACC 2014;63;747–62

Fig. 10.2 The dual risk factors of slow gait speed (>6 s to walk 5 m) and high Society of Thoracic Surgeons (STS) score (>15 % predicted mortality or major morbidity) identified patients at the highest risk. Among those with the dual risk factors, 43.2 % experienced a major morbidity or mortality compared with only 5.9 % of those without either risk factor. Reproduced with permission from Afilalo J, et al. Gait speed as an incremental predictor of mortality and morbidity in elderly patients undergoing cardiac surgery. JACC 2010; 56: 1668–76

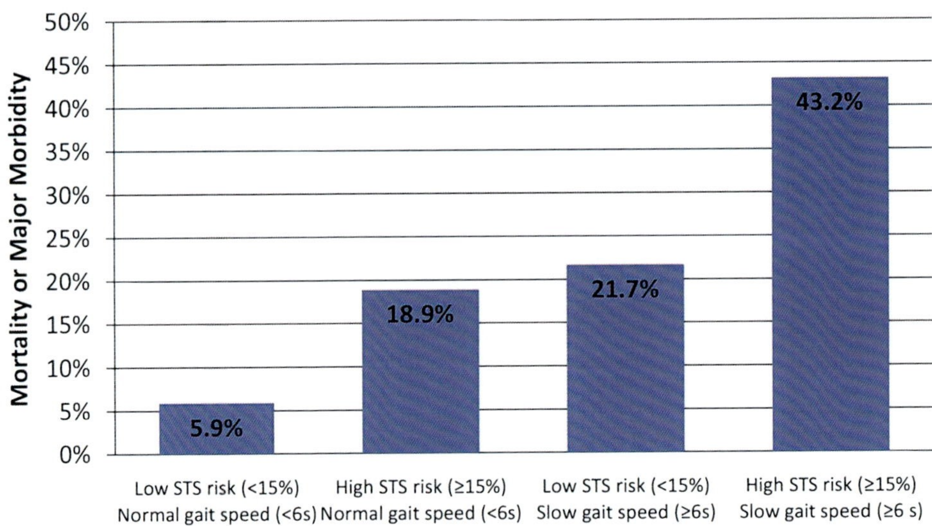

for certain, patients at increased risk for of a poor outcome from open surgery. For example, frail elderly females (assessed by gait speed) with prior coronary artery bypass surgery and reduced left ventricular ejection fraction with severe aortic stenosis will be very high-risk patients for open, surgical AVR and therefore should be considered for Transcatheter Aortic Valve Replacement (TAVR). Gait sped is now collected in the latest version of the STS Database and in the Transcatheter Valve Therapy (TVT) registry.

Frailty has a direct and strong association with excess mortality, morbidity, functional decline, and other adverse events following cardiac surgery. In a review of studies that objectively measured frailty in over 4700 patients collectively frailty was strongly associated with excess mortality, morbidity, and functional decline [8]. Not surprisingly, frailty was more pronounced in the older patients undergoing TAVR compared to younger patients undergoing coronary artery bypass or open AVR. Many studies point out the importance of identifying frailty preoperatively in patients proposed for open cardiac surgery for aortic value replacement or TAVR. Its presence predicts inferior outcomes in these interventions.

10.2 Coronary Artery Disease/Coronary Artery Bypass Grafting

The combination of the explosion of the population aged >70 and the strong association of the development of atherosclerotic coronary artery disease with advanced age has fueled a demographic shift in the surgical management of coronary artery disease. Indeed, while the total volume of coronary artery bypass procedures has decreased from 2001 to 2010, the number of elderly patients referred for bypass surgery has increased. In fact the percentage of octogenarians who receive coronary artery bypass grafting (CABG) has increased from 7 to 11 % [9]. Remarkably, the mortality risk for elderly patients undergoing CABG has decreased while the predicted risk for surgery has been gradually increasing. The reasons for this achievement are unknown; however, postulated explanations include increasing use of the left internal mammary in elderly patients, more use of off-pump CABG, and greater collective experience with CABG.

Percutaneous coronary intervention (PCI) and CABG have emerged as complementary rather than competing interventions for the management of multi-vessel coronary artery disease. The vast majority of randomized controlled trials, which have compared PCI to CABG included very few patients >75 years of age. Small, non-randomized trials before the advent of drug eluting stents (DES) favored CABG over medical therapy [10] and CABG over PCI [11]. The quality of this body of evidence, however, is insufficient to support a firm recommendation that CABG can be demonstrated to be superior to PCI or medical therapy in elderly patients. However, age alone should not preclude the consideration of CABG in the elderly cohort. A large Canadian registry, the APPROACH database, analyzed outcomes from over 21,000 patients who underwent coronary angiography for ischemic heart disease. Nearly 1000 of this patient cohort were >80 years of age. Four-year risk-adjusted survival was highest for CABG at 77.4 %, followed by 71.6 % for PCI and 60.3 % for medical therapy [12]. While a selection bias for patients who received intervention is unavoidable in this retrospective analysis, it suggests that the benefits of surgical revascularization extend to elderly patients.

Equally compelling as an outcome is functional status or quality of life (QOL) for elders who elect to undergo invasive procedures. The literature that addresses QOL following CABG suggests benefit for elderly patients undergoing CABG. A retrospective analysis reported favorable 1- and 2-year outcomes in octogenarians who underwent CABG [13]. Over 80 % of survivors were living in their own home, 74 % rated their health as good or excellent, and 82 % would undergo operation again. While frailty predicts poor outcomes, future research in this area should be directed towards answering important questions: are there long-term consequences from an episode of delirium following CABG; is longer-term quality of life—5–10 years—maintained in these patients?

What remains a central tenet in the evaluation of the elderly patient with ischemic heart disease being considered for an intervention is the evaluation and management by a dedicated team. This team should at a minimum consist of a cardiologist, surgeon, nurses, and potentially other allied specialties. With the patient as a focus, such a team is more likely to suggest wiser, thoughtful patient specific recommendations. Increasingly interdisciplinary teams consisting of a highly cohesive group of clinicians of different training backgrounds are especially effective in evaluating and caring for vulnerable seniors being treated with an invasive cardiac procedure.

10.3 Aortic Stenosis/Surgical Aortic Valve Replacement and Transcatheter Aortic Valve Replacement

The management of aortic stenosis in elderly patients has undergone a tremendous paradigm shift during the past 5 years. This transformation in care is the result of the introduction of transcatheter aortic valve replacement (TAVR). In the USA, there are at present two commercially available devices—the Edwards Sapien 3 and the Medtronic Corevalve Evolut R. Both TAVR devices are approved by the Food and Drug Administration (FDA) for the treatment of aortic stenosis in high-risk or inoperable patients and recently for treatment of failing aortic bioprosthetic valves—so-called valve in valve (ViV) indication. The pace of innovation for TAVR is astounding: there have been 3 new versions in 3 years.

The evidence supporting TAVR is derived from several studies. The PARTNER trial [14] is a landmark study which evaluated medical therapy, surgical AVR, and TAVR with a balloon-expandable valve and will be detailed here for clarity and guidance. This trial randomized 1057 patients in 2 arms. One arm examined patients deemed inoperable and compared TAVR to medical therapy (natural history of AS). The second arm randomized high-risk patients to TAVR or surgical AVR. The study included patients with severe, symptomatic aortic stenosis who were deemed inoperable ($n=358$) or high risk for surgical AVR ($n=699$). The inoperable 358 patients were randomized between TAVR and medical therapy for aortic stenosis. The 699 high-risk patients were randomized between TAVR and surgical AVR. Both arms met their predefined endpoints. In the inoperable arm, the TAVR patients had superior outcomes to medically treated patients—an absolute mortality difference favoring TAVR of 20 % at 1 year. Of note, the number of patients needed to treat (NNT) to achieve this outcome was remarkably low: 4. In the high-risk cohort, TAVR was found non-inferior to surgical AVR for mortality [15].

A similar positive experience was observed in a multi-center randomized trial comparing a self-expanding TAVR—the Medtronic CoreValve—to Surgical AVR [16]. The mean age of patients in this study was 83. Many of these patients had significant co-morbidities that predicted an operative mortality of at least 8 %.

One of the most important developments from the introduction of TAVR has been the development and maintenance of the Transcatheter Valve Therapy (TVT) Registry. The TVT registry was developed in collaboration by the American College of Cardiology (ACC) and the Society of Thoracic Surgeons (STS). The ACC measures outcomes after cardiac catheterization in the National Cardiovascular Data Registry (NCDR) and the STS measures the results from over 95 % of the cardiac surgery programs in the USA. The partnership of these two professional societies along with the FDA and the Centers for Medicare Medicaid Services (CMS) is a national and international respected collaboration. Increasingly, the preoperative assessment strategies mentioned in this chapter are captured in this database and will be of great help in defining the benefit and burdens of these interventions for aortic valve disease in seniors.

Further, insights from the PARTNER trial can help to delineate subsets of elderly patients with aortic stenosis who may not receive benefit from intervention [17]. The validity of the STS risk model was confirmed, as operative mortality, defined as in hospital or within 30 days was 10.5 %. Recalling that the STS risk model predicted an operative mortality of 15 % as a criterion for entry into the study. This small difference in observed versus expected (or predicted) mortality is likely the result of the inclusion of higher-volume and better performing AVR sites in the PARTNER trial. Important risk factors for short term and intermediate term mortality emerged from this analysis as well. A serum albumin of <3.0 g/dl was a factor that predicted early death. This risk factor can be viewed as reflective of a variety of factors—both catabolic situations such as advanced heart failure and factors such as weight loss and cachexia—which are traditional markers reflecting high peri-operative mortality. Two risk factors emerged that predicted mid-term death (median follow-up of 2.8 years). These factors were a BMI <22 kg/m^2, and a history of cancer—any cancer. While by definition these patients were all deemed "high risk" only 8 % of patients undergoing AVR had worse 1 year survival than patients deemed inoperable.

Most believe TAVR is less invasive and therefore a less stressful intervention for elderly high-risk patients. However, the impact of frailty upon patients undergoing TAVR is largely unknown. A single-center experience involving 159 patients with frailty as determined by an index combining the variables of gait speed, grip strength, serum albumin, and activities of daily living was associated with a longer hospital length of stay; but, surprisingly, frailty was not associated

with increased peri-procedural complications [18]. Frailty, as might be predicted, was independently and strongly associated with increased 1-year mortality [18]. Clearly additional research in this area is needed to clarify the real outcome risk of TAVR.

The pace of the use and evolution of TAVR for aortic stenosis is staggering. For example, within 3 years of commercial introduction, the vascular sheaths utilized to introduce the valves have gone from 24 French to 14 French in diameter, a development that has changed the delivery of the valve from a transapical (TA) approach in about 30 % of patients now to over 95 % delivered transfemorally (TF). Similarly, a 5 % rate of major vascular complications such as stroke related to these large sheaths has dropped to 1 %. Also, the latest generation valves, the Sapien 3 and the Evolt-R, have allowed the rate of moderate or severe perivalvular insufficiency to fall from 15 % to now less than 2 %. The Partner 3 intermediate risk trial (S3i) enrolled patients at intermediate risk (STS predicted risk of mortality of 4–8 %) for surgical AVR and treated them with a Sapien 3. The peri-procedural mortality dropped from 5 % to about 1 %, and major complications were few [19]. There is great relevance of these data for elderly patients as the vast majority of patients over 80 years meet criteria for intermediate risk. While at present, surgical AVR is still the standard therapy for most octogenarians it is likely that the paradigm for treating AS in the elderly will shift to TAVR as more data are developed and analyzed.

Now scholars must address the durability of TAVR. Currently follow-up data suggest these valves remain durable for at least 5 years but a septuagenarian may live on average another 7–15 years. The ongoing TVT registry will accumulate these data and the subsequent analyses will help clinicians select patients for this intervention. The ultimate goal is to select patients for TAVR who are **declining from** aortic stenosis and not patients who are **declining with** aortic stenosis

10.4 Conclusion

The rapid growth of the elderly population continues to challenge cardiothoracic surgeons to achieve high quality outcomes that consider a patient's quality of life and functional ability. It is imperative that surgeons, cardiologists, geriatricians, and other medical professionals collaborate in multi- and interdisciplinary teams to optimally evaluate frailty and other risk factors and then manage accordingly seniors with symptomatic CAD and AS. The current technological advances, clinical investigations, and access to increasingly valuable national registries will allow clinicians to improve the quality of interventions offered to elders with CAD and AS.

References

1. Mozaffarian D, Benjamin E, Go AS, et al. Heart disease and stroke statistics—2015 Update. Circulation. 2015;131:e29–322.
2. Bergman H, Ferrucci L, Guralnik J, et al. Frailty: an emerging research and clinical paradigm – issues and controversies. J Gerontol A Biol Sci Med Sci. 2007;62:731–7.
3. Walston J, McBurnie MA, Newman A, et al. Frailty and activation of the inflammation and coagulation systems with and without clinical comorbidities: results from the Cardiovascular Health Study. Arch Intern Med. 2002;162:2333–41.
4. BarzilayJI BC, Moore T, et al. Insulin resistance and inflammation as precursors of frailty: the Cardiovascular Health Study. Arch Intern Med. 2007;167:635–41.
5. Schaup LA, Pluijm SMF, Deeg DJH, et al. Low testosterone levels and decline in physical performance and muscle strength in older men: findings from two prospective cohort studies. Clin Endocrinol. 2008;68:42–50.
6. Howell K, Cleveland Jr JC, Meng X. Il-6 production during cardiac surgery correlates with increasing age. J Surg Res. 2016;201(1):76–81.
7. Afilalo J, Eisenberg MJ, Morin JF, et al. Gait speed as an incremental predictor of mortality and morbidity in elderly patients undergoing cardiac surgery. J Am Coll Cardiol. 2010;56:1668–76.
8. Sephehri A, Beggs T, Hassan A, et al. The impact of frailty on outcomes after cardiac surgery: a systematic review. J Thorac Cardiovasc Surg. 2014;148:3110–7.
9. Kurlansky P. Do octogenarians benefit from coronary artery bypass surgery: a question with a rapidly changing answer? Curr Opin Cardiol. 2012;27:611–9.
10. Krumhotz HM, Forman DE, Kuntz, et al. Coronary revascularization after MI in the very elderly: outcomes and long-term follow up. Ann Int Med. 1993;119:1084–90.
11. Kaul TK, Fields BL, Wyatt DA, et al. Angioplasty versus coronary artery bypass in octogenarians. Ann Thorac Surg. 1994;58:1419–26.
12. Graham MM, Ghali WA, Faris PD, et al. Survival after coronary revascularization in the elderly. Circulation. 2002;105:2378–84.
13. Fruitman DS, MacDougall CE, Ross DB, et al. Cardiac surgery in octogenarians: can elderly patients benefit? Quality of life after cardiac surgery. Ann Thorac Surg. 1999;68:2129–35.
14. Leon MB, Smith CR, Mack M, et al. Transcatheter aortic-valve implantation for aortic stenosis in patients who cannot undergo surgery. N Engl J Med. 2010;363:1597–607.
15. Smith CR, Leon MB, Mack MJ, et al. Transcatheter versus surgical aortic-valve replacement in high-risk patients. N Eng J Med. 2011;364:2187–98.
16. Adams DH, Popma JJ, Reardon MJ, et al. Transcatheter aortic-valve replacement with a self-expanding prosthesis. N Engl J Med. 2014;370:1790–8.
17. Szeto WY, Svensson LG, Rajeswaran J, et al. Appropriate patient selection or health care rationing? Lessons from surgical aortic valve replacement in the Placement of Aortic Transcatheter Valves I trial. J Thorac Cardiovasc Surg. 2015;150:557–68.
18. Green P, Woglom AE, Genereux P, et al. The impact of frailty status on survival after transcatheter aortic valve replacement in older adults with severe aortic stenosis. J Am Coll Cardiol Intv. 2012;5:974–81.
19. Kodali S. Early clinical and echocardiographic outcomes with the Sapien 3 transcatheter aortic valve replacement system in inoperable, high-risk, and intermediate-risk aortic stenosis patients. Presented at: American College of Cardiology/i2 Scientific Session; March 15, 2015; San Diego, CA.

Teresita M. Hogan and Thomas Spiegel

11.1 Introduction

The emergency department (ED) provides acute care to America's ill and injured; yet, the specifics of emergency care delivery are rapidly evolving as our nation ages and its health system changes. The ED is superficially understood by many as a "healthcare safety net" and the most rapid portal of entry for patients with acute and potentially life-threatening events [1]. Yet if you look deeper every day the ED serves as the nucleus for prehospital systems, as an acute diagnosis and treatment center, and as the manager presiding over one quarter of all acute care outpatient visits in the USA [2]. This is especially true for older adult patients. The determination of hospital admission versus discharge made in the ED establishes the course and cost of care for approximately 11 million older adults annually [2]. Non-emergency department providers who understand specifics of ED elder care can better navigate the system and optimize care when their patients utilize the ED.

The growing numbers of older adults requiring emergent care is disrupting business as usual for our nation's EDs. Today's ED model of care, design, and operations are based on principles from 1962. Unfortunately, this model no longer fits the demographics and complexity of our population, nor the rising expectations of efficient, effective, coordinated, and expert care now demanded from the ED. Outcomes of this traditional ED model of care show increased morbidity and mortality occurring in older adults despite their receiving more medical tests, increased admission rates, and concentrated physician attention [3, 4]. A model change is needed to improve emergency department care for older adults [5, 6].

Solutions for improving elder ED care range from enhanced geriatric training for ED staff, to providing specialized elder ED services, to the physical redesign of existing EDs with sections dedicated to elder patients. In some situations, entire EDs dedicated to older adult care have been suggested [7], and in 2008 the first specialized Geriatric Emergency Department (GED) was opened. Since this time there has been a surge in the development of entire GEDs or sections of EDs specifically dedicated to the older population. As of 2013 nearly 40 EDs self-identified as "geriatric" or "senior friendly" in a snowball sample [8]. Trends show that more GEDs and EDs with elder care enhancements are opening every year.

To facilitate enhanced geriatric ED care, the Society for Academic Emergency Medicine (SAEM), the American College of Emergency Physicians (ACEP), The American Geriatrics Society (AGS), and the Emergency Nurses Association (ENA) have collaborated on unprecedented joint recommendations for targeted elder ED improvements. The document they produced is termed the "Geriatric Emergency Department Guidelines" [9].

In this chapter we will discuss older adults as a special ED population, with unique needs, and detail specific topics in ED elder care. Finally we will discuss how the current ED model of care can shift to better fit the demands from the growing number and complexity of older adults in the ED.

T.M. Hogan, MD (✉)
Department of Medicine, Section of Emergency Medicine, and Section of Geriatrics & Palliative Care, University of Chicago Medicine & Biological Sciences, 5841 S. Maryland Avenue, Chicago, IL 60637, USA
e-mail: thogan@medicine.bsd.uchicago.edu

T. Spiegel, MD, MBA, MS
Department of Medicine, Section of Emergency Medicine, University of Chicago Medicine & Biological Sciences, 5841 S. Maryland Avenue, Chicago, IL 60637, USA

11.2 Epidemiology and Demographics

The baby boom generation of 1946–1964 generates approximately 10,000 new 65 year olds daily in the USA. From 2002 to 2010, the number of persons over age 65 years rose

© Springer International Publishing Switzerland 2017
J.R. Burton et al. (eds.), *Geriatrics for Specialists*, DOI 10.1007/978-3-319-31831-8_11

by 15 %, constituting 13 % of the population. By 2030, almost 20 % of the population will be over age 64 [10]. Due to this aging demographic, in 2010 nearly 20 million older adults visited US EDs. Many factors drive elder patients to seek ED care. Of course they come when they experience symptoms they perceive as an emergency. They come for acute injury and they come with slow deterioration in chronic conditions. Studies show older patients appropriately use emergency services and require ED care in high numbers [11, 12]. They come in spite of access to other sources of care. In fact, many elders are referred to the ED by their primary care physicians to undergo complex diagnostic evaluations, or to receive treatments not available in the office, same day sick visits, and off hours care [13]. Unfortunately, there are fewer EDs available every year. From 1993 to 2003 the number of US hospitals fell by 11 % decreasing the total number of EDs by 9 % [11].

Elders are more difficult to evaluate, stabilize, treat, and disposition than any other segment of the population. This means that in addition to the resource mismatch of more and more older patients presenting to fewer EDs, they present more frequently, sicker, and with a higher degree of complexity. Elder ED evaluations take 19–58 % longer, with admissions in up to 33 % for patients 65–74 years old, and reaching as high as 47 % for those over 75 [12, 14]. Those over 85 years' experience 823 ED visits per 1000 persons with an even higher rate of admission [10].

Equally important in the strain of older ED visits is the fact that ED expectations are increasing. EDs are expected to more fully evaluate and treat every patient, as part of the mandate to decrease hospital admissions. EDs are tasked to deliver definitive care discharge more patients, and when admitting, to more fully evaluate and to initiate earlier more comprehensive treatments. The traditional ED model of care developed for evaluation and treatment of one easily identifiable problem, with quick disposition to definitive care may be inadequate and obsolete for older patients. Yet we have not developed a new system and our evolution is slow. This is precipitating a crisis in the traditional model of ED care.

11.3   What the ED Is for Older Adult Care

The ED serves as a nucleus for prehospital systems otherwise known as Emergency Medical Systems (EMS). EDs receive ambulance transports from community, municipal, and private ambulance providers. Older adults use EMS services in high numbers and are at excess risk for adverse events [11]. Elders transported by EMS are often acutely ill and 30 % require high intensity care. The ED does not usually hire, train, or set the standards of practice for providers in the prehospital system. Yet, designated EDs offer teleme-

try radio communications with paramedics through which they direct options for care including recommending:

- the site for care, i.e. where the ambulance will take the patient
- specific medical interventions needed,
- activation of special paths of care such as stroke or myocardial infarction.

11.3.1   Centers of Excellence

Some hospitals and EDs provide centers of excellence in the care of specific problems. It is common for hospitals to carry designations such as Trauma, Stroke, or Chest Pain Centers. Various levels of intensity exist in each of these center designations signifying increasing levels of service. Examples:

- Acute ST segment elevation myocardial infarction (STEMI) centers are hospitals with a cardiac catheterization lab available following a protocol to speed care of acute STEMI patients from the ED door to opening of the vessel (door to balloon/stent time).
- Trauma centers are hospitals with protocols and personnel for rapid surgical treatment of the myriad of traumatic injuries such as rapid access to a neurosurgeon. Trauma center ED personnel are specially trained; they have specific equipment, policies, and protocols. Imaging modalities and surgical personnel are readily available, and access to operating rooms and intensive care units (ICUs) are prioritized.

Various subcategories or levels of centers of excellence exist such as level one or level two trauma centers that signify differing availability or access to different surgical specialists or procedures. Prehospital providers have protocols designating that specific types of patients must be taken to specific levels of care. Patients are often unaware of these stipulations and may be transported to unexpected/undesired institutions when protocols designate they should be transported to specific centers.

11.3.2 Ambulance Transport Issues

Older patients are far more likely to present to the ED via ambulance compared to younger patients [3], and EMS personnel are often the first point of contact for these patients. EMS workers, however, receive little to no specialty training for this older population compared to other unique populations such as children [5]. There are compelling reasons, however, to train EMS personnel in care for the elderly. Paramedics are the first point of contact for elderly patients and can bridge a vital communication gap given the correct tools. Hearing or visual impairment, dementia, and limited understanding of a complex history are a few confounding factors that make communicating an accurate history challenging for elderly patients. EMS providers may be the only personnel who can obtain history from caregivers and witnesses to events such as syncope/falls/seizures. They are often the only link to establish a baseline mental status, goals of care, and medication lists. When transporting from nursing or skilled facilities, EMS personnel obtain standardized transport forms, and portable health information that can decrease redundant tests and delays in diagnoses. EMS deficiencies in geriatric-specific education have been acknowledged. The AGS and the National Council of State EMS Training Coordinators has developed an optional course, "Geriatrics Education for EMS," which is now available to interested EMS providers [15].

11.3.3 The ED as an Acute Diagnosis and Treatment Center

The ED serves as an acute diagnosis and treatment center for its medical community. Complex elder patients often require advanced laboratory and imaging services unavailable in standard medical offices. Providers refer patients to the ED in large numbers to receive such services in a timely manner. Patients unwilling to wait for these services often present directly to the ED in an effort to receive immediate testing and treatment for their medical concerns. Treatments such as intramuscular or intravenous medications, blood transfusions, wound care, splinting, control of blood pressure, blood sugar, infectious symptoms, and pain management, to name a few, are often more available and accessible through the ED than in a clinic or private office setting. Some institutions are capable of obtaining subspecialist consultations in the ED. Sometimes the demand for ED evaluation and treatment is seen as more for convenience than necessity. However, even the most experienced emergency physicians are often unable to determine the urgency for care, until after significant evaluation and testing has been performed.

11.3.4 The ED as Governor of Disposition to Inpatient vs Outpatient Care

The ability to perform and the level of reimbursement for advanced diagnostics and treatments have shifted evaluations which historically took place in the inpatient setting, into the ED. Now a CT of the abdomen performed in the ED often prevents admission of patients for serial abdominal exams to exclude appendicitis, cholecystitis, or diverticular abscess. Initiation of IV antibiotics in the ED can prevent

admission for conditions from cellulitis to pneumonia. Advanced imaging can exclude acute stroke, spinal cord compression, and intestinal ischemia. Such determinations allow safer dispositions of patients to outpatient evaluation and care. This is a huge driver of reimbursement, and hospital administrators now utilize the ED to ensure best allocation of resources to reimbursement for populations of patients in a strategy termed population health [16].

11.4 Age-Related Issues and How They Impact Emergency Care

11.4.1 Age-Related Physiologic Changes

- Cardiac: as one ages, there are progressively fewer cardiac myocytes, decreased ventricular compliance, higher incidence of electrophysiologic abnormalities (sick-sinus syndrome, arrhythmias, bundle branch blocks, etc.), increased systolic blood pressure, and decrease in maximal heart rate and reduced cardiac output reserve [17]. These changes lead to a decreasing ability of older adults to compensate for increased cardiac demands, thus leaving older patients sensitive to volume, orthostatic, and stress changes. In the ED these changes alter our evaluation of syncope, dyspnea, weakness, and hypotension. They result in a higher burden of disease, chronic symptoms, and lack of reserve to what in younger patients would be minor events. See Chap. 21 Cardiology for additional information.

- Pulmonary: Chest wall changes such as kyphosis, vertebral compression, intercostal muscle weakness, costochondral cartilage calcification, and progressive respiratory-muscle strength decline can reduce inspiratory and expiratory force by as much as 50 %. Lung changes lead to decreases in ventilatory responses to hypoxia and hypercapnia by 50 and 40 %, respectively. Declines in T-cell function, mucociliary clearance, coordinated swallowing, and cough reflexes (especially in those with neurologic dysfunction) have a large impact on respiratory issues.

- These changes specifically affect trauma evaluation, dyspnea evaluation, and the severity and treatment of respiratory infections, such as pneumonia. More use of noninvasive respiratory support is called for in the elder population.

- Renal: Glomerular filtration rate declines by 45 % by age 80 which makes medication choices and dosing potentially precarious. Renal tubular function declines as well leading to an inability to conserve sodium and compensate for fluid losses resulting in a higher incidence of recurrent dehydration. The use of contrast agents for scanning can severely damage elder kidneys and must be evaluated prior to infusion of contrast adding to the both the time and cost of ED evaluations requiring these agents. Additionally, the evaluation of orthostatic hypotension and syncope are very common in elders seen in the ED provider education must ensure awareness of these physiologic changes.

Understanding these changes is critical in managing a geriatric patient's medication regimen, as well as underscoring the need to monitor hydration status.

Lower Urinary Tract: Increased collagen in the bladder, and benign prostatic hypertrophy in males lead to impaired bladder emptying in older adults. Urinary tract infections lead to 30–50 % of all community-acquired bacteremia in the elderly. These changes are impactful when seeking a source of infection in a febrile elderly patient.

- Gastrointestinal (GI): Constipation increases with age, from 4 % in the young, 19 % in middle-aged, and up to 34 % in the elderly. This is attributable to sedentary lifestyle, diet/dehydration, systemic illness, and medications. Therefore constipation management should focus on the external cause with appropriate modification or with addition to a patient's medication regimen.

Hepatobiliary: The liver realizes a decrease in the number of hepatocytes and hepatic blood flow up to 40 % after the age 60. The metabolism of some drugs is altered and elders may be increasingly sensitive to certain drugs requiring mediation regimen changes. Importantly, biliary disease is the most common reason for abdominal surgery in elders and up to 80 % of nursing home residents over 90 years have biliary stones.

- Body Composition: Lean muscle decreases by up to 40 % by age 80 with even greater declines in strength. Combining with decreases in activity, resting body energy expenditure also decreases. Elders are susceptible to protein-energy malnutrition when stressed. Finally, aging changes in the skin's dermis and epidermis make both wound repair and healing difficult.
- These changes make significant stresses such as infections, injuries, and/or surgeries potentially catastrophic. At best, emergency physicians need to take these changes into account when evaluating the treatment recommendations and prognosis of a given elder patient.
- Central Nervous System: The prevalence of dementia increases with age from 1.5 % in ages 65–70 and doubles every 5 years to at least 25 % by age 85. As discussed in the following section, both dementia and delirium have significant negative impacts on the quality-of-life of affected patients, both increase the need for and cost of care, and the length of hospital stays.

- Hematologic: While the steady state RBC and neutrophil counts are often in a normal range, the hematopoietic system's response is impaired during stresses that challenge the elder body to mount a proper WBC response and check infections. Unchecked bacterial growth may then advance resulting in elder patient presenting to the emergency department in extremis.

11.4.2 Age-Related Sensory Challenges (e.g., Sight, Hearing)

Visual acuity, depth perception, sound sensitivity at high frequencies, and speech discrimination all decrease with age. Put into unfamiliar surroundings, and the typical noisy ED with monotone walls, curtain dividers, and fluorescent lighting; and many older patients will become confused and either lethargic or agitated.

11.4.3 Atypical Disease Presentations

The older patient presents atypically compared to a younger adult with the same disease process. However, within the older group, these 'atypical' presentations become typical for them. These variations must be understood to take optimal care of this population. For example, many frail elders manifest alteration of mental status as the primary symptom of systemic infections [18]. Emergency providers need to know these presentations but most do not receive specific training or practice according to this paradigm.

11.4.4 Polypharmacy in Elders

Older ED patients often take from 6 to 8 concurrent prescription and over-the-counter medications [19]. From 7 to 10 % of elder ED visits involve an adverse drug event. Additionally, from 13 to 25 % of ED prescriptions to older patients pose a potential drug–drug or drug–disease interaction, and one-fifth of ED patients report mild to moderate adverse drug events from ED prescriptions [20]. This is critical for both identification of drug related problems in elders and ensuring ED prescription treatments do no harm.

The problem of controlling an acutely agitated elder patient is significant and sedatives from the ED often have unanticipated and long lasting effects. ED policies should include pathways for elder behavior control during acute change in mental status [21]. Use of Beers criteria improves risk of ED visit related adverse drug events. Targeting high-risk medications (e.g., warfarin, insulin, and digoxin) is also important in these patients [22]. See Chap. 5 Medication Management to learn more about managing this significant ED challenge.

resources and facilitate the most appropriate patient placement to home, SNF, rehab facility, observation, or admission. In discharged patients we can ensure appropriate follow-up ranging from simple telephone call back systems to telemedicine encounters [78]. These ancillary services can also prevent hospital admission for a patient who may need slightly closer monitoring or medication titration but may not need round-the-clock inpatient care [68]. GEDs create discharge protocols to appropriately communicate relevant clinical information to patients and/or caregivers and ensure this information is presented understandably.

The Follow-up/Transitions of Care category extends the Staffing/Administration discussion and formalizes it by reaching into the community, emphasizing the opportunity to coordinate and optimize care. The importance of this is underscored by the Institute of Medicine when it cited that "ineffective transitions of care put the patient's safety at great risk." [4] Inpatient/outpatient continuity of care is declining. In 1996, 44.3 % of admitted patients were seen by their PCP during their inpatient stay, while in 2006 only 31.9 % of admitted patients saw their PCP while inpatient [77]. This makes effective transitions of care all the more critical.

Whether returning patients to their home, nursing home, or a skilled nursing facility, ED providers need to improve communication of what occurred in the emergency department and help establish a safety net to prevent return visits. Care coordinators and geriatric advanced practice nurses provide invaluable communication between a patient's caregivers and PCP to ensure clear treatment goals and establish follow-up visits [79]. Any currently practicing ED physician understands the frustration of receiving a patient from a nursing home without any collateral information, and likewise physicians must anticipate the confusion of a caregiver who receives a patient with vague discharge instructions and possibly a new prescription.

11.8.7 Physical Design

The physical design of the ED provides opportunities for improved care. A patient with visual, hearing, or physical impairments benefits from improved lighting, quieter areas to communicate, more comfortable mattresses and modified lavatory facilities. Not only does this enhance patient satisfaction and safety but design prevents some never-events, promotes efficiency, and optimizes treatment [6].

In geriatric EDs the most common modifications include beds, mattresses, better lighting, skid-proof flooring, visual aids, handrails, corridor safety, assisted listening devices, and recliners. Additionally, observation units for patients whose evaluation goes beyond a typical ED stay, as is often the case for older patients, would improve satisfaction and reduce disorientation.

11.8.8 Equipment/Supplies

"Geriatric patient care requires equipment designed for a patient population with specific needs." [9] Physical and structural changes enhance safety and comfort and also reduce iatrogenic complications. Items such as extra soft or pressure-redistributing foam mattresses reduce skin breakdown and decubitus ulcer formation. Suggested starting point items include furniture such as reclining chairs with sturdy armrest to prevent falls. Equipment including body warmers, fluid warmers, non-slip fall mats and bedside commodes all assist with comfort and safety. Lighting is important and emphasizes contrast between walls and floors. Rooms should be private or have acoustically enhanced drapes and sound absorbing materials. Signs should be large and clear.

11.9 Summary: Improving Current and Future Care

Elders in the ED are a special population that is growing, has appropriate high utilization, and suffers significant morbidity and mortality despite high admission rates. A significant change in the current ED model is needed to meet the increasing demands for high quality and optimal performance expected of the modern ED. By developing, customizing, and deploying the above GED guidelines, an ED can effectively become more geriatric patient-friendly and thus enable comprehensive and quality care to the growing geriatric population. Access to an interprofessional team can enhance elder emergency care. Such a team can help ensure optimal protocols for: the planning and coordination of care during emergency evaluation and treatment, the availability of physical plant modifications and equipment, the education of optimal elder care for all ED staff, and the provision of quality transitions of care on ED discharge. This interprofessional collaboration can support the successful implementation of the GED guidelines and improve emergency care for older adults. We must respond quicky to implement known strategies improving care to the vulnerable elders in our EDs.

References

1. Taylor TB. Threats to the health care safety net. Acad Emerg Med. 2001;8(11):1080–7. http://doi.wiley.com/10.1111/j.1553-2712.2001.tb01119.x. Accessed 14 Oct 2015.
2. Schuur JD, Venkatesh AK. The growing role of emergency departments in hospital admissions. N Engl J Med. 2012;367(5):367:391–3. doi:10.1056/NEJMp1204431.
3. Aminzadeh F, Dalziel WB. Older adults in the emergency department: a systematic review of patterns of use, adverse outcomes, and effectiveness of interventions. Ann Emerg Med. 2002;39(3):238–47. doi:10.1067/mem.2002.121523.

4. Wilber ST, Gerson LW, Terrell KM, et al. Geriatric emergency medicine and the 2006 Institute of Medicine reports from the Committee on the Future of Emergency Care in the U.S. health system. Acad Emerg Med. 2006;13(12):1345–51. doi:10.1197/j.aem.2006.09.050.

5. Fitzgerald R. The future of geriatric care in our Nation's emergency departments: impact and implications. Dallas, TX: American College of Emergncy Physicians (ACEP); 2008.

6. Adams JG, Gerson LW. A new model for emergency care of geriatric patients. Acad Emerg Med. 2003;10(3):271–4.

7. Hwang U, Morrison RS. The geriatric emergency department. J Am Geriatr Soc. 2007;55(11):1873–6. doi:10.1111/j.1532-5415.2007.01400.x.

8. Hogan TM, Olade TO, Carpenter CR. A profile of acute care in an aging America: snowball sample identification and characterization of united states geriatric emergency departments in 2013. Acad Emerg Med. 2014;21(3):337–46. doi:10.1111/acem.12332.

9. Rosenberg MS, Carpenter CR, Bromley M, et al. Geriatric emergency department guidelines. Ann Emerg Med. 2014;63(5):e7–25. doi:10.1016/j.annemergmed.2014.02.008.

10. Albert M, McCaig LF, Ashman JJ. Emergency department visits by persons aged 65 and over: United States, 2009–2010. NCHS Data Brief. 2013;(130):1–8. http://198.246.124.29/nchs/data/databriefs/db130.pdf.

11. Wolinsky FD, Liu L, Miller TR, et al. Emergency department utilization patterns among older adults. J Gerontol A Biol Sci Med Sci. 2008;63(2):204–9.

12. Gruneir A, Silver MJ, Rochon PA. Emergency department use by older adults: a literature review on trends, appropriateness, and consequences of unmet health care needs. Med Care Res Rev. 2011;68(2):131–55. doi:10.1177/1077558710379422.

13. Hwang U, Shah MN, Han JH, et al. Transforming emergency care for older adults. Health Aff (Millwood). 2013;32(12):2116–20. doi:10.1377/hlthaff.2013.0670.

14. Downing A, Wilson R. Older people's use of accident and emergency services. Age Ageing. 2005;34(1):24–30. doi:10.1093/ageing/afh214.

15. American Geriatrics Society, National Council of State EMS Training Coordinators, and Jones and Bartlett Publishers. About GEMS: history of GEMS. Available at: http://www.naemt.org/about_us/history.aspx. Accessed 15 Dec 2015.

16. Kindig D, Stoddart G. What is population health? Am J Public Health. 2003;93(3):380–3. doi:10.2105/AJPH.93.3.380.

17. Rosenthal RA, Kavic SM. Assessment and management of the geriatric patient. Crit Care Med. 2004;32(4 Suppl):S92–105. doi:10.1097/01.CCM.0000122069.56161.97.

18. Adedipe A, Lowenstein R. Infectious emergencies in the elderly. Emerg Med Clin North Am. 2006;24(2):433–48. doi:10.1016/j.emc.2006.01.006.

19. Hustey FM, Wallis N, Miller J. Inappropriate prescribing in and older ED population. Am J Emerg Med. 2007;25(7):804–7. doi:10.1016/j.ajem.2007.01.018.

20. Hohl CM, Abu-Laban RB, Zed PJ, et al. Patient-reported adverse drug-related events from emergency department discharge prescriptions. CJEM. 2010;12(4):331–8.

21. Han JH, Zimmerman EE, Cutler N, et al. Delirium in older emergency department patients: recognition, risk factors, and psychomotor subtypes. Acad Emerg Med. 2009;16(3):193–200. doi:10.1111/j.1553-2712.2008.00339.x.

22. Budnitz DS, Shehab N, Kegler SR, Richards CL. Medication use leading to emergency department visits for adverse drug events in older adults. Ann Intern Med. 2007;147(11):755–65.

23. Heffner C. Diagnostic and statistical manual of mental disorders. 4th ed. Virginia: American Psychiatric Association; 2002.

24. Hustey FM, Meldon SW. The prevalence and documentation of impaired mental status in elderly emergency department patients. Ann Emerg Med. 2002;39(3):248–53. doi:10.1067/mem.2002.122057.

25. McCusker J, Cole M, Abrahamowicz M, et al. Delirium predicts 12-month mortality. Arch Intern Med. 2002;162(4):457–63. doi:10.1001/archinte.162.4.457.

26. Leslie DL, Marcantonio ER, Zhang Y, et al. One-year health care costs associated with delirium in the elderly population. Arch Intern Med. 2008;168(1):27–32. doi:10.1001/archinternmed.2007.4.

27. Han JH, Shintani A, Eden S, et al. Delirium in the emergency department: an independent predictor of death within 6 months. Ann Emerg Med. 2010;56(3):244–52.e1. doi:10.1016/j.annemergmed.2010.03.003.

28. Huff JS. Altered mental status and coma. In: Tintinalli JE, Stapczynski JS, Cline DM, et al., editors. Tintinalli's emergency medicine: a comprehensive study guide. New York: McGraw-Hill; 2010. p. 1135–42.

29. Han JH, Wilson A, Ely EW. Delirium in the older emergency department patient: a quiet epidemic. Emerg Med Clin North Am. 2010;28(3):611–31. doi:10.1016/j.emc.2010.03.005.

30. Qaseem A, Wilt TJ, Weinberger SE, et al. Diagnosis and management of stable chronic obstructive pulmonary disease: a clinical practice guideline update from the American College of Physicians, American College of Chest Physicians, American Thoracic Society, and European Respiratory Society. American College of Physicians; American College of Chest Physicians; American Thoracic Society; European Respiratory Society. Ann Intern Med. 2011;155(3):179–91. doi: 10.7326/0003-4819-155-3-201108020-00008.

31. Green SM, Martinez-Rumayor A, Gregory SA, et al. Clinical uncertainty, diagnostic accuracy, and outcomes in emergency department patients presenting with dyspnea. Arch Intern Med. 2008;168(7):741–8. doi:10.1001/archinte.168.7.741.

32. Singer AJ, Emerman C, Char DM, et al. Bronchodilator therapy in acute decompensated heart failure patients without a history of chronic obstructive pulmonary disease. Ann Emerg Med. 2008;51(1):25–34. doi:10.1016/j.annemergmed.2007.04.005.

33. Jelinek GA, Ingarfield SL, Mountain D, et al. Emergency department diagnosis of pulmonary embolism is associated with significantly reduced mortality: a linked data population study. Emerg Med Australas. 2009;21(4):269–76. doi:10.1111/j.1742-6723.2009.01196.x.

34. Pedersen SH, Galatius S, Hansen PR, et al. Field triage reduces treatment delay and improves long-term clinical outcome in patients with acute ST-segment elevation myocardial infarction treated with primary percutaneous coronary intervention. J Am Coll Cardiol. 2009;54(24):2296–302. doi:10.1016/j.jacc.2009.06.056.

35. Jauch EC, Saver JL, Adams Jr HP, et al. Guidelines for the early management of patients with acute ischemic stroke: a guideline for healthcare professionals from the American Heart Association/American Stroke Association. Stroke. 2013;44(3):870–947. doi:10.1161/STR.0b013e318284056a.

36. Adams HP Jr, del Zoppo G, Alberts MJ, et al. Guidelines for the early management of adults with ischemic stroke: a guideline from the American Heart Association/ American Stroke Association Stroke Council, Clinical Cardiology Council, Cardiovascular Radiology and Intervention Council, and the Atherosclerotic Peripheral Vascular Disease and Quality of Care Outcomes in Research Interdisciplinary Working Groups: the American Academy of Neurology affirms the value of this guideline as an educational tool for neurologist. Stroke. 2007;38(5):1655–711. doi:10.1161/strokeaha.107.181486.

37. Hanks N, Wen G, He S, et al. Expansion of U.S. emergency medical service routing for stroke care: 2000–2010. West J Emerg Med. 2014;15(4):499–503. doi:10.5811/westjem.2014.2.20388.

38. Goldstein MB, Simel DL. Is this patient having a stroke? 2005;293(19):2391–402. doi:10.1001/jama.293.19.2391.

39. Lin CB, Peterson ED, Smith EE, et al. Emergency medical service hospital prenotification is associated with improved evaluation and treatment of acute ischemic stroke. Circ Cardiovasc Qual Outcomes. 2012;5(4):514–22. doi:10.1161/circoutcomes.112.965210.

40. van Duin D. Diagnostic challenges and opportunities in older adults with infectious diseases. Clin Infect Dis. 2012;54(7):973–8. doi:10.1093/cid/cir927.

41. Garlington W, High K. Evaluation of infection in the older adult. [Online] UpToDate Dec 7, 2012 [cited 2013 March 12]. Available from: URL:http://www.uptodate.com.

42. Mellors JW, Horwitz RI, Harvey MR, et al. A simple index to identify occult bacterial infection in adults with acute unexplained fever. Arch Intern Med. 1987;147(4):666–71. doi:10.1001/archinte.1987.00370040048009.

43. Gallagher EJ, Brooks F, Gennis P. Identification of serious illness in febrile adults. Am J Emerg Med. 1994;12(2):129–33.

44. Marco CA, Schoenfeld CN, Hansen KN, et al. Fever in geriatric emergency patients: clinical features associated with serious illness. Ann Emerg Med. 1995;26(1):18–24. doi:10.1016/S0196-0644(95)70232-6.

45. Rivers E, Nguyen B, Havstad S, et al. Early goal-directed therapy in the treatment of severe sepsis and septic shock. N Engl J Med. 2001;345(19):1368–77. doi:10.1056/NEJMoa010307.

46. Sun BC, Emond JA, Camargo Jr CA. Characteristics and admission patterns of patients presenting with syncope to US emergency departments, 1992–2000. Acad Emerg Med. 2004;11(10):1029–34. doi:10.1197/j.aem.2004.05.032.

47. Marrison VK, Fletcher A, Parry SW. The older patient with syncope: practicalities and controversies. Int J Cardiol. 2012;155(1):9–13. doi:10.1016/j.ijcard.2010.10.055.

48. Kapoor W, Snustad D, Peterson J, et al. Syncope in the elderly. Am J Med. 1986;80(3):419–28. doi:10.1016/0002-9343(86)90716-3.

49. Hogan TM, Jin L. Syncope in the older adult. In: Kahn J, Magauran BG Jr, Olskaher JS, editors. Geriatric emergency medicine: principles and practice. Cambridge, UK: Cambridge University Press; 2014. p. 114–27.

50. Cunningham R, Mikhail MG. Management of patients with syncope and cardiac arrhythmias in an emergency department observation unit. Emerg Med Clin North Am. 2001;19(1):105–21.

51. Lane P, Sorondo B, Kelly J. Geriatric trauma patients—are they receiving trauma center care? Acad Emerg Med. 2003;10(3):244–50. doi:10.1197/aemj.10.3.244.

52. Haas B, Gomez D, Zagorski B, et al. Survival of the fittest: the hidden cost of undertriage of major trauma. J Am Coll Surg. 2010;211(6):804–11. doi:10.1016/j.jamcollsurg.2010.08.014.

53. Callaway DW, Wolfe R. Geriatric trauma. Emerg Med Clin North Am. 2007;25(3):837–60. doi:10.1016/j.emc.2007.06.005.

54. Phillips S, Rond 3rd PC, Kelly SM, et al. The failure of triage criteria to identify geriatric patients with trauma: results from the Florida trauma triage study. J Trauma. 1996;40(2):278–83.

55. Heffernan DS, Thakkar RK, Monaghan SF, et al. Normal presenting vital signs are unreliable in geriatric blunt trauma victims. J Trauma. 2010;69(4):813–20. doi:10.1097/TA.0b013e3181f41af8.

56. Martin JT, Alkhoury F, O'Connor JA, et al. 'Normal' vital signs belie occult hypoperfusion in geriatric trauma patients. Am Surg. 2010;76(1):65–9.

57. National Association of Ems Physicians And American College Of Surgeons-Committee On Trauma. Field triage of the injured patient. Prehosp Emerg Care. 2011;58(4):541. doi:10.3109/10903127.2011.598622.

58. Caplan GA, Brown A, Croker WD, et al. Risk of admission within 4 weeks of discharge of elderly patients from the emergency department—the DEED study. Discharge of elderly from emergency department. Age Ageing. 1998;27(6):697–702. doi:10.1093/ageing/27.6.697.

59. Colby SL, Ortman JM. Projections of the size and composition of the U.S. population: 2014 to 2060 current population reports. Curr Popul Reports. 2015;25–1143. http://www.census.gov/content/dam/Census/library/publications/2015/demo/p25-1143.pdf.

60. D'Arcy LP, Stearns SC, Domino ME, et al. Is geriatric care associated with less emergency department use? J Am Geriatr Soc. 2013;61(1):4–11. doi:10.1111/jgs.12039.

61. Singer AJ, Thode HC Jr, Viccellio P, et al. The association between length of emergency department boarding and mortality. Acad Emerg Med. 18(12):1324–29. doi:10.1111/j.1553-2712.2011.01236.x.

62. Carpenter CR, Heard K, Wilber S, et al. Research priorities for high-quality geriatric emergency care: medication management, screening, and prevention and functional assessment. Acad Emerg Med. 2011;18(6):644–54. doi:10.1111/j.1553-2712.2011.01092.x.

63. The Advisory Board Company. Designing geriatric emergency departments—selected case studies. 2011. https://www.advisory.com/research/market-innovation-center/original-inquiry/2012/02/designing-geriatric-emergency-departments.

64. American College of Emergency Physicians, Pediatric Committee; and American Academy of Pediatrics, Committee on Pediatric Emergency Medicine. Guidelines for preparedness of emergency departments that care for children: a call to action. Ann Emerg Med. 2001;37(4):389–91.

65. Sullivan AF, Rudders SA, Gonsalves AL, et al. National survey of pediatric services available in US emergency departments. Int J Emerg Med. 2013;6(1):13. doi:10.1186/1865-1380-6-13.

66. Better Care. Smarter Spending. Healthier People: Paying Providers for Value, Not Volume. https://www.cms.gov/Newsroom/MediaReleaseDatabase/Fact-sheets/2015-Fact-sheets-items/2015-01-26-3.html.

67. Platts-Mills TF, Glickman SW. Measuring the value of a senior emergency department: making sense of health outcomes and health costs. Ann Emerg Med. 2014;63(5):525–7. doi:10.1016/j.annemergmed.2013.12.007.

68. Ouslander JG, Lamb G, Perloe M, et al. Potentially avoidable hospitalizations of nursing home residents: frequency, causes, and costs. J Am Geriatr Soc. 2010;58(4):627–35. doi:10.1111/j.1532-5415.2010.02768.x.

69. Keyes DC, Singal B, Kropf CW, et al. Impact of a new senior emergency department on emergency department recidivism, rate of hospital admission, and hospital length of stay. Ann Emerg Med. 2014;63(5):517–24. doi:10.1016/j.annemergmed.2013.10.033.

70. Carpenter CR, Shelton E, Fowler S, et al. Risk factors and screening instruments to predict adverse outcomes for undifferentiated older emergency department patients: a systematic review and meta-analysis. Acad Emerg Med. 2015;22(1):1–21. doi:10.1111/acem.12569.

71. Ballabio C, Bergamaschini L, Mauri S, et al. A comprehensive evaluation of elderly people discharged from an emergency department. Intern Emerg Med. 2008;3(3):245–9. doi:10.1007/s11739-008-0151-1.

72. Sanders AB. Care of the elderly in emergency departments: conclusions and recommendations. Ann Emerg Med. 1992;21(7):830–4. doi:10.1016/S0196-0644(05)81030-3.

73. Phelan EA, Genshaft S, Williams B, et al. A comparison of how generalists and fellowship-trained geriatricians provide "geriatric" care. J Am Geriatr Soc. 2008;56(10):1807–11. doi:10.1111/j.1532-5415.2008.01942.x.

74. American Geriatrics Society, National Association of Emergency Medical Technicians, Snyder DR. Geriatric education for emergency medical services. Jones & Bartlett Learning, 2014.

75. Désy PM, Prohaska TR. The geriatric emergency nursing education (GENE) course: an evaluation. J Emerg Nurs. 2008;34(5):396–402. doi:10.1016/j.jen.2007.08.023.

76. Carpenter CR, Shelton E, Fowler S, Suffoletto B, Platts-Mills TF, Rothman RE, Hogan TM.Risk factors and screening instruments to predict adverse outcomes for undifferentiated older emergency department patients: a systematic review and meta-analysis. Acad Emerg Med. 2015;22(1):1–21.

77. Meldon SW, Mion LC, Palmer RM, et al. A brief risk-stratification tool to predict repeat emergency department visits and hospitalizations in older patients discharged from the emergency department. Acad Emerg Med. 2003;10(3):224–32. doi:10.1197/aemj.10.3.224.

78. Brignell M, Wootton R, Gray L. The application of telemedicine to geriatric medicine. Age Ageing. 2007;36(4):369–74. doi:10.1093/ageing/afm045.

79. Sinha SK, Bessman ES, Flomenbaum N, et al. A systematic review and qualitative analysis to inform the development of a new emergency department-based geriatric case management model. Ann Emerg Med. 2011;57(6):672–82. doi:10.1016/j.annemergmed.2011.01.021.

Bellal Joseph, Ahmed Hassan, and Mindy J. Fain

12.1 Overview

The US older population has been rapidly growing, a result of the aging baby boomers and increasing life expectancy. By the year 2030, elderly Americans are expected to constitute 19 % of the population [1]. As a result, trauma/acute care surgeons will frequently be faced with the care of older patients who often present with unique diagnostic and therapeutic challenges. Overall, trauma is a leading cause of morbidity and mortality in older adults, with falls, motor vehicle crashes, and burns constituting the most common mechanisms of injury. Geriatric emergency general surgery includes a diverse range of disorders with distinct disease processes, presentation and management issues. The most common conditions include acute diverticulitis, mesenteric ischemia, acute cholecystitis, and acute appendicitis.

12.2 Geriatric Trauma

Trauma is generally considered to affect primarily the young population and the older population is perceived as sedentary and less active. However, the traditional norm is changing, and older adults maintain their health, placing them at risk for trauma from an active lifestyle. These trends, in addition to falls, burns, and motor vehicle crashes that affect frail elders, result in trauma as a leading cause of morbidity and mortality in the elderly.

B. Joseph, MD, FACS (✉) • A. Hassan, MD
Department of Surgery, The University of Arizona,
1501 N. Campbell Avenue, Tucson, AZ 85724, USA
e-mail: bjoseph@surgery.arizona.edu

M.J. Fain, MD
Department of Medicine, Arizona Center in Aging, University of Arizona College of Medicine, 1821 E. Elm Street, Tucson, AZ 85719, USA

There is a debate regarding the exact age definition of a geriatric trauma patient, whether the cutoff should be as low as 50, or as high as 70 years old. Despite this, it is estimated that over 500,000 geriatric trauma patients (over the age of 65 years) are admitted to the hospital every year, accounting for one quarter of all trauma admissions in the USA [2]. The number of geriatric trauma patients is increasing [3] and is already having a significant impact on our health care system. Elderly trauma patients present unique challenges: the mechanism of injury is different, they have decreased physiological reserves, and they have comorbidities treated with multiple medications, further complicating their presentation, clinical course, and outcomes. As a group, they experience higher mortality, higher complication rates, and slower recovery. Trauma surgeons in sync with multidisciplinary teams must be prepared to provide geriatric-specific, high quality, and cost-effective trauma care for these older adults currently in need, and in the future. These service lines will be tailored to the geriatric trauma patient and exist within the trauma bay, intensive care units, and general ward. This infrastructure will allow transitions of care both for in-hospital and outpatient care resulting in overall better patient outcomes.

12.2.1 Mechanisms of Injury in Older Adults

The mechanisms of injury in the elderly population are distinctly different from their younger counterparts. The three leading mechanisms of injury in the elderly are falls, motor vehicle collisions, and burns. Falls are the most common mechanism of injury in geriatric trauma patients and account for over 50 % of all unintentional injuries in the elderly [4]. Although falls from a standing position on a level surface are considered to be a low impact or benign mechanism of injury, they are associated with a significant morbidity (e.g., hip fracture, cervical spine or head injury) and mortality reaching as high as 40 % [5, 6]. There are many reasons for the increased number of falls, including aging itself, vision impairments, comorbid conditions, and medications, and the etiology of a fall is often multifactorial [7].

© Springer International Publishing Switzerland 2017
J.R. Burton et al. (eds.), *Geriatrics for Specialists*, DOI 10.1007/978-3-319-31831-8_12

Elderly drivers suffer a higher mortality rate following motor vehicle collisions (MVC) [8]. MVC related mortality in geriatric patients is five times higher than their younger counterparts [4, 8, 9], and it is the most common cause of trauma-related mortality in older adults. The older driver has the second highest rate of MVC per mile driven, second only to teenagers despite adhering to low risk driving conditions (e.g., driving during the day, avoiding poor weather conditions). This high crash rate is attributed to several aging-related conditions, including decreased visual acuity and nighttime vision and slower cognitive-visual processing, as well as associated medical conditions (e.g., arthritis), cognitive impairment, and adverse medication effects (e.g., benzodiazepines). In contrast to young adults, speeding and alcohol use are uncommon causes of MVC in the elderly. Approximately 25 % of older adults involved in an MVC sustain a chest injury, most commonly rib fractures, which can be devastating and lead to pneumonia and respiratory failure. Following an MVC, older adults are also more likely to suffer fractures than younger crash victims, including the cervical spine, hips, and extremities.

Burn related injuries are the 3rd leading cause of mortality in geriatric trauma patients. Every year 2000 older adults die from burn related injuries in the USA [7]. Among all the burn patients, the highest mortality exists in geriatric patients, accounting for 13–20 % of overall admissions in burn units [10]. The most common causes of burns are smoking in bed, ignition of clothing, and immersion in hot water bath. Burns in the elderly occur primarily at home and most common locations are the kitchen, bathroom, and living room. Similar to all age-related injuries, sensory, cognitive, and physical impairments in the elderly are chiefly responsible for these injuries. Burns in the elderly also tend to be more severe as older adults may have a reduced ability to recognize the severity of the situation, as well as a limited ability to escape [10]. Importantly, the reduced body mass in the elderly results in deeper thermal injuries [7].

12.2.1.1 Key Points

- Minor trauma can cause major injuries and death
- Standing falls from a level surface are the most common mechanism of injury in the elderly population.
- MVC related mortality is five times higher in the elderly compared to the young adults.
- Among all burn patients, older adults suffer the highest mortality.

12.2.2 Impact of Age-Related Physiologic Changes and Comorbidities

Physiological changes secondary to aging combined with comorbidities significantly increase the trauma-related morbidity and mortality [11]. Age-related changes in the cardiovascular, respiratory, musculoskeletal, and neurocognitive systems directly impact on pre-hospital triage, primary survey, and management.

Aging-associated changes in the cardiovascular system include a decrease in cardiac function, and an increase in the stiffness in the aorta and peripheral vasculature. There is also a decrease in both maximum heart rate and tachycardic response, which may be due to slower conduction velocity and lower endogenous response to catecholamines [12]. These changes pose a major challenge to the management of trauma patients. Due to a lower tachycardic response in the elderly to hemorrhage, pain or anxiety, the heart rate may be a poor indicator of shock and hypoperfusion [13]. The elderly patients have a higher baseline blood pressure so a normal blood pressure may be falsely reassuring in geriatric trauma patients [14]. Elderly trauma patients also tend to collapse very quickly without any warning signs [4]. Therefore, a heart rate above 90 beats per minute (rather than 130 beats per minute) and a systolic blood pressure less than 110 mmHg (rather than 95 mmHg) are more sensitive indicators of serious injury in the older trauma patient.

With aging, there is a loss of lung and chest wall elasticity. Moreover, calcification of the intercostal cartilages and degeneration of intervertebral disc space restricts the thoracic volume that limits the ability of the lung to expand and function effectively [15]. The alveolar compliance decreases in the elderly due to collagen deposition and surfactant reduction. Older adults have diminished respiratory reserve, with lower forced expiratory volume (FEV1), and lower baseline p02. In face of these changes, even a simple pneumothorax or hemothorax in the elderly can be catastrophic. Administration of supplementary oxygen is necessary in elderly trauma patients and ICU admission of geriatric patients should be considered to allow for an early detection of respiratory failure [16]. Chest wall injuries with rib fractures in elderly are poorly tolerated and associated with a higher mortality rate [17]. Narcotics should be used with caution in these patients as even low doses may result in a severe respiratory depression. In summary, older adults have a blunted response to hypoxia, hypercarbia, and acidosis, and may be unable to compensate for these metabolic challenges. They may maintain a normal respiratory rate despite progression of hypoxia and hypercarbia, complicating clinical assessment and leading to a false sense of security.

Changes in musculoskeletal system begin after the age of 30 years and after the age of 50 there is a 10 % loss in muscle mass with every decade of life. Decreased anabolic hormones, malnutrition, and decreased activity are responsible for these changes [18]. Ligaments and joints become stiffer and less flexible leading to a decreased joint stability. Lower bone density and osteoporosis facilitates fractures and complicates bone healing. Cervical osteophytes secondary to osteoarthritic changes decrease the neck flexibility, which makes neck extension difficult for intubation. Therefore care in intubation, and early stabilization of fractures and mobilization is necessary in geriatric trauma patients to avoid devastating complications.

Aging-related changes in the dura and veins increase the risk of subdural hemorrhage from head injury in the elderly. Brain atrophy, which accompanies aging, results in a larger intracranial space for asymptomatic accumulation of blood, delaying the development of signs and symptoms. Age-related changes in cerebrovascular auto-regulation may compromise the brain's ability to protect itself from hypotension; this is particularly relevant when considering therapeutic hypotension. Lastly, the presence of cognitive impairment and/or delirium is more common in older adults, and further complicates assessment.

12.2.2.1 Key Points

- Aging is associated with a physiologic decline that affects all organ systems.
- With aging there is a decrease in cardiac reserve, lung and chest wall elasticity, a loss of musculoskeletal mass and mobility, and changes in the brain and dura.
- These changes predispose elderly trauma patients to subtle presentations of serious injury, rapid hemodynamic collapse, need for prolonged respiratory support, and difficulty in intubation.

12.3 Geriatric Trauma Assessment and Initial Management

12.3.1 Geriatric Trauma Triage

Appropriate triage of trauma patients is important because it allows for maximized benefit of available resources to achieve the best outcomes. Studies demonstrate that even with a mild injury, older trauma patients have a significantly higher mortality compared to their younger counterparts [19]. It is still unclear whether the decrease in physiological reserve related to aging, associated comorbidities, or other unidentified factors is responsible for this difference. However, it is well recognized that improved outcomes can be achieved with an aggressive trauma care in patients who have survivable injuries.

As noted, geriatric trauma patients are a unique population with distinct characteristics that pose a challenge for appropriate triage. Currently, older adults are under-triaged, likely a result of an apparent benign mechanism of injury (e.g., after a level fall), subtle presentation of injury, and the use of traditional triage tools which depend upon classic physiologic criteria (e.g., blood pressure, pulse) to activate the trauma team. Due to their inherent higher vulnerability to morbidity and mortality, and lack of triage criteria for older adults, several studies have suggested that all geriatric trauma patients should be transferred to high level trauma centers regardless of their injury severity. The potential result of this approach is that it may result in a significant over-triage and overwhelm current trauma centers [20]. The early identification of geriatric trauma patients who will benefit from aggressive therapy and early post-injury rehabilitation is a key step in matching resources to needs and improving outcomes, and geriatric-specific trauma guidelines are evolving.

According to the guidelines of the American College of Surgeons committee on Trauma, patients age 55 years and older are associated with higher mortality and morbidity rates and should be directly transported to a trauma center regardless of the severity of injury [21]. The latest version of the national trauma triage protocol (NTTP) has recommended that geriatric trauma patients age 65 and above with SBP < 110 mm of Hg should be triaged to a trauma center. The most accurate predictor of mortality in geriatric trauma patient is injury severity score (ISS); however, this variable cannot be used for the triage of geriatric patients because it is unavailable in the field. In its absence, physiologic parameters remain the only available measures for the field triage. More recently, shock index >1, which is a simple ratio of heart rate and systolic blood pressure, has been demonstrated to be an accurate predictor of mortality in geriatric trauma patients and may thus be appropriate for use in the field triage [22]. However, the impact of this change on triage performance is yet to be determined.

12.3.2 History

Obtaining a history is helpful, although in many instances it may be difficult. As possible, the following questions should be obtained: events immediately leading to the trauma, chronic conditions and medications, usual level of function and cognition, and the presence of advance directives. Although discussed later, an understanding of a patient's goals of care, preferences, and values is a critical component of geriatric trauma care.

12.3.3 Initial Assessment

It is important to maintain a high index of suspicion for significant injury in the geriatric trauma patient, and conduct a careful assessment and implement close monitoring. For initial assessment, the standard primary survey should be utilized, with special attention to the aging-related physiologic responses that may otherwise delay the recognition of serious clinical problems. In addition to blunted responses to hypoxia, hypercarbia, acidosis, and hemodynamic challenge, older adults may have diminished pain perception. This may hide from clinical view the presence of serious injuries, including chest, abdominal, and skeletal fractures. The impact of medications, such as anticoagulants and beta blockers, and comorbid conditions, including osteoarthritis, and heart failure should also be directly assessed and managed. For example, airway management can be complicated by cervical osteoarthritis, and preexisting conditions such as myocardial ischemia can be the cause of hypotension, rather than hemorrhage.

When evaluating an older adult with a fall, specific attention should be paid to the assessment of any other associated injuries, such as cervical, rib, or pelvic fracture, as well as an otherwise unrecognized condition that may have contributed to the fall. Falls may result from pneumonia, sepsis, cardiac disease, medications, or other conditions [23]. The presentation of acute illness in older adults may be very subtle and limited to a functional impairment (e.g., fall) or exacerbation of an underlying chronic condition (e.g., heart failure). Older adults may not be febrile with an acute infection, and may not complain of chest pain with acute cardiac ischemia. Therefore, even in patients with no signs of infection, sepsis or acute ischemia, a high index of suspicion should be maintained, and contributing etiologies for a fall should be evaluated.

One of the most dreaded complications of falls in older patients is a traumatic brain injury. Low threshold should be maintained for suspecting an intracranial injury, particularly in patients with headache, drowsiness, or confusion. Hip fracture is another major complication that carries significant morbidity and mortality. It is essential to promptly evaluate geriatric patients with falls for hip fractures while in the ED and if necessary to expedite emergency surgery. Although attention should be paid to correction of underlying electrolyte imbalances and stabilization of comorbidities, it is critical not to unnecessarily delay surgical repair of a hip fracture.

12.3.4 Risk Assessment in Trauma Patients

While it is well recognized that aging is associated with a physiological decline, this decline is not uniform across all individuals or even an individual's organ systems. The frailty index has recently emerged as an index of the physiological age and reserve of an individual and studies have demonstrated that frailty is an accurate predictor of morbidity and mortality in trauma patients. In fact, the use of age alone for clinical decision may be misleading, and in geriatric trauma patients the frailty index has been shown to be superior to age in predicting the outcomes [24, 25].

Several models have been developed and validated to assess the frailty score of an individual (see Chap. 1, Frailty). The most common ones include the Fried's frailty and the Rockwood's frailty model. While both these models have been well validated in the literature, the practicality of these indices in a trauma cohort of patients is questionable due to their cumbersome nature. To improve the practical applicability of frailty score, studies have derived a simple 15-variable Trauma-Specific Frailty Index (TSFI) that has been validated and shown to be as accurate as a 50-variable questionnaire in predicting the outcomes in geriatric trauma patients (Table 12.1) [25, 26]. The TSFI has been shown to predict mortality as well as discharge disposition in geriatric trauma patients [27].

Table 12.1 Trauma-specific frailty index

Fifteen-variable trauma-specific frailty index			
Comorbidities			
Cancer history	Yes (1)	No (0)	PCI (0.5)
Coronary heart disease	MI (1)	CABG (0.75)	
	Medication (0.25)	None (0)	
Dementia	Severe (1)	Moderate (0.5)	Mild (0.25)
	No (0)		
Daily activities			
Help with grooming	Yes (1)	No (0)	
Help managing money	Yes (1)	No (0)	
Help doing housework	Yes (1)	No (0)	
Help toileting	Yes (1)	No (0)	
Help walking	Wheelchair (1)	Walker (0.75)	Cane (0.5)
	No (0)		
Health attitude			
Feel less useful	Most time (1)	Sometimes (0.5)	Never (0)
Feel sad	Most time (1)	Sometimes (0.5)	Never (0)
Feel effort to do everything	Most time (1)	Sometimes (0.5)	Never (0)
Falls	Most time (1)	Sometimes (0.5)	Never (0)
Feel lonely	Most time (1)	Sometimes (0.5)	Never (0)
Function			
Sexual active	Yes (0)	No (1)	
Nutrition			
Albumin	<3 (1)	>3 (0)	

12.3.5 Management of Geriatric Trauma Patients

The ongoing management of geriatric trauma patients involves several domains, including identification of patient's baseline status (pre-injury), patient/family's goals of care, patient's anticipated prognosis and recovery, and early and ongoing discharge planning. Close monitoring is essential for early identification and management of associated injuries and impact of comorbidities and medications. Comprehensive delirium prevention and management protocols should be implemented (see Chap. 2, Delirium). Careful analgesia is important to optimize patient's functioning and reduce the incidence of delirium. Optimizing cognition, sleep, nutrition, managing constipation, and preventing skin breakdown are key elements of care. Collaboration with geriatricians (in consultation or co-management models) and/or palliative care teams offers the opportunity to optimize care and improve clinical outcomes for older adults.

12.3.6 Outcomes of Care for Geriatric Trauma Patients

During the past couple of decades, quality of healthcare services and outcomes has become increasingly important. Outcomes including in-hospital mortality (IHM), post-hospitalization mortality (PMH), in-hospital complications, functional status, and ICU and hospital length of stay have been extensively studied in geriatric patients. Multiple factors help determine these outcomes in geriatric trauma patients such as demographics, injury severity, and general clinical condition, which is a cumulative effect of age, comorbidities, decline in physiologic reserve, cognition, and functional ability of the patient. Elderly patients who are admitted to the hospital for an acute illness or after a traumatic injury are more prone to develop functional disability and be discharged to skilled nursing facilities for long-term care than younger adults. It has been reported that more than 90 % of geriatric trauma patients require skilled nursing care facilities at least 1 year after the injury. Complications resulting from a functional decline after injury include loss of independence, falls, incontinence, depression, malnutrition, and lack of socialization. Early evaluation of general clinical condition, injury severity, functional and cognitive impairments through a team assessment can enable a rapid and appropriate management utilizing geriatric principles to minimize the risk of adverse outcomes.

12.3.7 Transition of Care

The primary objective for any trauma patient admitted to the hospital is safe transition to a level of care that meets their needs and goals of care, and allows for the highest level of independence. The discharge site may be their home (often with family and home health services support) or an inpatient facility (including skilled nursing facility or rehabilitation hospital). A successful transfer requires comprehensive planning that should begin at the time of hospital admission and demands the early and ongoing assessment of patient's physical, cognitive, social, and financial situation by the physician, nurse, case manager, therapist, and the social worker. The discharge of these patients to these facilities is often limited by the financial restrictions, insurance coverage laws, reimbursement rules, and CMS regulations. These issues require a close communication among the health care providers, case manager, and social worker to allow a timely and appropriate discharge of these patients. An appropriate discharge plan is essential to ensure patient safety, to idealize patient outcomes, and to prevent readmissions.

A key element of the disposition of the patient is the assessment of functions associated with activities of daily life. The most commonly utilized tool to assess and document functional independence is Functional Independence Measure (FIM) instrument. It is composed of 18 elements which assesses 13 motor skills and 5 cognitive skills, each scaled from 1 to 7 with 1 meaning total assistance and 7 meaning total independence. This score is the most widely accepted and utilized of all functional assessment tools and also recognized by the CMS.

12.3.7.1 Key Points

- Transition of care from the hospital is challenging as a large number of geriatric patients require transfer to a rehab facility or a skilled nursing facility.
- Close communication and a strong working relationship among the health care providers are essential to ensure a safe and appropriate discharge of these patients.

12.3.8 End-of-Life Care in Older Adults

Withdrawal of care is a common occurrence in the geriatric trauma patients who are admitted to the ICU. Despite its frequency, it remains a complicated and challenging situation for health care providers. Most common causes for withdrawal of care include reduction of patient suffering, anticipated poor quality of life, and brain death [28]. It is important to understand that withdrawal of care should not always be viewed as a symbol of failure or defeat. Understanding the issues associated with end-of-life situations and palliative care is of paramount importance to improve the care of dying patients.

A patient-centered approach should be utilized to establish the goals of the treatment in geriatric patients. This requires an in-depth discussion with the patient and their families about the likely outcomes and subsequent quality of life. There are numerous prognostic models that predict mortality and may help in informed decision making, however none of these models are 100 % accurate. The decision for withdrawal of care should be based on risk-benefit analysis and patient's autonomy and wishes.

While advising patients and their families in arriving at a decision, there should be ongoing communication and a consensus should be achieved before reaching a final decision. One of the most significant concerns for patients and their families regards symptoms of pain, nausea, agitation, and respiratory decline in the final stages of life. While talking to the family, it is essential to understand what the family knows and what they wish to understand, and then communicate the information they need to make an informed decision. These decisions can cause significant distress and grief for the family so the physicians should understand their feelings, express empathy, and offer their support. The hallmark of palliative care is the relief of these symptoms to ensure that the patient is comfortable during the final days, and this should be discussed with patients and their families. Although all trauma/ acute care surgeons should be skilled in these conversations, collaboration with a palliative care team is strongly recommended. Chapter 6, Palliative Care and End of Life Issues, provides an in-depth discussion of this subject.

12.3.8.1 Key Points

- End-of-life decisions and withdrawal of care remains a challenge for geriatric patients.
- A patient-centered approach should be exercised to establish the goals of the treatment.
- An honest open communication between patients, their families, and caregivers is the cornerstone for high quality end-of-life care decisions.

12.4 Geriatric Emergency General Surgery

Emergency general surgery includes a diverse range of disorders that often presents a unique diagnostic and therapeutic challenge for the caregivers. Aging is associated with anatomical and physiological changes that further complicate the management of emergency general surgery in the elderly population. As the US population continues to age, the acute care surgeons are likely to see an increase number of these patients. It is essential for acute care surgeons to have a thorough understanding of the differences in the disease process, its presentation, and management to provide optimal care for these patients.

12.4.1 Clinical Presentation of Elderly Patients

Primary evaluation of the elderly patient with a suspected surgical emergency is challenging. Presentation of the elderly patients is often atypical, delayed, and vague.

Preexisting cognitive impairment or neurologic deficits (i.e., dementia, delirium, prior stroke, and neuropathy) are contributing factors for the atypical or delayed presentation of the patient or the ability to be detected by primary care providers [29]. Moreover, the history of present illness may be difficult to obtain as it is often complex, deficient, and imprecise. Physical examination similarly may be misleadingly benign and therefore not alert the surgeon to a serious underlying condition. Among patients hospitalized to an intensive care unit; altered mental status, absence of peritoneal signs, analgesics, antibiotics, and mechanical ventilation all contribute to delays and difficulties in surgical evaluation and treatment. All of these factors contribute to increased rates of morbidity and mortality among the elderly with surgical emergency conditions [30, 31].

12.4.2 Frailty and Emergency General Surgery

During the past few decades, quality of health care has become an important focus of outcomes research. The objective of such research is to bring to light best evidence-based practices that help improve patient outcomes. Countless studies have examined outcomes after general surgery in older adults. Predominantly, these studies have looked at mortality and complications as outcomes. The association of age and adverse outcomes is well established and validated. However, more recently the focus has shifted from age to functional status as a predictor of postoperative outcomes in patients undergoing general surgery. The use of objective measures of preoperative assessment helps in informed decision making, which is crucial for geriatric patients undergoing emergency general surgery and their families. The American College of Surgeons (ACS) has developed a surgical risk calculator based on multi-institutional NSQIP data that allows to accurately estimate the risk of most common surgical procedures and will help in informed decision making [32]. This risk calculator is based on 21 preoperative risk variables and also allows to adjust for surgeon's estimation of an increased risk using the Surgeon Adjustment Score (SAS). Several studies have shown that the NSQIP calculator reliably predicts the postoperative complication risk of surgical patients and aids clinicians and patients to make decisions using empirically derived patient-specific postoperative risks [33]. While accurate, the ACS NSQIP calculator does not incorporate several components of frailty that contribute significantly to the final postoperative outcomes of surgical patients. Studies have also shown that for patients undergoing emergency general surgery, frailty index better predicts complications and the addition of these additional variables to the NSQIP calculator may significantly improve the predictability of the NSQIP calculator [34].

Several models exist for the calculation of frailty index. The most comprehensive frailty questionnaire is the Rockwood frailty model based on 70 variables that assess the cognitive, physiological, physical, and social wellbeing of the individual. The Rockwood frailty index has been validated in patients undergoing an elective surgery. More recently a modified 50-variable Rockwood frailty index has been shown to reliably predict morbidity in patients undergoing emergency general surgery [35]. Interestingly, using the 15 strongest predictors out of the 50 variables, a similar predictability can be achieved. The use of this 15-variable EGS-specific frailty index allows for a more rapid yet accurate assessment of frailty status of patients undergoing emergency general surgery (see Table 12.1). For each question in the frailty index, a patient receives a score varying from 0 to 1. The sum of final score is then divided by 15 to calculate the frailty index of the patients. Patients with a frailty index of >0.325 are considered frail and are at high risk for morbidity following emergency general surgery.

12.4.2.1 Key Points
- Several risk assessment tools for geriatric patients undergoing emergency general surgery exist.
- Preoperative risk assessment aids the clinicians and patients in informed decision making.
- Frailty can be assessed in patients undergoing an emergency general surgery using a simple 15-variable EGS-specific frailty index.

12.4.3 Acute Diverticulitis

Diverticular disease is a common disorder in elderly resulting in 312,000 hospital admissions and 1.5 million days of inpatient care every year in the USA [36]. Over 75% of patients above 70 years of age in the western countries have colonic diverticulosis with left hemicolon being the most common site (sigmoid diverticulosis 95%) [37]. As individuals age, a variety of physiologic alterations manifest, many of which affect structural components of the colon, intraluminal pressure, colonic motility, and electrophysiology [38].

12.4.3.1 Age-Related Changes
Structural components of the extracellular matrix of the colonic wall are important in maintaining the strength and integrity of the colonic wall. Age-related changes take place in these components such as damage and breakdown of mature collagen and replacement with immature collagen. These changes decrease the compliance, leading to a stiffer tissue that is more vulnerable to tears especially under conditions of increased luminal pressures [39]. Age-related neural degeneration can lead to reduction of neurons in the mesenteric plexus and the intestinal cells of Cajal (the so called intestinal pacemaker cells), which induces smooth muscle dysfunction.

Age-related functional changes in the colon such as increased uncoordinated motor activity and high amplitude propagated tonic and rhythmic contractions result in segmentation, which significantly increases colonic intraluminal pressure. The pathogenesis of diverticulosis has also been associated with lack the dietary fiber. Other risk factors associated with diverticulosis are obesity, smoking, NSAID, and aspirin.

Up to 80% of diverticulosis patients are asymptomatic. Other symptoms vary from mild to severe fecal peritonitis with septic shock. In mild cases, patients present with lower abdominal pain and tenderness most commonly localized to the left side with loose stool or constipation. Elderly patients with intra-abdominal sepsis tend to present to physicians with less acute and delayed symptoms compared to younger patients. The classic triad of acute diverticulitis is lower abdominal pain, fever, and leukocytosis; however, this triad is only seen in less than half of cases. It is important to note that only 50% of elderly patients with intra-abdominal infection will present with nausea, vomiting, and fever. Cutaneous and visceral pain sensitivity decreases with age which can explain why elderly patients with abdominal sepsis present with a benign abdomen. The absence of definitive findings such as guarding and rigidity can decrease a physician's alertness to the presence of intra-abdominal sepsis. Thus, it is important that physicians maintain a high level of suspicion during physical examination of elderly patients [40].

The gold standard imaging test for the diagnosis of acute diverticulitis is computed tomographic (CT) scan which has a high sensitivity and specificity for the diagnosis of acute diverticulitis [41, 42]. The use of colonoscopy and sigmoidoscopy should be avoided in the acute stage of the disease as it may lead to perforation of the inflamed bowel. Colonoscopy is usually recommended 4–6 weeks after the acute phase of the inflammation to rule out other coexisting diseases such as cancer.

Conservative management for acute uncomplicated diverticulitis is successful in 70–100% of cases [43]. Geriatric patients with acute diverticulitis can be managed safely with outpatient therapy. For these patients the treatment of choice is 7–10 days of oral broad spectrum antibiotics [44]. Hospitalization is indicated only in patients that require analgesia, are unable to tolerate any diet, or in cases of complicated diverticulitis. The patient should be made NPO and broad spectrum antibiotics should be administered intravenously. These patients are followed serially with white cell counts, abdominal examination, and repeat CT scans (Fig. 12.1).

12.4.3.2 Key Points
- Several anatomical and physiological changes in the colon associated with advancing age predispose the elderly to diverticular disease.
- The presentation of acute diverticulitis in the elderly is subtle compared to the younger counterparts.

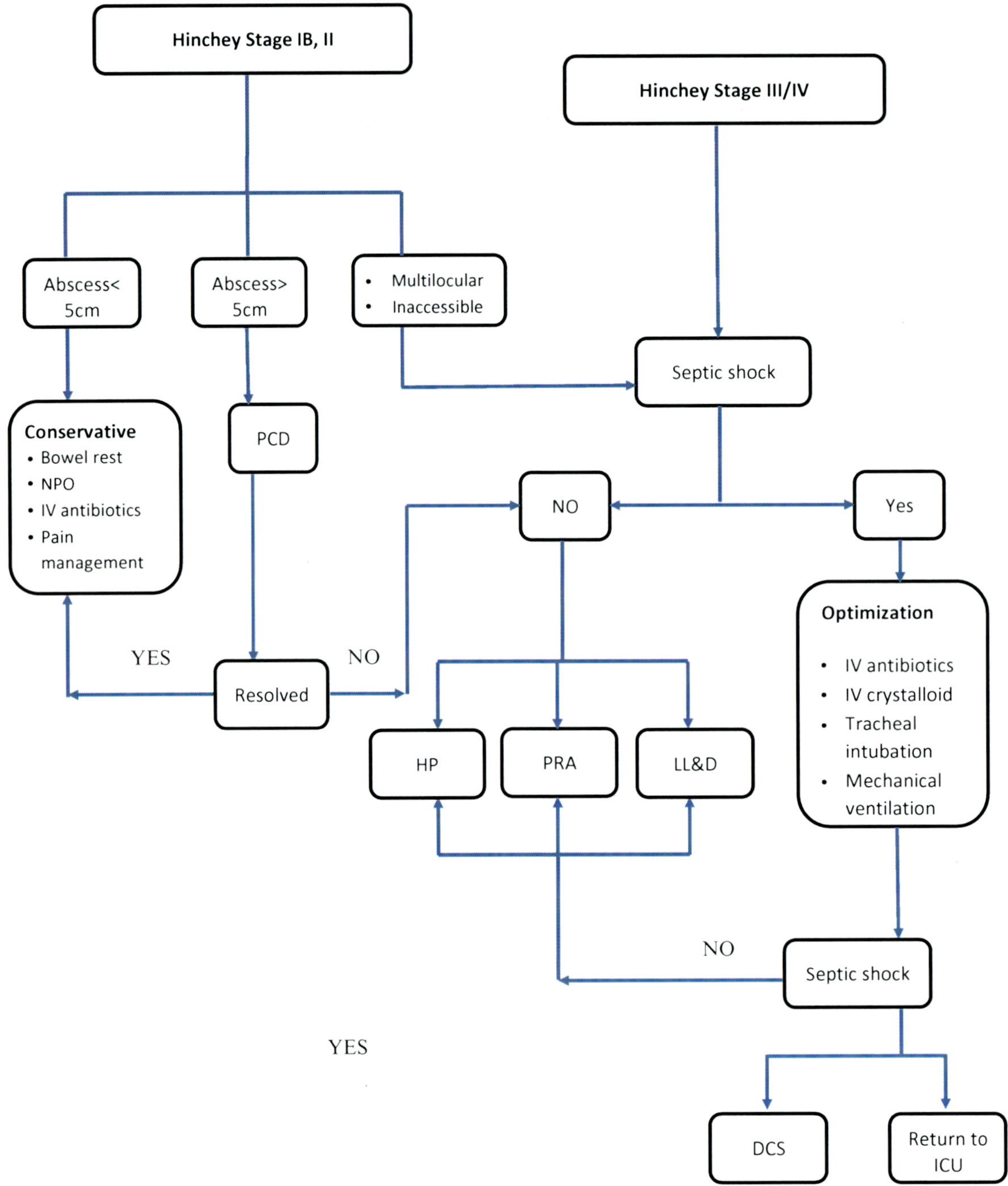

Fig. 12.1 Management of acute diverticulitis

- Medical management with bowel rest, analgesics, and antibiotics remain the corner stone treatment of acute diverticulitis.

12.4.4 Mesenteric Ischemia

Mesenteric ischemia is a rare but relatively common disorder in the elderly [45]. Despite the recent improvement in diagnosis and treatment, it is still associated with significant mortality rates around 60 % [46]. Approximately 50 % of elderly patients have a degree of atherosclerosis of the celiac, superior, and inferior mesenteric arteries which can precipitate acute mesenteric ischemia [47]. The superior mesenteric artery is most commonly implicated in acute mesenteric ischemia. Arterial embolism, arterial and venous thrombosis, and non-occlusive ischemia are the main causes of acute mesenteric ischemia [47]. Typically acute mesenteric ischemia presents with poorly localized severe abdominal pain classically described as "pain out of proportion" due to the absence of associated findings on physical examination [48]. The presence of these clinical features with pre-existing comorbidities such as atrial fibrillation, ischemic heart disease, and atherosclerosis should increase physicians' suspicion to consider mesenteric ischemia as a potential diagnosis. Of elderly patients, 30 % will present with nonspecific symptoms such as nausea, vomiting, or diarrhea that can mislead the diagnosis of mesenteric ischemia to a more benign disorder like gastroenteritis [48]. Ultimately, patients develop distention, shock, abdominal tenderness with guarding, and perforation [49]. Leukocytosis with a white blood cell count greater than $15,000/\mu$ is present in only 75 % of the patients. Metabolic acidosis and elevated serum lactate and amylase may be present if infarction has occurred. Fecal occult blood is reported in 50–75 % of the patients. Gross bleeding, however, occurs on rare occasions. As there is no definitive lab test and usually physical examination reveals nonspecific findings, physicians should maintain a high level of suspicion [50]. Plain X-rays films may initially be unremarkable but they may demonstrate intestinal distention and air-fluid levels. According to recent studies, CT angiography has a sensitivity of 80 % for diagnosing acute mesenteric infarction. Findings on CT scan indicative of mesenteric ischemia include thromboembolism in mesenteric vessels, portal venous gas, pneumatosis, diffuse bowel wall thickening, and mesenteric edema. Selective mesenteric angiography has a sensitivity of 90–100 % and is recommended if mesenteric ischemia is strongly suspected. However, due to the high prevalence of renal atherosclerosis in elderly, angiography can result in renal toxicity and should be kept in mind [47, 48].

12.4.4.1 Key Points
- Vague nonspecific clinical signs in geriatric patients can be deceiving.
- Comorbidities have a strong association with acute mesenteric ischemia.
- Early diagnosis and treatment of mesenteric ischemia in the elderly is crucial.

12.4.5 Acute Cholecystitis

Biliary tract disease including cholecystitis is the most common indication for abdominal surgery among elderly with abdominal pain [51]. The prevalence of gallstones increases sharply with age. About 15 % percent of men and 24 % of women have gallstones by the age 70. By age 90, this increases to 24 and 35 %, respectively [52]. Gallbladder disease in the elderly tends to be more severe compared to their younger counterparts as evidenced by the fact that a higher proportion of elderly patients undergo cholecystectomy for acute causes rather than elective cholecystectomy [53].

Biliary tract disease in the elderly is further complicated by the greater incidence of common bile duct stones. Common bile duct stones are found in patients undergoing cholecystectomy in up to 30 % of those in their 60s and in up to 50 % of those in their 70s [54]. Age-related changes in the biliary tract such as decrease bile salt secretion, increased cholesterol precipitation of the bile, increased common bile duct diameter, and decrease in gall bladder contractility are thought to account for the increased incidence of gallstone disease [55–57].

Acute cholecystitis presents a unique set of challenges in the elderly population. The typical presentation of acute cholecystitis includes severe right upper quadrant or epigastric pain, fever, nausea, and vomiting [53]. Laboratory values usually reveal leukocytosis with an increased number of band forms and may demonstrate a mild rise in transaminases, bilirubin, and alkaline phosphatase [58]. Diagnosis of acute cholecystitis in the elderly can be challenging as they commonly have a delayed and atypical clinical presentation. Abdominal pain remains a common presenting symptom but nausea, vomiting, fever, or leukocytosis is often absent. Symptoms are usually misleading and the clinical presentation is often blunted because of age-related physiological changes, mental illness, cognitive disability, dementia, or associated medications [59]. Around 40 % of elderly patients presenting with acute cholecystitis do not develop fever and more than 50 % may have negative peritoneal signs on examination. Absence of these signs does not indicate milder form of the disease as 40 % of the patients have severe complications [60]. The estimated diagnostic accuracy of clinical examination in acute abdominal pain in patients over the age of 80 is only 29 %, which is significantly low compared to younger patients [61]. Approximately 12 % of elderly patients with acute cholecystitis present in septic shock [62]. Surgical risks and complications of acute cholecystitis occur in more than 50 % of all patients older than 65 years. Complications include acute ascending cholangitis, gallbladder perforation, emphysematous cholecystitis, biliary peritonitis, carcinomatous changes, and gallstone ileus [63]. Acute ascending cholangitis is a disease of the elderly and rarely occurs before the age of 40. Most patients with acute ascending cholangitis present with Charcot's triad (i.e., fever, jaundice, and right upper quadrant pain) and occasionally as Reynold's pentad (i.e., Charcot's triad plus shock and mental status changes) [64].

Liver function tests remain the most important laboratory investigation in patients with suspected gall bladder disease. Patients with acute cholecystitis can present with a mild elevation in serum ALT and AST levels, however, the most significant abnormal laboratory values include the levels of bilirubin (total and fractionated) and alkaline phosphatase (AP). Ultrasound is the diagnostic gold standard for the diagnosis of acute cholecystitis.

Asymptomatic gallstones are a common feature in the elderly. Most patients with gallstones never develop acute cholecystitis. Among patients who experience a single episode of biliary colic, nearly half will never experience a second episode of colic within 5 years [65]. Based on these facts, conservative management of biliary colic may be considered appropriate for most elderly patients. Differentiating biliary colic from acute cholecystitis can be challenging in the elderly patients with diabetes mellitus. The presentation of acute cholecystitis in elderly patient with diabetes associated neuropathy is minimal. In such patients gangrenous cholecystitis can present with minimal symptoms and negative peritoneal signs can be misinterpreted as a recurrent attack of biliary colic [59]. Therefore, a very low threshold for suspicion should be maintained for these patients.

The gold standard for the management of acute cholecystitis is laparoscopic cholecystectomy. The rate of emergent cholecystectomy in patients older than age 65 is 37.6 % compared to 3.3 % in younger patients [66]. Postoperative morbidity, particularly cardiovascular and pulmonary complications, is significantly greater after emergent cholecystectomy compared to elective cholecystectomy in elderly patients [53]. For patients who are non-operative candidates or who cannot tolerate anesthesia in emergent settings, non-operative management with and antibiotics has shown to be effective.

12.4.5.1 Key Points

- The presentation of gall bladder disease in the elderly is extremely subtle compared to the younger counterparts.
- Early laparoscopic cholecystectomy is the gold standard treatment for acute cholecystitis across all age groups
- Biliary tract decompression with cholecystostomy and antibiotics has shown to be effective in non-operative candidates with acute cholecystitis.

12.4.6 Acute Appendicitis

Acute appendicitis is the most common emergent abdominal surgery performed with a lifetime incidence of 7 % [67]. Generally, appendicitis is considered to be a disease of the young with only 5–10 % of cases occurring in the elderly population. However, the incidence of the disease in the elderly is increasing due to an increase in the elderly population. Acute appendicitis is the third most common cause of abdominal pain in elderly [18]. The pathophysiology of appendicitis in the elderly is similar to the young however, there are several differences in the elderly that predispose them to increased progression and early perforation. The lumen of the appendix is narrowed and atherosclerosis compromises the blood flow to the appendix [68, 69]. As a result even mild increases in intraluminal pressure can lead to gangrene and perforation [67].

The reported incidence of perforation in elderly patients with acute appendicitis is as high as 70 % [70]. The blunted inflammatory response in the elderly prevents the development of significant clinical features of acute appendicitis and delays the presentation. This delay is further complicated by the delay in the time from presentation to the operating room and is associated with increased morbidity and perforation rates [71–73]. The diagnosis of acute appendicitis in the elderly is often delayed due to other suspected etiologies. Age-related physiological changes, atypical presentation, and a delay in seeking medical help lead to the delay in diagnosis and treatment. Due to these reasons, acute appendicitis is the leading cause of intra-abdominal abscess and fever of unknown origin in elderly. The prognosis of uncomplicated appendicitis in both the young and old age groups is equal, however, when perforated appendicitis occurs the elderly have a mortality rate of 33–50 % [67].

The use of scoring systems such as Alvarado score (a 10 point assessment using signs, symptoms and laboratory values) can aid in the diagnosis of acute appendicitis however, these scoring systems lack the sensitivity to safely exclude acute appendicitis. Therefore, there has been a recent trend in the use of imaging such as computed tomography (CT) scan and magnetic resonance imaging (MRI) for the diagnosis of acute appendicitis. The sensitivity of these diagnostic modalities for acute appendicitis is nearly 100 % and has been validated even in the elderly cohort of patients [74]. As the presentation of acute appendicitis in the elderly is significantly delayed, early use of imaging modalities may help reduce the time to the operating room in these patients.

Laparoscopic appendectomy is safe and remains the gold standard for the treatment of acute appendicitis in the elderly [75]. More recently antibiotics have gained popularity for the treatment of acute appendicitis. A recent randomized control trial demonstrated the antibiotics are a safe first line therapy in the treatment of acute appendicitis for all age groups [76]. Despite this, the morbidity and mortality associated with acute appendicitis in the elderly remains high. The elderly patients have significantly higher complications and mortality compared to their younger counter parts [77].

12.4.6.1 Key Points

- The presentation of acute appendicitis is delayed in the elderly and is associated with a higher incidence of gangrene and perforation.
- Laparoscopic appendectomy remains the gold standard treatment for acute appendicitis however, recent data suggests that the use of oral antibiotics for the treatment of acute appendicitis is safe and effective.
- The overall morbidity and mortality after acute appendicitis in the elderly is high compared to their younger counter parts.

12.5 Perioperative Care in Emergency Surgery

In recent years, interest has grown in the impact of surgery in the elderly. As the baby boomers continue to age, the number of geriatric patients undergoing surgery is increasing. It is therefore crucial that health care providers gain substantial knowledge and understanding of the care of the elderly patients. It is also important for health care providers to understand the differences in the elderly patients compared to their younger counterparts and how management needs to be modified to improve outcomes. Pre- and post-operative care is critical in elderly as they have higher rates of morbidity, which can alter the potential benefits of surgery in this population.

12.5.1 Preoperative Care

Preoperative assessment is performed to identify risk factors that lead to adverse outcomes. The pathophysiology of disease and the actual surgical procedure are important prognostic factors. However, the most important factors in the determination of postoperative morbidity and mortality are related to the general health and physiological reserve of the patient [78]. Diminished physiologic reserves have a direct impact on the patients' ability to bear the additional stress of surgery and the possible postoperative complications. In addition, comorbid status has a major impact on the surgical outcomes. The identification of these risk factors allows for optimization of these factors prior to surgery and has been shown to substantially improve the surgical outcomes in these patients.

12.5.2 Postoperative Care

12.5.2.1 Delirium

Delirium is defined as a state of temporary altered mental status. Two types of delirium usually present in the postoperative phase; emergence delirium (ED) and postoperative delirium (POD). ED is a benign cognitive disorientation that can occur during the transition from anesthesia to wakefulness and resolves within minutes or hours, while POD is an acute organic brain syndrome that usually develops within the first few postoperative days [79, 80]. POD is an acute disorder, but has been associated with a wide range of negative long-term outcomes for the elderly, despite that patients may initially recover completely. Approximately 15 % of all elderly patients experience POD after elective procedures with a higher incidence (30–70 %) among elderly undergoing emergency operations [81]. POD can prolong the hospital length of stay and the postoperative dependence of elderly people. It is also associated with reduced function

and independence, increased short- and long-term mortality, and prolonged cognitive impairment in survivors [78]. The definitive mechanism that underlies delirium is not clearly known; many hypotheses however agree that delirium is the final clinical consequence of complicated neurotransmitter abnormalities. Several associated factors for delirium have been identified which include infection, inflammation, metabolite disturbances, substance withdrawal, medications, discomfort, restraints, environmental disturbances including sleep disruption and severe pain with inadequate analgesia. There are several criteria to diagnose delirium: disturbed consciousness, cognitive changes, rapid onset and fluctuating course, presence of a causal medical condition, or change of substance usage [78, 82]. Delirium is discussed fully in Chap. 2.

12.5.2.2 Infection

Postoperative infections are an important cause of morbidity and mortality in elderly patients. Although the mechanism of how the aging process decreases the immunologic response is still unclear, it is well demonstrated in literature that elderly patients have diminished immune function that makes them more vulnerable to infection [83]. The most common sites of postoperative infection are the urinary tract, lungs, and surgical site [83]. Urinary tract infection (UTI) is typically due to prolonged bladder catheterization. Approximately 25 % of hospitalized patients undergo urinary bladder catheterization of these, 10–27 % develop UTIs [84]. Around 80 % of patients with nosocomial UTIs undergo urinary bladder catheterization. There is an increase in the need for urinary bladder catheterization in elderly patients for several reasons including medication side effects, neurogenic bladder, or obstruction secondary to spinal cord injury/ disease, multiple sclerosis, enlarged prostate, or cerebrovascular accident. Urinary catheters may also be used to provide supportive care for incontinent patients with open wounds located in the sacral or perineal regions (e.g. pressure ulcer). Although urinary tract infections and respiratory tract infections are the most common infections leading to delirium; the correlation with asymptomatic bacteriuria as a cause for delirium is still unknown and somewhat controversial. Elderly patients usually present with the classic symptoms of dysuria, fever, and frequency, which are commonly present in younger people, but they may present with more vague presentations such as an acute confusion state, decreased mobility, or newly developed urinary incontinence. Postoperative confusion may be the first and only sign of a UTI in elderly. It is important to recognize that diagnosis of UTI in the absence of dysuria, frequency or urgency is challenging. It is therefore necessary to examine the patient completely for other possible diagnoses and obtain objective laboratory data. The diagnosis should be made based on both the laboratory and clinical presentation of the patient.

One of the most important preventive strategies in the elderly patients is to minimize the use of urinary catheters and early removal of the catheters [83]. Many other strategies have been attempted to minimize bacterial colonization and subsequent infection such as disinfecting the skin regularly and using disinfectants in the collecting system. Hospitals should develop guidelines and protocolize the process of urinary catheterization regarding appropriate indications for insertion, maintenance techniques, and indications for removal and replacement. Hospital systems should also educate staff about these indications, and follow up via quality improvement programs.

Patients in the intensive care unit (ICU) are at risk for dying not only from their primary disease but also secondary to in-hospital complications such as nosocomial infections. Nosocomial pneumonia (NP) is the second most common nosocomial infection which occurs primarily in patients undergoing general surgery. Ventilator-associated pneumonia (VAP) is defined as pneumonia occurring more than 48 h after patients have been intubated and received mechanical ventilation. Diagnosing VAP requires a high clinical suspicion combined with bedside examination, radiographic examination, and microbiologic analysis of respiratory secretions. It is the leading cause of postoperative mortality in elderly patients [85]. Although NP has the same presentation and management in all age groups, certain risk factors including age and depleted physiological reserve make the elderly more vulnerable to develop NP. Also nasogastric tubes, tracheal intubation, dementia, aspiration, recent chest or abdominal surgery, and immobility can increase the risk for developing NP [85]. Underlying comorbidities, malnutrition, and impaired immune function increase the mortality associated with postoperative pneumonia in the elderly [83].

Surgical site infection (SSI) is an important postoperative complication and is the most common nosocomial infection in surgical patients, accounting for 38 % of nosocomial infections in this patient population [86]. It has a huge impact on morbidity and is also associated with substantial economic burden on the patients and the health care system [87]. Most significantly, the elderly patients with SSI have three times higher mortality than that of the elderly patients without infections [87, 88]. SSI can be defined as infection related to an operative procedure that occurs at or near the surgical incision within 30 days of the procedure or within 1 year if prosthetic material is implanted at surgery. It is related to the operative procedure and technique as well as patient-specific factors. Advanced age is considered a host-derived risk factor for surgical site infection [89]. SSI is caused by organisms introduced into the surgical wound at the time of the operative procedure [87]. Most of these organisms originate from the patient's own flora however, exogenous sources of bacteria can also lead to an infection. SSI can be prevented by the application of preventive practices such as appropriate antibiotic selection and administration, intraoperative maintenance of normothermia, the avoidance of shaving the surgical site until just prior to incising the skin, and ensuring perioperative euglycemia [89, 90]. Close monitoring of surgical wounds postoperatively is necessary to ensure the early detection and treatment of wound infections. Treatment of SSI involves opening the incision and allowing adequate drainage. The use of antibiotics should be guided by culture and sensitivity test [87]. Chapter 24, Infection and Immunity in Older Adults, provides a detailed discussion about the complexities of infections in seniors.

12.5.2.3 Cardiac Complications

Myocardial Ischemia and Infarction

Cardiac complications such as myocardial infarction and heart failure are the most common causes of postoperative morbidity and mortality that occur in 1–5 % of patients undergoing noncardiac surgery [91, 92]. At least 10 % of all perioperative deaths result from myocardial complications. The most common postoperative cardiac complications in the elderly patients are myocardial ischemia and myocardial infarction. The elderly are also more vulnerable to have post-myocardial infarction and heart failure [93]. The mortality associated with perioperative myocardial infarction is approximately 30 % [78]. Comorbid conditions such as hypertension, diabetes mellitus, and history of cardiac or renal failure are risk factors for higher incidence of perioperative myocardial infarction (5.1 %), cardiac death (5.7 %), or ischemia (12–17.7 %) in elderly patients [93].

The majority of perioperative myocardial infarctions occur during the first 3 days postoperatively and predominantly on the 1st postoperative day [94]. Although chest pain is the most common presenting symptom of myocardial ischemia in young patients, elderly patients may present with minimal chest pain which may be misleading. Myocardial ischemic events are silent in over 80 % of elderly patients [95]. Diagnosis of cardiac ischemic attacks during the postoperative period is often missed because of incisional pain, residual anesthetic effects, postoperative analgesia, and the lack of typical angina pain by elderly patients. Atypical presentation such as tachycardia hypotension, dyspnea, respiratory failure, syncope, confusion, nausea, and excessive hyperglycemia in diabetics are more common presentations of myocardial ischemia in the elderly.

Dysrhythmias

Postoperative arrhythmias are common and represent a major source of morbidity after both cardiac and noncardiac surgical procedures [96]. Postoperative atrial arrhythmias occur in 6.1 % of elderly patients undergoing noncardiac surgery [97]. Electrolyte disturbances and increased sympathetic nervous system activity postoperatively may lead to cardiac dysrhythmias, although myocardial ischemia or congestive heart failure should be taken in account [98].

The only proven preoperative risk factor for developing an atrial arrhythmia following surgery is age greater than 60 years [98]. Patients aged more than 60 years and undergoing elective thoracic surgery are independently associated with a higher risk for developing atrial fibrillation [97]. Cardiac arrhythmias may also be stimulated by pulmonary disease such as pneumonia or pulmonary embolism, volume overload, hyperthyroidism, or sympathomimetic drugs. Atrial arrhythmia-onset peaks 2–3 days following surgery. Perioperative atrial arrhythmias are usually well tolerated in younger patients, however in elderly can be associated with hemodynamic instability in elderly patients. The complications of atrial fibrillation include stroke and congestive heart failure. Atrial fibrillation is also associated with higher inpatient mortality when accompanied by myocardial infarction (25 vs. 16 %) [99]. Management of atrial fibrillation consists of heart rhythm and rate control and prophylaxis against thromboembolism.

Cardiac issues are discussed in depth in Chap. 21, Cardiovascular Disease.

12.5.2.4 Pulmonary Complications

Postoperative pulmonary complications are common especially in elderly patients with comorbidities. Nearly 5 % of all patients undergoing noncardiac surgery experience significant pulmonary complications, which are a common cause of postoperative morbidity and mortality. They account for up to 40 % of all postoperative complications and 20 % of potentially preventable deaths [100]. The most common pulmonary complications are lung collapse, hypoxemia, hypoventilation, acute respiratory distress syndrome, and pneumonia. Development of these complications can extend the intensive care unit stay and increase mortality. Patients of 70 years of age and above have a higher risk of respiratory complications including bacterial pneumonia, noncardiogenic pulmonary edema, and respiratory failure requiring intubation compared to younger patients [101]. Age-related alterations in pulmonary function combined with postoperative pulmonary pathophysiologic changes place the elderly patient at greater risk for complications. Clinical predictors of adverse pulmonary outcomes include site of surgery (chest, abdomen), duration and type of anesthesia, chronic obstructive pulmonary disease (COPD), asthma, preoperative hypersecretion of mucus, chest deformation, and perioperative nasogastric tube placement [102].

Aspiration

Aspiration is defined as the inhalation of oropharyngeal or gastric contents into the larynx and lower respiratory tract. Normal deglutition is a smooth coordinated process that involves a complex series of voluntary and involuntary neuromuscular contractions. Age-related changes affect each phase of the swallowing process, increasing the risk of aspiration in the elderly [103]. Other risk factors in the elderly that make them particularly vulnerable to oropharyngeal aspiration include dysphagia, poor oral hygiene, altered level of consciousness, and gastroesophageal reflux disease [103]. Dysphagia and recurrent pneumonia in elderly patients are alarming factors for the physicians. Patients found to be aspirating should undergo swallow therapy, modification of dietary consistency, training in specific swallowing techniques, and upright positioning while feeding. Surgery is rarely indicated.

Chapter 27 provides an in-depth discussion of pulmonary and critical care issues.

12.6 Geriatric Specialists and Geriatric Specialized Centers

The physiologic differences in the pediatric population compared to the adults led to the eventual recognition of pediatrics as a specialty and the establishment of pediatric centers including pediatric trauma centers. Similar to the pediatric population, geriatrics has matured as a specialty and the geriatric patient population is now being recognized as a specialized population that should receive care in the hands of specialists trained in taking care of these patients and at specialized geriatric centers dedicated to geriatric care [104]. Although currently there are no dedicated geriatric surgical centers in the USA, there is emerging evidence that suggests that centers which handle higher volume and higher proportion of geriatric patients have better outcomes [105]. Indeed, the American College of Surgeons (The Coalition for Quality In Geriatric Surgery Project) is launching in 2016 an investigation focused on developing criteria for Geriatric Surgical Centers. Many academic centers now have a geriatric program that provides a consultation service for inpatients. These geriatric programs rely on an interdisciplinary collaboration of physicians, surgeons, nurse practitioners, pharmacists, social workers, physical and occupational therapists, and geriatricians to meet the needs of geriatric patients. Some centers have dedicated geriatric units to provide care for elderly patients transferred from other services. Along with the inpatient care of elderly patients; these geriatric programs also emphasize and provide early rehabilitation services for these patients [106]. The effectiveness of these geriatric programs has been evaluated in several randomized controlled trials. The largest trial randomized over 1300 frail patients to receive geriatric inpatient care or usual inpatient care [107]. Patients who received geriatric inpatient care had significantly reduced morbidity and improved functional recovery quality of life at the time of discharge compared to the patients who received usual inpatient care.

The overall 1-year mortality and total costs were similar between the two groups.

As the US health system transitions from a fee-for-service model to a fee-for-quality model, comprehensive geriatric programs and appropriate follow-up services represent a promising approach that can yield substantial benefits without incurring extra costs to the overall health system.

12.6.1 Key Points

- Geriatric patients are a distinct patient population that require specialized care.
- Several hospitals have developed interdisciplinary geriatric programs to provide comprehensive geriatric assessment and care for elderly patients.
- The use of geriatric programs is associated with improved functional recovery and rehabilitation.

There are no conflicts of interests to report. The authors have no financial or proprietary interest in the subject matter or materials discussed in the manuscript.

References

1. Friese R, Wynne J, Joseph B, et al. Age and mortality after injury: is the association linear? Eur J Trauma Emerg Surg. 2014;40(5):567–72.
2. Rzepka SG, Malangoni MA, Rimm AA. Geriatric trauma hospitalization in the United States: a population-based study. J Clin Epidemiol. 2001;54(6):627–33.
3. Rhee P, Joseph B, Pandit V, et al. Increasing trauma deaths in the United States. Ann Surg. 2014;260(1):13–21.
4. Gillies D. Elderly trauma: they are different. Aust Crit Care. 1999;12(1):24–30.
5. Lord SR, Sherrington C, Menz HB, Close JC. Falls in older people: risk factors and strategies for prevention. Cambridge University Press; 2007. p. 3–26.
6. Joseph B, Pandit V, Khalil M, et al. Managing older adults with ground-level falls admitted to a trauma service: the effect of frailty. J Am Geriatr Soc. 2015;63(4):745–9.
7. Trauma ACoSCo. Advanced trauma life support student course manual. Chicago: American College of Surgeons; 2012.
8. Çevik Y, Doğan NÖ, Daş M, Karakayalı O, Delice O, Kavalcı C. Evaluation of geriatric patients with trauma scores after motor vehicle trauma. Am J Emerg Med. 2013;31(10):1453–6.
9. Sifrit KJ, Stutts J, Staplin L, Martell C. Intersection crashes among drivers in their 60s, 70s and 80s. Paper presented at: proceedings of the human factors and ergonomics society annual meeting, 2010.
10. Huang S-B, Chang W-H, Huang C-H, Tsai C-H. Management of elderly burn patients. Int J Gerontol. 2008;2(3):91–7.
11. Jacobs DG, Plaisier BR, Barie PS, et al. Practice management guidelines for geriatric trauma: the EAST Practice Management Guidelines Work Group. J Trauma Acute Care Surg. 2003;54(2):391–416.
12. Evers BM, Townsend Jr C, Thompson J. Organ physiology of aging. Surg Clin North Am. 1994;74(1):23–39.
13. Stamatos C. Geriatric trauma patients: initial assessment and management of shock. J Trauma Nurs. 1993;1(2):45–54. quiz 55-46.
14. Scalea TM, Simon HM, Duncan AO, et al. Geriatric blunt multiple trauma: improved survival with early invasive monitoring. J Trauma Acute Care Surg. 1990;30(2):129–36.
15. Morris JA, MacKenzie EJ, Edelstein SL. The effect of preexisting conditions on mortality in trauma patients. JAMA. 1990;263(14):1942–6.
16. Muse DA. Conscious and deep sedation. In: The Clinical Practice of Emergency Medicine, 3rd ed, Harwood-Nuss, A, Wolfson, AB (Eds), Lippincott, Williams and Wilkins, Philadelphia 2001. p.1761.
17. Battle CE, Hutchings H, Evans PA. Risk factors that predict mortality in patients with blunt chest wall trauma: a systematic review and meta-analysis. Injury. 2012;43(1):8–17.
18. Kacey DJ, Perez-Tamayo A. Principles and practice of geriatric surgery. JAMA. 2012;307(18):1981.
19. McGwin Jr G, MacLennan PA, Fife JB, Davis GG, Rue III LW. Preexisting conditions and mortality in older trauma patients. J Trauma Acute Care Surg. 2004;56(6):1291–6.
20. Caterino JM, Valasek T, Werman HA. Identification of an age cutoff for increased mortality in patients with elderly trauma. Am J Emerg Med. 2010;28(2):151–8.
21. Barie PS, Hammond JS, Holevar MR, Sinclair KE, Scalea TM, Wahl W. Practice management guidelines for geriatric trauma. 2001.
22. Pandit V, Rhee P, Hashmi A, et al. Shock index predicts mortality in geriatric trauma patients: an analysis of the National Trauma Data Bank. J Trauma Acute Care Surg. 2014;76(4):1111–5.
23. Ellis G, Marshall T, Ritchie C. Comprehensive geriatric assessment in the emergency department. Clin Interv Aging. 2014;9:2033.
24. Jokar TO, Rhee PM, Zangbar B, et al. Redefining the association between old age and poor outcomes after trauma: the impact of the frailty syndrome. J Am Coll Surg. 2015;221(4):S83–4.
25. Joseph B, Pandit V, Zangbar B, et al. Superiority of frailty over age in predicting outcomes among geriatric trauma patients: a prospective analysis. JAMA Surg. 2014;149(8):766–72.
26. Joseph B, Pandit V, Zangbar B, et al. Validating trauma-specific frailty index for geriatric trauma patients: a prospective analysis. J Am Coll Surg. 2014;219(1):10–7. e11.
27. Joseph B, Pandit V, Rhee P, et al. Predicting hospital discharge disposition in geriatric trauma patients: is frailty the answer? J Trauma Acute Care Surg. 2014;76(1):196–200.
28. Chang TT, Schecter WP. Injury in the elderly and end-of-life decisions. Surg Clin North Am. 2007;87(1):229–45. viii.
29. Kim PK, Kauder DR, Schwab CW. Acute care surgery and the elderly. In Britt LD, Trunkey DD, Feliciano DV, eds. Acute care surgery principles and practice. Springer; 2007. p. 187–93.
30. Levkoff SE, Cleary PD, Wetle T, Besdine RW. Illness behavior in the aged. J Am Geriatr Soc. 1988;36(7):622–9.
31. Watters JM, Blakslee JM, March RJ, Redmond ML. The influence of age on the severity of peritonitis. Can J Surg. 1996;39(2):142.
32. Bilimoria KY, Liu Y, Paruch JL, et al. Development and evaluation of the universal ACS NSQIP surgical risk calculator: a decision aid and informed consent tool for patients and surgeons. J Am Coll Surg. 2013;217(5):833–42.e831–3.
33. Faraklas I, Stoddard GJ, Neumayer LA, Cochran A. Development and validation of a necrotizing soft-tissue infection mortality risk calculator using NSQIP. J Am Coll Surg. 2013;217(1):153–60. e153; discussion 160-151.
34. Sadoum M, Zangbar B, Rhee PM, et al. NSQIP surgical risk calculator and frailty in emergency general surgery: a measure of surgical resilience. J Am Coll Surg. 2015;221(4):130.

35. Joseph B, Pandit V, Zangbar B, et al. Emergency general surgery in the elderly: too old or too frail? J Am Coll Surg. 2014;219(3): 53–4.

36. Matrana MR, Margolin DA. Epidemiology and pathophysiology of diverticular disease. Clin Colon Rectal Surg. 2009;22(3): 141–6.

37. Reisman Y, Ziv Y, Kravrovitc D, Negri M, Wolloch Y, Halevy A. Diverticulitis: the effect of age and location on the course of disease. Int J Colorectal Dis. 1999;14(4-5):250–4.

38. Thomson H, Busuttil A, Eastwood M, Smith A, Elton R. Submucosal collagen changes in the normal colon and in diverticular disease. Int J Colorectal Dis. 1987;2(4):208–13.

39. Stumpf M, Cao W, Klinge U, Klosterhalfen B, Kasperk R, Schumpelick V. Increased distribution of collagen type III and reduced expression of matrix metalloproteinase 1 in patients with diverticular disease. Int J Colorectal Dis. 2001;16(5):271–5.

40. Clinch D, Banerjee AK, Ostick G. Absence of abdominal pain in elderly patients with peptic ulcer. Age Ageing. 1984;13(2): 120–3.

41. Ambrosetti P, Grossholz M, Becker C, Terrier F, Morel P. Computed tomography in acute left colonic diverticulitis. Br J Surg. 1997;84(4):532–4.

42. Cho KC, Morehouse HT, Alterman DD, Thornhill BA. Sigmoid diverticulitis: diagnostic role of CT—comparison with barium enema studies. Radiology. 1990;176(1):111–5.

43. Kellum JM, Sugerman HJ, Coppa GF, et al. Randomized, prospective comparison of cefoxitin and gentamicin-clindamycin in the treatment of acute colonic diverticulitis. Clin Ther. 1992;14(3): 376–84.

44. Jacobs DO. Diverticulitis. N Engl J Med. 2007;357(20): 2057–66.

45. Kärkkäinen JM, Lehtimäki TT, Manninen H, Paajanen H. Acute mesenteric ischemia is a more common cause than expected of acute abdomen in the elderly. J Gastrointest Surg. 2015;1–8.

46. Shih M-CP, Hagspiel KD. CTA and MRA in mesenteric ischemia: part 1, role in diagnosis and differential diagnosis. Am J Roentgenol. 2007;188(2):452–61.

47. Ruotolo RA, Evans S. Mesenteric ischemia in the elderly. Clin Geriatr Med. 1999;15(3):527–57.

48. Greenwald DA, Brandt LJ, Reinus JF. Ischemic bowel disease in the elderly. Gastroenterol Clin North Am. 2001;30(2): 445–73.

49. Dupee RM. Case report: acute intestinal ischemia in the elderly. Ann Long Term Care. 2008;16(3):34.

50. Roth L, Greenberger NJ, Blumberg RS, Burakoff R. Current diagnosis & treatment: gastoenterology, hepatology, & endoscopy. 3rd ed. New York: McGraw Hill Companies Inc; 2009. ISSN 1946-3030. Can J Gastroenterol Hepatol. 2010;24(2):97.

51. Brunt L, Quasebarth M, Dunnegan D, Soper N. Outcomes analysis of laparoscopic cholecystectomy in the extremely elderly. Surg Endosc. 2001;15(7):700–5.

52. Riall TS, Zhang D, Townsend CM, Kuo Y-F, Goodwin JS. Failure to perform cholecystectomy for acute cholecystitis in elderly patients is associated with increased morbidity, mortality, and cost. J Am Coll Surg. 2010;210(5):668–77.

53. Wargo JA, Kahng KU. Benign disease of the gallbladder and pancreas. In: Rosenthal RA, Zenilman ME, Katlic MR, editors. Principles and practice of geriatric surgery. 2nd ed. New York: Springer; 2011. p. 361–76.

54. Krasman M, Gracie W, Strasius S. Biliary tract disease in the aged. Clin Geriatr Med. 1991;7(2):347–70.

55. Einarsson K, Nilsell K, Leijd B, Angelin B. Influence of age on secretion of cholesterol and synthesis of bile acids by the liver. N Engl J Med. 1985;313(5):277–82.

56. Jansen PL, Strautnieks SS, Jacquemin E, et al. Hepatocanalicular bile salt export pump deficiency in patients with progressive familial intrahepatic cholestasis. Gastroenterology. 1999;117(6): 1370–9.

57. Poston GJ, Singh P, Maclellan DG, et al. Age-related changes in gallbladder contractility and gallbladder cholecystokinin receptor population in the guinea pig. Mech Ageing Dev. 1988; 46(1–3): 225–36.

58. Parker LJ, Vukov LF, Wollan PC. Emergency department evaluation of geriatric patients with acute cholecystitis. Acad Emerg Med. 1997;4(1):51–5.

59. Cobden I, Venables C, Lendrum R, James O. Gallstones presenting as mental and physical debility in the elderly. Lancet. 1984;323(8385):1062–4.

60. Morrow DJ, Thompson J, Wilson SE. Acute cholecystitis in the elderly: a surgical emergency. Arch Surg. 1978;113(10):1149–52.

61. De Dombal F. Acute abdominal pain in the elderly. J Clin Gastroenterol. 1994;19(4):331–5.

62. Hafif A, Gutman M, Kaplan O, Winkler E, Rozin R, Skornick Y. The management of acute cholecystitis in elderly patients. Am Surg. 1991;57(10):648–52.

63. Lyon C, Clark DC. Diagnosis of acute abdominal pain in older patients. Am Fam Physician. 2006;74(9):1537–44.

64. Hanau LH, Steigbigel NH. Acute (ascending) cholangitis. Infect Dis Clin North Am. 2000;14(3):521–46.

65. Siegel JH, Kasmin FE. Biliary tract diseases in the elderly: management and outcomes. Gut. 1997;41(4):433–5.

66. Glenn F. Acute cholecystitis. Surg Gynecol Obstet. 1976;143(1): 56–60.

67. Omari AH, Khammash MR, Qasaimeh GR, Shammari AK, Yaseen MK, Hammori SK. Acute appendicitis in the elderly: risk factors for perforation. World J Emerg Surg. 2014;9(1):6.

68. Freund H, Rubinstein E. Appendicitis in the aged. Is it really different? Am Surg. 1984;50(10):573–6.

69. Paajanen H, Kettunen J, Kostiainen S. Emergency appendectomies in patients over 80 years. Am Surg. 1994;60(12):950–3.

70. Yamini D, Vargas H, Bongard F, Klein S, Stamos MJ. Perforated appendicitis: is it truly a surgical urgency? Am Surg. 1998;64(10): 970–5.

71. Eldar S, Nash E, Sabo E, et al. Delay of surgery in acute appendicitis. Am J Surg. 1997;173(3):194–8.

72. Segev L, Keidar A, Schrier I, Rayman S, Wasserberg N, Sadot E. Acute appendicitis in the elderly in the twenty-first century. J Gastrointest Surg. 2015;19(4):730–5.

73. Sherlock DJ. Acute appendicitis in the over-sixty age group. Br J Surg. 1985;72(3):245–6.

74. Pooler BD, Lawrence EM, Pickhardt PJ. MDCT for suspected appendicitis in the elderly: diagnostic performance and patient outcome. Emerg Radiol. 2012;19(1):27–33.

75. Guller U, Jain N, Peterson ED, Muhlbaier LH, Eubanks S, Pietrobon R. Laparoscopic appendectomy in the elderly. Surgery. 2004;135(5):479–88.

76. Hansson J, Körner U, Khorram-Manesh A, Solberg A, Lundholm K. Randomized clinical trial of antibiotic therapy versus appendicectomy as primary treatment of acute appendicitis in unselected patients. Br J Surg. 2009;96(5):473–81.

77. Hui TT, Major KM, Avital I, Hiatt JR, Margulies DR. Outcome of elderly patients with appendicitis: effect of computed tomography and laparoscopy. Arch Surg. 2002;137(9):995–8; discussion 999–1000.

78. Lagoo-Deenadayalan SA, Newell MA, Pofahl WE. Common perioperative complications in older patients. In: Rosenthal RA, Zenilman ME, Katlic MR, editors. Principles and practice of geriatric surgery. 2nd ed. New York: Springer; 2011. p. 361–76.

79. Radtke F, Franck M, Hagemann L, Seeling M, Wernecke K, Spies C. Risk factors for inadequate emergence after anesthesia: emergence delirium and hypoactive emergence. Minerva Anestesiol. 2010;76(6):394–403.

80. Young J, Inouye SK. Delirium in older people. BMJ. 2007; 334(7598):842.

81. Ansaloni L, Catena F, Chattat R, et al. Risk factors and incidence of postoperative delirium in elderly patients after elective and emergency surgery. Br J Surg. 2010;97(2):273–80.

82. Strøm C, Rasmussen L. Challenges in anaesthesia for elderly. Singapore Dent J. 2014;35:23–9.

83. Beliveau MM, Multach M. Perioperative care for the elderly patient. Med Clin N Am. 2003;87(1):273–89.

84. Cunha BA. Urinary tract infections in males. Conns Current Therapy. 2003:733–5.

85. Feldman C. Pneumonia in the elderly. Med Clin N Am. 2001; 85(6):1441–59.

86. Neumayer L, Hosokawa P, Itani K, El-Tamer M, Henderson WG, Khuri SF. Multivariable predictors of postoperative surgical site infection after general and vascular surgery: results from the patient safety in surgery study. J Am Coll Surg. 2007;204(6):1178–87.

87. Kirby JP, Mazuski JE. Prevention of surgical site infection. Surg Clin North Am. 2009;89(2):365–89.

88. Kaye KS, Anderson DJ, Sloane R, et al. The effect of surgical site infection on older operative patients. J Am Geriatr Soc. 2009; 57(1):46–54.

89. Barie PS. Surgical site infections: epidemiology and prevention. Surg Infect (Larchmt). 2002;3(S1):s9–21.

90. Dellinger EP, Hausmann SM, Bratzler DW, et al. Hospitals collaborate to decrease surgical site infections. Am J Surg. 2005; 190(1):9–15.

91. McGory ML, Maggard MA, Ko CY. A meta-analysis of perioperative beta blockade: what is the actual risk reduction? Surgery. 2005;138(2):171–9.

92. Auerbach AD, Goldman L. β-Blockers and reduction of cardiac events in noncardiac surgery: scientific review. JAMA. 2002; 287(11):1435–44.

93. Mehta RH, Rathore SS, Radford MJ, Wang Y, Wang Y, Krumholz HM. Acute myocardial infarction in the elderly: differences by age. J Am Coll Cardiol. 2001;38(3):736–41.

94. Ryder DL. The use of β-blockers to decrease adverse perioperative cardiac events. Dimens Crit Care Nurs. 2008;27(2):47–53.

95. Badner NH, Knill RL, Brown JE, Novick TV, Gelb A. Myocardial infarction after noncardiac surgery. Anesthesiology. 1998;88(3): 572–8.

96. Loran DB, Hyde BR, Zwischenberger JB. Perioperative management of special populations: the geriatric patient. Surg Clin N Am. 2005;85(6):1259–66.

97. Amar D, Zhang H, Leung DH, Roistacher N, Kadish AH. Older age is the strongest predictor of postoperative atrial fibrillation. J Am Soc Anesthesiol. 2002;96(2):352–6.

98. Ramsay JG. Cardiac management in the ICU. Chest J. 1999;115 Suppl 2:138S–44S.

99. Amar D. Prevention and management of perioperative arrhythmias in the thoracic surgical population. Anesthesiol Clin. 2008;26(2):325–35.

100. Ergina PL, Gold SL, Meakins JL. Perioperative care of the elderly patient. World J Surg. 1993;17(2):192–8.

101. Polanczyk CA, Marcantonio E, Goldman L, et al. Impact of age on perioperative complications and length of stay in patients undergoing noncardiac surgery. Ann Intern Med. 2001;134(8): 637–43.

102. McAlister FA, Bertsch K, Man J, Bradley J, Jacka M. Incidence of and risk factors for pulmonary complications after nonthoracic surgery. Am J Respir Crit Care Med. 2005;171(5):514–7.

103. Feinberg MJ, Knebl J, Tully J, Segall L. Aspiration and the elderly. Dysphagia. 1990;5(2):61–71.

104. Watters JM. Surgery in the elderly. Can J Surg. 2002;45(2): 104–8.

105. Zafar SN, Obirieze A, Schneider EB, et al. Outcomes of trauma care at centers treating a higher proportion of older patients: the case for geriatric trauma centers. J Trauma Acute Care Surg. 2015;78(4):852–9.

106. G 60 Geriatric Trauma Program Trauma Newsletter Methodist Dallas Medical Center Adult Level I Trauma Center and Emergency Care. 2015. http://www.methodisthealthsystem.org/ G60. Accessed 18 Nov 2015.

107. Cohen HJ, Feussner JR, Weinberger M, et al. A controlled trial of inpatient and outpatient geriatric evaluation and management. N Engl J Med. 2002;346(12):905–12.

Jana D. Illston, Joseph M. Malek, David R. Ellington, and Holly E. Richter

13.1 Introduction

A quarter of women in the USA have at least one pelvic floor disorder: urinary incontinence, fecal incontinence, or pelvic organ prolapse [1, 2]. This prevalence increases with age such that nearly half of women over age 80 have symptoms of one or more pelvic floor disorders, and 1 in 5 of these women over age 80 will have undergone at least one surgical procedure for prolapse or urinary incontinence [1–3]. With a projected 9 % increase in the proportion of the US population over age 65 by the year 2060, there will be an unprecedented number of older women with symptomatic pelvic floor disorders [4]. Providers must be prepared to treat these women and restore quality of life. Costs of ambulatory care for these disorders were estimated at more than $400 million per year in 2005–2006 and are increasing [5]. Good geriatric gynecological care is critical to optimizing outcomes for vaginal atrophy, pelvic organ prolapse, urinary incontinence, fecal incontinence, and perioperative management.

13.2 Atrophy/Genitourinary Syndrome of Menopause

The urogenital consequences of decreased estrogen levels affect approximately half of postmenopausal women [6–10]. Symptoms associated with the genitourinary syndrome of menopause include vaginal and vulvar complaints (e.g., itching, dryness, burning, malodorous discharge, feeling of pressure, dyspareunia, and post-coital bleeding) as well as urinary complaints of dysuria, urgency, frequency, nocturia, incontinence, hematuria, and recurrent urinary tract infections [9–12].

Many of the symptoms of pelvic floor disorders are related to estrogen withdrawal [6, 9]. Estrogenic stimulation of the vagina results in a thicker epithelium with increased glycogen. When these epithelial cells are sloughed as a part of normal exfoliation, the glycogen is hydrolyzed into glucose, which is then converted into lactic acid by lactobacilli [6, 9]. Lactic acid lowers vaginal pH to between 3.5 and 4.5 and is an essential component in vaginal health and defense against vaginal and urinary tract infection [6, 9]. Without estrogen, the vaginal epithelium thins, there are fewer lactobacilli, the pH rises, and other, less-desirable bacteria can proliferate more easily [6, 9]. Decreases in estrogen also result in decreased elasticity, vaginal blood flow, and lubrication [9]. This lack of lubrication is often the first symptom and can present even before other clinical symptoms and signs appear [6, 9].

Objective findings of atrophy (Fig. 13.1) include a pH >4.6, pale and smooth/shiny vaginal epithelium, petechiae, friability, dryness, ulceration, and poor rugation [6, 9, 13]. Urethral caruncles or eversion of urethral mucosa may appear [9]. The Vaginal Physical Examination Scale has been recommended, in combination with pH testing, for objective clinical evaluation and includes the findings of petechiae, vaginal wall friability, conization (decreased elasticity), and absence of rugae [13, 14]. These objective measures should be combined with subjective measures, specifically vaginal dryness, itching/irritation, and dyspareunia (components of the Most Bothersome Symptom tool) for complete clinical evaluation [13].

It is important to remember that age-related vaginal atrophy is a diagnosis of exclusion, and other etiologies including lichen sclerosis, lichen planus, sexually transmitted infections, and neoplasia must be considered before attributing symptoms, such as hematuria, postmenopausal bleeding, itching, or discharge, to estrogen deprivation [15]. Thorough history and physical examination are paramount to developing the correct diagnosis.

J.D. Illston, MD • J.M. Malek, MD • D.R. Ellington, MD, FACOG
(✉) • H.E. Richter, PhD, MD, FACOG, FACS
Division of Urogynecology and Pelvic Reconstructive Surgery,
Department of Obstetrics and Gynecology, University of Alabama
at Birmingham, 176F, Suite 10382, 619 19th Street South,
Birmingham, AL 35249-7333, USA
e-mail: dellington@uabmc.edu

© Springer International Publishing Switzerland 2017

J.R. Burton et al. (eds.), *Geriatrics for Specialists*, DOI 10.1007/978-3-319-31831-8_13

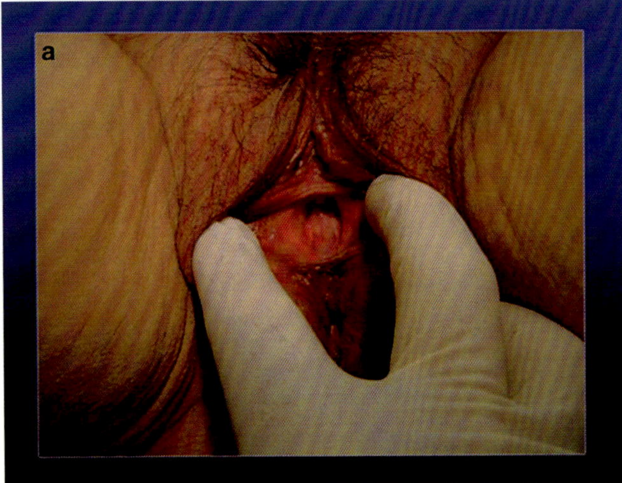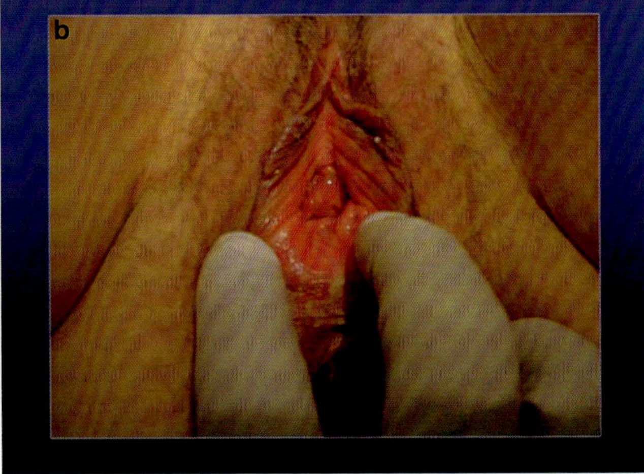

Fig. 13.1 Effect of topical estrogen therapy: Both images are from 64-year old G2P2002 women who underwent 2 vaginal deliveries. (**a**) Patient discontinued estrogen therapy 5 years previously. (**b**) Patient on estrogen continuously since menopause. Images courtesy of Dr. Murray A. Freedman © 2008

In addition to the effect on the vagina, lack of estrogen also impacts other tissues in the pelvis. Autonomic and sensory neurons in the vagina are responsive to estrogen, and treatment with topical estrogen has been shown to decrease innervation density, which may partially explain symptom improvement with estrogen therapy [16]. The female lower urinary and genital tracts are both embryologically derived from the urogenital sinus, and estrogen receptors have been found in the vagina, urethra, and bladder trigone [11]. These receptors may contribute to the impact of estrogen deprivation on lower urinary tract symptoms, and treatment with topical estrogen has been shown to improve nocturia, recurrent urinary tract infections, frequency, urgency, and incontinence, both urgency and stress urinary incontinence [11, 12].

Treatment improves symptoms of the genitourinary syndrome of menopause and can be either hormonal or non-hormonal [12, 15, 17]. Non-hormonal treatments, such as pH-balanced gels, water-based moisturizers, or hyaluronic acid, can work well for patients with few, minor complaints, whereas patients with more than two symptoms get better relief from vaginal estrogen therapy [12, 15]. Selective Estrogen Receptor Modulators (SERMs), like ospemifene, which is an estrogen agonist in the vagina but not the endometrium, and Tissue Selective Estrogen Complexes (TSEC), which combine an estrogen and a SERM, are effective in treating problems like moderate-to-severe dyspareunia (ospemifene) or vaginal symptoms and maturation index (Conjugated Equine Estrogens with bazedoxifene) [15, 18–21].

There are many commercially available preparations of vaginal estrogen in the USA, and all are considered safe and efficacious at the approved dose and frequency [12, 15, 22]. Delivery options such as vaginal creams, vaginal tablets, pessaries, and ovules/rings are available, and the hormones can include conjugated equine estrogens, estradiol, estriol, or promestriene [12, 15, 17]. Some conjugated equine estrogen products have been associated with slightly higher rates of side effects like bleeding, breast tenderness, and endometrial hyperplasia, but they are still considered safe and effective [12, 15, 17].

Concerns about hormone use have decreased the percentage of women using systemic estrogen therapy and have arguably been detrimental to the urogenital health of women [23]. While systemic estrogen levels are low and within the normal, postmenopausal range for women using low-dose vaginal estrogen, some studies have shown elevation in estrogen levels above pretreatment baselines, although systemic absorption decreases as the vagina becomes more estrogenic [12, 15, 17, 22, 24]. For many women, this change is likely insignificant; however, for women with a history of estrogen-sensitive cancer, particularly those taking aromatase inhibitors, vaginal estrogen is not recommended as a first-line therapy for genitourinary syndromes [12, 15, 17]. The risks and quality-of-life benefits can be discussed and balanced on an individual basis if non-hormonal treatments are insufficient for symptom relief [12, 15, 17].

While there are no long-term data to confirm endometrial safety for women with a uterus, most expert recommendations and current guidelines state that treatment with a progestin is not indicated for women using low-dose vaginal estrogen therapy [12, 17, 25]. Low-dose estrogen does not appear to increase the risk of endometrial pathology significantly and there are potential increased risks of thrombosis and breast cancer with the progestin [15]. As always, any postmenopausal vaginal bleeding should be thoroughly evaluated [25].

In spite of the prevalence of symptoms, adverse effect on quality of life, and the availability of effective treatments, vaginal atrophy is underreported [6, 9, 15, 17, 26]. Increasing awareness by asking about specific atrophy symptoms and consequently getting treatment to affected women is an important way of improving the urogenital health and general quality of life for older female patients [15].

13.3 Prolapse

Pelvic organ prolapse is a bothersome condition that has a significant negative impact on quality of life. By age 80, 12.6% of women will undergo surgical treatment for prolapse, and the actual prevalence is even higher when symptomatic women managed non-surgically are included [3]. Prolapse is undoubtedly a multifaceted problem with many different biological, lifestyle, and other inciting factors [27]. Older age, white race, higher parity, prior hysterectomy or prolapse/incontinence procedure, obesity, frequent heavy lifting, chronic constipation, chronic coughing, and smoking have all been linked with greater risk of prolapse [27].

Symptoms of prolapse tend to be related to the most advanced portion of the prolapse and are often pelvic pressure, heaviness, or feeling a bulge. Pelvic pain and low back pain are not associated with greater degree of prolapse and many women will not experience symptoms of prolapse until the leading edge is at the hymen or beyond [27].

13.3.1 Evaluation

Use of a Sims speculum or the posterior blade of a Graves speculum can allow the examiner to inspect the anterior and posterior compartments separately, and the apex can be examined digitally or by retracting the anterior and posterior compartments simultaneously. Rectovaginal examination can also be useful in evaluation of the posterior compartment, including differentiating between rectocele and enterocele [27].

The Pelvic Organ Prolapse Quantification (POPQ) System is widely used in the research setting as it allows for standardization of physical findings by defining the locations of points on the anterior, posterior, and apical vagina as well as genital hiatus and perineal body (see Fig. 13.2) [28]. While the entire POPQ does not necessarily need to be performed in the clinical setting, identification and recording of key attributes including the leading edge of the anterior, apical, and posterior compartments is important and clinically relevant [27]. Stages of prolapse are 0-IV based on the leading edge, e.g. most severe portion, of the prolapse with 0 being no prolapse (apex is within 2 cm of total vaginal length) and stage IV being total eversion within 2 cm of the total vaginal length [28].

Pelvic organ prolapse presents along a spectrum from asymptomatic women with minimal anatomic findings to severely bothered patients with total vaginal vault prolapse or uterine procidentia. Generally speaking, asymptomatic patients do not require treatment, and surgery should not be

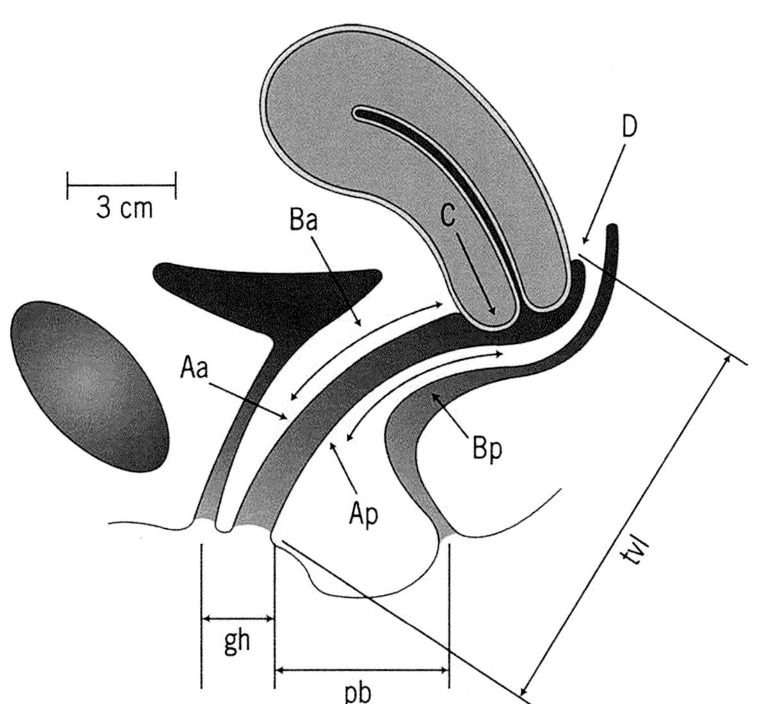

Fig. 13.2 Diagrammatic representation of the pelvic organ prolapse quantification system for staging prolapse by physical examination findings, showing the 6 sites (points Aa and Ba anteriorly, points Ap and Bp posteriorly, point C for the cervix or apex, and point D for the cul-de-sac), genital hiatus (gh), perineal body (pb), and total vaginal length (tvl) used for pelvic organ prolapse quantification. Reprinted from Weber AM, Richter HE. Pelvic Organ Prolapse. Obstet Gynecol 2005;106:615–34; modified from Bump RC, Mattiasson A, Bø K, Brubaker LP, DeLancey JOL, Klarskov P, Shull BL, Smith RB. The standardization of terminology of female pelvic organ prolapse and pelvic floor dysfunction. Am J Obstet Gynecol 1996;175:10–17

performed unless the patient's symptoms warrant the potential risks of intervention [27]. Whereas in the past, some thought that early surgical treatment of prolapse may prevent progression, observation of a cohort treated for stress urinary incontinence showed that only 2 % of asymptomatic women with stage II prolapse had any anatomic worsening of their disease and none underwent surgical treatment in the 5- to 7-year follow-up period [29].

13.3.2 Non-Surgical Treatment

For women who are symptomatic, non-surgical management options include pessaries and pelvic floor muscle training. These options can be very appealing for women who have less bothersome symptoms or significant surgical risk, but they should be considered and offered to all women. Adjunct therapies to optimize other aspects of disease should also be considered including lifestyle changes, like weight loss, as well as treatment of chronic constipation and defecatory dysfunction [27].

The pessary is a very useful device for the non-surgical treatment of prolapse, and most women can be successfully fit. Of Medicare beneficiaries with a prolapse diagnosis, 11–13 % were treated with a pessary [30]. While there are many different designs and sizes, the two main categories are support and space-filling, and the ring with support and Gellhorn pessaries are probably the most useful in each of these respective categories (see Fig. 13.3) [27, 31]. The ring with support is often the first choice because of its ease of use and ability for many patients to remove, clean, and manage it themselves. For women who cannot retain the ring with support, a Gellhorn is often an effective option, but it tends to require provider visits for removal and cleaning [31]. Women who are sexually active and use a pessary should be able to remove and reinsert the pessary themselves since most, if not

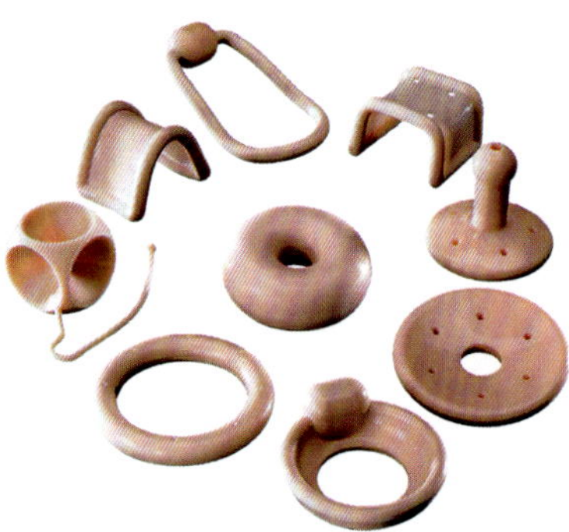

Fig. 13.3 Pessaries: (**a**) an assortment of pessaries, (**b**) Gellhorn pessaries, (**c**) ring and ring with support pessaries, (**d**) Gellhorn pessary in position, (**e**) Ring with incontinence knob pessary in position, (**f**) Ring pessary in position. **a, d, e, f**, Photographs provided by CooperSurgical Inc; Images **b, c**, Photographs provided by BIOTEQUE AMERICA, INC

all, pessaries are not compatible with vaginal intercourse [31]. Vaginal epithelial health is an important consideration with pessary use, and vaginal estrogen therapy should be considered if needed, although many women may not require it. Periodic inspection of the vagina for abrasions and ulcerations is essential, and compliance with follow-up is key to identifying problems before they result in severe complications [27, 31]. While there are no data-driven guidelines on follow-up intervals, typically every 3–6 months for a patient unable to remove her own pessary is reasonable, and that can be extended as long as 1 year for a woman who is able to remove and clean the pessary frequently herself [31, 32]. Usually minor abrasions or ulcerations can be resolved by leaving the pessary out and applying vaginal estrogen cream for several weeks. More significant complications, such as fistula formation, typically only result from extended neglect [31]. Vaginal discharge and unmasking of occult stress urinary incontinence can also be bothersome side effects of pessary use [31, 33].

Pelvic Floor Muscle Training (PFMT) can be effective in reducing symptoms for women with mild to moderate (usually stage I to II) prolapse [31]. This treatment usually involves working on isolation of pelvic floor muscles and doing exercises which strengthen and improve muscle bulk. Studies have shown both symptomatic and anatomic improvements with PFMT for patients with stages I, II, and III prolapse [31, 34]. Success of these treatments is likely dependent, however, on having motivated patients who are willing to comply with the exercise program.

For women who desire more than non-surgical management for their prolapse symptoms, there are many surgical treatment options available. These options include both obliterative and reconstructive procedures.

13.3.3 Surgical Treatment

Obliterative procedures, such as the Le Fort colpocleisis with levator plication and high perineorrhaphy, have many advantages for women who do not desire preservation of the ability for vaginal intercourse. These procedures tend to be shorter and less morbid than reconstructive repairs and are highly effective [27, 35–39]. Success rates range from 91 to 100 %, which is outstanding for efficacy of prolapse repair [38]. Patient-centered outcomes are excellent with 90–95 % of patients experiencing improved quality of life, satisfaction with outcome, and willingness to recommend the procedure to others [35, 36, 38]. Post-surgical regret, although very uncommon (approximately 5–10 %), is not zero risk [27, 35, 40]. Urinary tract infection is the most common postoperative complication, and women who underwent simultaneous colpocleisis and midurethral sling do not have increased complications in the immediate postoperative period [37].

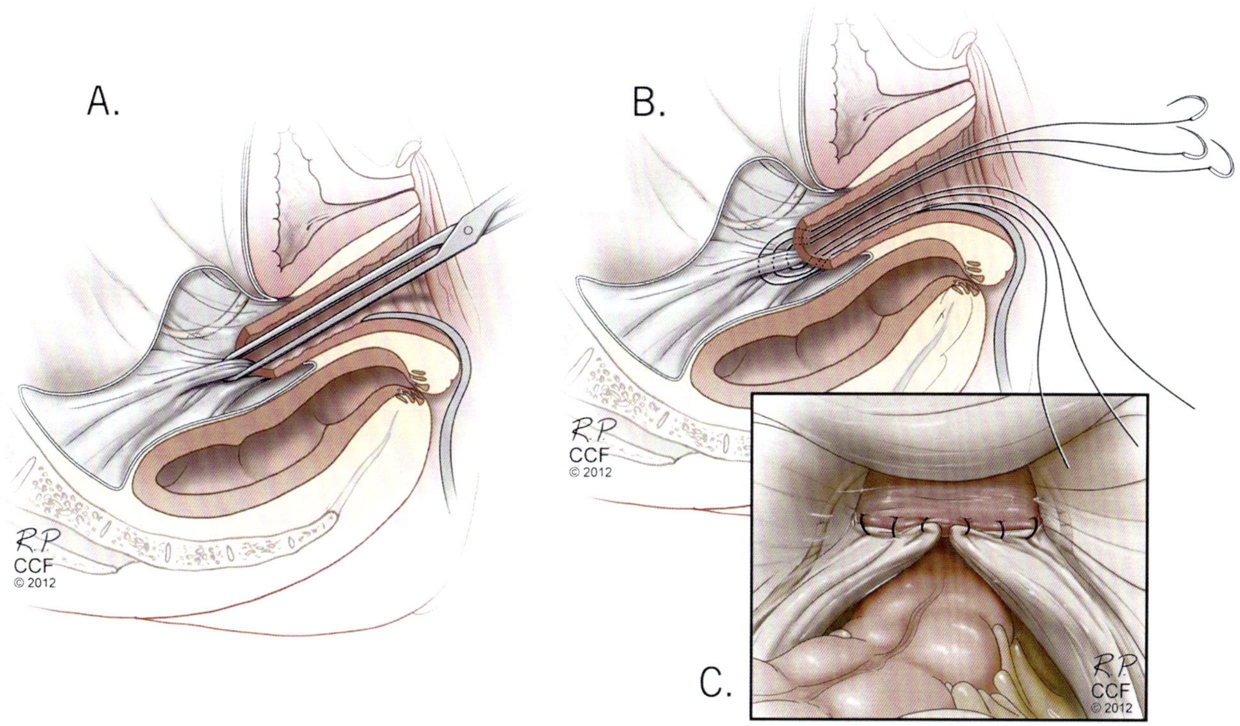

Fig. 13.4 High uterosacral ligament suspension technique. Reprinted with permission, Cleveland Clinic Center for Medical Art & Photography © 2004–2015 All Rights Reserved

Reconstructive repairs can be performed vaginally or abdominally, and can be performed with native tissue or using augmentation with mesh, fascia, or biologic grafts. Minimally invasive options include the vaginal, laparoscopic, and robotic approaches. Currently, no clinical trials have definitively shown which methods of prolapse repair are the most effective.

Vaginal native tissue or "traditional" repairs can be performed in all three compartments: apical, anterior, and posterior. The two most common methods used for apical support are the high uterosacral ligament suspension and sacrospinous ligament fixation (see Figs. 13.4 and 13.5) [41–44]. These methods were compared head-to-head in the Pelvic Floor Disorders Network's Operations and Pelvic Muscle Training in the Management of Apical Support Loss (OPTIMAL) trial and were shown to have similar outcomes for anatomic and functional success as well as adverse events [44]. The types of adverse events did differ, however, with ureteral obstruction being more likely with uterosacral suspension and buttock pain being more likely in the sacrospinous suspension groups. Usually ureteral obstructions can be identified on intraoperative cystoscopy and can be resolved without any lasting repercussions. The buttock pain from sacrospinous suspension generally resolves without intervention in most patients by 6 weeks postoperatively, however a small subset (<5 %) may require

interventions including physical therapy or trigger point injections for the pain [44, 45]. With the strict definition of success used for the OPTIMAL trial, approximately 60 % of patients were considered to have successful outcomes, 5 % of patients required repeat surgical treatment.

Suspension of the apex is critical to the success of prolapse repairs. In addition to appropriate apical suspension, other defects should also be addressed including enterocele, cystocele, and rectocele. Enterocele can be repaired with cephalad purse-stringing of the enterocele sac, with or without excision of the sac, and reapproximating the anterior and posterior apical vaginal connective tissue [27]. Anterior colporrhaphy is the preferred native tissue repair for the anterior compartment defects, but paravaginal repairs can also be considered when appropriate for surgeons with sufficient expertise [27]. Posteriorly, traditional colporrhaphy is recommended with perineorrhaphy as needed. Care must be taken not to overcorrect or narrow the vagina, which could cause pain or worsened sexual function [27].

Vaginal repairs augmented with mesh have been a recent topic of controversy. In light of apparent failure rates with native tissue repairs, there was keen interest in the possibility of improved results with mesh augmentation. Popularity of mesh augmentation grew more quickly than the data supporting its use, and concerns about safety and efficacy were raised [46, 47]. Many of the original vaginal mesh

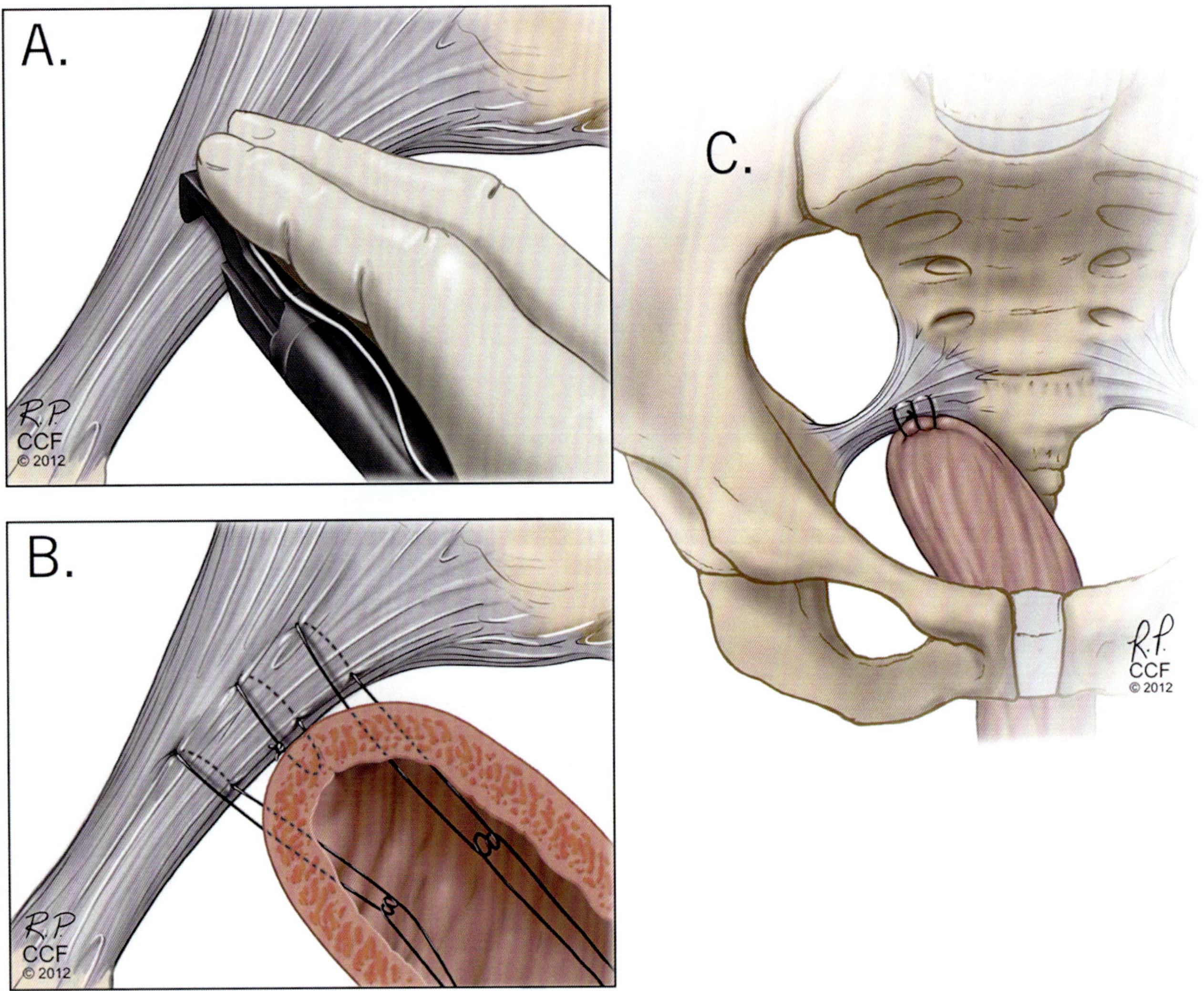

Fig. 13.5 Sacrospinous ligament suspension. Reprinted with permission, Cleveland Clinic Center for Medical Art & Photography © 2004–2015 All Rights Reserved

products have been discontinued, and those that remain are being rigorously investigated to assess their clinical outcomes.

From the existing data, it appears that mesh augmentation may improve outcomes in the anterior compartment, but further study is needed [46–48]. There are not currently data to support the use of vaginal mesh for apical and posterior support [46, 47, 49, 50].

Abdominal sacrocolpopexy, which can be performed open, laparoscopically, or robotically, is a procedure in which a graft is used to pull the vagina up to the sacrum, and it has been considered the most durable prolapse repair option (see Fig. 13.6). Longer-term studies have shown, however, that even with sacrocolpopexy, success rates decrease over time [51]. At 5 years, nearly a third of women in the eCARE trial met treatment failure criteria, but only 5 % had undergone a repeat procedure. Additionally, mesh exposure rate was about 10 % and exposures continued to occur throughout the extended study period. Minimally invasive abdominal sacrocolpopexy can be performed laparoscopically or robotically and has similar prolapse outcomes as an open abdominal procedure [52, 53]. Minimally invasive procedures have longer operating times but less blood loss and shorter hospital stays than open procedures [52, 54]. When comparing laparoscopic and robotic modalities, laparoscopy has been shown to offer decreased cost, shorter operative time, and less pain at 1 week postoperatively [55]. One study also showed less blood loss, lower rate of bladder injury, and decreased reoperation rate with laparoscopic as compared to robotic sacrocolpopexy [56].

Older patients undergoing urogynecologic surgery have been shown in some studies to have similar outcomes as younger women [57, 58]. Much like with midurethral slings, however, some studies did find higher rates of complications for older patients [59]. Even so, the overall rates of complications are low, and chronological age should not be the only factor in surgical decision making.

Fig. 13.6 Sacrocolpopexy with mesh attached to anterior and posterior vagina as well as sacrum. Reprinted with permission, Cleveland Clinic Center for Medical Art & Photography © 2004–2015 All Rights Reserved

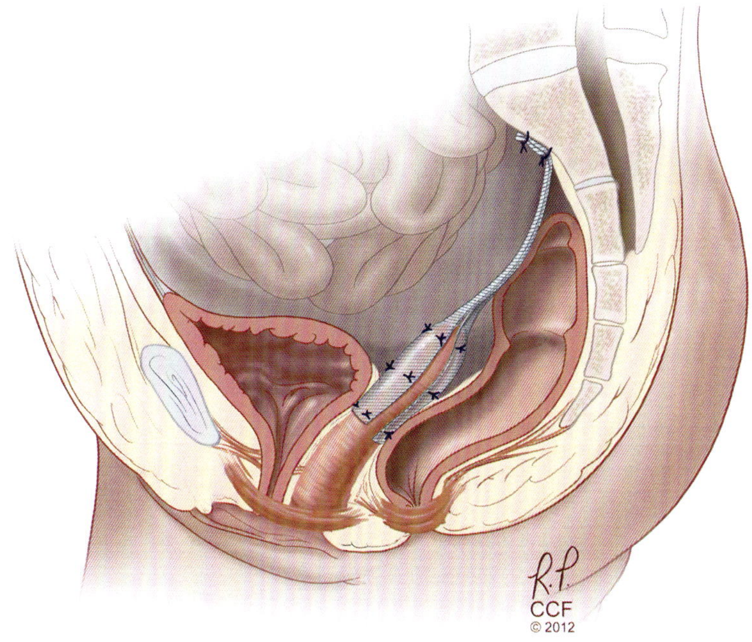

13.3.4 Urinary Function

Urinary incontinence (UI) is a common pelvic floor disorder which affects 49.2 % of adult women, and increases to above 60 % prevalence in women over age 70 [60]. Prevalence of incontinence starts off gradually in young adults, reaches a peak in mid-life, and climbs steadily in the older population [61, 62]. While the overall prevalence increases with age, the distribution of incontinence types changes from more stress incontinence in younger women to more urgency and mixed incontinence in older women [60]. Older women also tend to have more severe incontinence than younger women [60, 63]. Urinary incontinence is not considered a normal part of aging and has a huge impact on patients' lives [64]. UI has been associated with functional decline, fall risk, nursing home placement, depressive symptoms, and frailty [64, 65].

Even when incontinence is significantly bothersome, many women do not seek care [64, 66]. Patients are often reticent to mention these issues to providers, who must initiate the conversation.

The burden of disease for urinary incontinence is significant—economically and emotionally. UI severity has been associated with major depression, medical comorbidity, and decreased quality of life, particularly in those with nighttime and coital symptoms or comorbid fecal incontinence [66–70]. The financial cost of UI is estimated at more than $16 billion in 1995 dollars, $7.6 billion of which was for women over age 65 [71]. In spite of a 15 % decrease in the cost per capita, Medicare costs for female beneficiaries nearly doubled from 1992 to 1998, due to an increase in the number of patients requiring treatment [72].

13.3.5 Definitions

The terminology for urinary incontinence was standardized by the International Continence Society [73–78].

Urinary Incontinence The complaint of any involuntary leakage of urine.

Stress Urinary Incontinence (SUI) The complaint of involuntary leakage on effort or exertion, or on sneezing or coughing.

Urinary Urgency The complaint of a sudden, compelling desire to pass urine which is difficult to defer.

Urgency Urinary Incontinence (UUI) The complaint of involuntary leakage accompanied by or immediately preceded by urgency.

Mixed Urinary Incontinence (MUI) The complaint of involuntary leakage associated with urgency and also with exertion, effort, sneezing, or coughing; applies to people with symptoms of both SUI and UUI.

Overactive Bladder Syndrome (OAB) Urinary urgency, with or without urgency incontinence, usually with increased daytime frequency (e.g., the complaint by the patient of voiding too often by day) and nocturia (complaint of waking up once or more at night to void) in the absence of urinary tract infection or other obvious pathology.

Other pertinent types of incontinence include [77]:

Functional Incontinence Untimely urination due to physical disability, lack of access to a toilet, or problems in thinking that prevent a person from reaching a toilet.

Overflow Incontinence Unexpected and near continuous leakage of small amounts of urine because of a distended bladder which is not emptying properly; the etiology is from either outlet obstruction or inadequate detrusor contraction. Causes include neurologic impairment, fecal impaction, and medication adverse effects.

13.3.6 Impact of Age

Age-related changes are important contributors to urinary incontinence in older patients, but they can be difficult to delineate from comorbidities and confounding factors, like parity [79]. There are, however, many age-related changes in the anatomy and physiology of the lower urinary tract (LUT) [65, 79, 80]. Detrusor contractility weakens, urethral closure pressure decreases, urethral blood flow and vascular density decrease [65, 79, 80]. Older patients also tend to have more detrusor overactivity (DO), higher post-void residual (PVR) volume, lower volume voids, and decreased flow rate [79]. These changes accompany the previously discussed increases in urgency UI, frequency, and nocturia [79]. Additionally, medical comorbidities, neurologic/psychiatric status, functional and environmental issues, and medications impact UI and make it a multifactorial geriatric syndrome [65, 79]. This complexity is clinically relevant as addressing those components may improve symptoms without any other interventions [79, 81].

Other risk factors for UI include female gender, white race, and elevated body mass index (BMI) [60, 82, 83]. Hysterectomy, smoking, thyroid disease, depression, decreased physical activity, arthritis, diabetes, and childbirth have also been linked [60, 82, 83]. Both vaginal and cesarean delivery have been associated with an increased risk of UI, but the impact of parity is stronger in younger women and appears to dissipate by age 65 [84, 85]. Neurological status, chronic cough, menopause, collagen integrity, and medication use are also important factors [82]. Persistence of UI has been associated with increased age, white race, higher parity, elevated BMI, decreased physical activity, type 2 diabetes, stroke, and hysterectomy, yet the greatest increased odds of UI were associated with older age, white race, and obesity [86].

13.3.7 Evaluation

In the initial evaluation of UI, patient history is essential to differentiate the type of incontinence (SUI, UUI, MUI, overflow), and urinalysis is also recommended to rule out hematuria, pyuria, bacteriuria, and glycosuria [64]. Physical examination is useful for evaluation of anatomy, atrophy, pelvic floor tone, strength, and coordination. Post-void residual (PVR), simple cystometrics, and complex urodynamics can also be useful but are usually not needed in the initial evaluation of most patients [87].

13.3.8 Non-Surgical Treatment

13.3.8.1 Contributing Factors

Like other geriatric syndromes, UI often has more than one cause, and successful treatment often entails addressing several of these factors [65]. For many older women, especially those who are frail, simply addressing contributing factors regardless of UI type (SUI, UUI, MUI) will improve bladder control. Contributing factors include: ensuring there is adequate access to toilets which may mean improving the patient's mobility or adapting the environment; and if the patient is cognitively impaired, recommending prompted toileting. Prompted toileting differs from scheduled toileting because the patient is asked if they need to use the toilet on a schedule (typically every 2–3 h) but regardless of the response (yes or no) she is taken to the toilet and praised if able to void. Other contributing factors include comorbid disease and medications. Medical conditions that contribute to UI and may require referral to a primary provider to optimize treatment include: heart failure, chronic obstructive pulmonary disease, and chronic cough. Many medications contribute to UI (see Table 13.1) and should be reduced or minimized.

13.3.8.2 Urgency and Urgency Incontinence

Urinary urgency, overactive bladder syndrome, and urgency incontinence become increasingly prevalent with age and have a negative impact on quality of life [60, 88]. In many patients these irritative symptoms persist and necessitate management as a chronic disease process rather than as an acute illness [89]. First line management options include lifestyle modification and behavioral therapy; and then adding medications when symptoms are not adequately controlled.

Lifestyle modifications involve changing habits that may be contributing to urinary urgency or incontinence. Limiting caffeine, which is both a diuretic and a bladder irritant, discouraging extremes of fluid intake (too much or too little), and restricting fluid intake several hours before bedtime can be helpful [64, 88]. Constipation that places pressure on the urethral sphincter (obstruction) or places pressure on the bladder should be treated [65]. Smoking causes chronic cough and patients should be encouraged to quit. Studies in bariatric patients have shown that even a 5 % weight loss can bring a significant improvement in UI, with more weight loss conferring even greater benefit [90, 91].

Table 13.1 Medications commonly associated with urinary incontinence

Medication/Class	Adverse effects/Comments
ACE[a] inhibitors	Cough (stress UI)
Alcohol	Frequency, urgency, sedation
α Adrenergic agonists	Outlet obstruction
α Adrenergic blockers	Stress leakage
Anticholinergics	Impaired emptying, constipation
Cholinesterase inhibitors	Increased uninhibited contractions
Calcium channel blockers	Impaired detrusor contraction
Estrogen (oral, transdermal)	Stress and mixed UI
GABA[b]-ergics (gabapentin, pregabalin)	Edema, nocturnal diuresis
Loop diuretics	Polyuria, frequency, urgency
NSAIDs[c]/thiazolidinediones	Edema, nocturnal diuresis
Sedative hypnotics	Sedation, delirium, immobility
Opioid analgesics	Constipation, sedation, delirium
Antipsychotics	Anticholinergic effects, sedation

From Reuben DB, Herr KA, Pacala JT, Pollock BG, Potter JF, Semla RP, editors. Geriatrics at Your Fingertips. Seventeenth Edition. New York: American Geriatric Society; 2015:154

[a]Angiotensin-converting enzyme

[b]Gamma-aminobutyric acid

[c]Nonsteroidal anti-inflammatory drugs

Behavioral therapy involves teaching the patient techniques to reduce urgency and incontinence episodes. These can include isolating and strengthening appropriate muscle groups with Kegel exercises, learning stress strategies, urge suppression techniques like "freeze and squeeze," and using voiding schedules to increase the amount of time between voids [64]. Behavioral techniques can be very effective but do require a cognitively intact and motivated patient [64, 88, 92].

Antimuscarinic medical therapy, including oxybutynin, tolterodine, solifenacin, darifenacin, fesoterodine, and trospium can be effective, but side effects, cost, and drug interactions must all be considered [64]. The maximum dose of trospium, solifenacin and fesoterodine must be reduced for many older women based on creatinine clearance which frequently declines with age. Due to their anticholinergic properties (which inhibits detrusor contractions), antimuscarinics have significant side effects which contributes to low adherence (less than one third) one year after initiation of antimuscarinic therapy [93]. Side effects include dry mouth, constipation, blurry vision, and the potential for cognitive impairment. Cognitive side effects are a significant concern in the older population, particularly in patients who may already have some level of cognitive impairment. Most of the antimuscarinics have not been shown to cause impairment, however several studies have demonstrated cognitive changes with oxybutynin [88, 94–98]. When possible, use of extended release antimuscarinics is preferred over immediate release as the longer acting formulations have better efficacy with fewer side effects [99]. The impact of side effects on chronic issues like cognitive impairment, constipation, dry mouth, and mobility must be considered before starting antimuscarinic therapy in any patient, but especially in an older patient.

In addition to antimuscarinics, mirabegron, a β3-adrenoceptor agonist, has been shown to be effective and well tolerated in the older population with hypertension being the most common adverse effect; blood pressure should be monitored during initiation of therapy [100]. Other reported adverse events in mirabegron treated patients include headache, nausea, dizziness, and tachycardia (including atrial fibrillation). Mirabegron is renally excreted and the maximum dose must be reduced if creatinine clearance is less than 25 ml/min. Because it is not anticholinergic, the side effect profile of mirabegron may be preferable for some patients. Vaginal estrogen treatment can also improve lower urinary tract symptoms including urgency, frequency, nocturia, and incontinence, so treatment of vaginal atrophy should be considered [12, 64, 101].

13.3.9 Procedure-Based and Surgical Treatment

When urgency symptoms are refractory to first line therapy, behavioral therapy, lifestyle interventions, pharmacotherapy, and combinations thereof, other, more invasive options may be considered. These therapies include the neuromuscular toxin, Botulinum, and neuromodulation of sacral and tibial nerves.

Percutaneous tibial nerve stimulation (PTNS) involves using a small needle inserted near the ankle to stimulate

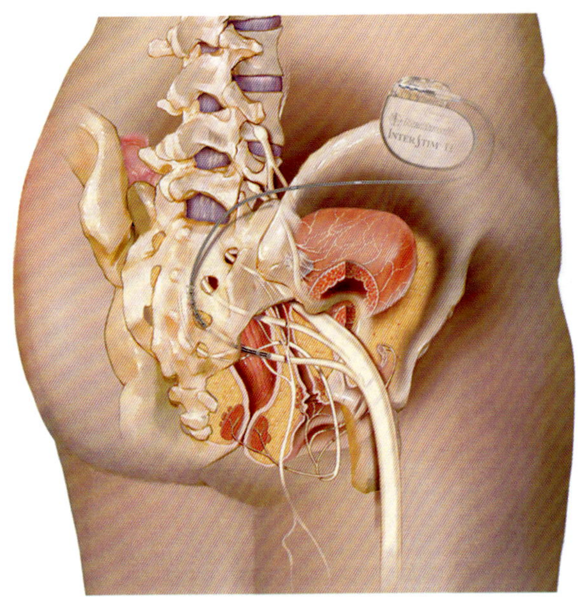

Fig. 13.7 Sacral neuromodulation device—permanent placement. Reprinted with the permission of Medtronic, Inc. © 2014

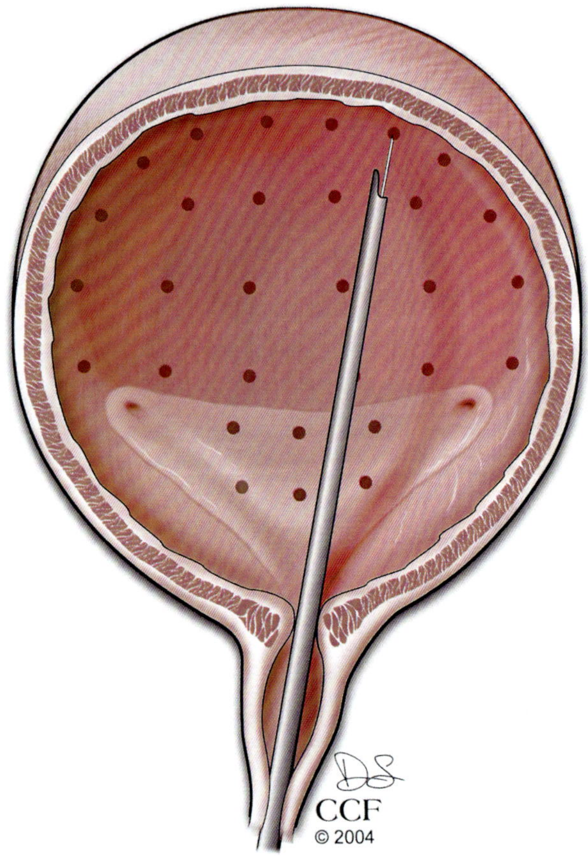

Fig. 13.8 Sites of Botulinum toxin injection during cystoscopy. Reprinted with permission, Cleveland Clinic Center for Medical Art & Photography © 2004–2015 All Rights Reserved

the posterior tibial nerve [102]. These 30-min stimulation treatments are performed weekly for 12 weeks and additional treatments can be repeated as needed [102]. This technique has been shown to improve OAB symptoms up to 24 months [102].

Sacral neuromodulation (SNM) involves a staged procedure where a lead is placed into the S3 foramen. Test stimulation is typically performed for 2 weeks, and if the patient has at least a 50 % improvement in symptoms, a permanent neurostimulator is implanted and connected to the lead [103, 104]. The neurostimulator provides continuous stimulation of sacral nerves to modulate neural signals to and from the bladder, anal sphincter, and pelvic floor (see Fig. 13.7) [105]. SNM is FDA approved for the treatment of OAB, urgency UI, non-obstructive urinary retention, and fecal incontinence (see section to follow), and appears to be as safe and effective in older patients as younger ones [64, 103, 104, 106].

Botulinum toxin is an FDA-approved treatment for refractory OAB, which has been shown to improve symptoms and quality of life [107–109]. Botulinum toxin works at the presynaptic cholinergic junction by inhibiting the release of acetylcholine and thus causing temporary detrusor muscle paralysis [110]. It is administered cystoscopically by injecting the toxin into multiple points in the detrusor or suburothelially (see Fig. 13.8) [109, 111]. Potential adverse events include urinary retention and urinary tract infection. Patients that receive this therapy must be willing to self-catheterize if needed [108]. Botulinum toxin has been shown to be effective in the older population [112]. The Refractory Overactive Bladder: Sacral NEuromodulation vs. BoTulinum Toxin Assessment (ROSETTA) trial, a comparative effectiveness trial between Botulinum toxin and SNM for patients with refractory OAB, is currently in follow-up [113].

13.4 Stress Urinary Incontinence

Stress urinary incontinence (SUI) affects 15–20 % of women over the age of 65 [60, 62]. It is very costly from an economic perspective [114, 115] with annual out of pocket costs per woman at nearly $750 (in 2006 dollars) [114].

13.4.1 Evaluation

Evaluation for SUI can be straightforward with a good history and physical examination. Leak with Valsalva maneuver on exam or simple cystometrics using a bladder fill and cough stress test can be sufficient, and complex urodynamic testing is not needed for women with uncomplicated, demonstrable SUI [116].

Fig. 13.9 Retropubic (*green*) and transobturator (*blue*) midurethral slings. From Retropubic versus Transobturator Midurethral Slings for Stress Incontinence, Richter HE, Albo ME, Zyczynski HM, et al., Volume 362, Supplement Page 14, Copyright © 2010 Massachusetts Medical Society. Reprinted with permission from Massachusetts Medical Society

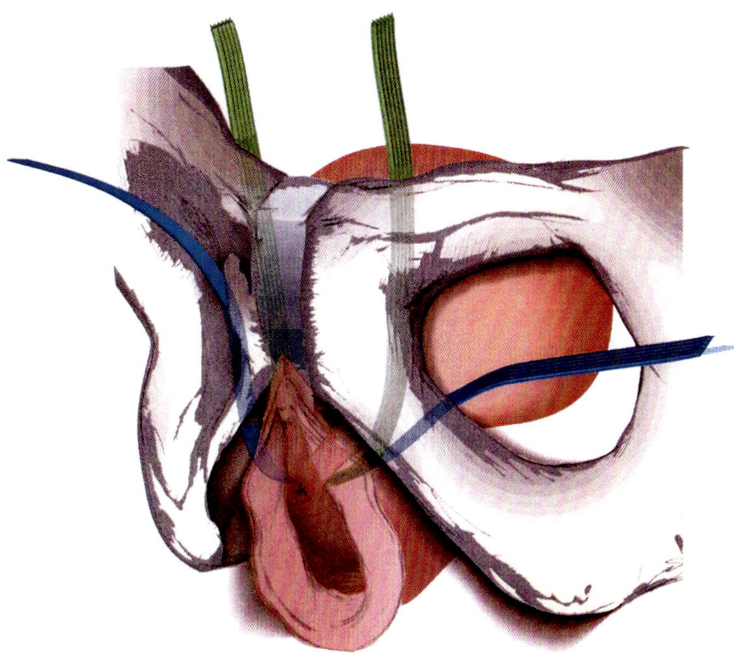

13.4.2 Non-Surgical Treatment

Conservative management options for SUI include behavioral therapy and urethral or vaginal inserts [117]. Some women have symptom improvement with continence pessaries, continence tampons, or urethral inserts, but the cure rates are lower than with behavioral therapy [117, 118]. Pelvic floor muscle training and bladder training have been shown to improve objective and subjective cure rates for SUI and are a good initial option for treatment [117]. If a woman does not improve with conservative therapy, she can consider more invasive options.

13.4.3 Surgical Treatment

SUI can be managed surgically with procedures such as polypropylene midurethral sling placement (Fig. 13.9), pubovaginal sling, Burch colposuspension, and periurethral bulking. Studies have shown trends with an increase in the number of total incontinence procedures performed per year in the USA as well as a shift from inpatient to outpatient procedures with the advent of the synthetic midurethral sling [119, 120]. These increases are notable in women over age 52 [121]. Women over age 75, however, do not appear to be getting the same treatment as rates of polypropylene midurethral sling in this population have increased much more slowly than in younger women [122]. This disparity may stem from concerns regarding surgical complications in older patients with more comorbidities or questions regarding

successful outcomes. In spite of comprising a significant proportion of the population suffering from UI, older women have been historically under-represented in clinical trials for SUI surgery [123]. More recently, however, many different studies have tried to evaluate the surgical treatment of SUI in older women [115, 124–148].

Results from studies of midurethral slings in older women have been inconsistent, which may be in part due to the heterogenous study populations and varied definitions of success. Some studies show greater risk of voiding dysfunction, outlet obstruction, de novo urinary urgency, urinary tract infection, need for catheterization, need for division of sling, and perioperative medical complications with lower rates of cure and satisfaction after midurethral sling in older patients, whereas others show no differences [115, 124, 125, 128–134, 136–138, 140–143, 145, 146, 148]. Older patients may also be more symptomatic than younger ones, and two studies showed that when differences in preoperative symptom bother were considered, age did not influence quality of life outcomes postoperatively [115, 124]. One prospective, randomized clinical trial comparing immediate midurethral sling versus expectant management for 6 months in older women found a significant improvement in satisfaction, symptoms, and quality of life in the immediate surgery group [147]. Another study showed that urethral hypermobility was an important predictor of midurethral sling treatment success in older women [139]. In summary, the overarching theme of the results is that older women do significantly benefit from midurethral slings and have improved quality of life postoperatively, although their improvements may be less pronounced than in younger women.

The pubovaginal sling (PVS) using autologous rectus fascia is another option for older patients [144, 149, 150]. Age has not been associated with worsened outcomes for PVS, however, menopausal status has [150]. At 2 years postoperatively, one study showed good short-term outcomes for PVS with 85 % of patients improved and satisfied, and another, smaller study showed 100 % of 19 geriatric women with resolved SUI [149, 151]. Long-term results from SISTEr (Stress Incontinence Surgical Treatment Efficacy Trial) were less promising for PVS with only 27 % continence at 7 years [150].

Treatment with Burch colposuspension was also studied in the SISTEr trial, which found that while patients who underwent the Burch procedure had lower success rates (38 % at 2 years to 13 % at 7 years) than those who underwent PVS they also had fewer urinary tract infections, less difficulty voiding, and less postoperative urgency incontinence [150, 152]. A sub-analysis of the older patients in the trial revealed that older women had similar perioperative outcomes and worse 2-year outcomes than younger women [144].

Periurethral bulking is another option for SUI treatment that is typically used either as a primary treatment in a patient who is a poor surgical candidate or as a secondary procedure after failure of another procedure. Two studies have evaluated bulking agents after failed midurethral sling and found

cure rates of 35–60 % with few complications [153, 154]. Even with these modest success rates, one study showed 77 % of patients were satisfied with the treatment and another showed negative pad tests (no leakage on a protective undergarment pad) in more than 70 % of patients [154, 155].

13.5 Fecal Incontinence

Fecal incontinence (FI) is defined as the unintentional loss of liquid or solid stool and anal incontinence (AI) includes the leakage of gas [156]. Estimating the number of people affected by this condition is difficult because only one third of patients discuss their incontinence with their physicians [157]. Fecal incontinence is common with prevalence rates ranging from 7 to 15 % in community-dwelling US populations [156]. The prevalence of FI is higher among care-seeking populations, home care populations, and adults in long-term care facilities [158]. In a study of community dwelling adults over the age of 65, the rate of FI over 4 years was 17 %. Controlling for age, comorbidity, and body mass index, significant independent risk factors for incident FI in women were white race, depression, chronic diarrhea, and urinary incontinence [159]. Other risk factors for FI are listed in Table 13.2 [160].

13.5.1 Evaluation

A thorough history and physical examination is essential to establishing the diagnosis of FI and tailoring treatment options. The history should include duration of symptoms, frequency of incontinence, time of day, quality of stool, control of flatus, frequency of bowel movements, constipation or diarrhea, use of pads, and impact on quality of life. Consistency of lost stool may correlate with the severity of incontinence since solid stool is easiest, liquid stool more difficult, and flatus most difficult to control [161]. Thus those patients with loss of solid stool have the most severe incontinence. A thorough obstetrical history should also be obtained including number of vaginal deliveries, weight of babies delivered, use of forceps, and significant tears, repairs, or episiotomies.

The physical examination should start with the inspection of the anal verge area looking for any scars or deformities. The patient should be asked to squeeze to simulate holding in a bowel movement to see if there is uniform contracture of muscles. Making the patient strain, as if having a bowel movement, can show perineal descent, hemorrhoids, vaginal prolapse, or even rectal prolapse [161]. Innervation can be crudely checked by touching the perineal area with a Q-tip and monitoring for an anal wink and also with pinprick sensation.

Table 13.2 Risk factors for fecal incontinence

Anal
- Injury
- Fistula
- Rectal prolapse
- Hemorrhoids
- Anal carcinoma
- Perianal infection
- Congenital

Rectal
- Proctitis
- Rectal carcinoma
- Rectal infection

Neurological
- Central nervous system (stroke, dementia, spinal cord injury, tumor, multiple sclerosis, cauda equina)
- Peripheral nervous system (pudendal neuropathy, diabetes mellitus)

Functional
- Fecal impaction
- Diarrhea
- Irritable bowel syndrome
- Physical disabilities
- Psychiatric disorders
- Metabolic, medication, malabsorption

With kind permission from Springer Science+Business Media: Curr Obstet Gynecol Rep, An Evidence-Based Approach to the Evaluation, Diagnostic Assessment and Treatment of Fecal Incontinence in Women, 3, 2014, 155–164, Meyer I, Richter HE

A digital rectal examination should be performed to check for masses, blood, fistula, or rectocele [162]. During the rectal examination baseline tone represents the internal anal sphincter and the patient should be asked to squeeze for assessment of the external anal sphincter. The accuracy of digital examination is operator dependent but overall, rectal exams have been proven as reliable as anal manometry in assessing anal resting and squeeze tone [163]. The reported positive predictive value of digital examinations to identify low resting and squeeze pressures by experienced clinicians was 67 and 81 %, respectively [164, 165].

Anorectal physiology testing involves manometry with rectal compliance testing, electromyography (EMG), and endoanal ultrasound (EAU). Manometry with rectal compliance testing is the preferred method for defining the functional weakness of the anal sphincter complex and for detecting abnormal rectal sensation [166, 167]. Rectal compliance is determined by inflating a balloon in the rectum and measuring the volume at the patient's first desire, strong desire, and maximum tolerable volume. Decreased compliance could represent a rectum that does not adequately store stool and may push the feces past the sphincter muscles even though sphincters are intact and supply adequate pressure, or it could be indicative of hypersensitivity in a woman sensitized by FI accidents. EMG assesses anal sphincter activity using a surface electrode or a concentric needle and can be helpful to distinguish between neurogenic and myogenic damage [160]. Endoanal ultrasound (EAU) assesses the structural integrity and morphology of the anal sphincters [160]. Whether a sphincter defect on EAU is the etiology of a patient's FI is still controversial as EAU has been shown to have low specificity for diagnosis [168, 169] and the degree of separation and size of tear shown on EAU may not correlate with symptom severity [170, 171].

13.5.2 Conservative Management

Conservative medical management for the treatment of fecal incontinence may include dietary modification with the use of bulking agents or antidiarrheal drugs, pelvic floor exercises, biofeedback, and bowel management strategies.

Fiber is frequently recommended to normalize stool consistency especially in patients with diarrhea-associated FI [172]. One small randomized controlled trial showed that fiber decreased FI in this group [173]. Restricting the fluid intake with these products may further enhance their ability to increase stool bulk. Antidiarrheal drugs are often used to treat FI and systematic reviews have shown they improve FI symptoms with loperamide being more effective than diphenoxylate (which is also to be avoided in older people related to its anticholinergic adverse effects) [174, 175].

Pelvic floor muscle exercises (PFME) are nearly always recommended to patients but there is little consensus on how they should be taught [172]. In general, they involve patients practicing squeezing their pelvic floor muscles with the goal of strengthening these muscles and the squeeze pressure of the anal sphincter. These exercises may particularly benefit patients who have early fatigue of the external sphincter muscle on digital examination [172]. Biofeedback is an adjunct to PFME and is performed using visual, auditory, or verbal feedback techniques with manometry or EMG probe inserted into the anorectum to display pressure changes [168]. The goal is to counteract the most common physiologic deficits contributing to FI by improving strength and isolation of pelvic floor muscle contractions, the ability to sense and contract pelvic floor muscles in response to minimal rectal distention, and the ability to tolerate greater rectal distention without experiencing uncomfortable urge sensations [172]. Randomized control trials comparing pelvic floor exercises and biofeedback have yielded inconsistent results with two larger studies showing no benefit for biofeedback compared to pelvic floor exercises taught by digital rectal exam [176, 177], while another study showed biofeedback to be superior compared to verbally taught pelvic floor exercises [178].

Bowel management strategies for patients focus on trying to schedule bowel movements at the same time each day in order to prevent FI. Daily enemas or suppositories can be used at the same time each day, such as right after eating breakfast, to induce a bowel movement and empty the rectum. Bulking agents and/or antidiarrheal medications can be used to reduce stooling between the timed bowel movements [161].

13.5.3 Surgical Management

13.5.3.1 Sphincteroplasty

Anal sphincter defects recognized during childbirth and repaired immediately are outside the scope of this chapter. Delayed sphincteroplasty is a surgical option for women being treated for FI who have disruption of the internal or external anal sphincter remote from delivery. The initial functional improvement after sphincteroplasty is good with studies reporting 70–80 % improvement [179]. However, long-term (≥5 years) success is disappointing with rates ranging from 20 to 58 % [168, 179]. Wound infection, occurring in 6–35 %, is the most common complication [179, 180]. Predictors of long-term failure include deep infection, longer duration of FI symptoms, and advanced age at the time of repair [179, 180].

13.5.3.2 Sacral Nerve Stimulation

Sacral nerve stimulation (SNS) was approved by the FDA in 2011 for the treatment of fecal incontinence, and results

a

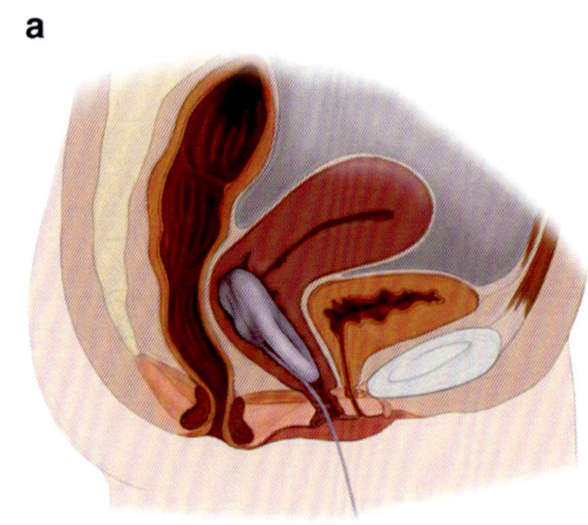

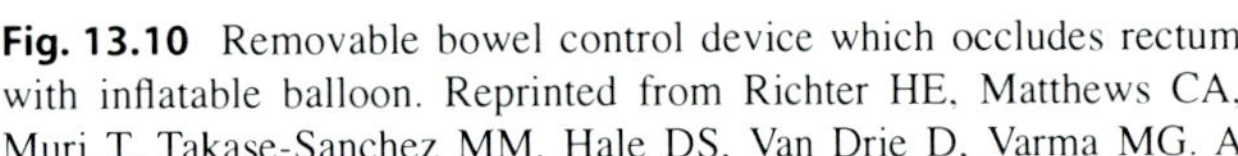

b

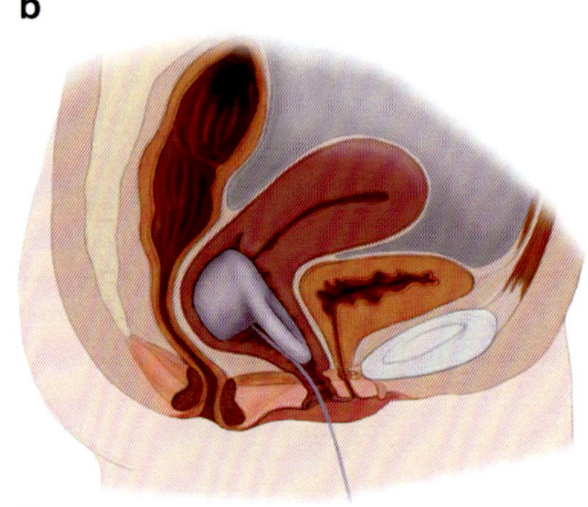

Fig. 13.10 Removable bowel control device which occludes rectum with inflatable balloon. Reprinted from Richter HE, Matthews CA, Muri T, Takase-Sanchez MM, Hale DS, Van Drie D, Varma MG. A vaginal bowel-control system for the treatment of fecal incontinence. Obstet Gynecol 2015;125:540-7. © 2015 by the American College of Obstetricians and Gynecologists. All rights reserved

from the FDA-monitored trial have been encouraging. In this trial, 285 patients were screened and 133 were eligible for stage I. Of those, 120 (90 %) proceeded to stage II permanent stimulation [181]. Results with follow-up over 5 years showed that 85 % of patients maintained their treatment goal and 36 % reported complete continence [182]. Other studies have demonstrated over 80 % of patients achieving a ≥50 % reduction in incontinence episodes per week with sustained long-term results up to 14 years [160]. The most commonly reported complications are pain and infection at the insertion site which have been reported in 3–11 % of patients [183, 184].

13.5.3.3 Colostomy

A colostomy is an option to eliminate all episodes of FI although mucus can still leak in patients with a retained rectum. These procedures are infrequently performed for FI, but for some patients with incapacitating FI who are afraid to leave their homes due to fear of incontinence, this may be a reasonable choice [161].

13.5.4 Further Treatment Options

There are other, less-commonly used and investigational treatment options. Injection of an inert bulking agent around the anal canal has been shown to decrease FI in some patients [172]. Anal plugs commonly cause discomfort in patients but when patients are able to tolerate the devices they report improvement [185]. A mesh sling that is tunneled beneath the puborectalis muscle via a transobturator approach is being investigated [172]. A removable bowel-control device has been designed to help women with FI. The device is placed intra-vaginally with an inflatable balloon which is

oriented posteriorly and can be connected to a hand-held pump. While inflated, the balloon occludes the rectum to help prevent unwanted stool from passing (see Fig. 13.10). Early studies have shown significant improvement at 4 and 12 weeks in FI by objective and subjective measures with the most common adverse event being vaginal cramping and discomfort. Further longer-term studies are being done to evaluate the device's efficacy [186].

13.6 Constipation

Constipation is a common contributing factor to both UI and FI that affects between 2 and 27 % of the population in Western countries. In the USA, it accounts for nearly 92,000 hospitalizations per year and 2.5 million physician office visits [187–189]. Constipation can be defined as less than two bowel movements per week or straining for at least a quarter of the time [190]. The etiology of constipation is multifactorial. The pelvic floor and anal sphincters, which should relax as the contents of the distal colon are propelled outward during evacuation, are intimately linked to defecatory function. Constipation may result from impairment of these coordinated efforts, or it may result from systemic illness, neurogenic disorders, or medications [191].

The mainstay of treatment for idiopathic constipation includes dietary modification, pharmacological agents, and behavioral therapy including biofeedback techniques. In general, a treatment pathway in recommended sequence is: 1. Exclude other pathologies and secondary causes (often medications). 2. Begin treatment with dietary and lifestyle modifications. 3. Move to osmotic laxatives or bulking agents—there is no consensus on order in which these should be tried. Note that bulking agents may cause fecal impaction

References

1. Bierman A, Spector W, Atkins D, et al. Improving the Health Care of Older Americans. A Report of the AHRQ task force on aging. Rockville: Agency for Healthcare Research and Quality; 2001. AHRQ Publication No. 01-0030.
2. Bailey IL. New procedures for detecting early vision losses in the elderly. Optom Vis Sci. 1993;70:299–305.
3. Castor TD, Carter TL. Low vision: physician screening helps to improve patient function. Geriatrics. 1995;50:51–2. 55–57; quiz 58–59.
4. Fletcher DC, Shindell S, Hindman T, Schaffrath M. Low vision rehabilitation. Finding capable people behind damaged eyeballs. West J Med. 1991;154:554–6.
5. Fletcher DC. Low vision: the physician's role in rehabilitation and referral. Geriatrics. 1994;49:50–3.
6. Klein BE, Klein R, Lee KE, Cruickshanks KJ. Performance-based and self-assessed measures of visual function as related to history of falls, hip fractures, and measured gait time. The Beaver Dam Eye Study. Ophthalmology. 1998;105:160–4.
7. Klein R, Klein BE, Linton KL, De Mets DL. The Beaver Dam Eye Study: visual acuity. Ophthalmology. 1991;98:1310–5.
8. Tielsch JM, Javitt JC, Coleman A, et al. The prevalence of blindness and visual impairment among nursing home residents in Baltimore. N Engl J Med. 1995;332:1205–9.
9. Tielsch JM, Steinberg EP, Cassard SD, et al. Preoperative functional expectations and postoperative outcomes among patients undergoing first eye cataract surgery. Arch Ophthalmol. 1995;113:1312–8.
10. American Academy of Ophthalmology. Preferred Practice Patterns. Cataract in the Adult Eye. 1996.
11. Applegate WB, Miller ST, Elam JT, et al. Impact of cataract surgery with lens implantation on vision and physical function in elderly patients. JAMA. 1987;257:1064–6.
12. Bruce DW, Gray CS. Beyond the cataract: visual and functional disability in elderly people. Age Ageing. 1991;20:389–91.
13. Cataract Management Guideline Panel. Clinical Practice Guideline Number 4. Cataract in adults: management of functional impairment. Rockville: Department of Health and Human Services, Public Health Service; 1993. AHCPR Pub 93-0542.
14. Crabtree HL, Hildreth AJ, O'Connell JE, et al. Measuring visual symptoms in British cataract patients: the cataract symptom scale. Br J Ophthalmol. 1999;83:519–23.
15. Javitt JC, Steinberg EP, Sharkey P, et al. Cataract surgery in one eye or both. A billion dollar per year issue. Ophthalmology. 1995;102:1583–92. discussion 1592–1583.
16. Lee AG, Beaver HA, Teasdale T. The aging eye (CD-ROM). Houston: Baylor College of Medicine; 2001.
17. Mangione CM, Orav EJ, Lawrence MG, et al. Prediction of visual function after cataract surgery. A prospectively validated model. Arch Ophthalmol. 1995;113:1305–11.
18. Mangione CM, Phillips RS, Lawrence MG, et al. Improved visual function and attenuation of declines in health-related quality of life after cataract extraction. Arch Ophthalmol. 1994;112:1419–25.
19. Monestam E, Wachtmeister L. Impact of cataract surgery on car driving: a population based study in Sweden. Br J Ophthalmol. 1997;81:16–22.
20. Owsley C, Stalvey B, Wells J, Sloane ME. Older drivers and cataract: driving habits and crash risk. J Gerontol A Biol Sci Med Sci. 1999;54:M203–11.
21. Powe NR, Schein OD, Gieser SC, et al. Synthesis of the literature on visual acuity and complications following cataract extraction with intraocular lens implantation. Cataract Patient Outcome Research Team. Arch Ophthalmol. 1994;112:239–52.
22. Powe NR, Tielsch JM, Schein OD, et al. Rigor of research methods in studies of the effectiveness and safety of cataract extraction with intraocular lens implantation. Cataract Patient Outcome Research Team. Arch Ophthalmol. 1994;112:228–38.
23. Schein OD, Steinberg EP, Cassard SD, et al. Predictors of outcome in patients who underwent cataract surgery. Ophthalmology. 1995;102:817–23.
24. Schein OD, Bass EB, Sharkey P, et al. Cataract surgical techniques. Preferences and underlying beliefs. Arch Ophthalmol. 1995;113:1108–12.
25. Steinberg EP, Tielsch JM, Schein OD, et al. National study of cataract surgery outcomes. Variation in 4-month postoperative outcomes as reflected in multiple outcome measures. Ophthalmology. 1994;101:1131–40. discussion 1140–1131.
26. Steinberg EP, Tielsch JM, Schein OD, et al. The VF-14. An index of functional impairment in patients with cataract. Arch Ophthalmol. 1994;112:630–8.
27. Bass EB, Steinberg EP, Luthra R, et al. Do ophthalmologists, anesthesiologists, and internists agree about preoperative testing in healthy patients undergoing cataract surgery? Arch Ophthalmol. 1995;113:1248–56.
28. Superstein R, Boyaner D, Overbury O. Functional complaints, visual acuity, spatial contrast sensitivity, and glare disability in preoperative and postoperative cataract patients. J Cataract Refract Surg. 1999;25:575–81.
29. Tobacman JK, Zimmerman B, Lee P, et al. Visual function impairments in relation to gender, age, and visual acuity in patients who undergo cataract surgery. Ophthalmology. 1998;105:1745–50.
30. Uusitalo RJ, Brans T, Pessi T, Tarkkanen A. Evaluating cataract surgery gains by assessing patients' quality of life using the VF-7. J Cataract Refract Surg. 1999;25:989–94.
31. Rumsey KE. Redefining the optometric examination: addressing the vision needs of older adults. Optom Vis Sci. 1993;70:587–91.
32. Rubin GS, Roche KB, Prasada-Rao P, Fried LP. Visual impairment and disability in older adults. Optom Vis Sci. 1994;71:750–60.
33. Rubin GS, West SK, Munoz B, et al. A comprehensive assessment of visual impairment in a population of older Americans. The SEE Study. Salisbury Eye Evaluation Project. Invest Ophthalmol Vis Sci. 1997;38:557–68.
34. American Academy of Ophthalmology. Preferred Practice Patterns. Age-related Macular Degeneration. Limited Revision. 2001.
35. American Academy of Ophthalmology. Preferred Practice Patterns. Primary Open Angle Glaucoma. 2000.
36. American Academy of Ophthalmology. Preferred Practice Patterns. Vision Rehabilitation for Adults. 2001.
37. Albrecht KG, Lee PP. Conformance with preferred practice patterns in caring for patients with glaucoma. Ophthalmology. 1994;101:1668–71.
38. Appollonio I, Carabellese C, Magni E, et al. Sensory impairments and mortality in an elderly community population: a six-year follow-up study. Age Ageing. 1995;24:30–6.
39. Brenner MH, Curbow B, Javitt JC, et al. Vision change and quality of life in the elderly. Response to cataract surgery and treatment of other chronic ocular conditions. Arch Ophthalmol. 1993;111:680–5.
40. Campbell VA, Crews JE, Moriarty DG, et al. Surveillance for sensory impairment, activity limitation, and health-related quality of life among older adults—United States, 1993–1997. Morb Mortal Wkly Rep CDC Surveill Summ. 1999;48:131–56.
41. Carter TL. Age-related vision changes: a primary care guide. Geriatrics. 1994;49:37–42. 45; quiz 46-37.
42. Collaborative Normal-Tension Glaucoma Study Group. Comparison of glaucomatous progression between untreated patients with normal-tension glaucoma and patients with thera-

peutically reduced intraocular pressures. Am J Ophthalmol. 1998;126:487–97.

43. Collaborative Normal-Tension Glaucoma Study Group. The effectiveness of intraocular pressure reduction in the treatment of normal-tension glaucoma. Am J Ophthalmol. 1998;126:498–505.

44. The Diabetes Control and Complications Trial/Epidemiology of Diabetes Interventions and Complications Research Group. Retinopathy and nephropathy in patients with type 1 diabetes four years after a trial of intensive therapy. N Engl J Med. 2000;342:381–9.

45. The Diabetic Retinopathy Study Research Group. Indications for photocoagulation treatment of diabetic retinopathy: Diabetic Retinopathy Study Report No. 14. Int Ophthalmol Clin. 1987;27:239–53.

46. The Diabetic Retinopathy Study Research Group. Photocoagulation treatment of proliferative diabetic retinopathy. Clinical application of Diabetic Retinopathy Study (DRS) findings, DRS Report No. 8. Ophthalmology. 1981;88:583–600.

47. The Early Treatment Diabetic Retinopathy Study Research Group. Photocoagulation for diabetic macular edema: Early Treatment Diabetic Retinopathy Study Report No. 4. Int Ophthalmol Clin. 1987;27:265–72.

48. The Early Treatment Diabetic Retinopathy Study Research Group. Early photocoagulation for diabetic retinopathy. ETDRS Report No. 9. Ophthalmology. 1991;98:766–85.

49. Klein BE, Klein R, Linton KL. Prevalence of age-related lens opacities in a population. The Beaver Dam Eye Study. Ophthalmology. 1992;99:546–52.

50. Klein R, Klein BE, Linton KL. Prevalence of age-related maculopathy. The Beaver Dam Eye Study. Ophthalmology. 1992;99:933–43.

51. Klein R. Age-related eye disease, visual impairment, and driving in the elderly. Hum Factors. 1991;33:521–5.

52. Tielsch JM, Sommer A, Katz J, et al. Socioeconomic status and visual impairment among urban Americans. Baltimore Eye Survey Research Group. Arch Ophthalmol. 1991;109:637–41.

53. Mangione CM, Gutierrez PR, Lowe G, et al. Influence of age-related maculopathy on visual functioning and health-related quality of life. Am J Ophthalmol. 1999;128:45–53.

54. Olsen CL, Kassoff A, Gerber T. The care of diabetic patients by ophthalmologists in New York State. Ophthalmology. 1989;96:739–45.

55. Perry DP. ARMD is robbing older people blind–and stealing their independence, too. J Am Optom Assoc. 1999;70:7–9.

56. Salive ME, Guralnik J, Christen W, et al. Functional blindness and visual impairment in older adults from three communities. Ophthalmology. 1992;99:1840–7.

57. Jette AM, Branch LG. Impairment and disability in the aged. J Chronic Dis. 1985;38:59–65.

58. Cummings SR, Nevitt MC, Browner WS, et al. Risk factors for hip fracture in white women. Study of Osteoporotic Fractures Research Group. N Engl J Med. 1995;332:767–73.

59. Cwikel J. Falls among elderly people living at home: medical and social factors in a national sample. Isr J Med Sci. 1992;28:446–53.

60. Kelsey JL, Browner WS, Seeley DG, et al. Risk factors for fractures of the distal forearm and proximal humerus. The Study of Osteoporotic Fractures Research Group (published erratum appears in Am J Epidemiol 1992 135:1183). Am J Epidemiol. 1992;135:477–89.

61. Lord SR, McLean D, Stathers G. Physiological factors associated with injurious falls in older people living in the community. Gerontology. 1992;38:338–46.

62. Melton 3rd LJ, Riggs BL. Risk factors for injury after a fall. Clin Geriatr Med. 1985;1:525–39.

63. Myers AH, Robinson EG, Van Natta ML, et al. Hip fractures among the elderly: factors associated with in-hospital mortality. Am J Epidemiol. 1991;134:1128–37.

64. Nevitt MC, Cummings SR, Kidd S, Black D. Risk factors for recurrent nonsyncopal falls. A prospective study. JAMA. 1989;261:2663–8.

65. Nevitt MC, Cummings SR, Hudes ES. Risk factors for injurious falls: a prospective study. J Gerontol. 1991;46:M164–70.

66. O'Loughlin JL, Robitaille Y, Boivin JF, Suissa S. Incidence of and risk factors for falls and injurious falls among the community-dwelling elderly. Am J Epidemiol. 1993;137:342–54.

67. Sattin RW, Lambert Huber DA, DeVito CA, et al. The incidence of fall injury events among the elderly in a defined population. Am J Epidemiol. 1990;131:1028–37.

68. Sattin RW. Falls among older persons: a public health perspective. Annu Rev Public Health. 1992;13:489–508.

69. Sorock GS. Falls among the elderly: epidemiology and prevention. Am J Prev Med. 1988;4:282–8.

70. Speechley M, Tinetti M. Falls and injuries in frail and vigorous community elderly persons. J Am Geriatr Soc. 1991;39:46–52.

71. Tinetti ME. Instability and falling in elderly patients. Semin Neurol. 1989;9:39–45.

72. Tinetti ME, Powell L. Fear of falling and low self-efficacy: a case of dependence in elderly persons. J Gerontol. 1993;48:35–8.

73. Tinetti ME, Doucette J, Claus E, Marottoli R. Risk factors for serious injury during falls by older persons in the community. J Am Geriatr Soc. 1995;43:1214–21.

74. Tinetti ME, McAvay G, Claus E. Does multiple risk factor reduction explain the reduction in fall rate in the yale FICSIT trial? Frailty and injuries cooperative studies of intervention techniques. Am J Epidemiol. 1996;144:389–99.

75. Tobis JS, Block M, Steinhaus-Donham C, et al. Falling among the sensorially impaired elderly. Arch Phys Med Rehabil. 1990;71:144–7.

76. Wilson MR, Coleman AL, Yu F, et al. Functional status and well-being in patients with glaucoma as measured by the Medical Outcomes Study Short Form-36 questionnaire. Ophthalmology. 1998;105:2112–6.

77. Wang JJ, Mitchell P, Smith W, et al. Impact of visual impairment on use of community support services by elderly persons: the Blue Mountains Eye Study. Invest Ophthalmol Vis Sci. 1999;40:12–9.

78. Wang JJ, Mitchell P, Smith W. Vision and low self-rated health: the Blue Mountains Eye Study. Invest Ophthalmol Vis Sci. 2000;41:49–54.

79. Branch LG, Horowitz A, Carr C. The implications for everyday life of incident self-reported visual decline among people over age 65 living in the community. Gerontologist. 1989;29:359–65.

80. Carabellese C, Appollonio I, Rozzini R, et al. Sensory impairment and quality of life in a community elderly population. J Am Geriatr Soc. 1993;41:401–7.

81. Keeffe JE, Lam D, Cheung A, et al. Impact of vision impairment on functioning. Aust N Z J Ophthalmol. 1998;26 Suppl 1:S16–8.

82. Keeffe JE, McCarty CA, Hassell JB, Gilbert AG. Description and measurement of handicap caused by vision impairment. Aust N Z J Ophthalmol. 1999;27:184–6.

83. Keller BK, Morton JL, Thomas VS, Potter JF. The effect of visual and hearing impairments on functional status. J Am Geriatr Soc. 1999;47:1319–25.

84. Kelly M. Consequences of visual impairment on leisure activities of the elderly. Geriatr Nurs. 1995;16:273–5.

85. Lee PP, Smith JP, Kington R. The relationship of self-rated vision and hearing to functional status and well-being among seniors 70 years and older. Am J Ophthalmol. 1999;127:447–52.

86. Lee PP, Spritzer K, Hays RD. The impact of blurred vision on functioning and well-being. Ophthalmology. 1997;104:390–6.

87. Lee PP, Whitcup SM, Hays RD, et al. The relationship between visual acuity and functioning and well-being among diabetics. Qual Life Res. 1995;4:319–23.

88. Thompson JR, Gibson JM, Jagger C. The association between visual impairment and mortality in elderly people. Age Ageing. 1989;18:83–8.

89. Sooriakumaran P. The evolution of the doctor-patient relationship. Int J Surg. 2007;5(1):57–65.

90. Livingston PM, Lee SE, McCarty CA, Taylor HR. A comparison of participants with non-participants in a population-based epidemiologic study: the Melbourne Visual Impairment Project. Ophthalmic Epidemiol. 1997;4:73–81.

91. Dargent-Molina P, Hays M, Breart G. Sensory impairments and physical disability in aged women living at home. Int J Epidemiol. 1996;25:621–9.

92. McClure ME, Hart PM, Jackson AJ, et al. Macular degeneration: do conventional measurements of impaired visual function equate with visual disability? Br J Ophthalmol. 2000;84:244–50.

93. Ware Jr JE, Sherbourne CD. The MOS 36-item short-form health survey (SF-36). I. Conceptual framework and item selection. Med Care. 1992;30:473–83.

94. Mangione CM, Berry S, Spritzer K, et al. Identifying the content area for the 51-item National Eye Institute Visual Function Questionnaire: results from focus groups with visually impaired persons. Arch Ophthalmol. 1998;116:227–33.

95. Mangione CM, Phillips RS, Seddon JM, et al. Development of the activities of daily vision scale. A measure of visual functional status. Med Care. 1992;30:1111–26.

96. Scott IU, Smiddy WE, Schiffman J, et al. Quality of life of low-vision patients and the impact of low-vision services. Am J Ophthalmol. 1999;128:54–62.

97. Cassard SD, Patrick DL, Damiano AM, et al. Reproducibility and responsiveness of the VF-14. An index of functional impairment in patients with cataracts. Arch Ophthalmol. 1995;113:1508–13.

98. Hart PM, Chakravarthy U, Stevenson MR, Jamison JQ. A vision specific functional index for use in patients with age related macular degeneration. Br J Ophthalmol. 1999;83:1115–20.

99. Horowitz A. Vision impairment and functional disability among nursing home residents. Gerontologist. 1994;34:316–23.

100. Parrish RK, Gedde SJ, Scott IU, et al. Visual function and quality of life among patients with glaucoma. Arch Ophthalmol. 1997;115:1447–55.

101. Ross CK, Stelmack JA, Stelmack TR, et al. Development and sensitivity to visual impairment of the Low Vision Functional Status Evaluation (LVFSE). Optom Vis Sci. 1999;76:212–20.

102. Turco PD, Connolly J, McCabe P, Glynn RJ. Assessment of functional vision performance: a new test for low vision patients. Ophthalmic Epidemiol. 1994;1:15–25.

103. Lawton MP, Brody EM. Assessment of older people: self-maintaining and instrumental activities of daily living. Gerontologist. 1969;9:179–86.

104. Rovner BW, Zisselman PM, Shmuely-Dulitzki Y. Depression and disability in older people with impaired vision: a follow-up study. J Am Geriatr Soc. 1996;44:181–4.

105. Rovner BW, Ganguli M. Depression and disability associated with impaired vision: the movies project. J Am Geriatr Soc. 1998;46:617–9.

106. Appollonio I, Carabellese C, Frattola L, Trabucchi M. Effects of sensory aids on the quality of life and mortality of elderly people: a multivariate analysis. Age Ageing. 1996;25:89–96.

107. Klein R, Cruickshanks KJ, Klein BE, et al. Is age-related maculopathy related to hearing loss? Arch Ophthalmol. 1998;116:360–5.

108. Bagley M. Helping older adults to live better with hearing and vision losses. J Case Manag. 1998;7:147–52.

109. Guralnik JM. The impact of vision and hearing impairments on health in old age. J Am Geriatr Soc. 1999;47:1029–31.

110. Rudberg MA, Furner SE, Dunn JE, Cassel CK. The relationship of visual and hearing impairments to disability: an analysis using the longitudinal study of aging. J Gerontol. 1993;48:M261–5.

111. Rubin GS, Bandeen-Roche K, Huang GH, et al. The association of multiple visual impairments with self-reported visual disability: SEE project. Invest Ophthalmol Vis Sci. 2001;42:64–72.

112. Heine C, Browning CJ. Communication and psychosocial consequences of sensory loss in older adults: overview and rehabilitation directions. Disabil Rehabil. 2002;24:763–73.

113. Bazargan M, Baker RS, Bazargan SH. Sensory impairments and subjective well-being among aged African American persons. J Gerontol B Psychol Sci Soc Sci. 2001;56:P268–78.

114. Wallhagen MI, Strawbridge WJ, Shema SJ, et al. Comparative impact of hearing and vision impairment on subsequent functioning. J Am Geriatr Soc. 2001;49:1086–92.

115. Uhlmann RF, Larson EB, Koepsell TD, et al. Visual impairment and cognitive dysfunction in Alzheimer's disease. J Gen Intern Med. 1991;6:126–32.

116. George J, Bleasdale S, Singleton SJ. Causes and prognosis of delirium in elderly patients admitted to a district general hospital. Age Ageing. 1997;26:423–7.

117. Steinman SB, Steinman BA, Trick GL, Lehmkuhle S. A sensory explanation for visual attention deficits in the elderly. Optom Vis Sci. 1994;71:743–9.

118. Reyes-Ortiz CA, Kuo YF, DiNuzzo AR, et al. Near vision impairment predicts cognitive decline: data from the Hispanic established populations for epidemiologic studies of the elderly. J Am Geriatr Soc. 2005;53:681–6.

119. Anstey KJ, Luszcz MA, Sanchez L. Two-year decline in vision but not hearing is associated with memory decline in very old adults in a population-based sample. Gerontology. 2001;47:289–93.

120. Kosnik WD, Sekuler R, Kline DW. Self-reported visual problems of older drivers. Hum Factors. 1990;32:597–608.

121. Kline DW, Kline TJ, Fozard JL, et al. Vision, aging, and driving: the problems of older drivers. J Gerontol. 1992;47:P27–34.

122. Ball K, Owsley C, Stalvey B, et al. Driving avoidance and functional impairment in older drivers. Accid Anal Prev. 1998;30:313–22.

123. McGwin G, Owsley C, Ball K. Identifying crash involvement among older drivers: agreement between self-report and state records. Accid Anal Prev. 1998;30:781–91.

124. Owsley C, Ball K, McGwin Jr G, et al. Visual processing impairment and risk of motor vehicle crash among older adults. JAMA. 1998;279:1083–8.

125. Shipp MD, Penchansky R. Vision testing and the elderly driver: is there a problem meriting policy change? J Am Optom Assoc. 1995;66:343–51.

126. Sloan JP. Primary care geriatrics, mobility failure. New York, NY: Springer; 1997. p. 35.

127. Lord SR, Dayhew J, Howland A. Multifocal glasses impair edge-contrast sensitivity and depth perception and increase the risk of falls in older people. J Am Geriatr Soc. 2002;50:1760–6.

128. Lord SR, Dayhew J. Visual risk factors for falls in older people. J Am Geriatr Soc. 2001;49:508–15.

129. de Boer MR, Pluijm SM, Lips P, et al. Different aspects of visual impairment as risk factors for falls and fractres in older men and women. J Bone Miner Res. 2004;19:1539–47.

130. Ivers RQ, Cumming RG, Mitchell P, et al. Visual risk factors for hip fracture in older people. J Am Geriatr Soc. 2003;51:356–63.

131. Buckley JG, Heasley KJ, Twigg P, Elliott DB. The effects of blurred vision on the mechanics of landing during stepping down by the elderly. Gait Posture. 2005;21:65–71.

132. Startzell JK, Owens DA, Mulfinger LM, Cavanagh PR. Stair negotiation in older people: a review. J Am Geriatr Soc. 2000;48:567–80.

133. Campbell AJ, Robertson MC, La Grow SJ, et al. Randomised controlled trial of prevention of falls in people aged > or =75 with severe visual impairment: the VIP trial. BMJ. 2005;331:817.

134. Coleman AL, Stone K, Ewing SK, et al. Higher risk of multiple falls among elderly women who lose visual acuity. Ophthalmology. 2004;111:857–62.

135. Tromp AM, Pluijm SM, Smit JH, et al. Fall-risk screening test: a prospective study on predictors for falls in community-dwelling elderly. J Clin Epidemiol. 2001;54:837–44.

136. Abdelhafiz AH, Austin CA. Visual factors should be assessed in older people presenting with falls or hip fracture. Age Ageing. 2003;32:26–30.

137. Salive ME, Guralnik J, Glynn RJ, et al. Association of visual impairment with mobility and physical function. J Am Geriatr Soc. 1994;42:287–92.

138. West SK, Munoz B, Rubin GS, et al. Function and visual impairment in a population-based study of older adults. The SEE project. Salisbury Eye Evaluation. Invest Ophthalmol Vis Sci. 1997;38:72–82.

139. Marx MS, Werner P, Cohen-Mansfield J, Feldman R. The relationship between low vision and performance of activities of daily living in nursing home residents. J Am Geriatr Soc. 1992;40:1018–20.

140. Pillar T, Gaspar E, Dickstein R. Physical rehabilitation of the elderly blind patient. Int Disabil Stud. 1990;12:75–7.

141. Maino JH. Visual deficits and mobility. Evaluation and management. Clin Geriatr Med. 1996;12:803–23.

142. Boter H, Mistiaen P, Duijnhouwer E, Groenewegen I. The problems of elderly patients at home after ophthalmic treatment. J Ophthalmic Nurs Technol. 1998;17:59–65.

143. Cate Y, Baker SS, Gilbert MP. Occupational therapy and the person with diabetes and vision impairment. Am J Occup Ther. 1995;49:905–11.

144. Gutierrez P, Wilson MR, Johnson C, et al. Influence of glaucomatous visual field loss on health-related quality of life. Arch Ophthalmol. 1997;115:777–84.

145. Javitt JC, Brenner MH, Curbow B, et al. Outcomes of cataract surgery. Improvement in visual acuity and subjective visual function after surgery in the first, second, and both eyes. Arch Ophthalmol. 1993;111:686–91.

146. Jayamanne DG, Allen ED, Wood CM, Currie S. Correlation between early, measurable improvement in quality of life and speed of visual rehabilitation after phacoemulsification. J Cataract Refract Surg. 1999;25:1135–9.

147. Lundstrom M, Fregell G, Sjoblom A. Vision related daily life problems in patients waiting for a cataract extraction. Br J Ophthalmol. 1994;78:608–11.

148. Bergner M, Bobbitt RA, Carter WB, Gilson BS. The sickness impact profile: development and final revision of a health status measure. Med Care. 1981;19:787–805.

149. Nelson P, Aspinall P, O'Brien C. Patients' perception of visual impairment in glaucoma: a pilot study. Br J Ophthalmol. 1999;83:546–52.

150. Phillips KE, Russello SM, Bonesi J, Garcon R. Functional visual problems: training home care aides to identify early signs. Caring. 1997;16:54, 56–60, 62–54.

151. Sherwood MB, Garcia-Siekavizza A, Meltzer MI, et al. Glaucoma's impact on quality of life and its relation to clinical indicators. A pilot study. Ophthalmology. 1998;105:561–6.

152. Swagerty DL. The impact of age-related visual impairment on functional independence in the elderly. Kans Med. 1995;96:24–6.

153. Wahl HW, Schilling O, Oswald F, Heyl V. Psychosocial consequences of age-related visual impairment: comparison with mobility-impaired older adults and long-term outcome. J Gerontol B Psychol Sci Soc Sci. 1999;54:P304–16.

154. Morse AR, Yatzkan E, Berberich B, Arons RR. Acute care hospital utilization by patients with visual impairment. Arch Ophthalmol. 1999;117:943–9.

155. Wenger NS, Shekelle PG. Assessing care of vulnerable elders: ACOVE project overview. Ann Intern Med. 2001;135:642–6.

156. Smeeth L, Iliffe S. Community screening for visual impairment in the elderly. Cochrane Data-Base Syst Rev. 2000:CD001054.

157. American Academy of Ophthalmology. Preferred Practice Patterns. Comprehensive Adult Medical Eye Evaluation. 2000.

158. U.S. Preventive Services Task Force. Recommendations for screening for visual impairment. In: Guide to clinical preventive services. 2nd ed. Baltimore: Williams & Wilkins; 1996. p 373–82.

159. Rahmani B, Tielsch JM, Katz J, et al. The cause-specific prevalence of visual impairment in an urban population. The Baltimore Eye Survey. Ophthalmology. 1996;103:1721–6.

160. Ariyasu RG, Lee PP, Linton KP, et al. Sensitivity, specificity, and predictive values of screening tests for eye conditions in a clinic-based population. Ophthalmology. 1996;103:1751–60.

161. Bernth-Petersen P. Visual functioning in cataract patients. Methods of measuring and results. Acta Ophthalmol (Copenh). 1981;59:198–205.

Geriatric Orthopedic Surgery

Stephen L. Kates and Jason S. Lipof

15.1 Introduction

Among older adults, musculoskeletal disorders are very common and often interfere with function and quality of life. These conditions include arthritic joints, fragility fractures, musculoskeletal infections, degeneration and tearing of tendons, tendinitis, and compressive disorders of the spine and peripheral nerves. Because patients are living longer, healthier lives and have higher expectations for the quality of their lives than previous generations, many older patients will seek musculoskeletal care to improve their function and quality of life. Older adults have tremendous variability in their health status and physiologic state, both of which must be carefully considered when providing musculoskeletal care. Simply stated, the older adult orthopedic patient is very different from younger adults and this chapter will focus on specific considerations, techniques, and approaches to care required by the older adult.

15.2 The Problem

People are living longer and often healthier lives into their 90s. Accompanying this aging of the population is the expectation that functional status will be maintained, a goal which frequently requires orthopedic intervention. In some cases, this enables older adults to continue working or participating in sports activities into old age. For others, the orthopedic interventions will enable individuals to live independently. Use of a thoughtful and detail oriented approach to geriatric patients enables the surgeon to correct these musculoskeletal issues successfully.

The older adult is frequently a better-educated patient, having not only studied their musculoskeletal condition online but also the background of their surgeon. Such research has been intensified by direct to consumer marketing of medications, surgical implants, and surgical techniques by device manufacturers, pharmaceutical companies, health systems, and individual physicians. It is common that patients will have watched videos of a surgery they may need, and studied the specific implant types and options available on the internet. Improved education of the patient and their family leads to higher expectations for their care and outcomes. Additionally, the free availability of information, combined with health reform measures has led to a perception that orthopedic care is a commodity for purchase similar to shopping for an item online. These new expectations will clearly shape the future practice of orthopedic surgery. Although Geriatric Orthopaedic Surgery is not yet a recognized specialty in orthopedics, surgeons are beginning to recognize that older adults have different needs, expectations, and a different paradigm of care is frequently required to successfully treat them. It is anticipated that Geriatric Orthopaedic Surgery will become a recognized and fellowship trained specialty over the next 10 years.

15.3 Epidemiology

The population is aging worldwide and is expected to create a significant increase in the demand for orthopedic surgery. Most subspecialties within orthopedic surgery will see an increased geriatric caseload as a result. Specific procedures that will be more prominent include total joint replacement,

Stephen L. Kates, MD (✉)
Department of Orthopaedic Surgery, Virginia Commonwealth University, West Hospital, 1200 East Broad Street, 9th Floor, Richmond, VA 23298, USA
e-mail: Stephen.Kates@vcuhealth.org

J.S. Lipof, MD
Department of Orthopaedic Surgery and Rehabilitation, University of Rochester Medical Center, 601 Elmwood Avenue, Box #665, Rochester, NY 14642, USA

© Springer International Publishing Switzerland 2017
J.R. Burton et al. (eds.), *Geriatrics for Specialists*, DOI 10.1007/978-3-319-31831-8_15

fracture care, hand and upper extremity surgery, spine surgery, and foot and ankle surgery. Total joint surgery, for example, has been growing rapidly [1]. This increase in case volume will require surgeons to develop enhanced skills to successfully manage the special needs of older adult patients. Additionally, there will likely be the need for an increase in the number of surgeons to manage this increased volume. Hospitals and health systems are developing enhanced care protocols, specialized inpatient units, and enhanced rehabilitation pathways to effectively care for their older adult patients [2].

## 15.4	Usual Care

In the past usual care for the older adult orthopedic patient involved single specialty management and in some cases, multidisciplinary management of the patient's medical problems. Without multidisciplinary, various health disciplines all contribute their advice and care management in a "silo" manner. This old care paradigm creates variability in outcomes and is quite prone to communication breakdown and a lack of coordination for the care. Duplication of efforts or ordering of unnecessary studies occurs. Each of the disciplines views the patient from their specific perspective and does its best to manage their specific area of focus. When that specific area appears to no longer be an issue, the service typically signs off the case. There is often a lack of clarity about which services write orders.

With single specialty management, the patient goes through the care process with management of only the primary orthopedics team. The patient, for example needing a joint replacement, may be seen preoperatively by their primary care physician for surgical clearance. After admission, they are only seen by the surgical and anesthesia teams. Medical co-management is only requested if a serious complication or adverse event occurs. Then it is sometimes too late to assuage the problem. Traditional management often results in adverse outcomes, increase in morbidity, mortality and hospital readmission.

Medical centers commonly utilize multidisciplinary care. With time, it will be necessary to change usual care to **interdisciplinary co-managed care**, particularly for the more complex older adult [3, 4]. Such a change will require culture change and manpower changes to effectively implement them. In interdisciplinary care, providers function as a cohesive team. Care coordination usually is undertaken with a nurse or mid-level provider care manager. Frequent respectful communication avoids unnecessary testing, builds collegiality, and decreases adverse events. This interdisciplinary approach is especially critical for the complex older adult patient undergoing major surgery.

## 15.5	Patient Presentation to the Orthopedic Surgeon

Older adults in a clinic setting are frequently accompanied by family members who are there to advocate for them. Such visits take more time and the observations, question and opinions of all are important to consider. The perspective of the family members is valuable especially when discussing living situation, help after surgery, cognitive status, prior interventions, history of falls and the wishes, fears and expectations of the patient and those also present must be considered. Many seniors alone with the physician avoid such important discussions. Learning about such issues after surgery precludes effective care.

Patients who reside in institutions are especially vulnerable as they may not have family at the visit and often accompanied by a nursing assistant unfamiliar with important care issues. In such a situation, one should call a family member, the institution nursing supervisor or the primary care provider for information to avoid problems in the consultation [5].

## 15.6	Assessment

Some specific areas include the following.

### 15.6.1	Functional Status

Functional impairments are prevalent in the geriatric population. One must determine the patient's baseline level of cognitive and physical function. Patients typically have multiple comorbidities and physiological loses associated with aging and these patterns are quite variable resulting in marked heterogeneity in this patient population; this situation mandates carefully planned and coordinated care to achieve high quality [6]. Chapter 8, Tools for Geriatric Assessment by Specialists, provides a review of the evaluation of physical function, cognitive status, frailty, and other measures.

### 15.6.2	Frailty

Frailty is an important predictor of surgical complications, longer lengths of stay, nursing home placement, and higher mortality and morbidity. One should be able to identify patients who are frail and plan an intervention accordingly. There are several methods to evaluate a patient for frailty [7–9]. The Fried Frailty Index [7] is one such method. Chapter 1—Frailty expand on these points.

15.6.3 Nutritional Issues

Proper nutrition is fundamental for the aging patient, especially for those healing after a fracture or recovering from major surgery. In a recent study, 48 % of patients sustaining a hip fracture were found to be malnourished [10]. A serum albumin level of less than 3 g/dL has been correlated with poor outcomes after hip fracture [10]. Screening tools for malnutrition have not been shown to be indicative of nutritional status. Complete nutritional assessment by the team or consulting dietician in geriatric patients with major orthopedic injuries should be routine [11, 12]. Oral feeding is preferred. Nasogastric feeding may precipitate delirium and lead to aspiration pneumonia. Parenteral nutrition should be avoided as it may contribute to metabolic derangement, delirium, and is associated with increased risk of sepsis.

The diet should consist of easily chewable high-caloric foods, delivered in small portions. Supplementation with liquid shakes or smoothies between, or in addition to, meals may also improve nutritional status. In sum, optimal nutrition is important for health maintenance, injury recovery, and is predictive of gait status and mortality after fragility fractures [13].

15.6.4 Comorbidities

Comorbid conditions are common in the aging population and make caring for any patient more complex. The validated Charlson Comorbidity Index (CCI) is widely used to predict inpatient and 1-year mortality in hospitalized patients. The CCI is based on comorbidities and severity [14, 15]. One study of CCI scores in over 1000 patients undergoing surgical treatment for proximal femur fractures found a 12 % increase in postoperative complications for every one point increase in the score [16].

15.6.5 Social Situation and Its Impact

The social and living situation of older orthopedic patients can have an impact on their care plan, rehabilitation potential and quality of life. It is important to determine the premorbid level of physical activity and independence to determine if a patient would even benefit from surgery. Older adults may find it difficult and overwhelming to make medical decisions, and may defer to family members for insight. It is imperative to know the patients advance directives and health care proxy. Patients without a strong support system likely will require nursing home care after hospitalization and a social worker should be involved early.

15.7 Surgical Decision-Making

The decision to proceed with surgical intervention always should be examined at length with the patient and their support system. Goals of care, expectations, and outcomes must be discussed. The benefits of surgery must be weighed against the risks on an individual basis. Alternatives to surgical intervention such as physical therapy, injection therapy, chronic pain management, and palliative care must be discussed for a fully informed decision.

15.8 Palliative Care

For patients who are poor surgical candidates, have poor prognoses, or are simply awaiting surgical intervention, a palliative care consult should be considered, if not already a part of an interdisciplinary team. An interdisciplinary team is skilled in managing pain, coordinating care, and maximizing quality of life and has a prominent palliative care focus.

15.9 Family Involvement and Communication

It is important that the patient's family be involved in medical decision-making, whether that is in the acute setting, or in the clinic. Determining if the patient has a designated power of attorney or a health care proxy is also necessary; as family members of this patient population often take a very active role in the patient's medical care. Often times, patient comorbidities such as dementia, delirium, or mild cognitive reserve may add a layer of complexity to a treatment plan. Involving close family members early on in the course of care may change the treatment plan and recovery of a patient. Creating open and honest channels of communication between the patient, family, physician, and health care team is essential to establishing rapport and the essential doctor–patient relationship [5].

A deeper understanding of a patient's support system and family dynamics is also essential in determining goals of care and likelihood of successful rehabilitation. A patient's treatment plan may also change based on the patient's health literacy, and that of their family [5]. In the modern practice of medicine, shared decision-making between the physician and patient has become commonplace. Though many older patients are able to share in the discussion of medical and surgical treatments, many will rely on their family to participate in decision-making. Care planning may also be influenced by family support. For example, if an individual has a strong family presence, they may advocate for early return to the home, visiting nursing, and home therapy with the assistance of family members. If there is a poor support network, long-term inpatient rehabilitation may be the best option. Investigation of the patient's support system is necessary in determining a patient's course of treatment.

15.10 Pre-Surgical Medical Assessment and Care Coordination

15.10.1 Elective Surgery

Planning an elective orthopedic procedure for the geriatric patient affords the surgeon and patient certain luxuries that urgent surgeries do not allow. The patient should visit their primary care provider to optimize management of comorbidities. The primary care provider may request other specialty consultation to idealize the preoperative management of chronic diseases. A preoperative office visit to the anesthesiologist is helpful for patient and increasingly a part of preoperative team assessments.

15.10.2 Urgent/Emergent Surgical Care

In the emergency department (ED), a problem-focused history and physical exam, review with the emergency room physician and family members by the orthopedist is imperative to determine the best plan and initiate any needed workup and arrange for quick bed assignment. It is important to determine if there were delays in seeking/receiving care and to understand the circumstances and mechanism of the injury. If the patient suffered a fall, contributing cardiac and neurological conditions should be sought. Stroke, myocardial infarction, arrhythmia, head injury, loss of consciousness, and syncope should be ruled out. Assessment of the patient's current and baseline cognitive function is also important—a mini-mental status examination is sufficient to determine amnesia and may be used to determine acute changes during the course of hospitalization. A current and accurate list of medical problems and medications should be reviewed. A social history including place and type of residence, level of independence, and pre-injury ambulation status should be obtained, along with smoking and alcohol use history. The patient's healthcare proxy or power of attorney should be contacted early in the admission process to support medical decision-making. Advanced directives and resuscitation (code) status should be determined and discussed with the patient upon admission.

The physical examination should include inspection for other injuries and then focus on the injured extremity. A detailed musculoskeletal and neurovascular exam should be completed with special physical exam tests, if necessary. Care should be taken not to excessively mobilize an injured extremity as it may cause bleeding, neurological damage, and increased pain for the patient.

The goal of preoperative assessment is to ensure that the patient is optimized for surgical intervention [4, 17]. Surgical repair, within 24 h of the injury, has been shown to decrease initial pain, length of hospitalization, rate of complications, and influence favorable long-term outcomes [18–22]. A care team is ideal to achieve avoiding delay in care [17, 23, 24].

15.11 Care Team Models

Organized and protocol-driven models of fracture care for seniors improve quality and decrease healthcare costs and are highly replicable in any institution [17, 23, 25–28]. The Rochester Model of co-managed care for fragility fractures is a comprehensive approach to the orthogeriatric patient [17]. Elderly orthopedic patients often have one or more medical comorbidities, which affect the outcome of surgery. Furthermore, polypharmacy is common in this aging population [27] contributing to complicated side-effect profiles and further pharmacotherapy. Involvement of a geriatrician is desirable in managing the intricacies of complex medical patients in the immediate perioperative period—thus the concept of a patient-centric, protocol driven model of care. The orthopedics and geriatric medicine services co-manage each patient, write their own orders, see the patient daily, and share responsibility [28]. The care team consists of orthopedics, geriatrics, anesthesiologists, mid-level providers, nurses, physical and occupational therapists, dieticians, and social workers [17]. This comprehensive approach allows for streamlined care delivery from admission to discharge, decreased redundancy and medical errors, implementation of evidence-based best practices, decreased cost of hospitalization, and fosters communication and collegial relationships [17, 28]. Though this model has proven to benefit patients, this care team model has been implemented in only select institutions across the USA. Some barriers to implementation of such team care are a lack of leadership, initial costs, and competing interests amongst colleagues and hospital administration [29]. However, the many benefits of implementing an orthogeriatric care program should overcome any barriers [4].

15.12 Anesthesia Considerations

The anesthesiologist has a variety of tools and techniques at their disposal to induce analgesia. In addition to general anesthesia, regional nerve blockade is commonly used in conjunction with orthopedic procedures. Though several studies have attempted to determine the optimal anesthesia approach, no study has found that one technique is superior to the other. However, regional anesthesia has been shown to have many benefits over general anesthesia in several studies [30, 31]. Patients receiving regional anesthesia for primary hip and knee replacements had an 80 % lower 30-day mortality rate compared to general anesthesia. Additionally, they had a 30–50 % lower risk of major complications such as pneumonia, renal failure, and stroke [32]. In a meta-analysis of over 2000 patients who had surgical fixation of hip fractures with general or regional anesthesia there was a lower incidence of thromboembolism and decreased 30-day mortality in the regional anesthesia group. General anesthesia was associated with a statistically significant decrease in operative time [33]. A similar meta-analysis found no statistically significant difference in cognitive dysfunction postoperatively [34].

Regional anesthesia can be helpful for acute pain relief and decreases perioperative oral and intravenous opioid use with improved pain scores [35–37].

The principles of anesthesia in older patients are discussed more thoroughly in Chap. 9.

15.13 Management of Anticoagulants

Anticoagulant medications confer an added complexity in acute orthopedic patients. One must balance the urgency of fracture fixation with the risks of anticoagulant reversal and adverse effects of a delay in time to surgery, especially a problem for hip fracture as early surgery decreases the development of pressure ulcers, delirium, pneumonia, and death [38–40].

Most believe that for patients on warfarin lowering an INR to 1.5 and below is safe for elective surgery. For patients therapeutic on warfarin, it takes about 4–5 days for the INR to reach 1.5 or below after discontinuation of the medication [41]. This is impractical for patients who require urgent surgery. Reversal of warfarin with Vitamin K has been extensively studied. Given intravenously, 1 mg of Vitamin K upon hospital admission significantly reduces the time to surgery and decreases INR [42]. Reversal of warfarin-associated

coagulopathy in hip fracture patients with fresh frozen plasma (FFP) and Vitamin K has been shown to be safe, based on a retrospective study [43]. Both oral and intravenous Vitamin K have equal or greater efficacy in lowering a high INR than subcutaneous administration. There is no optimal dose of Vitamin K to lower INR [44]. Oral administration of Vitamin K may be superior to the IV route due to rare fatal anaphylaxis [45]. Reversal of warfarin-associated coagulopathy with FFP, human donor plasma with coagulation factors and plasma proteins, has also effective. With FFP, there is a risk of an exacerbation of heart failure. A formula utilizing FFP for warfarin-associated coagulopathy is valuable: 1 unit of $FFP = 0.57 \times Pre\text{-}INR - 0.72$ [46].

The risk of reversal of warfarin is dependent on the original indication. Those with certain prosthetic heart valves or a hypercoagulable state have a near immediate risk of thrombosis. Those with a history of venous thrombosis or atrial fibrillation have a near-normal risk of thrombosis if they have taken warfarin for at least 6 months [47, 48].

A retrospective study compared outcomes of patients with hip fractures undergoing surgery. In the approximately 8 % of patients who were receiving warfarin, reversing their elevated INR using FFP, vitamin K or both compared to patients not on warfarin found no clear difference between operative time, time to surgery, in-hospital mortality, thrombotic or bleeding events, transfusion rates, or 30-day mortality with a slight increased length of stay for the warfarin group [49].

15.14 In-Surgery Considerations

A primary consideration when positioning an older adult for orthopedic surgery is to assure all bony prominences are carefully padded and the patient is securely strapped to avoid skin injury or movement (Fig. 15.1). Movement or even a fall

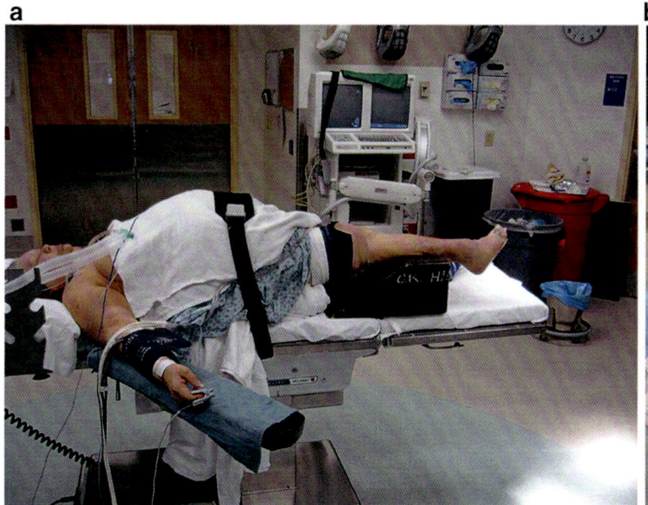
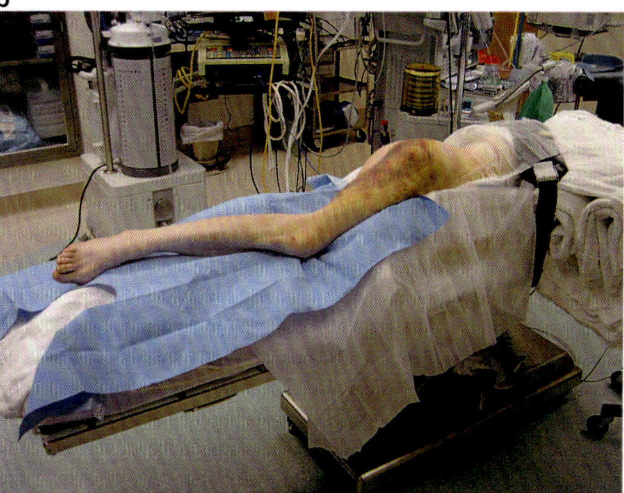

Fig. 15.1 Careful surgical positioning of the elderly patient is essential. (**a**) A patient with an ankle fracture is positioned with padding and safety straps. (**b**) Ecchymotic skin is frequently encountered in the elderly patient. Such skin must be handled gently

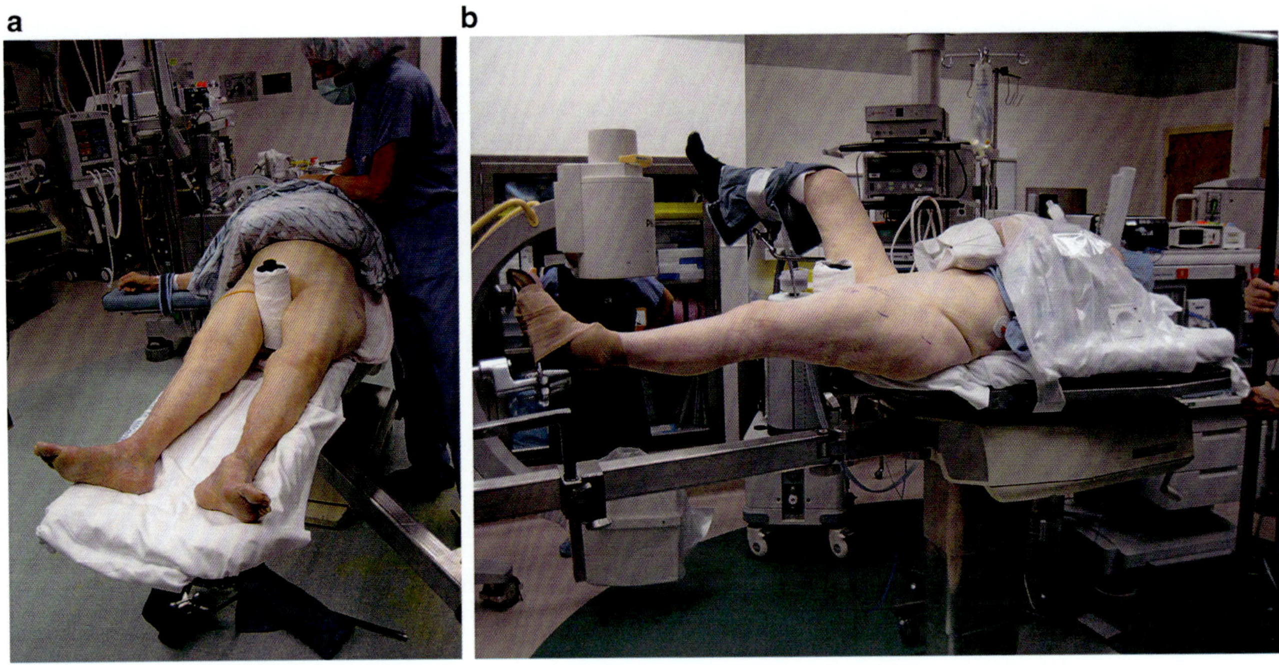

Fig. 15.2 (**a**) A patient is positioned on the fracture table with padding of bony prominences. (**b**) A warm air blanket keeps the patient's core body warm during surgery

Fig. 15.3 Surgical draping with iodine impregnated sticky drapes

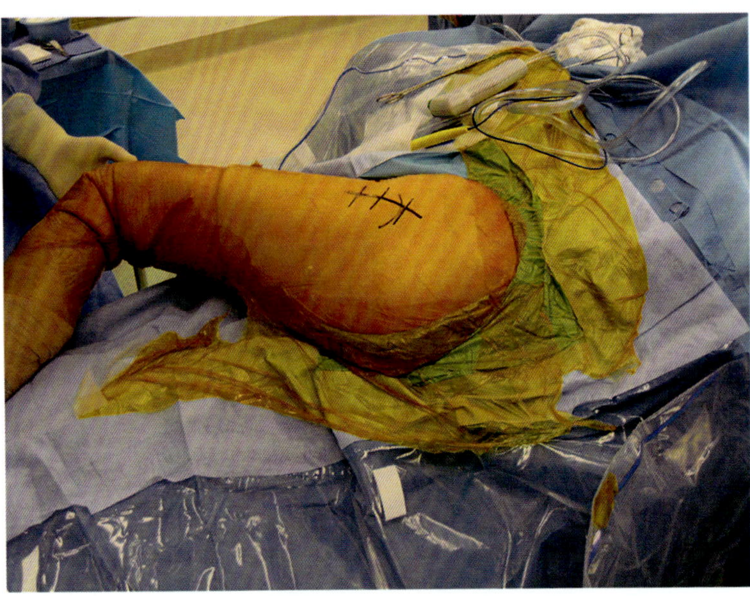

is problematic when using a fracture table (Fig. 15.2). The patient should be kept warm with a body temperature of 36–38 °C. Often times, older adults will have stiffened joints or limited range of mobility of their spine. This should be discussed with the patient prior to getting on the table and extremity positions and spine position should reflect the limited mobility the patient had prior to surgery.

Positioning should be done with the help of the attending physician to be certain that appropriate exposure is achieved and that the patient rests in a comfortable position during surgery. The drapes should be securely fixed to the patient, preferably with adhesive rather than staples or towel clamps (Fig. 15.3). Care in removing drapes is essential to avoid injury especially to age related skin atrophy; for example, circular bandages should be unrolled to avoid injury as is more likely if cut.

Shorter surgical time reduces the risk of wound infection, blood loss (Fig. 15.4), untoward effects of the anesthetic, and likely cognitive dysfunction (Fig. 15.5). Proper fluid management is vital to reduce complications [50–53].

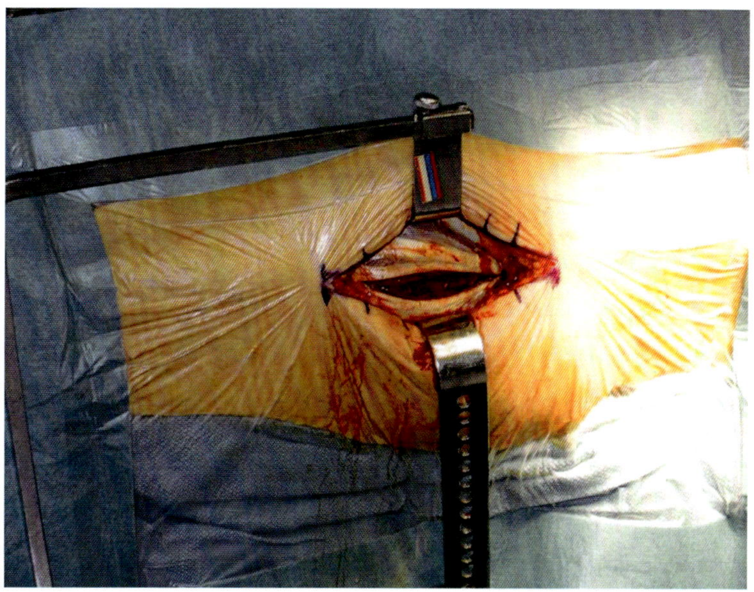

Fig. 15.4 Meticulous attention to hemostasis is suggested in elderly patients to help them remain in a state of medical equilibrium

Clinical assessment of the patient's volume and hemoglobin status is essential in every patient. Fluid depletion is best corrected with isotonic saline with caution to avoid over expansion. The NIH-sponsored FOCUS trial, Safety and Effectiveness of Two Blood Transfusion Strategies in Surgical Patients with Cardiovascular Disease, suggests maintaining hemoglobin levels at or above 8 g/dL for elderly patients with cardiac comorbidities [54].

Because of poor bone quality arthroplasty is valuable and a variety of cemented implants should be available.

Hip fracture, femur fracture, and periprosthetic fracture should be performed urgently for reasons noted earlier. Proximal humerus fracture and distal radius fracture surgery can be semi-elective. A detailed care pathway discussed early is able to improve outcome quality, patient satisfaction, and lower costs [3, 4, 17, 22].

15.15 Postoperative Care

Postoperative care should be standardized and protocol driven and ideally involving an interprofessional team.

Pain management is complex: under-reporting, especially in those with cognitive impairment, and analgesics have an increased side-effect profile in older people. Multimodal analgesia using narcotics, non-narcotic analgesics, and local nerve blocks is effective [55–58]. The combination of NSAIDs/acetaminophen with opiates produces synergistic pain relief and decreases the need for opioid medications. Intravenous, oral and subcutaneous morphine, fentanyl, and hydromorphone have no difference in the deterioration of cognitive function or incident delirium [57]. Meperidine causes delirium and should be avoided [58].

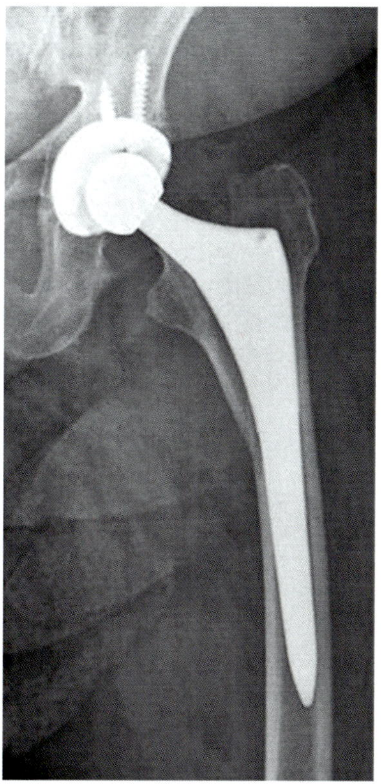

Fig. 15.5 A periprosthetic fracture occurred intraoperative in this 85-year-old patient

Intravenous patient-controlled analgesia (PCA) provides superior postoperative pain relief compared to nurse administered boluses but because of comorbidities, especially brain disease and hand arthritis it may not be effective in some seniors.

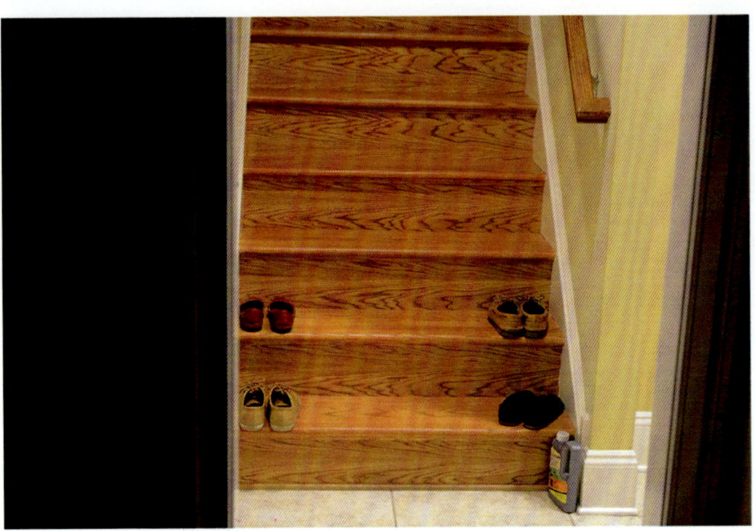

Fig. 15.6 Tripping hazards are present on these stairs: items such as shoes on the stairs, and slick stair treads

Meta-analyses found that local nerve blocks are effective and reduce complications in femur fracture [59, 60].

In most situations, the goal of orthopedic surgical intervention is to restore the patient to their prior level of activity and independence, or to an increased level of independence. A secondary goal of surgery is to prevent the complications of immobility and its sequelae—pressure sores, stiff joints, deconditioning, pneumonia, and delirium. In almost all cases, rehabilitation should begin soon after surgery. Every surgeon has his or her own preference in the initiation of mobility and physical therapy and these differences depend on the surgery performed (a patient with total knee arthroplasty may immediately bear weight as tolerated while one with a tibial plateau fracture may be non-weight bearing for some time). The surgeon must decide on this status, and engaging early physical and occupational therapists is most valuable to achieve the best outcomes, avoid complications, and achieve ideal analgesia [61–63].

Braces are best avoided but occasionally one is essential: tibial plateau fracture, some ankle fractures, and minor wrist fractures management. Complications of braces include delirium, pressure pain, tendon injury, and skin breakdown.

Orthopedic patients are especially vulnerable to skin injury. Pressure sores are serious complications and can lead to hospital readmission, sepsis, surgery, and death. With high quality care they are largely preventable. Doing so lies in careful bedside care. Skin must be checked several times a day for proper positioning, padding, redness, blisters, and ulcers. Sores most commonly are found at the hips, sacral region, heels, and elbows. Routine and frequent skin assessment and care by members of the multi- or interdisciplinary team is most valuable in avoiding or managing skin pressure problems. Such an approach is better than the common practice of the past, which included routine repositioning (an activity that can cause a shear injury, a precursor to an ulcer), pressure relieving mattresses or beds. Interdisciplinary team care and early mobilizations are effective strategies in reducing skin injury [64–67].

Evaluation tools for assessing risk of pressure ulcers include the Braden [68] and Norton [69] scales. The Norton scale may be better at identifying high-risk patients [69]. Grip strength (possibly as a surrogate for sarcopenia) predicts inpatient and 30-day risk of pressure ulcers [70].

Delirium is a common and serious complication in the postoperative affecting about half of patients after hip fracture and increasing mortality and length of stay [4, 71–74]. Certain medications sometimes used perioperatively (anticholinergics, benzodiazepines, skeletal muscle relaxants, and NSAIDs) are important precipitants and are best avoided. Other risk factors and strategies to minimize this complication are discussed in depth in Chap. 2.

Falls in the elderly are often multifactorial. Reducing the risk of a future fall is of utmost importance. A home safety evaluation should be considered when necessary, and proper modifications implemented (Fig. 15.6).

With the increasing popularity of bisphosphonates, atypical bisphosphonate-related femur fractures have become more common (Fig. 15.7). For patients undergoing osteoporosis treatment with this class of medication, it is important to determine the risk of fracture of the contralateral side in the postoperative period.

The risk of complications, poor outcomes, and mortality in older orthopedic patients requiring surgery is high, a result of many comorbidities, losses of physiological function and remarkable heterogeneity. Such patients are simply more vulnerable, and perioperative care requires a highly orchestrated interdisciplinary team to achieve the best outcomes [75–85].

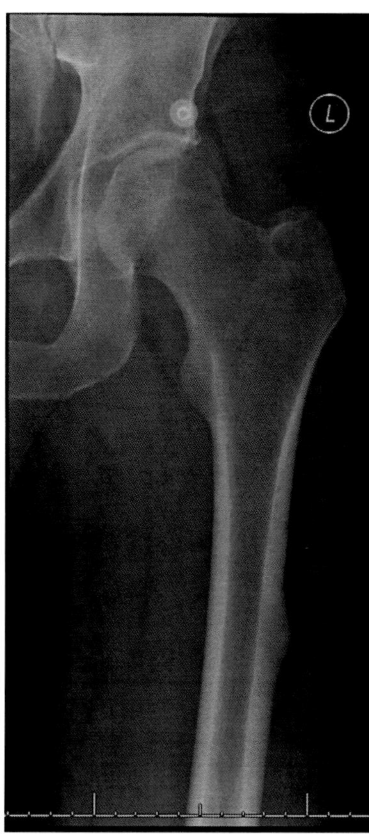

Fig. 15.7 A stage 1 atypical fracture on the lateral cortex of the femur was a result of excessive duration of bisphosphonate therapy

References

1. Cram P, Lu X, Kates SL, Singh JA, Li Y, Wolf BR. Total knee arthroplasty volume, utilization, and outcomes among Medicare beneficiaries, 1991–2010. JAMA. 2012;308(12):1227–36.
2. Cutler DM, Ghosh K. The potential for cost savings through bundled episode payments. N Engl J Med. 2012;366(12):1075–7.
3. Batsis JA, Phy MP, Melton 3rd LJ, Schleck CD, Larson DR, Huddleston PM, et al. Effects of a hospitalist care model on mortality of elderly patients with hip fractures. J Hosp Med. 2007;2(4):219–25.
4. Friedman SM, Mendelson DA, Bingham KW, Kates SL. Impact of a comanaged Geriatric Fracture Center on short-term hip fracture outcomes. Arch Intern Med. 2009;169(18):1712–7.
5. McNeil CK, K and r, M. Talking with your older patient – a clinician's handbook 208 [cited 2015 October 13, 2015]; 1: Available from: file:///C:/Users/Steve/Downloads/talking_with_your_older_patient.pdf.
6. Grigoryan KV, Javedan H, Rudolph JL. Orthogeriatric care models and outcomes in hip fracture patients: a systematic review and meta-analysis. J Orthop Trauma. 2014;28(3):e49–55.
7. Fried LP, Tangen CM, Walston J, Newman AB, Hirsch C, Gottdiener J, et al. Frailty in older adults: evidence for a phenotype. J Gerontol A Biol Sci Med Sci. 2001;56(3):M146–56.
8. Makary MA, Segev DL, Pronovost PJ, Syin D, Bandeen-Roche K, Patel P, et al. Frailty as a predictor of surgical outcomes in older patients. J Am Coll Surg. 2010;210(6):901–8.
9. Farhat JS, Velanovich V, Falvo AJ, Horst HM, Swartz A, Patton Jr JH, et al. Are the frail destined to fail? Frailty index as predictor of surgical morbidity and mortality in the elderly. J Trauma Acute Care Surg. 2012;72(6):1526–30. discussion 30-1.
10. Pioli G, Barone A, Giusti A, Oliveri M, Pizzonia M, Razzano M, et al. Predictors of mortality after hip fracture: results from 1-year follow-up. Aging Clin Exp Res. 2006;18(5):381–7.
11. Bell JJ, Bauer JD, Capra S, Pulle RC. Quick and easy is not without cost: implications of poorly performing nutrition screening tools in hip fracture. J Am Geriatr Soc. 2014;62(2):237–43.
12. Fiatarone Singh MA. Exercise, nutrition and managing hip fracture in older persons. Curr Opin Clin Nutr Metab Care. 2014;17(1): 12–24.
13. Gumieiro DN, Rafacho BP, Goncalves AF, Tanni SE, Azevedo PS, Sakane DT, et al. Mini Nutritional Assessment predicts gait status and mortality 6 months after hip fracture. Br J Nutr. 2013;109(9): 1657–61.
14. Charlson ME, Pompei P, Ales KL, MacKenzie CR. A new method of classifying prognostic comorbidity in longitudinal studies: development and validation. J Chronic Dis. 1987;40(5):373–83.
15. Poses RM, McClish DK, Smith WR, Bekes C, Scott WE. Prediction of survival of critically ill patients by admission comorbidity. J Clin Epidemiol. 1996;49(7):743–7.
16. Menzies IB, Mendelson DA, Kates SL, Friedman SM. The impact of comorbidity on perioperative outcomes of hip fractures in a geriatric fracture model. Geriatr Orthop Surg Rehabil. 2012;3(3): 129–34.
17. Kates SL, Mendelson DA, Friedman SM. Co-managed care for fragility hip fractures (Rochester model). Osteoporos Int. 2010;21 Suppl 4:S621–5.
18. Bottle A, Aylin P. Mortality associated with delay in operation after hip fracture: observational study. BMJ. 2006;332(7547):947–51.
19. Orosz GM, Magaziner J, Hannan EL, Morrison RS, Koval K, Gilbert M, et al. Association of timing of surgery for hip fracture and patient outcomes. JAMA. 2004;291(14):1738–43.
20. Simunovic N, Devereaux PJ, Sprague S, Guyatt GH, Schemitsch E, Debeer J, et al. Effect of early surgery after hip fracture on mortality and complications: systematic review and meta-analysis. CMAJ. 2010;182(15):1609–16.
21. Al-Ani AN, Samuelsson B, Tidermark J, Norling A, Ekstrom W, Cederholm T, et al. Early operation on patients with a hip fracture improved the ability to return to independent living. A prospective study of 850 patients. J Bone Joint Surg Am. 2008;90(7): 1436–42.
22. AAOS. Management of hip fractures in the elderly. 2014; September, [17]. Available from: http://www.aaos.org/Research/guidelines/HipFxSummaryofRecommendations.pdf.
23. Kates SL. Lean business model and implementation of a geriatric fracture center. Clin Geriatr Med. 2014;2014:30(2).
24. Fleisher LA, Beckman JA, Brown KA, Calkins H, Chaikof E, Fleischmann KE, et al. ACC/AHA 2007 guidelines on perioperative cardiovascular evaluation and care for noncardiac surgery: a report of the American College of Cardiology/American Heart Association Task Force on Practice Guidelines (Writing Committee to Revise the 2002 Guidelines on Perioperative Cardiovascular Evaluation for Noncardiac Surgery): developed in collaboration with the American Society of Echocardiography, American Society of Nuclear Cardiology, Heart Rhythm Society, Society of Cardiovascular Anesthesiologists, Society for Cardiovascular Angiography and Interventions, Society for Vascular Medicine and Biology, and Society for Vascular Surgery. Circulation. 2007; 116(17):e418–99.
25. Kates SL, Mendelson DA, Friedman SM. The value of an organized fracture program for the elderly: early results. J Orthop Trauma. 2011;25(4):233–7.
26. Kates SL, Blake D, Bingham KW, Kates OS, Mendelson DA, Friedman SM. Comparison of an organized geriatric fracture program to United States government data. Geriatr Orthop Surg Rehabil. 2010;1(1):15–21.

27. Baranzini F, Diurni M, Ceccon F, Poloni N, Cazzamalli S, Costantini C, et al. Fall-related injuries in a nursing home setting: is polypharmacy a risk factor? BMC Health Serv Res. 2009;9:228.

28. Friedman SM, Mendelson DA, Kates SL, McCann RM. Geriatric co-management of proximal femur fractures: total quality management and protocol-driven care result in better outcomes for a frail patient population. J Am Geriatr Soc. 2008;56(7):1349–56.

29. Kates SL, O'Malley N, Friedman SM, Mendelson DA. Barriers to implementation of an organized geriatric fracture program. Geriatr Orthop Surg Rehabil. 2012;3(1):8–16.

30. Neuman MD, Silber JH, Elkassabany NM, Ludwig JM, Fleisher LA. Comparative effectiveness of regional versus general anesthesia for hip fracture surgery in adults. Anesthesiology. 2012;117(1):72–92.

31. Neuman MD, Rosenbaum PR, Ludwig JM, Zubizarreta JR, Silber JH. Anesthesia technique, mortality, and length of stay after hip fracture surgery. JAMA. 2014;311(24):2508–17.

32. Memtsoudis SG, Stundner O, Rasul R, Sun X, Chiu YL, Fleischut P, et al. Sleep apnea and total joint arthroplasty under various types of anesthesia: a population-based study of perioperative outcomes. Reg Anesth Pain Med. 2013;38(4):274–81.

33. Urwin SC, Parker MJ, Griffiths R. General versus regional anaesthesia for hip fracture surgery: a meta-analysis of randomized trials. Br J Anaesth. 2000;84(4):450–5.

34. Mason SE, Noel-Storr A, Ritchie CW. The impact of general and regional anesthesia on the incidence of post-operative cognitive dysfunction and post-operative delirium: a systematic review with meta-analysis. J Alzheimers Dis. 2010;22 Suppl 3:67–79.

35. Gille J, Gille M, Gahr R, Wiedemann B. Acute pain management in proximal femoral fractures: femoral nerve block (catheter technique) vs. systemic pain therapy using a clinic internal organisation model. Anaesthesist. 2006;55(4):414–22.

36. Fletcher AK, Rigby AS, Heyes FL. Three-in-one femoral nerve block as analgesia for fractured neck of femur in the emergency department: a randomized, controlled trial. Ann Emerg Med. 2003;41(2):227–33.

37. Foss NB, Kristensen BB, Bundgaard M, Bak M, Heiring C, Virkelyst C, et al. Fascia iliaca compartment blockade for acute pain control in hip fracture patients: a randomized, placebo-controlled trial. Anesthesiology. 2007;106(4):773–8.

38. Juliebo V, Bjoro K, Krogseth M, Skovlund E, Ranhoff AH, Wyller TB. Risk factors for preoperative and postoperative delirium in elderly patients with hip fracture. J Am Geriatr Soc. 2009;57(8):1354–61.

39. Khan SK, Kalra S, Khanna A, Thiruvengada MM, Parker MJ. Timing of surgery for hip fractures: a systematic review of 52 published studies involving 291,413 patients. Injury. 2009;40(7):692–7.

40. Zuckerman JD, Skovron ML, Koval KJ, Aharonoff G, Frankel VH. Postoperative complications and mortality associated with operative delay in older patients who have a fracture of the hip. J Bone Joint Surg Am. 1995;77(10):1551–6.

41. White RH, McKittrick T, Hutchinson R, Twitchell J. Temporary discontinuation of warfarin therapy: changes in the international normalized ratio. Ann Intern Med. 1995;122(1):40–2.

42. Bhatia M, Talawadekar G, Parihar S, Smith A. An audit of the role of vitamin K in the reversal of International Normalised Ratio (INR) in patients undergoing surgery for hip fracture. Ann R Coll Surg Engl. 2010;92(6):473–6.

43. Vitale MA, Vanbeek C, Spivack JH, Cheng B, Geller JA. Pharmacologic reversal of warfarin-associated coagulopathy in geriatric patients with hip fractures: a retrospective study of thromboembolic events, postoperative complications, and time to surgery. Geriatr Orthop Surg Rehabil. 2011;2(4):128–34.

44. Dezee KJ, Shimeall WT, Douglas KM, Shumway NM, O'Malley PG. Treatment of excessive anticoagulation with phytonadione (vitamin K): a meta-analysis. Arch Intern Med. 2006;166(4):391–7.

45. Fiore LD, Scola MA, Cantillon CE, Brophy MT. Anaphylactoid reactions to vitamin K. J Thromb Thrombolysis. 2001;11(2):175–83.

46. Fakheri RJ. Formula for fresh frozen plasma dosing for warfarin reversal. Mayo Clin Proc. 2013;88(6):640.

47. Jaffer AK, Brotman DJ, Chukwumerije N. When patients on warfarin need surgery. Cleve Clin J Med. 2003;70(11):973–84.

48. Spandorfer J. The management of anticoagulation before and after procedures. Med Clin North Am. 2001;85(5):1109–16. v.

49. Gleason LJ, Mendelson DA, Kates SL, Friedman SM. Anticoagulation management in individuals with hip fracture. J Am Geriatr Soc. 2014;62(1):159–64.

50. Tote SP, Grounds RM. Performing perioperative optimization of the high-risk surgical patient. Br J Anaesth. 2006;97(1):4–11.

51. Tornetta 3rd P, Mostafavi H, Riina J, Turen C, Reimer B, Levine R, et al. Morbidity and mortality in elderly trauma patients. J Trauma. 1999;46(4):702–6.

52. Sinclair S, James S, Singer M. Intraoperative intravascular volume optimisation and length of hospital stay after repair of proximal femoral fracture: randomised controlled trial. BMJ. 1997;315(7113):909–12.

53. Davidson J, Griffin R, Higgs S. Introducing a clinical pathway in fluid management. J Perioper Pract. 2007;17(6):248–50. 55-6.

54. Carson JL, Terrin ML, Noveck H, Sanders DW, Chaitman BR, Rhoads GG, et al. Liberal or restrictive transfusion in high-risk patients after hip surgery. N Engl J Med. 2011;365(26):2453–62.

55. Strike SA, Sieber FE, Gottschalk A, Mears SC. Role of fracture and repair type on pain and opioid use after hip fracture in the elderly. Geriatr Orthop Surg Rehabil. 2013;4(4):103–8.

56. Elvir-Lazo OL, White PF. The role of multimodal analgesia in pain management after ambulatory surgery. Curr Opin Anaesthesiol. 2010;23(6):697–703.

57. Fong HK, Sands LP, Leung JM. The role of postoperative analgesia in delirium and cognitive decline in elderly patients: a systematic review. Anesth Analg. 2006;102(4):1255–66.

58. Marcantonio ER, Juarez G, Goldman L, Mangione CM, Ludwig LE, Lind L, et al. The relationship of postoperative delirium with psychoactive medications. JAMA. 1994;272(19):1518–22.

59. Abou-Setta AM, Beaupre LA, Rashiq S, Dryden DM, Hamm MP, Sadowski CA, et al. Comparative effectiveness of pain management interventions for hip fracture: a systematic review. Ann Intern Med. 2011;155(4):234–45.

60. Rashiq S, Vandermeer B, Abou-Setta AM, Beaupre LA, Jones CA, Dryden DM. Efficacy of supplemental peripheral nerve blockade for hip fracture surgery: multiple treatment comparison. Can J Anaesth. 2013;60(3):230–43.

61. Gialanella B, Prometti P, Monguzzi V, Ferlucci C. Neuropsychiatric symptoms and rehabilitation outcomes in patients with hip fracture. Am J Phys Med Rehabil. 2014;93(7):562–9.

62. Allen J, Koziak A, Buddingh S, Liang J, Buckingham J, Beaupre LA. Rehabilitation in patients with dementia following hip fracture: a systematic review. Physiother Can. 2012;64(2):190–201.

63. Buddingh S, Liang J, Allen J, Koziak A, Buckingham J, Beaupre LA. Rehabilitation for long-term care residents following hip fracture: a survey of reported rehabilitation practices and perceived barriers to delivery of care. J Geriatr Phys Ther. 2013;36(1):39–46.

64. Rich SE, Margolis D, Shardell M, Hawkes WG, Miller RR, Amr S, et al. Frequent manual repositioning and incidence of pressure ulcers among bed-bound elderly hip fracture patients. Wound Repair Regen. 2011;19(1):10–8.

65. Rich SE, Shardell M, Hawkes WG, Margolis DJ, Amr S, Miller R, et al. Pressure-redistributing support surface use and pressure ulcer

incidence in elderly hip fracture patients. J Am Geriatr Soc. 2011;59(6):1052–9.

66. Baumgarten M, Rich SE, Shardell MD, Hawkes WG, Margolis DJ, Langenberg P, et al. Care-related risk factors for hospital-acquired pressure ulcers in elderly adults with hip fracture. J Am Geriatr Soc. 2012;60(2):277–83.

67. Mears SC, Kates SL. A guide to improving the care of patients with fragility fractures, Edition 2. Geriatr Orthop Surg Rehabil. 2015;6(2):58–120.

68. Comfort EH. Reducing pressure ulcer incidence through Braden Scale risk assessment and support surface use. Adv Skin Wound Care. 2008;21(7):330–4.

69. Xakellis GC, Frantz RA, Arteaga M, Nguyen M, Lewis A. A comparison of patient risk for pressure ulcer development with nursing use of preventive interventions. J Am Geriatr Soc. 1992;40(12):1250–4.

70. Gumieiro DN, Rafacho BP, Gradella LM, Azevedo PS, Gaspardo D, Zornoff LA, et al. Handgrip strength predicts pressure ulcers in patients with hip fractures. Nutrition. 2012;28(9):874–8.

71. Marcantonio ER, Flacker JM, Michaels M, Resnick NM. Delirium is independently associated with poor functional recovery after hip fracture. J Am Geriatr Soc. 2000;48(6):618–24.

72. Marcantonio ER, Flacker JM, Wright RJ, Resnick NM. Reducing delirium after hip fracture: a randomized trial. J Am Geriatr Soc. 2001;49(5):516–22.

73. Inouye SK, Bogardus Jr ST, Charpentier PA, Leo-Summers L, Acampora D, Holford TR, et al. A multicomponent intervention to prevent delirium in hospitalized older patients. N Engl J Med. 1999;340(9):669–76.

74. Potter J, George J. The prevention, diagnosis and management of delirium in older people: concise guidelines. Clin Med. 2006;6(3):303–8.

75. Munin MC, Rudy TE, Glynn NW, Crossett LS, Rubash HE. Early inpatient rehabilitation after elective hip and knee arthroplasty. JAMA. 1998;279(11):847–52.

76. Perell KL, Nelson A, Goldman RL, Luther SL, Prieto-Lewis N, Rubenstein LZ. Fall risk assessment measures: an analytic review. J Gerontol A Biol Sci Med Sci. 2001;56(12):M761–6.

77. National Center for Injury Prevention and Control CfDCaPCfDCaP. Injury prevention & control: data & statistics (WISQARS). 2015 [cited 2015 10/15/2015]; Available from: http://www.cdc.gov/injury/wisqars/.

78. Tinetti ME, Ginter SF. Identifying mobility dysfunctions in elderly patients. Standard neuromuscular examination or direct assessment? JAMA. 1988;259(8):1190–3.

79. Tinetti ME, Kumar C. The patient who falls: "It's always a trade-off". JAMA. 2010;303(3):258–66.

80. Gillespie LD, Robertson MC, Gillespie WJ, Lamb SE, Gates S, Cumming RG, et al. Interventions for preventing falls in older people living in the community. Cochrane Database Syst Rev. 2009;2, CD007146.

81. Campbell AJ, Robertson MC, Gardner MM, Norton RN, Buchner DM. Falls prevention over 2 years: a randomized controlled trial in women 80 years and older. Age Ageing. 1999;28(6):513–8.

82. Foundation NO. America's bone health: the state of osteoporosis and low bone mass in our nation. Washignton: National Osteoporosis Foundation; 2002. [cited 2015 10/15/2015]. Available from: http://nof.org/files/nof/public/content/file/63/upload/49.pdf.

83. Services UDoHaH. Bone health and osteoporosis: a report of the surgeon general. In: Services HaH, editor. Rockville: Health and Human Services; 2004.

84. Colon-Emeric C, Kuchibhatla M, Pieper C, Hawkes W, Fredman L, Magaziner J, et al. The contribution of hip fracture to risk of subsequent fractures: data from two longitudinal studies. Osteoporos Int. 2003;14(11):879–83.

85. Cosman F, de Beur SJ, LeBoff MS, Lewiecki EM, Tanner B, Randall S, et al. Clinician's guide to prevention and treatment of osteoporosis. Osteoporos Int. 2014;25(10):2359–81.

Matthew Kashima

16.1 Introduction

Otolaryngology Head and Neck Surgery (OHNS) is a unique subspecialty that is defined by an anatomical region not confined to a single organ system as are many other specialties. Because of this, the subspecialties of OHNS deal with very different pathologies. OHNS is also a medical and surgical specialty. Unlike other surgical specialties, an otolaryngologist will often serve as their medical counterpart.

As the population continues to age, all clinicians will need to be aware of geriatric manifestations of otolaryngologic conditions and of unique presentations and manifestations of those conditions in an older population. Some patients will deal with conditions they have had since their youth while others may experience new episodes of a recurrent condition and others may have new onset of a disorder. Providers need to be familiar with how conditions present at an advanced age. Some of the complaints may be due to the aging process and not due to a specific pathologic disorder.

16.2 Otology

16.2.1 Hearing Loss

Hearing loss is common in the older population. Up to 25 % of individuals between 65 and 74 years have hearing loss and 50 % of individuals over 75 have hearing loss. This hearing loss, however, can begin at a younger age. Hearing loss associated with noise exposure can be seen. Presbycusis, age related hearing loss, is a bilateral progressive hearing loss that affects the higher frequencies more than the lower

M. Kashima, MD, MPH (✉)
Department of Otolaryngology Head and Neck Surgery,
Johns Hopkins Bayview Medical Center, 4940 Eastern Avenue,
A Building, Room 102, Baltimore, MD 21224, USA
e-mail: MKashim1@jhmi.edu

frequencies. Discrimination, the ability to understand sounds, is more pronounced in the elderly when compared with younger patients with a similar hearing loss. Routine audiograms are helpful in documenting and following progression of hearing loss as an individual ages [1].

16.2.2 Sudden Sensorineural Hearing Loss (SSNHL)

Sudden sensorineural hearing loss is an abrupt loss of hearing. It usually affects one ear, but rarely it will affect both ears. It can be complete or partial, affecting some or all frequencies. Discrimination or understanding can also be affected. Patients with this presentation should be seen promptly and have an audiogram performed. Workup should include an imaging study of the temporal bone and internal auditory canal, MRI is preferable to evaluate the VIIIth cranial nerve for abnormalities/growths. Laboratory studies looking for metabolic, inflammatory, autoimmune, or infectious causes can be ordered but the cost and low yield has led to the recommendation that they not be ordered routinely. Treatment can be based on cause if known, but often empiric treatment with oral or intratympanic steroids is used [2]. The earlier the treatment begins, the better the chance of recovery of hearing [3, 4].

16.2.3 Hearing Aids

Hearing aids can be helpful to people with hearing loss. Hearing aids will amplify sounds and can be programmed to fit an individual's hearing loss. Hearing aids will not improve discrimination. Hearing aids are amplifiers and make sounds louder including background noise which may limit their utility in certain circumstances. Managing expectations is important in patients considering hearing aids. Patients must accept that they have hearing loss and be motivated to use them. Often frequent visits to an audiologist are necessary at first to maximize benefit and use. Cost can be a factor in

© Springer International Publishing Switzerland 2017
J.R. Burton et al. (eds.), *Geriatrics for Specialists*, DOI 10.1007/978-3-319-31831-8_16

obtaining hearing aids as they are not covered by many insurers including Medicare. There are a variety of devices on the market which are more affordable than hearing aids that can improve the ability to hear. Personal amplifiers range in size, price, and programmability. As technology continues to evolve, more sophisticated devices are becoming available. These devices can be purchased from independent retailers as well as from audiologists [5]. For patients with profound hearing loss cochlear implantation is available. Age alone, however, is not a contraindication to surgery.

16.2.4 Tinnitus

Tinnitus is the perception of sound that is not present in the environment. It is a common phenomenon with some estimates that it affects 10 % of the population. Tinnitus can be divided into two categories: objective tinnitus, which can be heard by others, and subjective tinnitus, noise perceived by patients that cannot be heard by others. Tinnitus can be described as buzzing, hissing, ringing, tapping, or humming sounds. It can also be a pulsatile. It can be unilateral or bilateral. It can be constant or intermittent.

Objective tinnitus can be caused by blood flow through normal vessels or arteriovenous malformations. Pulsatile tinnitus can be evaluated with a radiographic study. Angiogram, CT angiogram, and MRI/MRA/MRV are studies that can be ordered to diagnose cases of pulsatile tinnitus. A clicking sound between 40 and 200 beats per minute can be heard with palatal myoclonus. Sometimes this is described as the sound of an insect flapping its wings.

Subjective tinnitus can be related to hearing loss, medications, metabolic causes, psychological factors, neurologic issues, or dental issues. Workup includes an audiogram with tympanometry. Laboratory studies may also be performed to look for treatable causes of tinnitus.

Treatment consists of correcting any underlying condition. Review of medications with attention toward avoiding medications known to have a strong association with tinnitus can be helpful (Table 16.1). Avoidance of caffeine can be helpful. Masking sounds (a white noise generator, a fan or even a radio tuned between stations) can also be helpful in blocking the tinnitus. Reassuring patients that the sound is not unusual and is not indicative of a serious underlying problem can help alleviate anxiety in some patients [6].

Table 16.1 Medications potentially causing tinnitus

Aspirin
Nonsteroidal anti-inflammatory drugs
Aminoglycosides
Caffeine
Heterocycline antidepressants

For patients who cannot accommodate to tinnitus, treatment with anxiolytics can be helpful but their use in seniors is risky because of serious side effects such as confusion and falls. Chapter 5, Medication Management, reviews the use of these and other drugs in seniors.

16.2.5 Cerumen Impaction

Ear wax is normally produced by the lateral one-third of the external auditory canal. Ear wax is a mixture of products form cerumen and sebaceous glands, desquamated skin and hair. Its color can vary from white to dark brown and it can vary in consistency from moist, soft, sticky cerumen to dry, hard cerumen. Cerumen is protective. It mechanically traps dirt and debris from getting deep into the external auditory canals. There is evidence that cerumen has antimicrobial properties as well. Normally, cerumen is cleared from the ear canal by a combination of epithelial growth which is toward the external auditory meatus and mechanical movement of the ear canal during chewing [7].

Impactions can cause varying complaints ranging from no issues to hearing loss, itching, pain, tinnitus, vertigo, and otitis externa. It has been estimated that close to one-third of geriatric patients have cerumen impactions [8]. Cerumen removal can improve these symptoms. Coarse hairs that grow in the lateral ear canals of men become coarser and more prominent with age and can trap cerumen in the ear canal. Instrumenting the ear canal with cotton swabs, fingers, etc. can push cerumen medially in the ear canal leading to impactions. Hearing aids and ear buds can have the same effect.

There are a variety of techniques that can be used to remove cerumen. Irrigation is a frequently employed technique used by primary care and otolaryngology practices. Commercial systems are available but a syringe with an angiocatheter can be just as effective. The idea is to inject the irrigant past the impaction and allow the flow of fluid to propel the impaction laterally out of the ear canal. Irrigation should not be performed in the setting of a known perforation. Care must be taken to avoid injecting the irrigant directly onto the tympanic membrane as this could cause a tympanic membrane perforation. Caloric stimulation of the vestibular system can occur if fluids used are not at body temperature. If irrigation is not successful, cerumenolytics can be used. There is not one definitive cerumenolytic. Alcohol, hydrogen peroxide, acetic acid, docusate sodium, mineral oil, antibiotic drops, and over the counter preparations have all been used. If these preparations and irrigations fail to gain the desired result, mechanical removal by a skilled clinician is necessary. Complications of cerumen removal include otitis externa and ear drum perforation. Use of topical antibiotic drops after cerumen removal can prevent otitis externa from developing [9, 10].

16.2.6 Vestibular Disorders

Balance issues are common complaints in the elderly population. It has been estimated that over 12 million people over 65 are affected by balance disorders. The cause of difficulty can be multifactorial involving the vestibular system, proprioception, vision, and strength. The differential diagnosis for balance disorders is extensive and varied ranging from infectious, central and peripheral neurologic causes, metabolic, cardiovascular etiologies and side effects from medications. Balance issues can manifest in difficulty walking and driving as well as result in falls with resultant morbidity. This can limit the independence of individuals and lessen their quality of life. Vertigo is a sensation of spinning either of the individual or their surroundings. History will help to differentiate patients with vertigo from those presenting with unsteadiness or lightheadedness. Patients frequently have a difficult time describing their symptoms. It is important to remember that not all dizziness is vertigo and not all vertigo is otologic in etiology. A few common otologic causes of vertigo are discussed below [1].

16.2.7 Benign Paroxysmal Positional Vertigo (BPPV)

BPPV is caused when otoconia, small crystals, are dislodged from the macula and enter the semicircular canals. With changes in position, the otoconia travel through the semicircular canal stimulating the hair cells, which in turn activate the vestibulo-ocular reflex (VOR). The VOR causes eye movements that compensate for head motion. When the VOR is activated by misplaced otoconia the resulting eye movements without changes in head position are responsible for the intense sensation of vertigo. The vertigo lasts for seconds to a few minutes and is associated with changes in head position. It is often induced by getting into or out of bed, rolling over in bed, or turning the head. The patient will have nystagmus that begins after changes in position after a short latent period. The Dix–Hallpike maneuver will cause vertigo with the associated nystagmus in patients with BPPV. Patients with BPPV may have a history of head trauma. Episodes of BPPV can resolve on their own or continue to occur with changes in position. Episodes of BPPV can recur ofter period of no vertigo that can be variable in length. Treatment is canalith repositioning exercises by a skilled clinician, usually a physical therapist. It is helpful to have the patient learn these exercises to treat BPPV themselves if it recurs [11, 12].

16.2.8 Meniere's Disease

Meniere's disease, also known as endolymphatic hydrops, typically presents in adulthood with waxing and waning symptoms of hearing loss, tinnitus, aural fullness, and vertigo. The vertiginous symptoms last for hours. Over time, the hearing loss will be progressive and the tinnitus and vestibular weakness will persist. Evaluation includes focused history and physical examination, audiograms, and electroneuronography (ENG). Meniere's disease is often treated with low salt diet, avoiding caffeine and tobacco. Hydrochlorothiazide is also used. Vestibular suppressants such as meclizine or benzodiazepines (must be used with great caution in seniors) can be helpful during an acute attack [12]. For patients whose disease is not controlled by medical therapy intratympanic therapy is an alternative. Intratympanic treatments with aminoglycosides to effect a chemical labyrinthectomy can be used. Intratympanic gentamycin includes a risk of hearing loss and for that reason intratympanic steroids are also used to control vertiginous symptoms without the risk of hearing loss. Potential complications of intratympanic therapies are discomfort, need for multiple injections, caloric stimulation during injection, and persistent tympanic membrane perforation. Intratympanic steroids have been shown to be less effective in controlling symptoms. Surgical treatment including endolymphatic sac surgery and labyrinthectomy can be done although this surgery is performed less frequently with the development of intratympanic therapy [13, 14].

16.2.9 Vestibular Neuronitis

Vestibular neuronitis is an inflammation affecting the vestibular nerve. It often follows an upper respiratory infection. It presents with severe vertigo that comes on rapidly and lasts for days. The vertigo is exacerbated by movement. The vertigo can be associated with nausea and vomiting. It can be difficult to read or watch television. Symptoms are best controlled by laying still with eyes closed. Treatment consists of vestibular suppressants such as meclizine and benzodiazepines (used with caution in the geriatric population), hydration and vestibular rehabilitation with a physical therapist [12].

16.3 Rhinology

As the nose ages, the structure and function are altered. These alterations can result in nasal congestion, drainage, changes in smell and taste, difficulty breathing and sleeping. The bony structure of the nose is static but the cartilage is more subject to change over time. With aging the cartilage of the septum, which is confined by bones of the septum, can continue to grow. Since it is restricted by the bone, it can buckle leading to deviations of the septum which can cause nasal obstruction, congestion, trigger rhinorrhea and predispose to nasal and sinus infections.

16.3.1 Rhinitis

Rhinitis is an inflammatory condition of the nose characterized by nasal congestion and secretions. Rhinitis is often allergic. Non-allergic rhinitis describes conditions where no allergic etiology can be identified. Rhinitis affects millions of Americans. Patients with allergic rhinitis present with nasal congestion, rhinorrhea, sneezing, and itching in response to exposure to an environmental allergen. On examination they often have edematous nasal mucosa with clear drainage. Treatment involves identifying and trying to limit exposure to the allergen as well as medical treatment. Nasal saline spray can be beneficial by keeping the mucosa moist and facilitating clearance of allergens and irritants. Saline should be used frequently to gain maximal benefit. The only time not to use saline spray is after application of a medicated spray as the saline will rinse out the medication. Oral and topical antihistamines can be effective in controlling symptoms of itching, sneezing, and rhinorrhea but these agents must be used with great caution in seniors because of their association with delirium, falls, and other burdens (Chap. 5 provides details). Decongestants work by decreasing mucosal edema. Topical decongestants are potent vasoconstrictors, however, they can cause rhinitis medicamentosa (rebound swelling with withdrawal) with daily use for more than 5 days. For this reason, they should be used judiciously. They generally do not cause tachycardia or hypertension. Oral decongestants do not have a dramatic effect on nasal mucosal edema and are more likely to have systemic effects such as tachycardia, palpitations, and irritability. Topical nasal steroids are anti-inflammatory medications. They have very limited systemic absorption. Daily use is needed to have maximal effect due to the low dose. These sprays should be directed posteriorly and laterally to have maximal effect. Oral steroids are potent anti-inflammatory medications but they have serious side effects and should not be used indiscriminately. Anticholinergic medication such as ipratropium bromide topical spray can be used as drying agents. They are particularly helpful for patients with rhinorrhea as a chief complaint or vasomotor rhinitis [15].

16.3.2 Epistaxis

Nosebleeds are common and affect men and women equally. Dry conditions and upper respiratory infections make nosebleeds more frequent in the winter. Most nosebleeds occur anteriorly (around 90 %) and are easily controlled with direct pressure. Use of non-humidified oxygen via nasal cannula can dry out the nose and increase the risk of epistaxis. Posterior nosebleeds are more common in the elderly population than in younger patients but still account for only 10 % of nosebleeds in the geriatric population. Posterior nosebleeds are more commonly arterial and harder to control. Use of blood thinners can make epistaxis more difficult to control.

When epistaxis occurs, the patient should sit down and try to be calm. They should sit slightly forward and apply direct pressure to the fleshy portion of the nose. Pressure should be held continuously for 15 min to allow a clot to form. Any blood that drains into the mouth should be expectorated and not swallowed to prevent gastrointestinal upset, nausea, and vomiting. If the bleeding persists, the patient should blow their nose to remove and clot and apply a topical decongestant spray such as oxymetazoline and again hold pressure for 15 min. If the bleeding continues, urgent medical attention should be sought. Packing the nose can stop bleeding and stabilize the patient. Patients whose noses have been packed should be placed on antibiotics covering Staphylococcus to prevent infection from developing. The packing should be left in place for 3–5 days. Patients with persistent bleeding may require cauterization, embolization, and/or ligation of feeding vessels [16].

16.3.3 Smell and Taste Disorders

Multiple investigations have demonstrated age related decreases in smell and taste. Loss of smell can be an early sign of Alzheimer disease and Parkinson disease. Patients with olfactory dysfunction may not complain of olfactory issues as they are unaware of the loss [17]. The etiology of this loss is a combination of loss of olfactory neurons as well as changes in central processes [18]. Evaluation of patients presenting with olfactory and taste complaints should include a physical examination looking for physical reasons that can prevent odorants from getting to the olfactory epithelium—nasal obstruction due to nasal valve collapse, septal deviation, or secretions. If there is not obvious anatomical abnormality on examination, imaging studies can be obtained—CT scan of the sinuses. Olfactory testing can be done in the clinic setting using a standardized smell test such as the University of Pennsylvania Smell Identification Test [19]. MRI can be used to examine the olfactory bulb and tract as well as identify intracranial causes of olfactory dysfunction. Treatment of olfactory disorders consists of treating causes of nasal obstruction (managing allergies, treating infections). Educating patients to be vigilant when eating foods that could be spoiled and to be careful with personal hygiene can be useful when dealing with severe dysosmia.

16.4 Laryngology

16.4.1 Aging Voice

The larynx changes anatomically with aging. The vocal folds become thinner and the thyroarytenoid muscles atrophy. These changes lead to bowing of the vocal folds. These anatomic changes lead to physiologic changes—incomplete glottic closure, air escape, altered vocal fold tension and fundamental frequency, and decreased endurance. The voice tends to get higher pitched and strained as attempts are made to get better closure for phonation. The goal of treatment is to improve vocal loudness and reduce effort. The first line treatment is vocal therapy with a speech language pathologist. This intervention is noninvasive and works well for many individuals. For those who do not get the desired results from voice therapy vocal cord injections may be performed. A variety of materials have been used in injections, most injections achieve temporary improvement lasting for months. They can be repeated. They have the advantage of improving glottic closure immediately. Many injections can be done in the clinic avoiding the need for general anesthesia. Medialization thyroplasty is a surgical procedure where an implant is placed in the larynx to bulk up the vocal fold medializing the free edge making glottic closure easier. The procedure is done under local anesthesia with sedation allowing the patient to talk with the surgeon as the implant is placed. This allows the surgeon to gage how much to medialize the vocal fold to get the desired result of glottic closure to improve voice quality but not over correct deficit leading to difficulty breathing and poor vocal quality [20]. Its results are considered permanent [21].

16.4.2 Dysphagia

Dysphagia is difficulty in swallowing. It can be caused by dysfunction from the mouth to the stomach. A variety of disorders can cause dysphagia including neurologic, rheumatologic, endocrinologic, infectious, and anatomic disorders. Presbyphagia is disordered swallowing in otherwise healthy older individuals. Evaluation and treatment of swallowing disorders can involve otolaryngologists, neurologists, gastroenterologists, rehabilitation physicians, radiologists, speech language pathologists, dieticians, and nutritionists. Changes in dentition, dry mouth, and reduced strength of the tongue and muscles of mastication can lead to difficulty preparing the bolus and clearing it from the oral cavity. The oral phase of swallowing is the voluntary. The remainder of the swallow is involuntary [22, 23].

Evaluation of a patient presenting with difficulty swallowing guides interventions and treatment. Physical examination should include mental status, vocal quality and ability to handle secretions, evaluation of tongue and palate strength and movement, laryngeal examination and evaluation of the neck. Fiberoptic evaluation of the larynx as well as fiberoptic swallowing studies can be performed in the office or clinic. Radiographic studies including barium swallow studies with and without speech language pathologist and CT scans can demonstrate anatomic and functional causes of dysphagia. Obstruction from extrinsic masses (e.g., thyroid nodules/goiters, cervical osteophytes and neoplasms) can be

demonstrated on CT or fluoroscopic studies. Weakness, paralysis, hypo- or hyper-functioning of muscles can be seen on fluoroscopic or fiberoptic evaluation. Laryngeal penetration and penetration can be seen on fluoroscopic or fiberoptic evaluation [23].

Treatment is determined by what is found during the evaluation. The goal can be compensatory—developing strategies to deal with the deficit identified, or rehabilitative—to regain function that was lost. Swallowing therapy can help patients with coping strategies to overcome weakness and other changes from aging. Procedural intervention may be needed to deal with structural abnormalities [22].

16.5 Head and Neck Oncology

16.5.1 Neck Masses

Neck masses can represent a variety of pathology ranging from benign to life threatening. Neck masses are often categorized as congenital, inflammatory, and neoplastic. Although geriatric patients are unlikely to present with congenital neck masses, they occasionally occur and need to be considered in the differential. These include thyroglossal duct cysts, branchial cleft cysts, and lymphatic malformations. Inflammatory conditions in reactive lymphadenopathy, sialadenitis, and granulomatous lymphadenopathy. Neoplastic lesions can be benign—thyroid nodule/goiter, salivary neoplasm, lipoma, or malignant—thyroid cancer, salivary cancer, metastatic cancer in a lymph node, lymphoma.

Evaluation of a neck mass includes history of presentation, how long it has been present, change in size over time, tenderness, difficulty in breathing, change in voice or swallowing. Presence of risk factors—smoking, alcohol use, personal history of head and neck cancer, family history of cancers. Physical examination should include the location, size, and characteristics of the mass—soft/firm, mobile/fixed. Imaging with CT with contrast or MRI with contrast can help to define the location and anatomic origin of the mass. They can also identify other masses in the head and neck region. For example, a patient with an enlarged neck node found on exam may be found to have a base of tongue lesion on imaging. Imaging can demonstrate additional enlarged lymph nodes useful in staging cancers. Fine needle aspiration biopsies (FNAB) are able to diagnose many lesions based on cytology. Ultrasound guidance can help to ensure that the biopsy is of the specific abnormality palpated on exam. Limitations of FNAB are that histological architecture is not seen and evidence of invasion needed to diagnose well-differentiated thyroid cancers is not seen. Core needle biopsies can sometimes be done, obtaining tissue for evaluation in addition to cytology. In cases where FNAB is not feasible, excisional biopsies may be necessary for diagnosis [24].

Treatment is based on the diagnosis. Many benign lesions can be followed expectantly. Symptomatic benign lesions may be treated with surgical excision. Inflammatory lesions are best treated medically with anti-inflammatory medications or antibiotics as appropriate. Malignant lesions can be treated with surgery, radiation therapy, and/or chemotherapy depending on the type and stage of cancer.

16.6 Facial Plastic and Reconstructive Surgery

16.6.1 Facial Fractures

The facial skeleton undergoes changes with aging; the most prominent change is resorption of the alveolar bone in the maxilla and mandible. This problem is magnified in edentulous patients, in whom up to 50 % of the mandibular height may be lost. The bone of the facial skeleton becomes brittle, and decreased metabolic activity in the bone makes healing times prolonged. Resorption of bone and its fragility can make placing fixation plates difficult. Planning for repairing facial fractures in the elderly must take these facts into account to ensure the best possible outcome. Evaluation of facial fractures involves physical examination with attention to any soft tissue injury and nerve entrapment. CT scans will demonstrate the location and extent of fractures. Some fractures can be managed with observation. Non-displaced or minimally displaced, nonload bearing fractures can be successfully managed without intervention [25]. The health of the patient and risk of surgery need to be weighed against the risks of observation—poor cosmesis and function [26].

16.6.2 Cosmetic Surgery

Cosmetic surgery is common and many people seek to have signs of an aging face treated surgically. Veslev et al. [27] reviewed 183,914 cosmetic procedures and found complication rates to be similar between younger and older patients when stratified by medical comorbidities. Decisions about who is an acceptable surgical candidate for elective cosmetic surgeries has less to do with age and relies on the health of the individual [28].

References

1. Marple B, Meyerhoff W. Aging and the auditory and vestibular system. In: Bailey B, editor. Head and neck surgery-otolaryngology. 2nd ed. Philadelphia: Lippincott-Raven; 1998. p. 2217–23.
2. Rauch S, et al. Oral vs intratympanic corticosteroid therapy for idiopathic sudden sensorineural hearing loss. JAMA. 2011;305(20):2071–9.
3. Hasisaki G. Sudden sensory hearing loss. In: Bailey B, editor. Head and neck surgery-otolaryngology. 2nd ed. Philadelphia: Lippincott-Raven; 1998. p. 2193–8.
4. Shin J, Rauch S. Sudden sensorineural hearing loss. In: Shin J, Hartnick C, Randolph G, editors. Evidence – based otolaryngology. Springer; 2008. p. 273–92.
5. Chicchis A, Bess F. Hearing aids and assistive listening devices. In: Bailey B, editor. Head and neck surgery-otolaryngology. 2nd ed. Philadelphia: Lippincott-Raven; 1998. p. 2247–58.
6. Parnes S. Tinnitus in the elderly patient. In: Calhoun K, Eibling D, editors. Geriatric otolaryngology. New York: Taylor and Francis; 2006. p. 91–9.
7. Kelly KE, Mohs DC. The external auditory canal. Anatomy and physiology. Otolaryngol Clin North Am. 1996;29(5):725–39.
8. Lewis-Cullinan C, Jaken JK. Effect of cerumen removal on the hearing ability of geriatric patients. J Adv Nurs. 1990;15(5):594–600.
9. Jabor M, Gianoli G. Cerumen impaction. In: Calhoun K, editor. Expert guide to otolaryngology. Philadelphia: American College of Physicians; 2001. p. 75–85.
10. Torchinsky C, Davidson M. Cerumen impaction. In: Calhoun K, Eibling D, editors. Geriatric otolaryngology. New York: Taylor and Francis; 2006. p. 43–57.
11. Furman J. Benign paroxysmal positional vertigo. In: Calhoun K, Eibling D, editors. Geriatric otolaryngology. New York: Taylor and Francis; 2006. p. 155–64.
12. Miller A, Gianoli G. Dizziness. In: Calhoun K, editor. Expert guide to otolaryngology. Philadelphia: American College of Physicians; 2001. p. 102–131.
13. Kutz W, Slattery W. Meniere disease surgical labyrinthectomy versus other procedures: chance of decreased vestibular complaints. In: Shin J, Hartnick C, Randolph G, editors. Evidence – based otolaryngology. Springer; 2008. p. 347–50.
14. Miller M, Agrawal Y. Intratympanic therapies for Meniere's disease. Curr Otorhinolaryngol Rep. 2014;2(3):137–43.
15. Vining E. Rhinitis. In: Bailey B, editor. Head and neck surgery-otolaryngology. 2nd ed. Philadelphia: Lippincott-Raven; 1998. p. 349–58.
16. Barlow D. Epistaxis. In: Calhoun K, editor. Expert guide to otolaryngology. Philadelphia: American College of Physicians; 2001. p. 202–17.
17. Deems D, Doty R, Hummel T, Kratskin I. Olfactory function and disorders. In: Bailey B, editor. Head and neck surgery-otolaryngology. 2nd ed. Philadelphia: Lippincott-Raven; 1998. p. 317–31.
18. Schiffman SS. Taste and smell in disease (first of two parts). N Engl J Med. 1983;308:1275.
19. Doty RL, Frye RE, Agrawal U. Internal consistency reliability of the fractionated and whole University of Pennsylvania smell identification test. Precept Psychophs. 1998;(45):381–4.
20. Smith R. Complications of laryngeal surgery. In: Eisele D, Smith R, editors. Complications in head and neck surgery. 2nd ed. Philadelphia: Mosby; 2009. p. 387–403.
21. Bradley J, Hapner E, Johns M. What is the optimal treatment for presbyphonia? Laryngoscope. 2014;124:2439–40.
22. Di Pede C, Mantovani M, Del Felice A, Masiero S. Dysphagia in the elderly: focus on rehabilitation strategies. Aging Clin Exp Res. Epub ahead of print. November 2015.
23. Kashima H, Gaylor R. Upper digestive tract evaluation and imaging. In: Bailey B, editor. Head and neck surgery-otolaryngology. 2nd ed. Philadelphia: Lippincott-Raven; 1998. p. 589–95.
24. Kost K. Neck masses. In: Calhoun K, editor. Expert guide to otolaryngology. Philadelphia: American College of Physicians; 2001. p. 383–428.

25. Ross A, Wang T. Reconstruction in the elderly patient. In: Calhoun K, Eibling D, editors. Geriatric otolaryngology. New York: Taylor and Francis; 2006. p. 555–79.
26. Leach J, Dierks E. Mandibular fractures. In: Bailey B, editor. Head and neck surgery-otolaryngology. 2nd ed. Philadelphia: Lippincott-Raven; 1998. p. 977–88.
27. Veslev M, et al. Safety of cosmetic procedures in the elderly and octogenarian patients. Aesthet Surg J. 2015;35(7):864–73.
28. Friedman O, Wang T, Cook T. Cosmetic surgery int eh elderly patient. In: Calhoun K, Eibling D, editors. Geriatric otolaryngology. New York: Taylor and Francis; 2006. p. 581–601.

Rehabilitation

17

Dale C. Strasser

17.1 Introduction

Rehabilitation consists of a broad set of practical interventions and targeted medical management to promote function and quality of life particularly in the context of disabilities. Common rehabilitation approaches include therapeutic exercises, assistive technologies, compensatory strategies, orthotic devices, and environmental modifications—all delivered by a team of rehabilitation providers with complementary skill sets. Physicians provide medical direction and manage health care issues that directly impact function like pain, spasticity, cognitive impairment, and neurogenic bladders. For elderly individuals, this approach is modified on principles pioneered in Geriatric Medicine including the recognition and management of geriatric syndromes. The medical specialties of Physical Medicine and Rehabilitation (PM&R) and Geriatric Medicine share practical, patient-centered orientations to promote function and quality of life, which reflect a synergy between PM&R and Geriatric Medicine. Physicians collaborate closely with other health professionals, such as physical therapists and social workers, and the effectiveness of their work is influenced by the quality of communication, care coordination, and patient–caregiver goal setting. In this chapter, the context of Geriatric Rehabilitation is presented, along with practical suggestions on keeping this service delivery model active and relevant in an era of financial constraints and fragmentation of services.

17.2 Geriatric Rehabilitation: How Is It Different?

With a bit of respectful exasperation, the elderly woman looked up at the occupational therapist (OT) and stated "Honey, I have been peeling potatoes since I was twelve years old and I am tired of it." Even though the stroke had impaired her ability to do the task, the 84-year-old woman did not see much use for a one-handed potato peeling technique despite the sincere encouragement of her young therapist. I learned something profound in this exchange in my second year of residency. The patient desired some independence on her own terms, and she wanted to go home with her family. She worked hard to achieve these goals and her actions engaged her family to be effective caregivers. The lesson learned—rehabilitation activities should be personally meaningful to achieve patient participation and positive outcomes. Each patient is unique and the marked heterogeneity among seniors demands that clinicians identify the specific goals and aspirations of their recovery after any disabling perturbation.

The themes of rehabilitation are so interwoven with the principles of geriatric medicine that all clinicians working with older adults can be considered *rehabilitationist.* Broadly speaking, we seek to optimize function and quality of life for this rapidly expanding but too often inadequately treated group. The best treatments are customized to the desires and needs of individual patients and framed in practical, feasible terms.

In this chapter salient aspects of rehabilitation services for the geriatric population are presented. The discussion offers a framework ("a travel guide") for effective services, reviews the interface of frailty, rehabilitation, and common geriatric syndromes, describes services in the USA including the idiosyncrasies of post acute care (PAC), discusses the historical convergences of Geriatric Medicine and Physical Medicine

D.C. Strasser, MD (✉)
Department of Rehabilitation Medicine, Emory University
Medical School, Emory Rehabilitation Hospital, 1441 Clifton Rd,
NE, Atlanta, GA 30322, USA
e-mail: dstrass@emory.edu

© Springer International Publishing Switzerland 2017
J.R. Burton et al. (eds.), *Geriatrics for Specialists*, DOI 10.1007/978-3-319-31831-8_17

and Rehabilitation (PM&R), and comments on the future trends in the field.

A major impetus for this chapter, and more broadly for this book, arises from disparate themes. The cup is half empty and the cup is half full. On the one hand, over the last quarter of a century, significant progress has been made in the care of the geriatric patient through the incorporation of the principles of geriatric medicine across medical and surgical specialties in training, research, and the development of service delivery models. On the other hand, many colleagues appear to embrace these principles in an abstract and superficial manner; financial constraints and efforts to improve value can have unintended negative consequences on the care of these individuals; and further research on underlying mechanisms is needed.

Physicians advocating for distinctive services for a geriatric population encounter skepticism from colleagues who assert that specific emphasis on geriatric patients is not warranted. A version of "we don't need geriatric specialists in our field since we already treat many older patients" is a common reframe heard not only from PM&R physicians, but also across the spectrum of adult medical and surgical specialties. In the 1990s, my colleagues and I showed that older patients did not perceive the acute inpatient rehabilitation as positively as younger [1]. A few years later in a study of cognitive abilities and hip fracture rehabilitation outcomes, we found while demented patients began rehabilitation at lower functional levels, they made comparable gains as non-demented patients [2]. Many rehabilitation colleagues were surprised to learn that elderly patients were not as positive about acute rehabilitation as younger patients, and that rehabilitation could benefit elderly patients even those with varying degrees of cognitive impairments.

17.3 Geriatric Rehabilitation: How Is It Effective?

Over the last 25 years increasing evidence has emerged that geriatric patients who receive rehabilitation services targeted to their particular circumstances have improved outcomes. In a systematic review and meta-analysis of 17 randomized controlled clinical trials with nearly 5000 patients, Bachman concluded that rehabilitation programs designed specifically for geriatric patients have the potential to improve functional outcomes, decrease nursing home admissions, and improve life expectancy in this population compared with general rehabilitation services [3]. In 88 % of the geriatric rehabilitation units (or 15 of the 17 clinical trials), a comprehensive multidisciplinary geriatric assessment was performed while none were performed in the general rehabilitation groups. While the review was not able to examine the mechanisms underlying these differences, it is reasonable to conclude that this geriatric evaluation framed the rehabilitation interven-

tions to the distinctive needs of this patient group and incorporated issues of frailty, and geriatric syndromes.

Observations that general rehabilitation services are not optimally attuned to the needs of older patients preceded these clinical trials. The mismatch of acute inpatient rehabilitation and the dynamics of effective services for the frail and elderly patients was a source of frustration and made more poignant as geriatric medicine emerged in the 1980s and 1990s in the USA. This mismatch continues today. Spurred by the identification of functional impairments through the comprehensive geriatric assessment units, concerned professionals sought interventions including rehabilitation. Even though the field of PM&R had pioneered medical rehabilitation (primarily for a younger population), issues of pacing, goal setting, and rehabilitation therapies in the context of frailty and common geriatric syndromes were unfamiliar to many in general rehabilitation. And perhaps even more frustrating, individual rehabilitation practitioners did not appreciate the inadequacies of the current delivery model. Financial constraints and regulatory guidelines also impeded the incorporation of frail elderly patients into acute rehabilitation services.

17.4 Geriatric Rehabilitation: A Travel Guide Through Patient-Centered Care

Geriatric rehabilitation can be thought of as a journey culminating in the delivery of effective services. At the top of this pyramid is the destination (goals) of rehabilitation. The arrival at the planned destination depends on the development of a road map (or geriatric assessment) to establish the pathways. Drawing the map builds on knowledge of the terrain and driving conditions (principles of geriatric medicine). And finally, the foundation of the pyramid represents the specifics of service delivery (treatments, processes of care, and quality), or where the rubber meets the road (see Fig. 17.1).

Meaningful goals anchor geriatric rehabilitation efforts. A shared, collaborative process among providers, patients, families, and their caregivers is mandatory and should result in feasible goals, which are important to the patient. The process of goal setting is arguably more important than any specific objective. If you don't know where you are going, you are unlikely to get there. The starting point revolves around the patient's preferences with input from their families and social network. Without this essential buy-in, well-intentioned efforts, as in the example above, have limited chances of success.

A comprehensive geriatric assessment frames the development of goals and the means to achieve them and consists of medical, mental, physical, and environmental domains. For the rehabilitation specialist, the principles of geriatric medicine and common geriatric syndromes represent a necessary starting point is described elsewhere in this chapter in the cross

Fig. 17.1 A travel guide to patient-centered geriatric rehabilitation

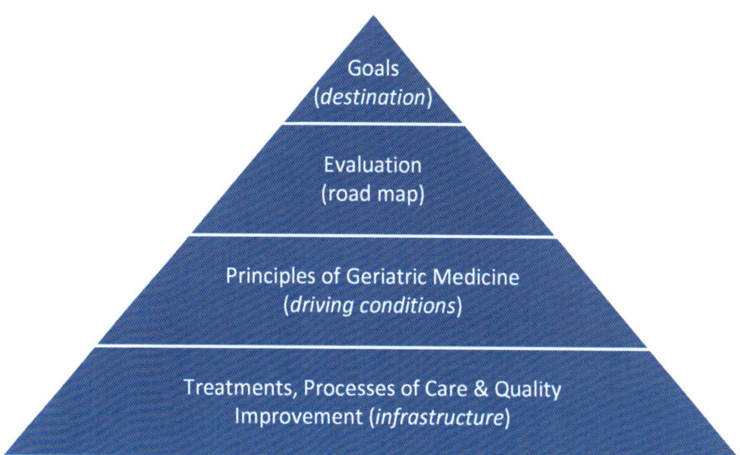

cutting issues of this book. Rehabilitation specialists delve in particular into function. Common domains of assessment of function include physical (e.g., ADLs, mobility, swallowing), cognitive (e.g., memory, judgment, language, and communication), and socio-environmental (housing, barriers social support, and resources). Only by evaluating all these factors can one gain an accurate road map for the "trip." For example, an individual's capabilities and potential with ADLs, gait, coping, and cognition within a particular social and physical environment can be pivotal in impacting the ability to live alone, navigate stairs, drive, and manage finances.

The specific treatments of geriatric rehabilitation are the final determinates of a successful arrival at the desired destination and represent the base of the pyramid. Specific treatments include not only the individual activities of a spectrum of rehabilitation professionals such as physical therapy or PT (mobility),occupational therapy or OT (self-care), speech language pathology or SLP (practical cognition), nurses (bladder management) and physicians (symptom management), but recent evidence points to the profound impact of care coordination and team functioning on treatment effectiveness [4]. Higher functioning teams predict improved patient outcomes and staff training interventions were shown to improve patient outcomes in a cluster randomized clinical trial [5]. Recent work to develop process of care measures of team effectiveness is encouraging that such tools could be applicable to Quality Improvement [6]. Process of care measures which capture meaningful interactions between staff and patients hold tremendous potential in the evaluation and improvement of treatment effectiveness, particularly in the relationship oriented areas of rehabilitation and geriatrics.

17.5 Navigating Uncertain Waters of Service Delivery

A common challenge encountered by health care providers is knowing what needs to be done, but an inability to figure out how to get the services in an era of increasing financial con-

straints. Much has been written about the ballooning health care costs in the USA. The fastest growing expenses for the Center for Medicare and Medicaid Services (CMS) are the post acute care (PAC) costs, which includes acute rehabilitation facilities sub-acute (SNF), home health (HH), outpatient therapies, and durable medical equipment (DME). CMS outlays for AC have doubled in the past 14 years. Forty percent of the growth of CMS expenses comes from increasing PAC costs. Understandably, this situation has resulted in close scrutiny of all PACs with subsequent increasing financial and administrative constraints. Ideas under consideration to address this situation include bundling of services and payment neutrality across sites. Under bundling a health care system is paid a lump sum per episode (e.g., hip fracture, stroke, or pneumonia) and has the flexibility to utilize the resources as they deem best. Payment neutrality refers to comparable payments across settings (e.g., sub-acute versus acute rehabilitation).

Many rehabilitation professionals are concerned about the potential deleterious effects of either of these changes primarily through a shift from "acute" rehabilitation to "sub-acute" rehabilitation along with decreasing payments for acute services. Sub-acute services are provided in skilled nursing facilities (SNFs), while acute rehabilitation is provided in acute inpatient rehabilitation facilities (IRFs). Services in both settings are reimbursed by Medicare, so it is understandable why CMS is keenly interested in the relative cost-effectiveness. Patients treated in sub-acute rehabilitation have longer lengths of stay, lower intensity of services, less physician involvement, and lower per diem costs than patients treated in acute rehabilitation. Physicians with documented rehabilitation expertise, usually in PM&R, manage care in acute settings including daily physician visits and weekly team conferences, while geriatricians or other generalists provide medical oversight in sub-acute settings with a minimum of a monthly visit. Comparisons of outcomes are challenging because of the different, but overlapping patients served and the lack of common functional outcome measures across the two settings. In addition, influential trade organizations for the respected entities advocate for their constituencies creating even more difficulties in meaningful outcome evaluations.

In principle, these settings serve different populations with distinct services. The primary criterion for admission to a sub-acute rehabilitation is a need for skilled level of services, which can be provided by either nursing, PT, or OT. Admission criterion for acute rehabilitation includes the patient's ability to participate in a minimum of three hours of therapy services a day, justification for two of three rehabilitation therapies (i.e., PT, OT, SLP), and the need for ongoing medical and nursing services . In addition, CMS stipulates that a minimum of 60 % of the patients fall into 1 of 13 diagnostic categories (such as stroke, Parkinson's disease, or brain injury). Of note, severe debility from a protracted hospitalization and elective joint replacements are not included in one of these categories even though these patients can be admitted within the other 40 % if they meet the other requirements. Hence acute rehabilitation provides more intensive services with greater physician involvement, more effort devoted to care coordination, and shorter lengths of stay at significantly higher per diem costs and total costs.

Practically speaking, this arrangement can be problematic in several ways. A patient may not fit well into any PAC category. For example, a medically complex patient may benefit from daily physician monitoring and proximity to medical specialists found in acute rehabilitation, but not have the physical endurance to tolerate the required intensity of rehabilitation therapies. A medically tenuous patient may not be accepted in acute or sub-acute rehabilitation, and still not meet the criteria for Long Term Acute Care (LTAC). The wide variations in services and outcomes found in both acute and sub-acute facilities further complicate post acute care discharge planning. It seems that the better the sub-acute facility, the lower chance of a bed availability! These circumstances put the acute hospital discharge planner in an awkward situation as he or she is pressured to take the first available bed. Likewise acute rehabilitation facilities vary in their knowledge and skills in managing the frail, elderly patient. Also, there are patients who would benefit more from the intensity of acute rehabilitation after a period of recuperation and an initial lower intensity of exercise such as acute trauma with activity restrictions or profound debility. However, planned transitions from sub-acute to acute rehabilitation are uncommon and likely due, in part, to financial disincentives for the skilled nursing facility.

An ideal SNF patient could be someone who may not have the endurance to participate in the 3 h a day of therapy, and for whom an extended, slower pace rehabilitation course would likely prove more beneficial. LOS restrictions are more flexible and can extend up to 100 days, provided clinical improvement can be documented under CMS guidelines (though full coverage ends at 3 weeks). An IRF patient would be expected to benefit from a more intense and focused medical, nursing, and rehabilitation therapies, and would be able to achieve desirable goals in a relatively short period of time, such as 2–3 weeks. In general, payors are attracted to the SNF services because of the costs.

An ongoing debate exists in comparing acute versus sub-acute facilities. Discussions on this topic get convoluted as CMS places SNFs, IRFs, LTACs, and Home Health Services (HH) all in the category of post acute care (PAC). For Medicare beneficiaries, services provided in PAC settings are the fastest growing segment of healthcare in the USA. For example, Medicare payments to PAC providers reached $59 billion in 2013, more than doubling the costs since 2001. Faced with concerns on health care costs, CMS has pursued actions under Federal mandates to contain the costs of PACs. For example, IRFs have seen stricter admission criteria, payment cuts, and audit processes to monitor and recoup costs deemed unnecessary or not covered. Concurrent with these constraints has been a steady decline in the number of IRFs. The crux of the discussion is whether and to what extent rehabilitation services can be shifted to less expensive SNF settings.

Comparisons of patient outcomes between acute and sub-acute settings are complicated for a variety of reasons. While the two settings share some similar patients, the populations between the two differ as does the intensity of services, nursing staffing levels, and physician involvement. The two settings use different patient outcomes measurements, and there is tremendous variability among rehabilitation programs. In interpreting analyses between SNF and IRFs, any potential conflict of interests by payors, physician groups, and advocacy groups are salient. The per diem cost of sub-acute rehabilitation is approximately 1/3 to 1/2 of acute rehabilitation, a fact that demands an analysis of clinical quality outcomes in both settings.

With these caveats, there is reasonable evidence that for comparable patients outcomes are superior in acute settings, particularly for the diagnoses of stroke and hip fracture [7, 8]. In a study commissioned by the ARA Research Institute, an affiliate of the American Medical Rehabilitation Providers Association (AMRPA), Dobson DaVanzo & Associates, LLC examined the impact of the revised classification criterion for IRFs (acute rehabilitation), which were introduced in 2004 [9]. This study was commissioned in an environment of active discussions with CMS and nationally for site-neutral payment proposals and bundling demonstration projects, both of which were felt likely to shift patients from IRFS to SNFs. As an industry sponsored study which has not been published in peer-reviewed journals, readers are advised to examine the methods closely (link listed in reference [9]). With this caveat, the study merits a discussion given its apparent methodological rigor and consistency with findings from other published work.

The study examined over 100,000 matched pairs of patients with the same condition treated between 2005 and

Table 17.1 Comparisons of hip fracture outcomes: acute versus subacute rehabilitation*

• 13.3 vs 32.7 days length of stay
• 8.3 percentage point decrease in mortality rate
• 55.1 day increase in average days alive
• 53.1 fewer hospital readmissions per 1000 patients per year
• 52.8 more days residing at home (2-year period)
• Cost of $9.77 more per day (2-year period)

Reprinted with permission of the American Medical Rehabilitation Providers Association for The ARA Institute and Dobson DaVanzo & Associates, LLC. All Rights Reserved [8]

*$p < 0.0001$; $n = 20,970$

2009 (or 89.6% of IRF patients and 19.6% of SNF patients during the study period) with two analyses—cross-sectional and longitudinal. As expected, the cross-sectional analyses found a shift in to IRFs for patients with stroke, brain injury, major medical complexity, neurological disorders, and brain injury and to SNF for patients with elective joint replacements. Compared to the SNF patients, IRF patients had better clinical outcomes on five of six measures in the longitudinal analysis. The sixth measure was hospital readmission and IRF patients had fewer hospital readmissions than SNF patients for amputation, brain injury, hip fracture, major medical complexity, and pain syndrome. See Table 17.1 for one sub-group analysis—hip fracture.

17.6 The Convergence of PM&R and Geriatric Medicine

Rehabilitation is an attitude and an orientation towards the maintenance and promotion of function. In the early to mid-twentieth century, rehabilitation techniques emerged as concerned health care providers addressed functional loss and disability with exercise, wheelchairs, prosthetics, compensatory strategies, and specific medical interventions for disable groups. In the process, a function oriented service delivery model incorporating multidisciplinary interventions within a biopsychosocial framework emerged to optimize a disabled individual's function. This approach contrasted radically with the traditional medical model at that time of physician dominated authoritative director of health care. This new approach emphasized the interactive role of patients, physicians, and other providers and was a marked departure from the typical model and represented a precursor to the contemporary emphasis on patient-centered care. Like students in school, success is viewed in terms of a skill performance. Can the disabled individual safely bathe, toilet, dress, climb stairs, live alone, or return to work?

Physical Medicine and Rehabilitation (PM&R) coalesced as a medical specialty in the USA and other countries in response to large numbers of injured soldiers associated with twentieth century armed conflicts. During World War I, specialty hospitals were developed for disabled soldiers, including for the treatment of spinal cord injuries. Taking advantage of recent advancements in engineering and manufacturing, concerned individuals, including friends and relatives of injured soldiers developed more useful canes, crutches, orthotics, and wheelchairs for the disabled. In the 1920s and 1930s, "physical therapy" physicians and other health professionals expanded on the therapeutic use of physical agents such as light, diathermy, hydrotherapy, electricity, and magnetism. In World War II, Howard Rusk in the USA and others developed effective models of service delivery for disabled soldiers [10]. The team based models of service delivery and the use of physical agents in medical care were precursors to the formal recognition of PM&R as a medical specialty in the USA.

Around the same time period in the UK, another young physician, Marjorie Warren, confronted a hospital full of patients with chronic conditions and disabilities where the expectation was long-term institutionalization. Dr. Warren discarded this warehouse attitude and pioneered a practical, patient-centered approach to address functional disabilities. She recruited diverse health care providers (e.g., aids, nurses, physiotherapists) and coordinated their efforts to train and mobilize her patients. Along the way, she developed new approaches such as the "shuffle board transfer" which is known in the USA as the "sliding board transfer." Between 1935 and 1939, 80% of the patients in the "Hospital of the Incurables" were successfully transitioned to the community. Dr. Warren played a pivotal role in the development of the medical specialty of Geriatric Medicine and was instrumental in the incorporation of Geriatric principles into the UK. National Health Service (NHS) in the late 1940s [11].

With advances in healthcare, the establishment of Medicare, and an aging population of baby boomers and their parents, the common interests of the medical specialties of PM&R and Geriatric Medicine became increasingly obvious. Beginning in the 1980s, seminal work on Geriatric Assessment Units documented the benefits of a comprehensive, functionally oriented geriatric assessments and multidisciplinary team interventions. The commonalities between the medical specialties were obvious to anyone who looked. With support of the John A. Hartford Foundation, the American Geriatrics Society spearheaded an exhaustive effort to articulate and support geriatrics principles among ten surgical and related medical specialties. Representatives of the American Academy of PM&R were active participants in this process which is reflected in a 2002 editorial entitled "Geriatrics and Physical Medicine and Rehabilitation: Common Principles, Complementary Approaches, and Twenty-First Century Demographics" [12].

The confluence of PM&R and Geriatrics reveals a basic insight—the value of a patient-centered approach with an emphasis on function and practical interventions delivered by multidisciplinary teams. In PM&R and Geriatrics, the service delivery model is a dynamic interaction of providers and patients to promote function, in contrast to a traditional and more passive model of a physician, a patient, and a prescribed intervention. Even though this dynamic patient-centered and team approach has proven highly effective, the maintenance of such an approach remains challenging and must adapt to changing circumstances and financial pressures of contemporary health care.

17.7 Frailty, Geriatric Syndromes, and Rehabilitation

Frailty is an example of a syndrome emerging in recent years. This syndrome is important for all rehabilitation clinicians to understand and learn to diagnose. Frailty can be thought of as increased vulnerability or decreased functional reserves to stress including social, physical, or psychological. Frail elder individuals are susceptible to major health and functional status changes caused by relatively minor perturbations. In fact, frailty is a powerful predictor of increased risk of adverse outcomes and mortality from nearly any significant perturbation such as major surgical procedure, stroke, fall, or fracture. It now can be easily recognized by any clinician using simple tools of assessment. Chapter 1 Frailty provides a thorough discussion of this syndrome.

Geriatric and rehabilitation frameworks are useful tools in the diagnosis and management of other geriatric syndromes. Falls, delirium, dementia, incontinence, polypharmacy, and pressure sores present as symptom complexes with multifactorial and overlapping causes and are usually associated with functional impairments. The presenting symptoms and associated risk factors are targeted with broad based biopsychosocial interventions to mitigate the symptom complexes. Not only does the interface of rehabilitation and geriatric syndromes reveal similarities in content and approach, a synergy emerges where insights from one informs the other.

A rehabilitation team can provide comprehensive input into the management of geriatric syndromes. Typically, the physician spends 5–15 min a day with a patient while various rehabilitation team members interact with patients 24 h a day across the spectrum of human activities. Nurses care for patients 24 h a day/7 days a week. They play a major role in setting the tone of the treatment environment that represents a transition from a dependent and passive role of acute care to a self-determining and active participation in rehabilitation. The PT works on gait, mobility, and balance; the OT addresses self-care, personal hygiene, and activities of daily living (ADLs), and the SLP treats disorders of swallowing, attention, and practical cognitive functioning. The impact of geriatric syndromes occurs in the practical world of daily living and members of the rehabilitation have the skills to intervene comprehensively in a coordinated manner.

17.7.1 Falls

Falls represent the quintessential geriatric syndrome [13]. They occur with increasing frequency such that an 80-year-old has an eight times greater risk of falls compared with a 65-year-old. A history of falls predicts increases in morbidity, mortality, disability, and early institutionalization. Falls have multifactorial risk factors which are categorized as intrinsic (e.g., polypharmacy, dementia, gait abnormalities), environmental (e.g., stairs, lighting, furniture), and situational (e.g., inattention, poor safety awareness, unfamiliar setting). The recognition of falls as a geriatric syndrome is paramount in rehabilitation. Effective interventions arise from a comprehensive biopsychosocial framework to address risk factors, promote healthy behaviors, and to develop interventions for identified issues of mobility (e.g., gait, balance, endurance), ADLs (e.g., toileting, dressing, meal preparation), neurocognition (e.g., attention, judgment, and safety awareness), and the social and physical environment (e.g., social support and physical barriers). A recent review of fall risk assessment tools in rehabilitation can be a helpful resource in the evaluation and treatment of falls [14].

17.7.2 Incontinence

For the elderly patient, successful interventions for bladder and bowel management commonly have a behavioral component. The acts of micturition and defecation are complex tasks involving the autonomic and conscious nervous systems—gross and fine motor skills are needed for toileting, while neurocognitive skills such as attention, communication, and visual spatial perceptions are utilized to ready the individual for continence. An interdisciplinary rehabilitation team should play an important role in bladder and bowel assessment and treatment by targeting the specific functional activities to promote continence, such as toilet transfers, clothing management, caregiver communication, and problem-solving. In one clinical trial in an acute rehabilitation setting, a staff awareness and skills training intervention on bladder management was associated with improved bladder continence and overall functional improvement [15]. Furthermore, measures of rehabilitation team functioning correlate with bladder management. Rehabilitation patients treated by higher functioning teams are associated with greater levels of bladder continence [16]. Bladder and bowel management are enhanced by an interdisciplinary rehabilitation team which targets specific deficits associated with the problem. Other sections of this book describe in detail medical and surgical interventions to promote bladder and bowel continence (Chaps. 19 and 21 provide this information).

17.7.3 Dementia

Neurocognitive decline in elderly individuals often is first noted by their children and others following relatively minor medical events like a frozen shoulder or an Emergency Department visit following a fall. In the rehabilitation setting, clinicians must be attuned to these comments and observations as underlying cognitive impairment in a senior profoundly influences risk for adverse outcomes and care planning. For example, major medical or surgical events like a stroke, hip fracture, coronary artery bypass procedure, or hospitalization for pneumonia can unmask cognitive decline, which in turn has implications for an individual's independence, living situation, and quality of life. Such patients are frequently referred for rehabilitation therapies and too often the cognitive impairment has not been recognized by clinicians in the acute care setting whose focus was on the acute illness. Recognizing even subtle cognitive impairment is critical in the assessment and management of specific deficits (e.g., money management, safety in the home and community, and learning new skills such as the use of a specialized wheelchair). For an elderly individual with recently apparent cognitive impairment, questions to be addressed during rehabilitation include hygiene, independent living, and safety with meal preparation, community activities or driving. Details on the diagnosis and management of dementia are available in Chap. 4, Psychiatry. A rehabilitation clinician must be expert in recognizing patients with even mild dementia and doing so helps greatly in their providing a practical, real-world plan to rehabilitation goals. Even for the patient not in a rehabilitation unit, the rehabilitation consulting team can add greatly to the management of patients with dementia by implementing interventions to optimize functional outcomes.

17.7.4 Delirium

A robust literature documents the extent of delirium in elder patients in acute hospitals and most other inpatient venues and that delirium is commonly not diagnosed especially in seniors where the common presentation is hypoactive as opposed to the typical hyperactive state of younger individuals. While the literature is not as robust as it is in the general hospital setting (where delirium is missed in up to 40 % of cases), the clinical impression in rehabilitation settings is that delirium is more common than generally thought. The recognition of delirium should refocus the efforts of medical and rehabilitation professionals towards risk reduction including the potential contributions of medications, sleep hygiene, and environmental factors. A patient with a reversible delirium may be inappropriately denied intensive services based on an erroneous interpretation of current symptoms. All rehabilitation clinicians should be expert in preventing, recognizing, and treating delirium in their patients. Chapter 2, Delirium, provides a detailed account of this common problem.

17.7.5 Polypharmacy

Common conditions impacting rehabilitation include pain, affect, agitation, neuropathy, spasticity, impairments of attention and memory, orthostasis, and bladder and bowel incontinence. Medications used for these conditions have disturbing side effect profiles, including especially those with anticholinergic properties. There are many non-pharmacological interventions that are effective for these problems. Rehabilitation professionals must be vigilant to medication side effects (including those from effectively agents used in younger patients) in the highly vulnerable senior population, and choose drugs wisely. A high functioning team can assist in identifying non-pharmacological treatments for many of these conditions such as pain, agitation, and spasticity. In addition, the interdisciplinary team can assist in assessing the impact of certain trials of medication for a spectrum of common rehabilitation issues cited above while at once monitoring for side effects. In a comprehensive review on the topic in PM&R, Geller et al. identified strategies modified from geriatric medicine and public health such as physician engagement, accurate assessment of medication lists, patient-centered process, using explicit and implicit criteria for guidance, practicing medication debridement when appropriate, and using technology and computer-assisted tools to identify problem areas and offer practical solutions [17]. Chapter 5 Medication Management provides a thorough review of this subject and detailed information of the popular Beer's list of drugs best avoided in seniors.

17.8 Heading to the Future

Substantive progress has been made in addressing the needs of our aging population through education, training, service delivery, and critical inquiry over the last 25 years. Support from private foundations (i.e., John A Hartford Foundation and Atlantic Philanthropies), professional organizations (i.e., AGS and AAPMR) and Federal agencies (i.e., NIA/NIH, AHRQ, and CMS) to name a few will continue to play pivotal roles. The Geriatrics for the Specialist Initiative (GSI) of the AGS typifies the impact of a targeted program to support the principles of geriatric medicine across medical and surgical specialties. (Information on this 20-year effort of the GSI is available on the web site of the American Geriatric Society). Insights gained through the work of Marjorie Warren in Geriatric Medicine and Howard Rusk in PM&R still resonate in the twenty-first century—an emphasis on function through comprehensive evaluations, interdisciplinary team treatments, and practical interventions directed at patient-centered goals. Ongoing broad based efforts across medical specialties and health care professionals will continue to address intertwined health and rehabilitative needs of our aging population.

Opportunities and challenges characterize the future of Geriatrics Rehabilitation. Current research across a range of areas such as sarcopenia, neuroplasticity, bone metabolism, gait and balance, and implementation science portend further progress, while efforts to improve cost-effectiveness, service delivery changes and related financial constraints can result in deterioration of services (so-called unintended consequences). The need for truly cost effective services is unassailable. For years, rehabilitation researchers and policy analyst describe the "black box" of rehabilitation. Rehabilitation works, but we have limited understanding of how the goals are achieved. More recent work on the active ingredients of rehabilitation services [6], rehabilitation team functioning [5], and the role of medical leadership in rehabilitation team effectiveness are promising avenues [4].

Gazing into a crystal ball, this author offers an optimistic perspective and envisions an evolution of rehabilitation akin to geriatrics and the relationship Geriatric Medicine has with primary care and other medical specialties. The need for rehabilitation services for this population exceeds the capacity of one or even a few medical specialties. From a foundation in the diagnosis and management of geriatric syndromes and frailty, rehabilitation providers develop and implement individualized interventions to optimized function. Further cross-fertilization among PM&R, Geriatric Medicine, and other specialties (e.g., psychiatry, neurology) brings important knowledge and skills to achieve the goals. PM&R physicians are active in sub-acute settings collaborating with other medical specialties and health care providers. Permeable membranes across PAC settings allow for the right service to the right patient at the right time. PM&R leaders spearhead formal Geriatric Rehabilitation Fellowship training programs.

A basic behavioral science of rehabilitation effectiveness reveals inside the "black box" of rehabilitation. Knowledge on the active ingredients of services, rehabilitation team effectiveness, and the optimal role of physician engagement leads to the development of valid and reliable measures suitable for evaluation and monitoring service delivery. As the values and perspectives of patients, families, and caregivers are incorporated into rehabilitation services and measured through standardized techniques, the spectra of unintended consequences of changes in service delivery lessens. PM&R physicians and other rehabilitation professionals are now seen as experts in team medicine, exercise medicine, and the optimization of function, and they work collaboratively across a range of medical, surgical, and health care professionals to achieve the common goals. While this rosy future is not pre-ordained, it does offer goals and a framework to progress. With the passion and commitment of our forbearers such as Marjorie Warren and Howard Rusk, real progress will continue.

References

1. Strasser DC, Falconer JA, Martino-Saltzman D. The relationship of patient's age to the perceptions of the rehabilitation environment. J Am Geriatr Soc. 1992;40(5):455–8.
2. Goldstein FC, Strasser DC, Woodward JL, Roberts VJ. Functional outcome of cognitively impaired hip fracture patients on a geriatric rehabilitation unit. J Am Geriatr Soc. 1997;45(1):35–42.
3. Bachmann S, Finger C, Huss A, et al. Inpatient rehabilitation specifically designed for geriatric patients: systematic review and meta-analysis of randomised controlled trials. BMJ. 2010;340:c1718. doi:10.1136/bmj.c1718.
4. Smits SJ, Bowden DE, Falconer JA, Strasser DC. Improving medical leadership and teamwork: an iterative process. Leadership in health services. Leadersh Health Serv. 2014;27(4):299–315. doi:10.1108/LHS-02-2014-0010.
5. Strasser DC, Falconer JA, Stevens AB, Uomoto JM, Herrin J, Bowen SE, Burridge AG. Team training and stroke rehabilitation outcomes: a cluster randomized trial. Arch Phys Med Rehabil. 2008;89(1):10–5.
6. Strasser DC, Burridge AB, Falconer JA, Uomoto JM, Herrin J. Toward spanning the quality chasm: an examination of team functioning measures. Arch Phys Med Rehabil. 2014;95(11):2220–3. doi:10.1016/j.apmr.2014.06.013.
7. Deutsch A, Granger CV, Heinemann AW, et al. Poststroke rehabilitation: outcomes and reimbursement of inpatient rehabilitation facilities and subacute rehabilitation programs. Stroke. 2006;37(6):1477–82. Epub 2006 Apr 20.
8. SNF, IRF. Assessment of patient outcomes of rehabilitative care provided in inpatient rehabilitation facilities (IRFs) and after discharge: study highlights for hip fracture patients. https://www.amrpa.org/newsroom/HipFractureSummary.pdf (2014). Accessed 24 Jan 2016.
9. Assessment of Patient Outcomes of Rehabilitative Care Provided in Inpatient Rehabilitative Facilities (IRFs) and After Discharge. Dobson DaVanzo & Associates LLC. Report Commissioned by the ARA Research Institute, an affiliate of the American Medical Rehabilitation Providers Association (AMPRA). https://www.amrpa.org/newsroom/Dobson%20DaVanzo%20Final%20Report%20-%20Patient%20Outcomes%20of%20IRF%20v%20%20SNF%20-%207%2010%2014%20redated.pdf (2014). Accessed 22 Jan 2016.
10. Rusk HA. A world to care for: the autobiography of Howard A. Rusk. New York: A Reader's Digest Press Book, Random House; 1977.
11. St John PD, Hogan DB. The relevance of Marjory Warren's writings today. Gerontologist. 2014;54(1):21–9. doi:10.1093/geront/gnt053. Epub 2013 Jun 7.
12. Strasser DC, Solomon DH, Burton JR. Geriatrics and physical medicine and rehabilitation: common principles complementary approaches, and 21st century demographics. Arch Phys Med Rehabil. 2002;83(9):1323–4.
13. Means KM. Neurologic: falls. In: Means K, Kortebein P, editors. Geriatrics – rehabilitation quick reference. New York: Demos Medical Publishing LLC; 2013. p. 159–61.
14. Lee J, Geller AI, Strasser DC. Analytical review: focus on fall screening assessments. PMR. 2013;5(7):609–21.
15. Vaughn S. Efficacy of urinary guidelines in the management of post-stroke incontinence. Int J Urol Nurs. 2009;3(1):4–12.
16. Strasser D, Stevens A, Herrin J, et al. Staff attitudes and continence management in rehabilitation. Presented at the American Geriatric Society National Meeting, Orlando, FL, May 2005 (Poster # A138). J Am Geriatr Soc. 2005;53(4. Supplement S1–S244):S65.
17. Geller AI, Nopkhun W, Dows-Martinez MN, Strasser DC. Polypharmacy and the role of physical medicine and rehabilitation. PMR. 2012;4(3):198–219.

Urology

18

Tomas L. Griebling

Geriatric care forms a large portion of most general urologic practice. Indeed, many of the most common urologic conditions occur with increasing incidence and prevalence among older adults. However, these should not necessarily be considered an inevitable or normal part of aging. Examples include urinary incontinence, pelvic organ prolapse, urinary tract infections, sexual dysfunction in both men and women, benign prostatic hyperplasia, and the various genitourinary malignancies. In addition, urologic conditions frequently influence the development of several geriatric syndromes such as falls, pressure ulcers, and polypharmacy. Many urologic conditions can be treated both medically and surgically, and decisions for care must be made within the framework of overall health including consideration of comorbidity, frailty, potential for improvement, and goals of care. Continued population growth among older adults will lead to future increases in urologic health needs in the geriatric age group. This will likely translate into an increased rate of the need for surgical care among older adults [1].

A number of anatomic and physiological changes occur in the genitourinary system that predispose to development of urologic disorders. A major challenge in clinical urology is differentiating these normal alterations from conditions that require active intervention. This is typically based on the development of symptoms that influence clinical function or quality of life. For example, the ratio of smooth muscle to collagen and supportive tissue in the bladder decreases with advancing age. These structural changes can lead to alterations in contraction strength and bladder compliance [2].

These changes can be associated with increased urinary frequency and urgency, nocturia, and a decreased ability to efficiently empty the bladder. Electron microscopy of bladder tissues in older adults has shown these structural changes and also development of 'dense bands' and loss of caveolae [3, 4]. Involuntary detrusor contraction may occur as well as decreased voluntary bladder contraction strength and velocity. Functional innervation to the bladder may decrease over time in response to chronic outlet obstruction and detrusor overactivity [5]. Over time this may lead to loss of compliance and muscle elasticity which can manifest as decreased urinary storage and impaired bladder emptying. With advancing age, bladder capacity tends to remain relatively stable or may decrease only slightly [6]. Also, alterations in neurotransmitters or epithelium may cause sensory changes with bladder filling so the sense of fullness is altered. Oxidative stress may damage tissues in the urothelium and detrusor and lead to symptomatic bladder dysfunction [7].

With aging, there are also progressive anatomic changes that tend to decrease pelvic floor muscle strength and soft tissue support which can lead to increased rates of pelvic organ prolapse in elderly women. Cadaveric studies using tissue biopsies have shown a generalized decrease in striated muscle tissue relative to connective tissue in the pelvic floor [8]. Other risk factors include increased parity and history of vaginal delivery. Bony support of the pelvis may influence these changes, and could be altered by some types of skeletal disease in elderly women including osteopenia or osteoporosis [9, 10]. Apoptotic cellular changes may lead to changes in soft tissue support in the pelvic floor structures [11]. Similarly, apoptosis of the rhabdosphincter can lead to an increased risk for development of stress urinary incontinence [12]. This can be associated with loss of normal circumferential anatomy and decreased urethral resistance and closure pressures which in turn lead to worsening incontinence [13]. Although pelvic floor muscle exercise may be helpful clinically for a variety of conditions, many older women may not be able to generate adequate voluntary muscle contraction on initial physical examination [14].

T.L. Griebling, MD, MPH (✉)
Department of Urology, The Landon Center on Aging,
The University of Kansas School of Medicine,
Mailstop 3016, 3901 Rainbow Boulevard,
Kansas City, KS 66160, USA
e-mail: tgriebling@kumc.edu

© Springer International Publishing Switzerland 2017
J.R. Burton et al. (eds.), *Geriatrics for Specialists*, DOI 10.1007/978-3-319-31831-8_18

18.1 Urinary Incontinence

Urinary incontinence (UI) is defined as the involuntary loss of urine [15]. UI can be classified as both a specific diagnosis and also a geriatric syndrome. Both incidence and prevalence of UI increase with advancing age, but UI should not be considered a normal or inevitable part of aging. UI can be transient or established, and various types have been recognized. It is important to diagnose the specific type of UI a patient experiences because this will guide therapeutic options. See also Chap. 13 Gynecologic Care: Pelvic Floor Disorders for additional information related to the older female patient.

18.1.1 Transient Urinary Incontinence

The term 'transient urinary incontinence' refers to UI that is generally caused by factors other than the bladder itself, and is typically reversible if the underlying etiology is addressed. In most cases, transient UI occurs relatively suddenly in a person who has previously been continent of urine or as sudden worsening of mild UI. It is estimated that about 30 % of new cases of UI in community dwelling older adults may be caused by a transient condition [16]. A wide variety of different clinical conditions have been linked to development of transient UI. Urinary tract infections are associated with urinary urgency, frequency, and urgency incontinence and may require antibiotic therapy. Atrophic vaginitis and urethritis may occur in elderly women and can often be effectively treated with vaginal estrogens [17]. Severe constipation can slow transit time and lead to increased water reuptake with subsequent development of polyuria; while low fecal impaction may cause bladder outlet obstruction.

Many medications can cause transient incontinence. The most common include diuretics, antipsychotics, benzodiazepines, calcium channel blockers, and medications with strong anticholinergic properties. Polypharmacy itself may also be associated with increased risk of UI [18]. Alcohol and other substance abuse may contribute to UI in some older adults. Polydipsia, peripheral edema, and congestive heart failure may produce polyuria and/or nocturia leading to transient UI. Psychological and behavioral disorders, delirium, and mobility impairment may also be linked to increased risk of UI. Normal pressure hydrocephalus (NPH) is associated with a classic triad of symptoms including UI, gait ataxia, and cognitive dysfunction. Sleep apnea can lead to nocturia and nocturnal polyuria that can cause UI and other bothersome lower urinary tract symptoms.

18.1.2 Established Urinary Incontinence

Established or chronic UI is quite commonly seen in geriatric patients. Population studies show that up to 44 % of all people over 65 years of age report some history of urinary leakage [19] and about 12 % of community dwelling older women reported severe or very severe UI. Rates in those living in nursing homes and those receiving home care services were much higher at about 37 % and 40 %, respectively. Several different types of established or chronic UI are recognized.

Urgency UI is the most common form of established incontinence in the geriatric population. Symptoms include urinary urgency and frequency, and some people are unable to reach toilet facilities before they experience loss of urine. This is often caused by detrusor overactivity with associated sensory and motor changes in the bladder. The etiology is complex and often multifactorial [20]. The term 'overactive bladder' has been used clinically to describe this condition. Many neurological disorders including stroke, Parkinson disease, multiple sclerosis, and spinal injury are associated with detrusor overactivity and urgency UI [21]. Increased white matter hyperintensities on brain MRI have been identified as a correlate of increased detrusor overactivity and associated urgency UI in older adults [22]. Some patients with urgency UI may also experience fecal incontinence due to an overlap in neural control mechanisms [23]. Detrusor hyperactivity with impaired contractility (DHIC) is a unique form of bladder dysfunction that is seen more commonly in geriatric patients. In this condition, patients experience urinary urgency due to the detrusor overactivity; however, they do not completely empty the bladder when they urinate due to impaired bladder contractility during the voiding effort. Effective treatment must address both components of storage and voiding dysfunction [24].

Stress UI is also very common in older adults including both men and women. In men, it is often associated with prior treatment for prostate disease including radical prostatectomy for prostate cancer, or transurethral resection for benign prostatic hyperplasia (BPH). In women, stress UI is most commonly caused by either urethral hypermobility or intrinsic sphincter deficiency. In all cases, the pressure in the bladder exceeds the urethral outlet resistance and leakage occurs with activities that increase intraabdominal pressure such as coughing, laughing, lifting, or sneezing.

Overflow incontinence is associated with incomplete emptying of the bladder due to either outlet obstruction or detrusor underactivity with poor contractility. There has recently been an increased interest in the concept of 'underactive bladder' including analysis of potential causes and treatments [25, 26]. Various neurogenic and myogenic factors associated with development of underactive bladder include poorly controlled diabetes, bladder ischemia from vascular disease, and chronic bladder obstruction from prostate enlargement in men or severe pelvic organ prolapse in women.

Functional incontinence is a term used to describe UI that is caused by factors other than the bladder itself. The most common associated causes include impairments in cognition or mobility. If the underlying problem can be corrected or improved, the functional UI may also resolve or improve. Mixed incontinence refers to a condition in which a patient experiences more than one type of UI. The most common combination is urgency and stress UI, although other combinations are also possible. This can make successful treatment of UI more challenging in affected patients.

Clinical evaluation requires careful history and physical examination to guide therapy. Evaluation should include assessment of the level of independence for performing activities of daily living as well as baseline cognitive status and mobility. Alterations in functional status, including increased dependence on others for ADLs have been linked to increased prevalence of UI [27]. Impaired mobility with reduced walking speed and poor balance contribute to increased risk of ADL decline and UI [28]. See Chap. 8 Tools for Assessment for information on ADL, IADL, and gait assessment.

A pelvic examination in women and genitourinary examination in men should be part of this routine evaluation. Assessment of prior therapies tried and level of success is important. In addition, evaluation of caregiver support and environmental factors including the living environment are useful. In addition, several other tests can be included in the assessment which may be useful, particularly in elderly patients. Urinalysis is used to evaluate for hematuria, UTI, proteinuria, or glucosuria that could indicate renal disease or diabetes. Voiding diaries help to identify voiding patterns and factors that may trigger UI. They can be particularly helpful in cases of nocturia to differentiate between nocturnal polyuria and other causative factors [29, 30].

Assessment of post-void residual volume either by bladder ultrasound or simple catheterization is helpful to check for incomplete bladder emptying associated with overflow incontinence, bladder outlet obstruction, or underactive bladder [31].

Urodynamic testing is useful in evaluation of UI for select geriatric patients. The main indications include underlying neurological or other comorbid conditions, failed prior therapy for UI, or planned genitourinary surgery [32]. The test is designed to reproduce symptoms if possible in order to help differentiate clinical issues and guide therapy. For example, it is helpful to distinguish between patients who don't empty the bladder due to outlet obstruction versus those with an underactive and poorly contractile bladder.

18.1.3 Negative Impacts of Urinary Incontinence

UI is associated with negative outcomes on overall and health-related quality of life for many older adults. People with chronic UI often experience increased rates of depression, social isolation, and stigmatization and embarrassment [33, 34]. It tends to limit ability to participate in social activities and interact with others outside of the home [35]. Health problems include increased skin irritation or infection, pressure ulcers, UTI, and falls.

Urinary incontinence is common in residents of nursing homes and other long-term care settings. Reported prevalence ranges from about 46% in short-term nursing home resident to over 75% among long-term residents [19]. UI in nursing home residents has been linked to decreased sense of dignity, autonomy, and blunted mood [36]. Organizational and staffing factors are important variables that contribute to rates of UI in nursing homes [37]. Targeted treatment and organizational process change can reduce rates of UI in these settings [38]. Prompted and assisted toileting programs, sometimes combined with assessment of bladder volumes using diaries or ultrasound, can be quite useful to help individual resident improve their continence status [39, 40].

18.1.4 Treatments for Urinary Incontinence

Treatments for UI should be tailored to individual patient needs and goals. Different types of UI require different treatments, and therapy should be based on overall goals of care, functional status, and comorbidities. Treatment often requires multiple components or approaches. The options include behavioral therapies, devices, medications, and surgeries (Table 18.1).

18.1.4.1 Behavioral Therapies

Behavioral therapies form the mainstay of treatment for UI in most patients. Avoiding dietary components that increase bladder irritation and urinary urgency and frequency can be useful. This includes caffeine, alcohol, highly acidic foods, and carbonated beverages [41]. Fluid restriction is generally not helpful, and can worsen urinary urgency and frequency in some patients due to increased urinary concentration; however, limiting fluids after dinner can reduce nocturia. Timed or scheduled urination can be useful, particularly among those with urinary urgency and urgency UI. Timed voiding is often combined with learning to delay voiding by controlling urge symptoms; this behavioral technique is called 'urge control' [42].

Pelvic floor muscle exercises are useful for many patients with stress UI and urgency UI. Patients generally need targeted instruction, and may benefit from working with a physical therapist or nurse for individualized coaching. Such behavioral treatments typically require 3–4 visits to

Table 18.1 Treatments for urinary incontinence

Behavioral therapies
Timed voiding
Prompted toileting
Assisted toileting
Diet modification (avoid caffeine, alcohol, carbonation, etc.)
Pelvic floor muscle exercises
Urge suppression strategies

Device therapies
Condom catheters (penile sheaths)
Pessaries (intravaginal support devices)
Indwelling catheters (urethral or suprapubic)
Absorbent pads and other products

Pharmacotherapies	Dosage
Antimuscarinic agents[a]	
Darifenacin (time released)	7.5 mg or 15 mg orally once daily
Fesoterodine (time released)	4 mg or 8 mg orally once daily
Oxybutynin	5 mg two or three times orally daily (maximum daily dose 30 mg)
Oxybutynin (time released)	5 mg, 10 mg, or 15 mg orally once daily
Oxybutynin (transdermal patch)	One patch (3.9 mg daily) topically, changed every 3 days
Oxybutynin (transdermal gel)	One packet topically once daily
Tolterodine	1 mg or 2 mg orally twice daily
Tolterodine (time released)	4 mg orally once daily
β-3 Agonist agents[b]	
Mirabegron (time released)	25 mg or 50 mg orally once daily

Surgical therapies
Stress urinary incontinence
Sling cystourethropexy (bladder neck)
Mid-urethral sling
Bladder neck suspensions
Bulking agent injection (bladder neck)
Urgency urinary incontinence
Chemodenervation (botulinum toxin injection)
Neuromodulation
Augmentation cystoplasty
Urinary diversion

[a]Main side effects of antimuscarinic agents: dry mouth, dry eyes, constipation, confusion, headache, blurred vision, tachycardia, QT interval prolongation on electrocardiogram, bradycardia and urinary retention

[b]Main side effects of β-3 agonist agents: hypertension, headache, nausea, dizziness and tachycardia

gain confidence in proper techniques and then a periodic review for reinforcement. Older adults using this type of behavioral therapy must be motivated to continue pelvic floor exercise, and understand how to use them at appropriate times. Pelvic floor muscle exercise has been shown to work well in both men and women, and can improve UI more than simple bladder training and timed voiding alone [43, 44].

18.1.4.2 Device Therapies

Many people use devices such as condom catheters or absorbent pads and products to manage urinary leakage. There are a variety of intravaginal pessaries that can be used for management of stress urinary incontinence (see Chap. 13 Gynecology). Penile clamps for men, or urethral plugs and inserts for women can be used in cases with stress incontinence, particularly with physical exercise or other activities. In general, devices are considered options for management of symptoms rather than definitive treatment of UI.

18.1.4.3 Pharmacotherapies

Medications are widely used for treatment of UI in both younger and older patients but should be initiated only after a trial of behavioral therapy. Most medications are targeted at overactive bladder and are used to treat urinary urgency, frequency, and urgency UI. Most are antimuscarinic, anticholinergic agents which block muscarinic receptors in the bladder and reduce involuntary detrusor contractions. Side effects of this class of medications include urinary retention, constipation, dry mouth, dry eyes, headache, and confusion [45]. Newer agents include beta-3 agonists that also work to reduce bladder overactivity, but avoid the typical anticholinergic effects; side effects for this agent include hypertension, headache, nausea, dizziness, and tachycardia (including atrial fibrillation). The route of administration may be an important consideration, particularly in geriatric patients. Transdermal preparations applied as either a skin patch or gel may be useful in those with swallowing problems. Time-released medications may improve adherence and efficacy. Liquid preparations may also be useful in patients with swallowing difficulties or in those who require use of a feeding tube.

Studies examining use of antimuscarinics in cohorts of older patients have shown efficacy, safety, and tolerability [46, 47]. Using the lowest effective drug dose is recommended, and patients should be monitored carefully and continuously for drug interactions or other adverse effects. Discontinuation of medication due to side effects or limited perceived efficacy is common, and several different medications may need to be tried to find one that works best for an individual patient [48–50]. Cost is also a factor when considering medication therapy for elderly patients [51]. Insurance coverage is variable and may differ substantially between medications for a given payment plan.

18.1.4.4 Surgical Therapies

Surgical therapy can be useful for treatment of UI in older adults, particularly if more conservative therapies such as behavioral options or medications have not been successful. In carefully selected patients surgical options improve outcomes for treatment of UI [52]. Age itself should not be the deciding factor of whether someone is a candidate for surgical intervention. Instead, overall health, comorbidity, and goals of care should be the guiding variables [53]. Development of less invasive surgery has increased surgical options for many older adults with UI and other lower urinary tract conditions [54].

Injection of bulking agents at the bladder neck to increase urethral outlet resistance is minimally invasive, and may be effective in elderly women with stress urinary incontinence [55]. A variety of materials have been used for this purpose. Results are generally good, and the procedure offers the advantage of being easily repeatable if needed. This type of therapy may be particularly useful in elderly women with stress UI who may not be good surgical candidates for more involved procedures.

Sling procedures include those that place grafts either under the mid-urethra or the bladder neck. Various graft materials are available including synthetic mesh, autologous fascia, and other biological grafts either from cadaver tissue donors or animal xenografts. Outcomes in carefully selected elderly women are generally good with complication rates similar to those in younger patients [56, 57]. However, other reports suggest that older women may have less overall clinical success with slings, and are at higher risk of complications [58, 59]. Sling procedures for treatment of male stress UI have also been developed, although outcome data specific to elderly men is limited. In men with stress UI, implantation of an artificial urinary sphincter is also an option. Good cognitive status and hand dexterity are needed to correctly operate the device after implantation. In select patients, this therapy can be extremely effective [60].

For patients with urinary urgency, frequency or urgency UI, neuromodulation and chemodenervation are minimally invasive surgical therapies that can help treat symptoms. Neuromodulation uses electrical stimulation of the nerves that control bladder contractility. Sacral neuromodulation is performed by implanting an electrode in the third sacral foramen (S3). This is connected to a programmable generator that provides impulses to the nerve. Success rates up to 83.3 % have been reported in selected elderly patients who underwent stimulator placement [61]. The most common complication is device infection or erosion that may require surgical removal. However, overall complication rates are similar in older and younger patients and age itself should not influence decisions for treatment with this therapy [62, 63]. Chemodenervation of the bladder detrusor muscle is also used for treatment of urgency UI and symptomatic urinary urgency and frequency. The most commonly used agent is onabotulinum toxin A. Studies have demonstrated clinical efficacy and safety even in elderly patients [64]. The main side effect of this treatment is urinary retention which may require clean intermittent catheterization at least temporarily in order to drain the bladder.

In highly select patients, urinary diversion may be considered for treatment of intractable UI. This could include reconstructive procedures with either creation of a urinary stoma such as an ileal conduit, or a continent catheterizable pouch. In some patients, management of a stomal device may be preferable to UI. However, these are major surgical procedures, and care through careful preoperative assessment (see Chap. 3) must be taken to weigh the risks and benefits for a given patient before selecting this type of therapy [65, 66].

18.2 Urinary Catheters

Urinary catheters are sometimes used in the management of urological and non-urological conditions. For example, patients with perineal skin breakdown or sacral pressure ulcers may require temporary indwelling catheter drainage to keep the affected area dry and allow for tissue healing. Temporary urinary catheter drainage is also used after reconstructive surgery with flap placement in order to keep the surgical site dry during healing.

However, in older adults, chronic indwelling catheters should be avoided if at all possible [67]. Indwelling catheters are associated with substantial complications including urinary tract infections, bacterial colonization, urosepsis, and stone formation [68]. Catheters should be removed when feasible, and patients should be monitored for signs or symptoms of infection. Tissue irritation from chronic catheterization can lead to squamous metaplasia of the bladder epithelium, and development of squamous cell carcinoma. If chronic catheter use is needed, suprapubic tube drainage is generally preferred over urethral catheterization. This reduces the risk for urethral and bladder neck erosion. In addition, it is often more comfortable for patients. It may be easier for caregivers to change compared to urethral catheterization, particularly in men, and also gets the catheter out of the genital tract which is beneficial for older adults who remain sexually active.

Persistent urinary leakage around an indwelling catheter is typically due to either bladder spasms or catheter blockage. Irrigation of the catheter with sterile saline can be helpful to relieve obstruction of the tube from urinary sediment. Clinicians should avoid placing larger caliber catheters, which will only serve to dilate the tract and will not solve the underlying problem of detrusor overactivity. If used in the urethra, larger catheters increase the risk of tissue erosion which can lead to severe urinary incontinence and can require advanced surgical reconstruction even bladder removal. Use of antimuscarinic medications to reduce bladder contractions can be very useful in patients who experience urinary incontinence associated with indwelling catheter drainage.

A variety of devices are available to manage urinary leakage including absorbent pads and condom catheters. These are useful for select patients. For example, they can be used when someone wants to participate in social activities that they might otherwise avoid due to UI. Numerous designs are available, and recent improvements have helped enhance odor control, fluid absorbency, and other associated factors [69–71]. Condom catheters are useful for men with UI. These disposable devices are designed to surround the penis and are connected to a urinary collection device. They can be particularly helpful for management of bothersome nocturia or if UI prevents men from participating in activities outside their home. Proper sizing and skin hygiene are important to prevent skin irritation or breakdown.

18.3 Urinary Tract Infections and Asymptomatic Bacteriuria

Urinary tract infection (UTI) is one of the most common urologic conditions that occur in older adults. Although both males and females experience UTIs, they tend to be more common in older women. It can sometimes be challenging to differentiate symptomatic UTIs, which need treatment and asymptomatic bacteriuria that does not require antibiotic therapy. Urine cultures are strongly recommended to confirm infection, help identify the associated bacterial organisms, and guide therapy. Antibiotic susceptibility patterns are in constant flux, and it is crucial to identify drug resistance and select appropriate treatment. Although empiric antibiotic therapy may be started based on clinical symptoms and dipstick urine results, antibiotics may need to be changed depending on results of antibiotic susceptibility testing. Catheterized urine samples may be needed if older adult patients have difficulty producing an adequate clean-catch specimen [72].

The most common symptoms of UTI include urinary urgency and frequency, dysuria, bladder pain, and fever. Cloudy and foul-smelling urine are common, but this can also be due to causes other than a UTI. Many older adults may not show these typical symptoms [73]. Instead, they may exhibit 'atypical symptoms' including confusion, lethargy, anorexia, agitation, UI, and behavioral changes [74]. Delirium may occur in some patients with UTIs [75]. Upper tract involvement with pyelonephritis or other complex forms of UTI are often associated with comorbidity such as stone disease, diabetes, or anemia [76]. Urosepsis in elderly patients may be serious, and is associated with increased risk of mortality due to decreased physiological reserve. Factors that increase the risk of mortality in older adults with urosepsis include advanced age (≥85 years), hypothermia, severe cognitive impairment, and chronic renal disease [77]. Hospital acquired UTIs are also associated with an increased risk of mortality compare to community acquired infections [78]. Management with fluid resuscitation and appropriate antibiotic therapy is crucial. Fungal UTIs are less common, and tend to occur with advanced age in patients with reduced immune status including those with a prior history of organ transplant on immunosuppressive therapy, those with HIV disease or AIDS, and in those with poorly controlled diabetes. Treatment may require antifungal agents such as fluconazole [79].

In contrast, asymptomatic bacteriuria with or without pyuria is a very common condition in older adults and should not be treated with antibiotics unless there are special considerations such as planned genitourinary surgery. In community dwelling older adults, asymptomatic bacteriuria occurs in about 10 % of men and 10–20 % of elderly women [80, 81]. Extensive data supports that asymptomatic bacteriuria does not require antibiotic therapy [82]. See also Chap. 24 Infection and Immunity in Older Adults for diagnosis and discussion of asymptomatic bacteriuria.

A number of clinical factors increase the risk of UTIs among older adults. Catheter associated UTIs are highly prevalent in acute care hospitals and other inpatient settings [68, 83]. Clean intermittent catheterization can reduce infection rates in patients with retention, and risk is lower compared to chronic indwelling catheter use. Obesity and significant underweight body mass index have both been linked to higher rates of UTI in older patients [84].

Several different therapies have been used to try to prevent UTIs in older adults. Administration of vaginal estrogens can reduce symptomatic UTI rates in elderly women by causing reacidification of the vaginal fluid milieu. This allows growth of Lactobacillus sp., the normal flora in the vagina. These bacteria act as an important host defense by killing bacteria associated with UTIs. Contraindication to vaginal estrogen use includes a personal history of breast or uterine cancer. Ingestion of cranberry juice or cranberry supplements is popular for UTI prevention. Proanthocyandidins in cranberry interact with fructose in bacterial cell walls and potentially prevent adherence of bacteria to the urothelium. However, data on clinical efficacy has been mixed. Recent evidence from a double-blind, randomized, placebo-controlled clinical trial in nursing home residents showed reductions in infection rates, but these statistically significant changes were limited to those with prior high rates of UTI [85]. In general, chronic antibiotic use for prophylaxis should be avoided unless no other options are available. Although it can be useful in select patients, it is also associated with an increased risk of drug resistant bacterial infection which makes treatment more challenging.

Evaluation and treatment of UTIs in nursing homes and other chronic care settings requires special consideration. Differentiation between symptomatic UTIs and asymptomatic bacteriuria can be particularly challenging in this setting, and overuse of antibiotic is common [86, 87]. Drug selection should be guided if possible by local antibiogram data based on local prevalence of specific organisms and resistance patterns [88]. Environmental contamination in nursing home and other chronic care settings may be associated with certain types of infection including methicillin-resistant *Staphylococcus aureus (MRSA)* [89]. Strict hand-washing and other infection prevention protocols can help to reduce this risk.

The overall costs associated with the evaluation and treatment of UTIs is staggering, and in the USA surpasses the cost of almost all other major genitourinary disorders [90, 91]. The high incidence of UTI certainly contributes, but overtreatment of asymptomatic bacteriuria and care provided in emergency rooms and urgent care centers are also important factors.

18.4 Hematuria

Hematuria is defined as the presence of blood in the urine. This is almost always abnormal, and clinical evaluation is generally indicated to identify potentially serious underlying causes [92]. Common etiologies for hematuria include urolithiasis, malignancies such as kidney cancer or urothelial tumors in the bladder, ureter or kidney, or trauma. Men with severe benign prostatic hyperplasia (BPH) may have bleeding from prostatic capillaries. The use of anticoagulation is common in geriatric patients for treatment of cardiac arrhythmias for stroke prevention. Both normal and supratherapeutic levels of anticoagulation can cause bleeding from a lesion in the urinary tract. All patients with hematuria, including those who develop hematuria after the initiation of anticoagulation, should undergo appropriate clinical evaluation [93]. This includes both cystoscopy and some type of contrast based imaging such as CT urogram or retrograde pyelography.

18.5 Sexual Health

Sexuality and sexual health remain an important part of life for many older adults who wish to remain sexually active if possible [94]. Survey data demonstrates that up to 20–30 % of all older adult men and women remain sexually active well into their 80s [95]. Urologic care providers can help to evaluate and treat sexual health issues in this population. Many common comorbid conditions including diabetes, hypertension, peripheral vascular disease, and heart disease can negatively impact sexual health in geriatric patients. In addition urinary incontinence and treatments for prostate cancer or other malignancies can substantially reduce sexual health in this population [96, 97]. Those with better overall health and less comorbidity tend to remain more sexually active with advancing age [98, 99]. Sexual health changes may also be signs or symptoms of underlying comorbid disease. Frailty has been shown to negatively affect sexual health status, and is associated with multiple changes in both physical and psychosocial domains [100]. Other gynecological disorders such as pelvic organ prolapse or atrophic vaginitis can also impair sexual function in elderly women. Impaired sexual health in older adults is also associated with higher rates of depression and other forms of mental health issues [101, 102].

Partner availability may limit sexual activity, and masturbation may become a primary form of sexual expression for some older people. Other forms of sexual expression may change with aging including a reduction in the emphasis on penetrative sexual activity and increased attention to intimacy with close physical and emotional contact [103]. The living environment may also influence sexual expression, particularly for those living with extended family caregivers or in nursing homes. Increased awareness of sexual health needs has led many nursing homes to work to better accommodate these residents [104]. Inappropriate sexual behavior may be problematic for older adults with cognitive impairment or dementia, and may be particularly challenging for caregivers [105]. Screening and treatment for sexually transmitted diseases may be indicated in some patients depending on sexual activity, and if signs or symptoms of infection are present [106].

A wide variety of therapies are available for sexual health dysfunction in older adults ranging from sexual therapy and counseling, to medications and surgeries designed to improve erectile function in men and sexual response in women. Treatments should be targeted on the patient's specific goals and outcomes, and should be selected within the scope of overall health and comorbidity. Chapter 22—Endocrinology provides a thorough discussion of the endocrine evaluation and treatment of hormonal deficiencies related to sexual dysfunction.

18.6 Urolithiasis and Stone Disease

Stone disease affects about 20 % of all adults at some point in their lives. Rates of stone formation are similar among older and younger adults, and those with a prior history are at risk for recurrence. Poor hydration status is one of the strongest risk factors for stone formation, and older adults often have a reduced sensation of thirst, or may have difficulty swallowing which can lead to inadequate fluid intake. Recent Medicare data suggest that compared to younger adults, older patients have a 2.5 to 3-fold increased rate of inpatient hospitalization for stone disease [107].

Stone composition may change with age, and older adults more often have uric acid stones compared to younger people [108]. This may particularly affect older patients with diabetes who may have impairments in urinary ammoniagenesis and produce abnormally high levels of uric acid with a low urinary pH [109]. Age-related alterations in vitamin D and calcium metabolism may also affect urolithiasis risk in older adults. Hyperuricosuria and hypercalcuria appear to be common in older patients with recurrent stone disease [110].

Small stones (<5 mm) often pass spontaneously with hydration and oral analgesics. Oral selective alpha-blockers such as tamsulosin may be helpful to enhance ureteral relaxation. Cystoscopy with ureteral stent placement is indicated to bypass the obstruction in cases of larger stones, particularly if the patient experiences intractable nausea, vomiting, or pain. Other indications for ureteral stent insertion include baseline renal insufficiency, a solitary functioning kidney, or significant urinary infection or bacteriuria. Surgical therapy with ureteroscopic stone fragmentation and extraction, extracorporeal shock wave lithotripsy, or percutaneous nephrostolithotomy may be required. The overall success rates for these procedures are similar in geriatric and younger patients [111, 112].

18.7 Benign Prostate Diseases

18.7.1 Benign Prostatic Hyperplasia

One of the most common urologic disorders in aging men is benign prostatic hyperplasia (BPH). Symptoms typically begin around 40–50 years of age [113]. Proliferation of epithelial and stromal elements occurs in response to serum testosterone. The effect of prostate enlargement is variable, and some men have no symptoms while others develop voiding difficulty. Typical symptoms include a decreased urinary stream with urgency, frequency, and nocturia. Severe cases may be associated with acute or chronic urinary retention and incomplete bladder emptying. Prostate size does not necessarily correlate with the degree of symptoms. The voiding symptoms associated with BPH can have a negative impact on overall and health-related quality of life for many men [114]. A useful symptom severity questionnaire is presented in Chap. 8—Tools for Assessment.

There are a variety of treatments available for BPH including both medical and surgical therapies. The most commonly used medications are α-adrenergic antagonists and 5-α-reductase inhibitors (Table 18.2). The α-adrenergic antagonists include terazosin (Hytrin), doxazosin (Cardura), tamsulosin (Flomax), and alfuzosin (Uroxatral). These drugs block α-adrenergic receptors in the prostatic urethra and bladder neck. This causes smooth muscle relaxation in these tissues, which in turn reduces outlet resistance. These medications have good overall efficacy [115]. The main adverse effect is orthostatic hypotension, which is more common with the older, less selective agents (terazosin, doxazosin).

Table 18.2 Medications for treatment of benign prostatic hyperplasia (BPH)

α-Adrenergic antagonist agents[a]	Dosage
Nonselective agents	
Doxazosin (Cardura)	1–8 mg orally once daily at bedtime (must titrate dose)
Terazosin (Hytrin)	1–10 mg orally once daily at bedtime (must titrate dose)
Selective agents	
Alfuzosin (Uroxatral)	10 mg orally once daily at bedtime
Tamsulosin (Flomax)	0.4 mg or 0.8 mg orally 30 min after the same meal once daily
5-Alpha reductase inhibitor agents[b]	Dosage
Dutasteride (Avodart)	0.5 mg orally once daily
Finasteride (Proscar)	5 mg orally once daily

[a]Main potential side effects of α-adrenergic antagonist agents: orthostatic hypotension, dizziness (these tend to be more pronounced with the nonselective agents)
[b]Main side effects of 5-alpha reductase inhibitor agents: decreased libido and erectile dysfunction

These drugs, particularly tamsulosin, may cause the intraoperative 'floppy iris syndrome' (leading to potential intraocular surgical complications). Although not generally reversible, the operating ophthalmologist should be made aware of the patient's use of this agent prior to cataract or other ocular surgery. In addition, intraocular surgery if indicated could be performed before starting the agent [116].

The 5-α-reductase inhibitors act by blocking the enzymatic catalysis of the conversion of testosterone into dihydrotestosterone (DHT). Reductions in circulating DHT lead to shrinking of the prostate gland and improvement in urinary outflow. It can take several months for these medications to reach full effect [117]. The two main drugs in this group are finasteride (Proscar) and dutasteride (Avodart). These medications generally work better in men with larger prostate volumes. Potential side effects include decreased libido and development of gynecomastia or breast tenderness. The drugs also cause an approximately 50 % reduction in circulating serum PSA. Prior to initiating these medications, a PSA level can be checked. After initiating a 5-α-reductase inhibitor, measured serum PSA levels should be doubled to estimate the actual PSA level. Several studies suggest that combination therapy with both an α-adrenergic antagonist and a 5-α-reductase inhibitor has better efficacy compared to monotherapy, particularly in men with more severe voiding symptoms or larger prostate glands [118, 119]. However, increased cost and potential side effects need to be carefully considered. Although phytotherapies are popular among older patients with BPH, to date there has been relatively limited research on their efficacy.

Surgical therapy for BPH may be required if medical treatment fails, options including both open and endoscopic procedures. Open suprapubic prostatectomy is typically reserved for patients with very large prostate gland volumes (>100 g). For the majority of men, transurethral surgeries have replaced open surgery and are associated with improved morbidity and good clinical outcomes. Transurethral resection of the prostate (TURP) remains the gold standard to which other forms of surgery are compared. Newer treatments use laser energy to vaporize or resect prostate tissue, or various forms of energy including radiofrequency, high-intensity focused ultrasound, or microwave thermotherapy [120, 121]. These ablate tissues and lead to necrosis and sloughing of affected tissues. Intraurethral prostatic stents have also been used to treat BPH, particularly in men with severe comorbidity who may be poor surgical candidates for even minimally invasive options [122, 123].

Many of the current minimally invasive options for treatment of BPH offer some potential advantages for elderly patients. In some cases, these can be done in an outpatient office setting under local anesthetic or sedation which obviates some of the risks associated with more involved anesthesia. Most have minimal risk of bleeding and can be advantageous for men on anticoagulation therapy.

18.7.2 Prostatitis

The overall prevalence of prostatitis among adult men ranges from 2 to 10 % [124, 125]. Prostate infections are either acute or chronic. The condition tends to occur more commonly in older men, and rates of hospitalization are 2–2.5 times higher in this population compared to younger men [91, 126]. Acute bacterial prostatitis is characterized by rapid onset of symptoms with fever, chills, urinary frequency and urgency, dysuria, and pelvic or perineal pain. Findings may be subtle in older men due to a reduction in overall immune response associated with aging. Physical examination may reveal an enlarged and tender prostate. Care should be taken to avoid vigorous prostate massage as this may lead to urosepsis. Urine cultures are useful to pinpoint the specific organism and guide choice of antibiotics. Inpatient care with intravenous antibiotics may be necessary if the patient is severely ill. If a prostate abscess is identified on CT imaging, surgical drainage is usually indicated. Acute urinary retention often occurs in cases of acute prostatitis and may require suprapubic tube insertion for bladder drainage. Urethral catheterization should be avoided to prevent bacterial seeding and urosepsis. Extended antibiotic therapy (>4 weeks) with an agent which achieves good tissue penetration such as doxycycline or a fluoroquinolone is often required.

Chronic prostatitis is more common than acute prostatitis in elderly men, and is usually associated with urinary urgency, frequency, nocturia, scrotal or perineal pain or referred pain in the low back and suprapubic region [127]. The physical findings are variable and the prostate may or may not be abnormal on rectal examination. Expressed prostatic secretions and urine culture are helpful in diagnosis and guiding therapy. Treatments include targeted antibiotic therapy and dietary modification to avoid urinary irritants such as alcohol, caffeine, or carbonated beverages.

18.8 Genitourinary Cancers

Cancers of the genitourinary tract increase in incidence and prevalence with advancing age. Depending on the type of cancer and the grade and stage, treatment ranges from surgical excision to chemotherapy, radiation therapy, or immunotherapy. Consideration of overall health, quality of life, and goals of care are important, and treatment choices must be made in the context of associated comorbidities. For a discussion of the general approach to the older patient with cancer, please see Chap. 26 Oncology. This section will review selected relevant issues associated with cancer diagnosis and treatment in the older adult population.

18.8.1 Kidney Cancer

Kidney cancers are frequently diagnosed in geriatric patients who have undergone abdominal imaging for other symptoms or conditions. The overall incidence of kidney cancer has been increasing over the past 30 years at a rate of 2–3 % annually [128]. In fact, the largest increases are in patients in their seventh and eighth decades. Age over 75 is a risk factor for more advanced disease, although in older adults with very small tumors, active surveillance is a feasible option, which may obviate the need for invasive surgical therapy [129]. Assessment of underlying comorbidity (see Chap. 3) may be particularly useful to guide therapeutic options for small kidney cancers in older patients [130].

In those who do require surgery, comorbidity is more important than chronological age in overall outcomes from either radical or partial nephrectomy [131, 132]. Outcomes and complications from laparoscopic and robotic partial nephrectomy appear similar to those observed in younger patients [133, 134]. Despite this observation, overall rates of partial nephrectomy in geriatric patients still lag the use in younger people [135]. The exact reasons for this are unclear, but may reflect clinician bias against using these techniques in older or frail (see Chap. 1) individuals. Cytoreductive surgery may be considered in some patients with more advanced disease, although complication rates including need for blood transfusion are higher among older adults [132, 136]. Immunotherapy may be considered, but can be difficult for some older adults to tolerate, particularly if they have associated functional impairments or worse overall performance status. In patients with upper tract urothelial cancers, radical nephroureterectomy may be considered, although the cancer-specific survival in this population >80 years of age is lower than in younger patients [137].

18.8.2 Bladder Cancer

Bladder cancer is one of the most common urologic malignancies, and occurs predominantly in older adults. Prevalence and incidence both increase substantially with advancing age. The primary risk factor is cigarette smoking, although exposure to certain chemicals such as aniline dyes also increases risk. Overall, the median age at diagnosis is >70 years due to the long latency of carcinogen exposure [138]. The most common associated symptom is hematuria. Diagnosis is typically made through a combination of imaging and direct visualization with cystoscopy. Tumor resection is required for tissue diagnosis and to determine the grade and stage of the cancer. It is important to clearly identify whether the tumor is superficial or invades the muscle of the wall of the bladder because this influences selection of therapy. Tumor restaging with repeat resection, especially in cases of incomplete initial resection or where there is a lack of muscularis propria in the sample, can be extremely useful. Adjuvant therapy with intravesical administration of mitomycin C or bacillus-Calmette-Guerin (BCG) may be considered in patients with superficial bladder cancer. However, it has been shown that BCG therapy has a somewhat decreased efficacy in older compared to younger adults [139]. This may be due to diminished immune response with aging.

The standard therapy for muscle-invasive bladder cancer has been surgical treatment with radical cystectomy and urinary diversion. This is one of the most invasive and complex surgical procedures performed in urology. Risk of morbidity and mortality is compounded by the fact that many of these patients have substantial underlying comorbidity and chronic health problems. For example, bladder cancer is frequently linked to a history of cigarette smoking and patients may have lung disorders such as chronic obstructive pulmonary disease (COPD) or restrictive airway disease that puts them at increased anesthetic risk. Despite this fact, multiple studies have demonstrated that with appropriate preoperative planning, intraoperative and postoperative care, radical cystectomy and urinary diversion is safe even in elderly patients [140, 141] Survival benefits have been demonstrated, but must be considered within the overall context of comorbidity and other health issues [142, 143]. There is an increase in perioperative complications in older patients undergoing this procedure, likely due to associated comorbid conditions [144, 145]. Reduced performance status, frailty, and sarcopenia predict complications in patients undergoing radical cystectomy [146, 147]. See Chap. 1 Frailty for information on this important geriatric syndrome.

Bladder sparing surgery in some elderly patients with muscle-invasive cancer using endoscopic resection followed by adjuvant radiation and/or chemotherapy shows similar overall survival to radical surgery in some studies with increased overall time in the hospital [148, 149]. Other studies show worse overall performance status and comorbidity and those who are very elderly tend to have worse outcomes in terms of both overall and cancer-specific survival [150, 151]. The most common indication for radiation therapy in patients with bladder cancer is for treatment of intractable bleeding in those who are not candidates for other surgical intervention [152].

18.8.3 Prostate Cancer

Prostate cancer is one of the most common solid tumor malignancies seen in adult men. This section will selectively focus on issues specific to geriatrics and elderly men.

Routine prostate cancer screening is controversial, but most agree that when it is used, screening should generally be discontinued once men have reached 70–75 years of age. This is because use of definitive therapy for prostate cancer with either radical prostatectomy or radiation therapy is generally reserved for men with an estimated remaining life expectancy of at least 10 or more years [153]. Mean life expectancy for men in the USA is approximately 82–84 years. In contrast to screening, targeted diagnostic assessment in selected patients at risk for development of prostate cancer may be useful to guide therapy in light of their overall health status. This may be true even if it is not done with curative intent [154].

Treatment decisions for elderly men with prostate cancer must be made with consideration of overall health and other comorbid conditions. Evaluation of functional status using activities of daily living (ADLs) and instrumental activities of daily living (ADLs) may be useful in this regard [155, 156]. In addition to functional status, information on disease burden and estimated remaining life expectancy can be useful in making clinical decisions in this population. In many cases, prostate cancer is a relatively slow growing and indolent tumor, and many elderly men may die of other conditions such as cardiovascular or pulmonary disease [157, 158]. However, some cases of prostate cancer may be more aggressive and develop into metastatic disease [159, 160].

Treatment of organ-confined prostate cancer includes radical prostatectomy or radiation with either external beam treatment or brachytherapy. While some studies show clinical outcomes equivalent to those in younger men, [161, 162] other studies suggest that elderly men are at higher risk for upgrading or upstaging of disease, biochemical recurrence of disease, urinary incontinence, or sexual dysfunction [163–165].

Some clinicians recommend radiation therapy in geriatric patients to avoid the risks associated with radical surgery. However, radiation therapy can be associated with complications including sexual dysfunction, radiation injury to other pelvic organs, or urinary incontinence [166]. Urinary incontinence following radical prostatectomy can have negative effects on quality of life including physical and social activities and mood in elderly men [167, 168]. Although cryotherapy has been suggested as a less invasive option for some men with organ-confined prostate cancer, long-term outcomes of this therapy are unclear [169].

Treatment of metastatic prostate cancer often involves use of hormonal therapy or chemotherapy in order to reduce disease and symptom progression, although they are not used with curative intent. The chemotherapeutic agent docetaxel has increased overall survival in early clinical trials [170]. Androgen deprivation therapy is more commonly used, and is beneficial in many patients although there are risks including cardiovascular disease and diabetes [171]. Because it blocks testosterone production, hormonal therapy is associated with gynecomastia, hot flashes, loss of libido, reduced sexual function, and sarcopenia which is part of the frailty phenotype [172]. Because this therapy is also associated with bone loss [173], men treated with hormonal therapy should be evaluated with imaging for bone disease before and during treatment. Bisphosphonates including alendronate and zoledronic acid slow bone resorption during anti-androgen therapy [174, 175]. The high cost of hormonal treatment may be a barrier for some patients and must be considered when making treatment decisions [176].

18.8.4 Testis Cancer

Primary germ cell tumors are relatively rare in elderly men, and occur most commonly between 15 and 35 years of age. Lymphoma is the most common testicular malignancy seen in the geriatric population [177]. In most cases, this represents a manifestation of systemic disease, and should be evaluated and treated in this context. If geriatric patients do present with a primary germ cell tumor, evaluation and treatment should follow accepted guidelines generally used in younger men. It may be necessary to adjust chemotherapy regimens based on age-related changes in renal hepatic or pulmonary function, or due to other underlying comorbidity. Overall life expectancy following successful treatment approaches that of other elderly men without a history of testis cancer [178].

18.9 Influence of Urologic Conditions on Geriatric Syndromes

The 'geriatric syndromes' are conditions that occur more commonly among older adults, are complex and typically multifactorial, and often have a substantial negative impact on outcomes for affected patients. Prevention is a key consideration, and urologic conditions may be associated with a number of these conditions. There is often overlap between conditions such as the association between urinary incontinence, falls, and frailty. These conditions may have both direct and direct effects on urologic health in older adults [179]. The Health and Retirement Study involved 11,000 older adults living either in the community or in nursing homes, and found that 49.9 % had at least one geriatric syndrome, and many had more than one [180]. The presence of one or more geriatric syndromes led to an increased need for assistance with activities of daily living (ADLs), even after controlling for other demographic factors and chronic diseases. Presence of one geriatric syndrome led to an adjusted risk ratio of 2.1 (95 % CI, 1.9–2.4). For two syndromes this increased to 3.6 (95 % CI, 3.1–4.1), and for three or more syndromes 5.6 (95 % CI, 5.6–7.6).

18.9.1 Falls

Falls are one of the most common conditions seen in elderly people, and are often associated with substantial injury including hip or long bone fractures and diminished mobility. Both indwelling urinary catheters and urinary incontinence are risk factors for injurious falls [181–183]. Overactive bladder and other lower urinary tract symptoms may also contribute to this risk [184, 185]. Nocturia is particularly problematic and has been linked to an increased risk of falls in the older population [186]. This can be due to a number of factors including postural hypotension, gait and balance problems, poor lighting, visual and other sensory impairments, and environmental trip hazards between the bed and toilet. Nocturia is also often associated with urinary urgency and older adults may fall when trying to rush to the toilet. Delirium and dementia have also been associated with an increased risk of falls in those with incontinence [187]. Targeted interventions in long-term care settings decrease the rate of falls and injuries among older adults with urinary incontinence [188]. Urinary catheters are physical restraints and should be avoided if at all possible.

Androgen deprivation therapy for metastatic prostate cancer in elderly men is associated with diminished bone mineral density and increased risk of fractures and other injuries due to falls in this population [189]. Careful attention to bone health is important in this population. Other studies have shown that older men with BPH and other conditions causing lower urinary tract symptoms have higher rates of falls and fractures compared to men without these urinary symptoms [190].

18.9.2 Pressure Ulcers

A pressure ulcer is an area of localized skin and tissue necrosis which most typically occurs over bony prominences. This is caused by prolonged pressure of the tissues against a hard surface, or from shearing forces with movement and transfers. Older adults are at increased risk for pressure ulcers due to a number of anatomic and physiological changes in the skin including decreased elastic tissue and changes in collagen and other connective tissue structures. Alterations in immune function and skin integrity also increase the risk of superficial skin infections. Urinary incontinence is a common factor that can lead to increased risk of pressure ulcer formation in elderly people. Tissue maceration due to chronic moisture from urinary leakage can exacerbate these issues, particularly for development of perineal and sacral ulcers. Careful positioning and transfer of older adults is especially important. This includes transfers of patients on and off operating tables during surgery. Adequate padding is essential to help reduce the risk of developing pressure ulcers during surgical care. Early physical mobilization and activity after surgery are also important. Prolonged bed rest increases the risk for pressure ulcers and many other serious conditions including deep vein thrombosis, pneumonia, pulmonary embolus, and deconditioning [191]. Frequent turning and repositioning of patients or use of specialized equipment such as air mattresses or other pressure reduction methods can be very useful to prevent injury. Overall prevalence of pressure ulcers among hospitalized older adults has been reported to be as high as 8.9 % [192]. Urinary, fecal, and dual incontinence are among the strongest risk factors for development of pressure ulcers in the geriatric population. Careful physical examination should be part of the routine care for elderly patients with urinary and/or bowel incontinence. Among hospitalized geriatric patients, increased waiting time in the emergency room, intensive care unit stays, and immobilizing procedures or medications increase the risk of pressure ulcers [193].

18.9.3 Elder Mistreatment

Screening for elder mistreatment is a responsibility of all health care professionals, and is subject to mandatory reporting in the USA and many other countries. Professionals who report suspected abuse are protected from liability or retaliation. Urologic care providers are in a unique position because they often see older adults on an ongoing basis for care of chronic health care conditions. They may be particularly able to identify cases of neglect or sexual abuse because of the nature of the conditions they treat such as urinary incontinence and pelvic floor disorders. Warning signs for abuse and neglect include poor hygiene, nervous interactions with accompanying caregivers, social withdrawal, or physical signs such as lacerations, abrasions, or bruises. Physical findings out of proportion to a reported mechanism of injury are also indications of potential abuse.

Urinary incontinence and associated depression and social isolation are risk factors for psychosocial abuse toward older adults by their caregivers [194]. Neglect by caregivers and self-neglect have also been associated with urinary incontinence among older adults [195]. Greater physical disability is also associated with self-neglect among elderly people [196]. Future research will help to identify if successful treatment of urinary incontinence may reduce rates of abuse and neglect for affected older adults.

Identification of sexual abuse or mistreatment among older adults is within the realm of urologic care. The National Center on Elder Abuse defines this as 'nonconsensual sexual contact of any kind.' [197]. Evaluation should include detailed history and examination, including pelvic examination. Screening for sexually transmitted diseases should also be considered in appropriate situations of increased risk derived from the sexual history.

18.10 End of Life Care and Urology

Urologic care of geriatric patients may include aspects of palliative and end of life care. This includes direct care for urologic conditions associated with terminal illness such as metastatic cancers of the genitourinary system or severe urosepsis. It may also include provision of urologic care for conditions seen more commonly near end of life including urinary incontinence or urinary tract infection [198]. Symptom management and high quality treatment within the overall goals of care for the patient and their loved ones is the main focus of palliative care. This includes pain and symptom relief and coordination of care [199]. Surgical therapy may be indicated in select cases where cytoreductive treatment for a large tumor burden or treatment for intractable bleeding or pain may be of benefit. Integrated care delivery with providers from multiple specialties and disciplines is particularly useful in palliative care settings [200]. Also see Chap. 6 Palliative Care.

18.11 Conclusions

Care of older adults forms a large portion of most general urologic practice. The incidence and prevalence of the majority of conditions treated by urologists increase with advancing age. Urinary incontinence is considered both a common diagnosis in older adults, and a common geriatric syndrome. It also contributes to other geriatric syndromes such as falls and pressure ulcers. Most of the genitourinary malignancies also occur predominantly in an older adult population. Increased understanding of general principles of geriatrics, and how these influence urologic care in this population will help urologists to provide enhanced care to older adult patients and may lead to better overall clinical outcomes.

References

1. Takao T, Tsujimura A, Kiuchi H, et al. Urological surgery in patients aged 80 years and older: a 30-year retrospective clinical study. Int J Urol. 2008;15:789–93.
2. DuBeau CE. The aging lower urinary tract. J Urol. 2006;175:S11–5.
3. Elbadawi A, Yalla SV, Resnick NM. Structural basis of geriatric voiding dysfunction. II. Aging detrusor: normal versus impaired contractility. J Urol. 1993;150:1657–67.
4. Lowalekar SK, Cristofaro V, Radisavljevic ZM, et al. Loss of bladder smooth muscle caveolae in the aging bladder. Neurourol Urodyn. 2012;31:586–92.
5. Fry CH, Bayliss M, Young JS, Hussain M. Influence of age and bladder dysfunction on the contractile properties of isolated human detrusor smooth muscle. BJU Int. 2011;108:E91–6.
6. Pfisterer MH, Griffiths DJ, Rosenberg L, et al. The impact of detrusor overactivity on bladder function in younger and older women. J Urol. 2006;175(5):1777–83. discussion 1783.
7. Aybek H, Aybek Z, Abban G, Rota S. Preventive effects of vitamin E against oxidative damage in aged diabetic rat bladders. Urology. 2011;77:508 e510-504.
8. Betschart C, Scheiner D, Maake C, et al. Histomorphological analysis of the urogenital diaphragm in elderly women: a cadaver study. Int Urogynecol J Pelvic Floor Dysfunct. 2008;19:1477–81.
9. Weemhoff M, Shek KL, Dietz HP. Effects of age on levator function and morphometry of the levator hiatus in women with pelvic floor disorders. Int Urogynecol J. 2010;21:1137–42.
10. Richter HE, Morgan SL, Gleason JL, et al. Pelvic floor symptoms and bone mineral density in women undergoing osteoporosis evaluation. Int Urogynecol J. 2013;24:1663–9.
11. Saatli B, Kizildag S, Cagliyan E, et al. Alteration of apoptosis-related genes in postmenopausal women with uterine prolapse. Int Urogynecol J. 2014;25:971–7.
12. Strasser H, Tiefenthaler M, Steinlechner M, et al. Age dependent apoptosis and loss of rhabdosphincter cells. J Urol. 2000;164:1781–5.
13. Kurihara M, Murakami G, Kajiwara M, et al. Lack of complete circular rhabdosphincter and a distinct circular smooth muscle layer around the proximal urethra in elderly Japanese women: an anatomical study. Int Urogyencol J Pelvic Floor Dysfunct. 2004;15:85–94.
14. Talasz H, Jansen SC, Kofler M, Lechleitner M. High prevalence of pelvic floor muscle dysfunction in hospitalized elderly women with urinary incontinence. Int Urogynecol J. 2012;23:1231–7.
15. Abrams P, Cardozo L, Fall M, et al. The standardisation of terminology of lower urinary tract function: report from the Standardisation Subcommittee of the International Continence Society. Neurourol Urodyn. 2002;21:167–78.
16. Herzog AR, Fultz NH. Prevalence and incidence of urinary incontinence in community-dwelling populations. J Am Geriatr Soc. 1990;38:273–81.
17. Goldstein I, Dicks B, Kim NN, et al. Multidisciplinary overview of vaginal atrophy and associated genitourinary symptoms in postmenopausal women. Sex Med. 2013;1:44–53.
18. Talasz H, Lechleitner M. Polypharmacy and incontinence. Z Gerontol Geriatr. 2012;45(6):464–7.
19. Gorina Y, Schappert S, Bercovitz A, et al. Prevalence of incontinence among older Americans. US Department of Health and Human Services, Centers for Disease Control and Prevention, National Center for Health Statistics. Vital Health Stat. 2014;3(36):1–24.
20. Smith PP. Aging and the underactive detrusor: a failure of activity or activation? Neurourol Urodyn. 2010;29:408–12.
21. Markinovic SP, Badlani G. Voiding and sexual dysfunction after cerebrovascular accidents. J Urol. 2001;165:359–70.
22. Wehrberger C, Jungwirth S, Fischer P, et al. The relationship between cerebral white matter hyperintensities and lower urinary tract function in a population based, geriatric cohort. Neurourol Urodyn. 2013;33:431–6.
23. Kovindha A, Wattanapan P, Dejpratham P, et al. Prevalence of incontinence in patients after stroke during rehabilitation: a multicentre study. J Rehabil Med. 2009;41:491.
24. Taylor 3rd JA, Kuchel GA. Detrusor underactivity: clinical features and pathogenesis of an underdiagnosed geriatric condition. J Am Geriatr Soc. 2006;54(12):1920–32.
25. Chancellor MB. The overactive bladder progression to underactive bladder hypothesis. Int Urol Nephrol. 2014;46 Suppl 1:S23–7.
26. Griebling TL, DuBeau CE, Kuchel G, et al. Defining and advancing education and conservative therapies of underactive bladder. Int Urol Nephrol. 2014;46 Suppl 1:S29–34.
27. Khatusky G, Walsh EG, Brown DW. Urinary incontinence, functional status, and health-related quality of life among Medicare beneficiaries enrolled in the program for all-inclusive care for the elderly and dual eligible demonstration special needs plans. J Ambul Care Manage. 2013;36:35–49.

28. Fritel X, Lachal L, Cassou B, et al. Mobility impairment is associated with urge but not stress urinary incontinence in community-dwelling older women: results from the Osségo Study. BJOG. 2013;120:1566–74.

29. Weiss JP, Blaivas JG. Nocturia. J Urol. 2000;163:5–12.

30. Udo Y, Nakao M, Honjo H, et al. Sleep duration is an independent factor in nocturia: analysis of bladder diaries. BJU Int. 2009;104:75–9.

31. Shimoni Z, Fruger E, Froom P. Measurement of post-void residual bladder volumes in hospitalized older adults. Am J Med. 2015;128(1):77–81.

32. Winters JC, Dmochowski RR, Goldman HB, et al. Urodynamic studies in adults: AUA/SUFU guideline. J Urol. 2012;188:2464–72.

33. Dugan E, Cohen SJ, Bland DR, et al. The association of depressive symptoms and urinary incontinence among older adults. J Am Geriatr Soc. 2000;48(4):413–6.

34. Laganà L, Bloom DW, Ainsworth A. Urinary incontinence: its assessment and relationship to depression among community-dwelling multiethnic older women. Sci World J. 2014;2014:708564.

35. Kwong PW, Cumming RG, Chan L, et al. Urinary incontinence and quality of life among older community-dwelling Australian men: the CHAMP Study. Age Ageing. 2010;39:349–54.

36. Xu D, Kane RL. Effect of urinary incontinence on older nursing home residents' self-reported quality of life. J Am Geriatr Soc. 2013;61:1473–81.

37. Yoon JY, Lee JY, Bowers BJ, Zimmerman DR. The impact of organizational factors on the urinary incontinence care quality in long-term care hospitals: a longitudinal correlational study. Int J Nurs Stud. 2012;49:1544–51.

38. Grabowski DC, O'Malley AJ, Afendulis CC, et al. Culture change and nursing home quality of care. Gerontologist. 2014;54: S35–45.

39. Iwatsubo E, Suzuki M, Igawa Y, et al. Individually tailored ultrasound-assisted prompted voiding for institutionalized older adults with urinary incontinence. Int J Urol. 2014;21:1253–7.

40. Schnelle JF, MacRae PG, Ouslander JG, et al. Functional Incidental Training, mobility performance and incontinence care with nursing home residents. J Am Geriatr Soc. 1995;43: 1356–62.

41. Gleason JL, Richter HE, Redden DT, et al. Caffeine and urinary incontinence in US women. Int Urogynecol J. 2013;24:295–302.

42. Burgio KL, Goode P, Johnson II TM, et al. Behavioral versus drug treatment for overactive bladder in men: the Male Overactive Bladder Treatment in Veterans (MOTIVE) Trial. J Am Geriatr Soc. 2011;59:2209–16.

43. Sherburn M, Bird M, Carey M, et al. Incontinence improves in older women after intensive pelvic floor muscle training: an assessor-blinded randomized controlled trial. Neurourol Urodyn. 2011;30:317–24.

44. Goode PS, Burgio KL, Johnson 2nd TM, et al. Behavioral therapy with or without biofeedback and pelvic floor electrical stimulation for persistent postprostatectomy incontinence: a randomized controlled trial. JAMA. 2011;305:151–9.

45. Moga DC, Carnahan RM, Lund BC, et al. Risks and benefits of bladder antimuscarinics among elderly residents of veterans affairs community living centers. J Am Med Dir Assoc. 2013;14: 749–60.

46. DuBeau CE, Kraus SR, Griebling TL, et al. Effect of fesoterodine in vulnerable elderly subjects with urgency incontinence: a double-blind, placebo-controlled trial. J Urol. 2014;191: 395–404.

47. Chapple C, DuBeau C, Ebinger U, et al. Darifenacin treatment of patients>or=65 years with overactive bladder: results of a randomized, controlled, 12-week trial. Curr Med Res Opin. 2007; 23(10):2347–58.

48. Sicras-Mainar A, Rejas J, Navarro-Artieda R, et al. Antimuscarinic persistence patters in newly treated patients with overactive bladder: a retrospective comparative analysis. Int Urogynecol J. 2014; 25:485–92.

49. Wagg A, Compion G, Fahey A, Siddiqui E. Persistence with prescribed antimuscarinic therapy for overactive bladder: a UK experience. BJU Int. 2012;110:1767–74.

50. Sears CL, Lewis C, Noel K, et al. Overactive bladder medication adherence when medication is free to patients. J Urol. 2010;183:1077–81.

51. Armstrong EP, Malone DC, Bui CN. Cost-effectiveness analysis of antimuscarinic agents for the treatment of overactive bladder. J Med Econ. 2012;15 Suppl 1:35–44.

52. Chow WB, Rosenthal RA, Merkow RP, et al. Optimal preoperative assessment of the geriatric surgical patient: a best practices guideline from the American College of Surgeons National Surgical Quality Improvement Program and the American Geriatrics Society. J Am Coll Surg. 2012;215:453–66.

53. Griebling TL. Incontinence guidelines: is lack of adherence a form of ageism? Nat Rev Urol. 2011;8:655–7.

54. Atiemo H, Griebling TL, Danishgari F. Advances in geriatric female pelvic surgery. BJU Int. 2006;98 Suppl 1:90–4.

55. Keegan PE, Atiemo K, Cody J, et al. Periurethral injection therapy for urinary incontinence in women. Cochrane Database Syst Rev. 2007;3, CD003881.

56. Jun KK, Oh SM, Choo GY, et al. Long-term clinical outcomes of the tension-free vaginal tape procedure for the treatment of stress urinary incontinence in elderly women over 65. Korean J Urol. 2012;53:184–8.

57. Serati M, Braga A, Cattoni E, et al. Transobturator vaginal tape for the treatment of stress urinary incontinence in elderly women without concomitant pelvic organ prolapse: is it effective and safe? Eur J Obstet Gyencol Reprod Biol. 2013;166:107–10.

58. Groutz A, Cohen A, Gold R, et al. The safety and efficacy of the "inside-out" trans-obturator TVT in elderly versus younger stress-incontinent women: a prospective study of 353 consecutive patients. Neurourol Urodyn. 2011;30:380–3.

59. Kim J, Lucioni A, Govier F, Kobashi K. Worse long-term surgical outcomes in elderly patients undergoing SPARC retropubic midurethral sling placement. BJU Int. 2011;108:708–12.

60. O'Connor RC, Nanigian DK, Patel BN, et al. Artificial urinary sphincter placement in elderly men. Urology. 2007;69(1):126–8.

61. Angioli R, Montera R, Plotti F, et al. Success rates, quality of life, and feasibility of sacral nerve stimulation in elderly patients: 1-year follow-up. Int Urogynecol J. 2013;24:789–94.

62. Chughtai B, Sedrakya A, Isaacs A, et al. Long term safety of sacral nerve modulation in Medicare beneficiaries. Neurourol Urodyn. 2014 [Epub ahead of print].

63. Peters KM, Killinger KA, Gilleran J, et al. Does patient age impact outcomes of neuromodulation? Neurourol Urodyn. 2013;32:30–6.

64. White WM, Pickens RB, Doggweiler R, et al. Short-term efficacy of botulinum toxin A for refractory overactive bladder in the elderly population. J Urol. 2008;180:2522–6.

65. Osborn DJ, Dmochowski RR, Kaufman MR, et al. Cystectomy with urinary diversion for benign disease: indications and outcomes. Urology. 2014;83:1433–7.

66. Gowda BD, Agarwal V, Harrison SC. The continent, catheterizable abdominal conduit in adult urological practice. BJU Int. 2008;102:1688–92.

67. Parsons BA, Narshi A, Drake MJ. Success rates for learning intermittent self-catheterisation according to age and gender. Int Urol Nephrol. 2012;44(4):1127–31.

68. Averch TD, Stoffel J, Goldman HB, et al. AUA white paper on catheter associated urinary tract infections: definitions and significance in the urological patient. Urol Pract. 2015;2:321–8.

69. Fader M, Cottenden AM, Getliffe K. Absorbent products for light urinary incontinence in women. Cochrane Database Syst Rev. 2007;2, CD001406.

70. Fader M, Cottenden AM, Getliffe K. Absorbent products for moderate-heavy urinary and/or faecal incontinence in women and men. Cochrane Database Syst Rev. 2008;4, CD007408.

71. White CF. Engineered structures for use in disposable incontinence products. Proc Inst Mech Eng H. 2003;217:243–51.

72. Gordon LB, Waxman MJ, Ragsdale L, Mermel LA. Overtreatment of presumed urinary tract infection in older women presenting to the emergency department. J Am Geriatr Soc. 2013;61:788–92.

73. Arinzon Z, Shabat S, Peisakh A, et al. Clinical presentation of urinary tract infection (UTI) differs with aging in women. Arch Gerontol Geriatr. 2012;55:145–7.

74. Juthani-Mehta M, Quagliarello V, Perrelli E, et al. Clinical features to identify urinary tract infection in nursing home residents: a cohort study. J Am Geriatr Soc. 2009;57:963–70.

75. Eriksson I, Gustafson Y, Fagerstrom L, Olofsson B. Urinary tract infection in very old women is associated with delirium. Int Psychogeriatr. 2011;23:496–502.

76. Kang SC, Tsao HM, Liu CT, et al. The characteristics of acute pyelonephritis in geriatric patients: experiences in rural northeastern Taiwan. Tohoku J Exp Med. 2008;214:61–7.

77. Rebelo M, Pereira B, Lima J, et al. Predictors of in-hospital mortality in elderly patients with bacteraemia admitted to an internal medicine ward. Int Arch Med. 2011;4:33.

78. Chin BS, Kim MS, Han SH, et al. Risk factors of all-cause in-hospital mortality among Korean elderly bacteremic urinary tract infection (UTI) patients. Arch Gerontol Geriatr. 2011;52:e50–5.

79. Fraisse T, Crouzet J, Lachaud L, et al. Candiduria in those over 85 years old: a retrospective study of 73 patients. Intern Med. 2011;50:1935–40.

80. Varli M, Guruz H, Aras S, et al. Asymptomatic bacteriuria among the elderly living in the community: prevalence, risk factors and characteristics. Eur Geriatr Med. 2012;3:87–91.

81. Juthani-Mehta M, Tinetti M, Perrelli E, et al. Diagnostic accuracy of criteria for urinary tract infection in a cohort of nursing home residents. J Am Geriatr Soc. 2007;55:1072–7.

82. American Geriatrics Society (AGS) choosing Wisely Workgroup. American Geriatrics Society identifies five things that healthcare providers and patients should question. J Am Geriatr Soc. 2013;61:622–31.

83. Daniels KR, Lee GC, Frei CR. Trends in catheter-associated urinary tract infections among a national cohort of hospitalized adults, 2001-2010. Am J Infect Control. 2014;42:17–22.

84. Dorner TE, Schwarz F, Kranz A, et al. Body mass index and the risk of infections in institutionalised geriatric patients. Br J Nutr. 2010;103:1830–5.

85. Calijouw MA, van den Hout WB, Putter H, et al. Effectiveness of cranberry capsules to prevent urinary tract infections in vulnerable older persons: a double-blind randomized placebo-controlled trial in long-term care facilities. J Am Geriatr Soc. 2014;62:103–10.

86. D'Agata E, Loeb MB, Mitchell SL. Challenges in assessing nursing home residents with advanced dementia for suspected urinary tract infections. J Am Geriatr Soc. 2013;61:62–6.

87. Kistler CE, Sloane PD, Platts-Mills TF, et al. Challenges of antibiotic prescribing for assisted living residents: perspectives of providers, staff, residents, and family members. J Am Geriatr Soc. 2013;61:565–70.

88. Fagan M, Maehlen M, Lindbaek M, Berild D. Antibiotic prescribing in nursing homes in an area with low prevalence of antibiotic resistance: compliance with national guidelines. Scand J Prim Health Care. 2012;30:10–5.

89. Murphy CR, Eells SJ, Quan V, et al. Methicillin-resistant staphylococcus aureus burden in nursing homes associated with environmental contamination of common areas. J Am Geriatr Soc. 2012;60:1012–8.

90. Griebling TL. Urologic diseases in America project: trends in resource use for urinary tract infections in women. J Urol. 2005;173:1281–7.

91. Griebling TL. Urological diseases in America project: trends in resource use for urinary tract infections in men. J Urol. 2005;173:1288–94.

92. Davis R, Jones JS, Barocas DA, et al. Diagnosis, evaluation and follow-up of asymptomatic microhematuria (AMH) in adults: AUA guideline. J Urol. 2012;188:2473–81.

93. Lim AK, Campbell DA. Haematuria and acute kidney injury in elderly patients admitted to hospital with supratherapeutic warfarin anticoagulation. Int Urol Nephrol. 2013;45:561–70.

94. Hyde Z, Flicker L, Hankey GJ, et al. Prevalence of sexual activity and associated factors in men aged 75 to 95 years: a cohort study. Ann Intern Med. 2010;153:693–702.

95. Schick V, Herbenick D, Reece M, et al. Sexual behaviors, condom use, and sexual health of Americans over 50: implications for sexual health promotion for older adults. J Sex Med. 2010;7 Suppl 5:315–29.

96. Tannenbaum C, Corcos J, Assalian P. The relationship between sexual activity and urinary incontinence in older women. J Am Geriatr Soc. 2006;54:1220–4.

97. Griebling TL. The impact of urinary incontinence on sexual health in older adults. J Am Geriatr Soc. 2006;54:1290–2.

98. Lindau ST, Gavrilova N. Sex, health, and years of sexually active life gained due to good health: evidence from two U.S. population based cross sectional surveys of ageing. BMJ. 2010;340:c810.

99. Bach LE, Mortimer JA, Vandeweerd C, Corvin J. The association of physical and mental health with sexual activity in older adults in a retirement community. J Sex Med. 2013;10:2671–8.

100. Lee DM, Tajar A, Ravindrarajah R, et al. Frailty and sexual health in older European men. J Gerontol A Biol Sci Med Sci. 2013;68:837–44.

101. Korfage IJ, Pluijm S, Roobol M, et al. Erectile dysfunction and mental health in a general population of older men. J Sex Med. 2009;6:505–12.

102. Cheng JY, Ng EM, Ko JS. Depressive symptomatology and male sexual functions in late life. J Affect Disord. 2007;104:225–9.

103. Lindau ST, Schumm LP, Laumann EO, et al. A study of sexuality and health among older adults in the United States. N Engl J Med. 2007;357:762–74.

104. Mroczek B, Kurpas D, Gronowska M, et al. Psychosexual needs and sexual behaviors of nursing care home residents. Arch Gerontol Geriatr. 2013;57:32–8.

105. Bardell A, Lau T, Fedoroff JP. Inappropriate sexual behavior in a geriatric population. Int Psychogeriatr. 2011;23:1182–8.

106. Wilson MM. Sexually transmitted diseases. Clin Geriatr Med. 2003;19:637–55.

107. Pearle MS, Calhoun EA, Curhan GC, et al. Urologic diseases in America project: urolithiasis. J Urol. 2005;173:848–57.

108. Daudon M, Doré JC, Jungers P, et al. Changes in stone composition according to age and gender of patients: a multivariate epidemiological approach. Urol Res. 2004;32:241–7.

109. Wong YV, Cook P, Somani BK. The association of metabolic syndrome and urolithiasis. Int J Endocrinol. 2015;[e-pub ahead of print]. doi:10.1155/2015/570674.

110. Usui Y, Matsuzaki S, Matsushita K, et al. Urolithiasis in geriatric patients. Tokai J Exp Clin Med. 2003;28:81–7.

111. Akman T, Binbay M, Ugurlu M, et al. Outcomes of retrograde intrarenal surgery compared with percutaneous nephrolithotomy in elderly patients with moderate-size kidney stones: a matched-pair analysis. J Endourol. 2012;26:625–9.

112. Anagnostou T, Thompson T, Ng CF, et al. Safety and outcome of percutaneous nephrolithotomy in the elderly: retrospective comparison to a younger patient group. J Endourol. 2008;22:2139–45.

113. Fitzpatrick JM. The natural history of benign prostatic hyperplasia. BJU Int. 2006;97 Suppl 2:3–6.

114. Perchon LFG, Pintarelli VL, Bezerra E, Thiel M, Dambros M. Quality of life in elderly men with aging symptoms and lower urinary tract symptoms (LUTS). Neurourol Urodyn. 2011;30:515–9.

115. Resnick MI, Roehrborn CG. Rapid onset of action with alfuzosin 10 mg once daily in men with benign prostatic hyperplasia: a randomized, placebo-controlled trial. Prostate Cancer Prostatic Dis. 2007;10:155–9.

116. Friedman AH. Tamsulosin and the intraoperative floppy iris syndrome. JAMA. 2009;301:2044–5.

117. Roehrborn CG, Bruskewitz R, Nickel JC, et al. Sustained decrease in incidence of acute urinary retention and surgery with finasteride for 6 years in men with benign prostatic hyperplasia. J Urol. 2004;171:1194–8.

118. Roehrborn CG, Siami P, Barkin J, et al. The effects of dutasteride, tamsulosin and combination therapy in lower urinary tract symptoms in men with benign prostatic hyperplasia and prostatic enlargement: 2-year results from the CombAT Study. J Urol. 2008;179:616–21.

119. Wang X, Wang X, Li S, et al. Comparative effectiveness of oral drug therapies for lower urinary tract symptoms due to benign prostatic hyperplasia: a systematic review and network meta-analysis. PLoS One. 2014;9(9), e107593.

120. Hoffman RM, Monga M, Elliot SP, MacDonald R, Wilt TJ. Microwave thermotherapy for benign prostatic hyperplasia. Cochrane Database Syst Rev. 2007;17, CD004135.

121. Aagaard MF, Niebuhr MH, Jacobsen JD, Krøyer Nielsen K. Transurethral microwave thermotherapy treatment of chronic urinary retention in patients unsuitable for surgery. Scand J Urol. 2014;48(3):290–4.

122. Bozkurt IH, Yalcinkaya F, Sertcelik MN, et al. A good alternative to indwelling catheter owing to benign prostate hyperplasia in elderly: Memotherm prostatic stent. Urology. 2013;82:1004–7.

123. Ogiste JS, Cooper K, Kaplan SA. Are stents still a useful therapy for benign prostatic hyperplasia? Curr Opin Urol. 2003;13:51–7.

124. Krieger JN, Riley DE, Cheah PY, Liong ML, Yuen KH. Epidemiology of prostatitis: new evidence for a world-wide problem. World J Urol. 2003;21:70–4.

125. Nickel JC, Teichman JMH, Gregore M, Clark J, Downey J. Prevalence, diagnosis, characterization, and treatment of prostatitis, interstitial cystitis, and epididymitis in outpatient urologic practice: the Canadian PIE Study. Urology. 2005;66:935–40.

126. Suskind AM, Berry SH, Ewing BA, et al. The prevalence and overlap of interstitial cystitis/bladder pain syndrome and chronic prostatitis/chronic pelvic pain syndrome in men: results of the RAND Interstitial Cystitis Epidemiology male study. J Urol. 2013;189(1):141–5.

127. Wagenlehner FM, Weidner W, Pilatz A, Naber KG. Urinary tract infections and bacterial prostatitis in men. Curr Opin Infect Dis. 2014;27(1):97–101.

128. Chow WH, Devesa SS, Warren JL, et al. Rising incidence of renal cell cancer in the United States. JAMA. 1999;281:1628–31.

129. O'Malley RL, Godoy G, Phillips CK, Taneja SS. Is surveillance of small renal masses safe in the elderly? BJU Int. 2010;105:1098–101.

130. O'Connor KM, Davis N, Lennon GM, et al. Can we avoid surgery in elderly patients with renal masses by using the Charlson comorbidity index? BJU Int. 2009;103:1492–5.

131. Roos FC, Pahernik S, Melchior SW, Thuroff JW. Renal tumour surgery in elderly patients. BJU Int. 2008;102:680–3.

132. Sun M, Abdollah F, Schmitges J, et al. Cytoreductive nephrectomy in the elderly: a population-based cohort from the USA. BJU Int. 2012;109:1807–12.

133. Hillyer SP, Autorino R, Spana G, et al. Perioperative outcomes of robotic-assisted partial nephrectomy in elderly patients: a matched-cohort study. Urology. 2012;79:1063–7.

134. Guzzo TJ, Allaf ME, Pierorazio PM, et al. Perioperative outcomes of elderly patients undergoing laparoscopic renal procedures. Urology. 2009;73:572–6.

135. Kates M, Badalato G, Pitman M, McKiernan J. Persistent overuse of radical nephrectomy in the elderly. Urology. 2011;78:555–9.

136. Kader AK, Tamboli P, Luongo T, et al. Cytoreductive nephrectomy in the elderly patient: the M.D. Anderson Cancer Center experience. J Urol. 2007;177:855–60. discussion 860-861.

137. Shariat SF, Godoy G, Lotan Y, et al. Advanced patient age is associated with inferior cancer-specific survival after radical nephroureterectomy. BJU Int. 2010;105:1672–7.

138. Shariat SF, Sfakianos JP, Droller MJ, et al. The effect of age and gender on bladder cancer: a critical review of the literature. BJU Int. 2010;105:300–8.

139. Margel D, Alkhateeb SS, Finelli A, Fleshner N. Diminished efficacy of Bacille Calmette-Guerin among elderly patients with non-muscle invasive bladder cancer. Urology. 2011;78:848–54.

140. Guillotreau J, Miocinovic R, Game X, et al. Outcomes of laparoscopic and robotic radical cystectomy in the elderly patients. Urology. 2012;79:585–90.

141. May M, Fuhrer S, Braun KP, et al. Results from three municipal hospitals regarding radical cystectomy on elderly patients. Int Braz J Urol. 2007;33:764–73. discussion 774-766.

142. Tyritzis SI, Anastasiou I, Stravodimos KG, et al. Radical cystectomy over the age of 75 is safe and increases survival. BMC Geriatr. 2012;12:18.

143. Donat SM, Siegrist T, Cronin A, et al. Radical cystectomy in octogenarians: does morbidity outweigh the potential survival benefits? J Urol. 2010;183:2171–7.

144. Lund L, Jacobsen J, Clark P, et al. Impact of comorbidity on survival of invasive bladder cancer patients, 1996-2007: a Danish population-based cohort study. Urology. 2010;75:393–8.

145. Liberman D, Lughezzani G, Sun M, et al. Perioperative mortality is significantly greater in septuagenarian and octogenarian patients treated with radical cystectomy for urothelial carcinoma of the bladder. Urology. 2011;77:660–6.

146. Smith AB, Deal AM, Yu H, et al. Sarcopenia as a predictor of complications and survival following radical cystectomy. J Urol. 2014;191:1714–20.

147. Weizer AZ, Joshi D, Daignault S, et al. Performance status is a predictor of overall survival of elderly patients with muscle invasive bladder cancer. J Urol. 2007;177:1287–93.

148. Martini T, Mayr R, Wehrberger C, et al. Comparison of radical cystectomy with conservative treatment in geriatric (>/=80) patients with muscle-invasive bladder cancer. Int Braz J Urol. 2013;39:622–30.

149. Wehberger C, Berger I, Marszalek M, et al. Bladder preservation in octogenarians with invasive bladder cancer. Urology. 2010;75:370–5.

150. Tran E, Souhami L, Tanguay S, Rajan R. Bladder conservation treatment in the elderly population: results and prognostic factors of muscle-invasive bladder cancer. Am J Clin Oncol. 2009;32:333–7.

151. Kohjimoto Y, Iba A, Shintani Y, et al. Impact of patient age on outcome following bladder-preserving treatment for non-muscle-invasive bladder cancer. World J Urol. 2010;28:425–30.

152. Kouloulias V, Tolia M, Kolliarakis N, et al. Evaluation of acute toxicity and symptoms palliation in a hypofractionated weekly schedule of external radiotherapy for elderly patients with muscular invasive bladder cancer. Int Braz J Urol. 2013;39:77–82.

153. Hoffman KE, Hguyen PL, Ng KA, D'Amico AV. Prostate cancer screening in men 75 years old or older: an assessment of self-reported health status and life expectancy. J Urol. 2010;183:1798–802.

154. Paterson AL, Sut MK, Khan AR, Sharma HK. Prostatic biopsies in selected men aged 75 years and older guide key clinical management decisions. Int Urol Nephrol. 2013;45:1539–44.

155. Thompson I, Thrasher JB, Aus G, et al. Guideline for the management of clinically localized prostate cancer: 2007 update. J Urol. 2007;177:2106–31.

156. Droz JP, Balducci L, Bolla M, et al. Management of prostate cancer in older men: recommendations of a working group of the International Society of Geriatric Oncology. BJU Int. 2010;106:462–9.

157. Ketchandji M, Kuo YF, Shahinian VB, Goodwin JS. Cause of death in older men after the diagnosis of prostate cancer. J Am Geriatr Soc. 2009;57:24–30.

158. Jeong CW, Ku JH, Kwak C, et al. Chronic pulmonary disease negatively influences the prognosis of patients with advanced prostate cancer. World J Urol. 2009;27:643–52.

159. Kunz I, Musch M, Roggenbuck U, et al. Tumour characteristics, oncological and functional outcomes in patients aged >/= 70 years undergoing radical prostatectomy. BJU Int. 2013;111:E24–9.

160. Scosyrev E, Messing EM, Mohile S, et al. Prostate cancer in the elderly: frequency of advanced disease at presentation and disease-specific mortality. Cancer. 2012;118:3062–70.

161. Namiki S, Ishidoya S, Kawamura S, et al. Quality of life among elderly men treated for prostate cancer with either radical prostatectomy or external beam radiation therapy. J Cancer Res Clin Oncol. 2010;136:379–86.

162. Pierorazio PM, Humphreys E, Walsh PC, et al. Radical prostatectomy in older men: survival outcomes in septuagenarians and octogenarians. BJU Int. 2010;106:791–5.

163. Trinh QD, Schmitges J, Sun M, et al. Open radical prostatectomy in the elderly: a case for concern? BJU Int. 2012;109:1335–40.

164. Ko J, Falzarano SM, Walker E, et al. Prostate cancer patients older than 70 years treated by radical prostatectomy have higher biochemical recurrence rate than their matched younger counterpart. Prostate. 2013;73:897–903.

165. Richstone L, Bianco FJ, Shah HH, et al. Radical prostatectomy in men aged > or = 70 years: effect of age on upgrading, upstaging, and the accuracy of a preoperative nomogram. BJU Int. 2008;101:541–6.

166. Mirza M, Griebling TL, Kazer MW. Erectile dysfunction and urinary incontinence after prostate cancer treatment. Semin Oncol Nurs. 2011;27:278–89.

167. Kopp RP, Marshall LM, Wang PY, et al. The burden of urinary incontinence and urinary bother among elderly prostate cancer survivors. Eur Urol. 2013;64:672–9.

168. Park SW, Kim TN, Nam JK, et al. Recovery of overall exercise ability, quality of life, and continence after 12-week combined exercise intervention in elderly patients who underwent radical prostatectomy: a randomized controlled study. Urology. 2012;80:299–305.

169. Dhar N, Ward JF, Cher ML, Jones JS. Primary full-gland prostate cryoablation in older men (> age of 75 years): results from 860 patients tracked with the COLD registry. BJU Int. 2011;108:508–12.

170. Miyake H, Sakai I, Harada K, et al. Significance of docetaxel-based chemotherapy as treatment for metastatic castration-resistant prostate cancer in Japanese men over 75 years old. Int Urol Nephrol. 2012;44:1697–703.

171. Keating NL, O'Malley AJ, Freedland SJ, Smith MR. Does comorbidity influence the risk of myocardial infarction or diabetes during androgen-deprivation therapy for prostate cancer? Eur Urol. 2013;64:159–66.

172. Reis C, Liberman S, Pompeo AC, et al. Body composition alterations, energy expenditure and fat oxidation in elderly males suffering from prostate cancer, pre and post orchiectomy. Clinics. 2009;64:781–4.

173. Shao YH, Moore DF, Shih W, et al. Fracture after androgen deprivation therapy among men with a high baseline risk of skeletal complications. BJU Int. 2013;111:745–52.

174. Campbell SC, Bhoopalam N, Moritz TE, et al. The use of zoledronic acid in men receiving androgen deprivation therapy for prostate cancer with severe osteopenia or osteoporosis. Urology. 2010;75:1138–43.

175. Planas J, Trilla E, Raventos C, et al. Alendronate decreases the fracture risk in patients with prostate cancer on androgen-deprivation therapy and with severe osteopenia or osteoporosis. BJU Int. 2009;104:1637–40.

176. Krahn M, Bremner KE, Tomlinson G, et al. Androgen deprivation therapy in prostate cancer: are rising concerns leading to falling use? BJU Int. 2011;108:1588–96.

177. Shih HJ, Shih LY, Chang H, et al. Clinical features of testicular lympyhoma. Acta Haematol. 2014;131:187–92.

178. Wheater MJ, Manners J, Nolan L, et al. The clinical features and management of testicular germ cell tumours in patients aged 60 years and older. BJU Int. 2011;108:1794–9.

179. McRae PJ, Peel M, Walker PJ, et al. Geriatric syndromes in individuals admitted to vascular and urology surgical unites. J Am Geriatr Soc. 2014;62:1105–9.

180. Cigolle CT, Langa KM, Kabeto MU, et al. Geriatric conditions and disability: the health and retirement study. Ann Intern Med. 2007;147(3):156–64.

181. Foley AL, Loharuka S, Barrett JA, et al. Association between the geriatric giants of urinary incontinence and falls in older people using data from the Leicestershire MRC incontinence study. Age Ageing. 2012;41:35–40.

182. Brown JS, Vittinghoff E, Wyman JF, et al. Urinary incontinence: does it increase risk for falls and fractures? J Am Geriatr Soc. 2000;48:721–5.

183. Chiarelli PE, Mackenzie LA, Osmotherly PG. Urinary incontinence is associated with an increase in falls: a systematic review. Aust J Physiother. 2009;55(2):89–95.

184. Kurita N, Yamazaki S, Fukumori N, et al. Overactive bladder syndrome severity is associated with falls in community-dwelling adults: LOHAS study. BMJ Open. 2013;3, e002413.

185. Hunter KF, Voaklander D, Hsu ZY, Moore KN. Lower urinary tract symptoms and falls risk among older women receiving home support: a prospective cohort study. BMC Geriatr. 2013;13:46.

186. Galizia G, Langellotto A, Cacciatore F, et al. Association between nocturia and falls-related long-term mortality risk in the elderly. J Am Med Dir Assoc. 2012;13:640–4.

187. Hasegawa J, Kuzuya M, Iguchi A. Urinary incontinence and behavioral symptoms are independent risk factors for recurrent and injurious falls, respectively, among residents in long-term care facilities. Arch Gerontol Geriatr. 2010;50:77–81.

188. Min LC, Reuben DB, Adams J, et al. Does better quality of care for falls and urinary incontinence result in better participant-reported outcomes? J Am Geriatr Soc. 2011;59:1435–43.

189. Bylow K, Dale W, Mustian K, et al. Falls and physical performance deficits in older patients with prostate cancer undergoing androgen deprivation therapy. Urology. 2008;72:422–7.

190. Parsons JK, Mougey J, Lambert L, et al. Lower urinary tract symptoms increase the risk of falls in older men. BJU Int. 2009;104(1):63–8.

191. Kortebein P, Symons TB, Ferrando A, et al. Functional impact of 10 days of bed rest in healthy older adults. J Gerontol A Biol Sci Med Sci. 2008;63:1076–81.

192. Barrios B, Labalette C, Rousseau P, et al. A national prevalence study of pressure ulcers in French hospital inpatients. J Wound Care. 2008;17:373–9.

193. Baumgarten M, Margolis DJ, Localio AR, et al. Extrinsic risk factors for pressure ulcers early in the hospital stay: a nested case-control study. J Gerontol A Biol Sci Med Sci. 2008;63:408–13.

194. Garre-Olmo J, Planas-Pujol X, Lopez-Pousa S, et al. Prevalence and risk factors of suspected elder abuse subtypes in people aged 75 and older. J Am Geriatr Soc. 2009;57:815–22.

195. Heath JM, Brown M, Kobylarz FA, et al. The prevalence of undiagnosed geriatric health conditions among adult protective services clients. Gerontologist. 2005;45:820–3.

196. Dong X, de Leon CFM, Evans DA. Is greater self-neglect severity associated with lower levels of physical function? J Aging Health. 2009;21:596–610.

197. U.S. Department of Health and Human Services. Administration on Aging, National Center on Elder Abuse. www.ncea.aoa.gove/index.aspx. Accessed 10 Apr 2014.

198. Sinclair CL, Kalender-Rich J, Griebling TL, Porter-Williamson K. Palliative care of urologic patients at end of life. Clin Geriatr Med. 2015;31:667–78.

199. Agar M, Currow D, Plummer J, et al. Changes in anticholinergic load from regular prescribed medications in palliative care as death approaches. Palliat Med. 2009;23:257–65.

200. Bergman J, Ballon-Landa E, Lorenz KA, et al. Community-partnered collaboration to build an integrated palliative care clinic: the view from urology. Am J Hosp Palliat Care. 2014;[e-pub ahead of print].

Vascular Surgery

Jason Johanning

Man is as old as his arteries

Sir William Osler

Vascular surgery involves surgical and nonsurgical interventions related to arterial, venous, and lymphatic pathophysiology throughout all ages, but the average age of a vascular surgeon's patient is that of the Medicare population and thus dominantly an elderly population. With the expected increase in our elderly population, the diagnosis and treatment of arterial disease will become must have knowledge for the vascular surgeon and generalists alike. Vascular surgeons therefore will be disproportionately impacted by the upcoming population shift and therefore must not only know the treatment of vascular disease but must also incorporate a knowledge of the role aging plays in relation to our surgical treatment and outcome. Although a working knowledge of the most common sites of disease, the initial diagnostic tests, treatment options and outcomes are necessary to provide optimal guidance for vascular patients. The goals of care in these patients must be focused on insuring the maximum possible ambulation, independence in old age and quality of life.

The vascular surgeon is tasked with establishing a diagnosis using primarily non-invasive tests, treating the patient initially medically with, for example, anticoagulants and drugs focused on atherosclerosis. If indicated, the surgeon may consider a therapeutic plan to include both minimally invasive and open surgical treatment. As vascular patients nearly always have multiple co-morbidities associated with advanced age, it is clear that vascular surgeons must be adept at recognizing and caring for the associated changes that occur in the aging patient and determining the best course of action: medical management and/or major surgical

intervention. The ultimate question becomes which of the actions will lead to the best outcome including extending and providing optimal quality of life.

19.1 Biology of Aging

Repetitive pulsation of the arterial system leads to fracture of the elastic lamella of the larger arteries specifically the aorta and its proximal branches leading to stiffening of the arterial tree and tendency towards dilation. This is reflected by the fact that young arteries in the aortic distribution will dilate by approximately 10 % with pulsatile flow in comparison with the aged aorta that dilates only 2–3 %, thus markedly reducing capacitance of the arterial tree. This arterial stiffening results in a rise in aortic systolic and a lowering of diastolic pressures and subsequent widening of the pulse pressure. These events in combination lead to increased pulse wave velocity in the smaller vasodilated vessels creating increased stress in distal organs as a result of aging arterial dynamics. Although there can be age related structural changes in the microcirculation, they are usually attributed to diseases such as diabetes, renal dysfunction, and atherosclerotic changes. However one must consider the relative breakdown of larger artery function and subsequent increased pulsatile flow. Pulsatile flow has been shown over time to result in damage to downstream tissues including thrombosis, edema, and inflammation. Thus one should consider that treatment aimed at reducing arterial stiffness and limiting aortic pressure fluctuations will likely improve end organ function in the elderly. Treatment of the aging patient should thus be focused on the stiffened central arteries creating the pulse wave propagation and the muscular arteries that remain functional. Thus drugs including ACE inhibitors, ARBs, and calcium channel blockers have been shown to reduce the pulse wave and demonstrate survival benefits in major trials including REASON and CAFÉ. The mechanism behind the beneficial effect of these medications in the older patient is understandable when the reduction in muscular effects of the

J. Johanning, MD, MS (✉)
Department of Surgery, University of Nebraska
Medical Center, Nebraska Western Iowa VA Medical Center,
983280 Nebraska Medical Center, Omaha, NE 68198-3280, USA
e-mail: jjohanning@unmc.edu

© Springer International Publishing Switzerland 2017
J.R. Burton et al. (eds.), *Geriatrics for Specialists*, DOI 10.1007/978-3-319-31831-8_19

small and medium sized arteries is blunted allowing the elastin within the artery to absorb the pulse wave, thus transferring the job of dissipating the pulsatility from the large to small and medium sized arteries [1].

19.2   Vascular Surgery and Frailty

Vascular surgeons are well aware that advanced chronologic age and the ability to perform a successful vascular operation are not mutually exclusive. The literature is replete with case series from individual institutions documenting the ability to take octogenarians and nonagenarians through complex vascular operations including carotid endarterectomy, open abdominal aortic aneurysm operations as well as femoral to pedal bypasses. However the literature is also clear in documenting that age in and of itself is an independent predictor of mortality and adverse outcomes after vascular surgical procedures. The research challenge remaining is to identify what factors can best be utilized preoperatively to predict a successful or unsuccessful outcome in vascular surgery patients with advanced age. Frailty is a syndrome that appears to be a powerful predictor of a markedly elevated risk for postoperative mortality and morbidity and is a likely candidate for future investigations given there now are reliable measures of frailty and increasingly these tools are being used preoperatively to establish risk. Chapter 1—Frailty provides an in-depth discussion of this syndrome and strategies to assess its presence. The concept of frailty applied to vascular surgery is just beginning to appear in the literature and little data exist examining frailty in the preoperative assessment of vascular surgery patients. However, the evidence from studies of non-vascular surgical patients shows that frailty assessment preoperatively has the potential to markedly improve the ability to risk stratify patients.

Retrospective frailty assessments suggest that geriatric measures may be ideal tools to assess the vascular surgical patient preoperatively. Arya et al. assessed patients undergoing both endovascular and open elective aortic aneurysm operations in the NSQIP database utilizing the modified frailty index (mFI) [2]. They noted that frail patients were more likely to suffer severe complications after both open and endovascular aortic repair. Importantly, frail patients experiencing complications were also noted to have a higher rate of failure to rescue [2]. Utilizing the same mFI assessment tool, Karam et al. demonstrated that an elevated mFI carried an odds ratio of 2.14 for 30-day mortality in vascular surgery patients [3]. Lee et al. have assessed the psoas muscle dimensions on CT scans as an indicator of frailty. They demonstrated that muscle area correlated significantly with postoperative mortality through all time points up to 90 days after elective aortic aneurysm repair [4]. Srinivasan et al.

assessed patients with ruptured abdominal aortic aneurysms and utilizing geriatric tools including the Katz functional independence score, Charlson score, number of admission medicines, visual impairment, hearing impairment, hemoglobin, and statin use as predictors [5]. They found that the geriatric variables were highly predictive of outcome compared to standard co-morbidity and they were able to construct a receiver operating characteristic curve to assess the ability of geriatric variables to assist in predicting outcomes. This curve is a plot of sensitivity/specificity pair corresponding to the decision threshold. The area under the curve generated is a measure of how well a parameter can distinguish two diagnostic outcomes such as presence or absence of poor outcome. An ideal test is that with a value of 1.00 with the current study having a very good level of 0.84. They thus determined that geriatric variables have significant predictive ability for poor outcomes compared to traditional co-morbidity focused tools [5]. For carotid surgery, Melin et al. assessed the utility of a deficit accumulation index tool called the Risk Analysis Index to assess frailty of patients undergoing carotid artery operations in the American College of Surgeons National Surgical Quality Improvement Program (NSQIP) database. It was noted that patients who scored frail had a markedly increased risk of stroke, myocardial infarction, death, and length of stay after carotid endarterectomy [6]. Clearly the early literature suggests that preoperative assessment using frailty can provide significant prognostic value to patients aside from classic medical co-morbidities. Chapter 8—Tools of Assessment provides information on many tools (including a frailty score) valuable in assessing seniors for geriatric focused co-morbidities that could put a patient at increased risk of poor outcomes after a surgical procedure.

Frailty, functional impairment and multiple co-morbidities have been shown to be predictors of poor outcomes in several recent trials confirming the previous retrospective studies suppositions that frailty and geriatric variables will play a large role in risk stratification of vascular patients. Partridge et al. used the Edmonton frail scale, MoCA, functional status including gait speed, timed up and go, and hand grip strength to assess 125 vascular surgery patients. They noted a high incidence of impaired physical functional and cognitive status. This combination of impairments was associated with a significantly increased hospital length of stay as well as adverse postoperative outcomes [7]. Ambler et al. used a deficit accumulation index model of frailty to follow 413 patients (median age 77) for a median of 18 months. They demonstrated, respectively, a receiver operating curve of 0.83, 0.78, and 0.74 for 1 year mortality, discharge to a care institution, and prolonged length of stay [8]. Both studies clearly attest to the strength and potential of using geriatric variables and assessment to risk stratify patients and convey operative risk in the preoperative setting.

The current data suggest that identifying frailty has the ability to assist in preoperative decision-making especially in complex and elderly patients. Both retrospective and prospective studies confirm that frail patients and those with other functional impairments are at an increased risk of immediate postoperative mortality and morbidity as well as long-term mortality. Future studies need to confirm these findings in larger cohorts of vascular patients. Until more risk assessment studies are available, vascular surgeons currently will need to use available preoperative risk assessment tools to be fully informed when counseling patients and their families about perioperative risk and goals of care.

19.3 Specific Vascular Surgical Considerations for Elderly Patients

History and physical examination for vascular disease is based on standard findings known to all clinicians caring for seniors. Briefly, symptoms of carotid embolization, the presence of an asymptomatic pulsatile abdominal mass at the umbilicus, and symptoms of claudication with loss of hair and decreased or absent pulses satisfy the bulk of assessing for the presence or absence of significant arterial pathology. Given the high prevalence of vascular disease in the geriatric population, a high index of suspicion should be present and lead all clinicians to the documentation of the presence or absence of vascular disease by history and physical examination.

The majority of conditions of arterial pathology in the carotid, infrarenal aorta, and lower extremities can be assessed using standard measures available in the vascular laboratory. The majority of vascular disease including retroperitoneal and supraclavicular structures can be imaged with the increasing resolution of ultrasonography. With the proximity of the arteries to the skin surface, the lack of exposure to radiation or need for potentially nephrotoxic dye, ultrasonography in conjunction with physiological pressure studies (Ankle Brachial Index) is now considered the primary assessment tool for most vascular surgeons for the initial and subsequent assessments of patients with peripheral arterial disease. Using this approach the vascular laboratory is able to reliably document the presence and extent of carotid, upper extremity, mesenteric, renal, infrarenal aortic, and lower extremity disease and differentiate the presence of atherosclerosis and conditions such as thrombosis and embolization both at a macro and micro level.

Recently with advancements in radiologic imaging, noninvasive head to toe assessment of the larger and medium arterial tree has become commonplace. Rather than supplanting the vascular laboratory, the use of advanced imaging serves to confirm or refute findings of the vascular laboratory, and provide detailed assessment for the surgeon prior to intervention. CT scanning of the arterial tree has become so good that for the most part it has reduced angiography for diagnostic purposes to highly selected situations such as determining the patency of tibial artery stenosis or occlusions or assessment of challenging cervicocerebral anatomy. Additionally the presence of calcium, which previously limited the ability of CT scans to provide diagnosis, has now been overcome and assessment of calcium and plaque characteristics is now easily assessed with detailed CT scanning. Magnetic resonance imaging (MRI) has become less popular than CT scanning due to cost, imaging time constraints, patient reluctance, and the potential for nephrogenic systemic dermatopathy in renal failure patients. However, MRI is still important in instances of markedly reduced flow in the carotid circulation. In that situation it may help determine the presence of a patent internal carotid artery.

Similar to non-invasive imaging, there has been a marked focus on providing vascular disease treatment with minimally invasive interventions. In general, all vascular patients have four specific options in order of increasing invasiveness. First is medical management, which all patients should receive and for some is all that is warranted. Second is a purely endovascular percutaneous catheter based approach provided either under conscious sedation or general anesthesia to treat arterial disease using balloons, stents, and devices designed to improve arterial flow. Third is a combination of open and endovascular procedures with the open component of the procedure usually limited to a small incision of limited bypass with the endovascular component serving to improve outflow or inflow and thus reduce the total magnitude of the operation. Fourth is a purely open operative approach that consists of standard incisional approach and intervention employing common surgical techniques without the need for advanced radiologic imaging. It is important to remember that there are usually two or three treatment options for patients with complex arterial pathology especially in the lower extremity. Thus one should consider for the elderly patient his or her goals of care, life expectancy, and then the surgeon should guide the patient using judgment that balances the expected long-term outcome of the intervention against the potential morbidity and loss of quality of life that may be incurred [9].

19.4 Carotid Artery Occlusive Disease

Stroke is the third leading cause of death in the USA, and results in significant disability. Approximately 80 % of strokes are ischemic and 20 % hemorrhagic. And of those 80 % of ischemic strokes, 20–30 % are attributed to athero-embolic disease due to stenosis of over 50 % of a carotid artery [10]. Proper diagnosis, management and treatment of carotid stenosis is important for reducing risk of ischemic stroke in elderly patients (75 % of strokes occur in patients older than 65 years of age). With the recent advent of carotid stenting and ability to treat formerly considered non-operable patients, a renewed focus had been placed on risk stratification for proper selection of appropriate treatment. Especially in the asymptomatic senior, treatment decisions must include considerations of vascular variables such as the degree of stenosis, presence of subtle symptoms, medical comorbid conditions, and patient goals of care with a careful assessment of life expectancy and potential risk reduction in the asymptomatic patient.

A focused history is important to identify those patients at increased risk for carotid disease and perioperative stroke especially in the asymptomatic patient. Risk factors for carotid disease are similar to those of atherosclerosis in other peripheral arteries: smoking history, advanced age, male gender, and positive family history. Risk factors for stroke risk are multifactorial, but for patients with carotid disease, the most important are a history of neurologic symptoms, the degree of carotid stenosis and the plaque characteristics. Patients with prior or current cardiovascular disease are at increased risk for concurrent carotid disease and given that myocardial infarction is the most common complication leading to death after a carotid intervention, it is imperative to know a patient's cardiac history. Neurologic symptoms such as unilateral weakness, numbness or paresthesias, aphasia or dysarthria, history of transient ischemic attack (TIA), prior stroke, or amaurosis fugax are all significant historical findings that, if present in the last 6 months, define a symptomatic state. Symptoms not usually associated with carotid disease are vertigo, ataxia, diplopia, nausea, vomiting, decreased consciousness, or generalized weakness. The importance of identifying symptoms cannot be over emphasized. Surgeons often must evaluate patients who have had a carotid scan (ultrasound and/or CTA) performed in a patient with vague symptoms that reveals an underlying lesion. Very careful assessment of such patients is critical to avoid an operative or endovascular intervention for an incidental and clinically non-significant finding.

A physical examination is important to document any pre-intervention deficits that have incurred from a remote stroke and in a patient with a history of a TIA to ensure full recovery of neurological function or identify subtle residual deficits. If assessing the patient for a bruit, one must recognize that a carotid bruit is typically present when the stenosis is 50–70 %, and it is often absent in patients truly at risk with a >70 % stenosis. Additionally, the examination should focus on (a) the heart assessing for irregular rhythm or murmur, which could portend an embolic stroke, (b) palpation of distal pulses to assess systemic nature of the disease, and (c) the cranial nerve examination to establish the baseline. A formal ophthalmologic examination should be obtained in the setting of amaurosis fugax or any associated visual symptoms to identify Hollenhorst plaques and/or cholesterol emboli from the offending plaque.

The initial diagnostic study of choice for the vascular surgeon is duplex ultrasonography performed in an ICAVL accredited laboratory. The degree of stenosis is determined by peak velocity through a narrowed lumen and is useful for determining plaque morphology. This procedure requires substantial operator experience and excellence and can only assess the extra cranial carotid arteries. An accredited laboratory will be able to correlate their ultrasound findings with more detailed and advanced imaging such as angiography, CTA, and MRA. Currently in the emergency department or in any urgent care venue, typically a CTA is done initially (except in patients with contrast allergy or renal failure) in the evaluation of a patient with symptoms suggestive of a stroke. Both the carotid vessels and the brain are imaged satisfactorily with this technique such that many surgeons now forego duplex examination. Modern scanners have impressive resolution and allow full examination of neck cervico-cerebral and intracranial arteries. High calcium content in plaque previously obscuring arterial flow has been essentially obviated with the current increase in CTA imaging capability. CTA, while non-invasive, does expose the patient to ionizing radiation and can be expensive. MRA is an option for non-invasive vessel imaging but is less often utilized because of time constraints, potential patient anxiety, and the known problem of over diagnosing the degree of stenosis because of interference from calcific lesions. In contrast, the MRI of the brain is ideal in assessing ischemic damage and in this regard it is more sensitive than CT. The effectiveness of the non-invasive imaging options has limited diagnostic angiography to situations where there is marked discrepancy between non-invasive images. The importance of this cannot be overstated: the patient avoids an invasive procedure for diagnosis only and foregoes the 1.0–1.5 % risk of stroke from angiography.

Once a patient is determined to have a lesion, the surgeon must determine the critical issue of whether the patient is symptomatic from the lesion or asymptomatic. The data have clarified that patients with a significant stenosis in the carotid artery ipsilateral to the symptomatic hemisphere benefit from carotid intervention performed by experienced surgeons or interventionists using open or endovascular techniques, respectively. Ideally all patients should have outcomes entered into an appropriate quality registry to confirm benefit to the patient and institution providing care. Randomized trials both with NASCET and CREST have documented an acceptable rate of perioperative stroke and death for patients undergoing intervention for stroke risk reduction that far outweighs treating the symptomatic patient with medical management alone [11, 12]. The two invasive options for management are either endovascular or open procedures. Carotid artery endovascular stenting is usually reserved for patients who are thought to be poor operative candidates such as those with cranial nerve deficits, prior head neck radiotherapy, difficult to access carotid lesions and in patients with contralateral occlusion. Additionally carotid artery stenting has been shown to reduce the perioperative myocardial infarction rate by half and thus may be the best choice for those patients with known severe cardiac disease. However open endarterectomy remains the gold standard for intervention. It has the lowest rate of perioperative stroke in acceptable operative candidates. Complications associated with both interventions include stroke, myocardial infarction, and death. The risk of myocardial infarction is higher with endarterectomy as are the rates of cranial nerve injury. Thirty-day stroke and death rates for endarterectomy by a highly experienced surgeon in symptomatic patients should be less than 6 %. Indeed, the majority of single centers and Vascular Quality Initiative registry report 30-day stroke and death on the order of 2–3 % [11].

The more contentious issue currently in the area of carotid artery stenosis is what to do with the patient with positive imaging who is thought to be asymptomatic from the lesion. Some believe these patients would benefit from intervention based upon randomized studies such as the ACAS trial. However, there are several caveats that must be considered as a surgeon evaluates such asymptomatic patients: (1) screening for asymptomatic carotid artery disease has not shown any benefit in stroke risk reduction (the United States Preventative Task Force has concluded that the harms of screening for asymptomatic carotid artery stenosis outweigh the benefits even in the setting of coexistent atherosclerotic disease, a carotid bruit, or prior head and neck radiotherapy); (2) the initial ACAS trial included only patients with an estimated life expectancy of over 5 years; (3) the trial demonstrated that the beneficial effect of endarterectomy is conferred only after approximately 4 years and if the perioperative stroke and death rate is less than 3 %; (4) current data suggest in Medicare recipients that asymptomatic carotid intervention is not acceptable with approximately 30 % of patients dying within 3 years after undergoing asymptomatic carotid artery intervention; and (5) elderly females are the least likely to benefit from asymptomatic carotid artery intervention based on a post hoc analysis of the ACAS trial [13–16]. To further investigate the role of asymptomatic carotid artery intervention, the currently active CREST II trial will investigate the role of intervening on asymptomatic carotid artery disease utilizing either carotid endarterectomy or carotid artery stenting with medical management versus best medical management alone in a two parallel randomized trial design.

The most important concern in considering a procedural intervention in a patient with asymptomatic carotid artery stenosis is that the surgeon must understand and fully explain the risk and benefit of an intervention so the patient can make a fully informed decision. In communications with patients, a surgeon must fully understand the patient's goals of care and

Table 19.1 Poor survival of patients in "real world" populations undergoing both symptomatic and asymptomatic CEA[a]

Time	Cumulative mortality risk %	
	Symptomatic	Asymptomatic
1 year	10	6.2
2 year	18.8	13.1
3 year	27.1	19.8
4 year	36.3	27.9

Data from Jalbert JJ, Nguyen LL, Gerhard-Herman MD, Jaff MR, White CJ, Rothman AT, et al. Outcomes after carotid artery stenting in Medicare beneficiaries, 2005 to 2009. JAMA Neurol. 2015 Mar;72(3):276–286

[a]A survival of a minimum of 5 years for asymptomatic patients based on the ACAS trial is needed for patients to benefit from asymptomatic endarterectomy

then, and only then, can a judgment concerning an intervention be wisely made. The surgeon can only advise a patient fully after an assessment of risk factors known to negatively impact short and long-term outcomes of an intervention. Strong arguments can be made for withholding CEA in the setting of dialysis and life limiting conditions where the data clearly show both short and long-term mortality does not reduce the risk of future stroke. More importantly, long-term survival studies have demonstrated that performance of CEA on asymptomatic patients may have acceptable perioperative stroke and death rates but does not achieve acceptable long-term survival. To emphasize this point, Wallaert et. al. demonstarated an overall 5-year survival of 80% in patients with asymptomatic disease; however those with high risk, for example, age >80, dialysis dependence, insulin dependent diabetes or sever contralateral disease are unlikely to survive long enough to benefit from CEA [17]. Graphical evidence of long-term survival for patients with both symptomatic and asymptomatic carotid disease and those at the extreme of age is noted in Table 19.1. Identifying frailty preoperatively helps stratify patients in the older age groups who will likely have poorer surgical outcomes (Fig. 19.1).

19.5 Abdominal Aortic Aneurysm

Abdominal aortic aneurysm (AAA) is a disease of the elderly most commonly in men who have smoked. AAA is an inflammatory disease of the aorta in which progressive remodeling of arterial wall initiated by smoking with a strong genetic component. The destruction of the aortic wall is caused by the end effector matrix metalloproteinase, which leads to loss of the elastin within the aorta and subsequent dilation of the wall. The presence of an aneurysm is defined by increase in vessel diameter by more than 50 % (usually a diameter over 3.0 cm). Over 95 % of aneurysms are located in the infrarenal location. Once present, aneurysms do not grow longitudinally but rather dilate over time. This growth

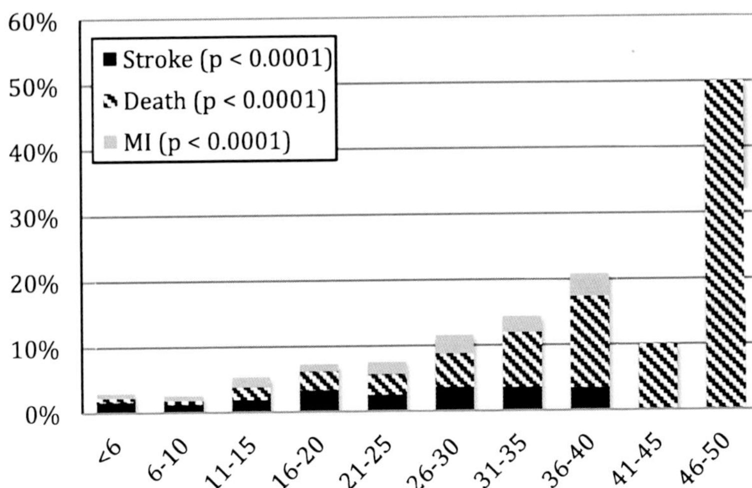

Fig. 19.1 Frailty has the potential to significantly improve patient selection in the preoperative period for patients undergoing carotid endarterectomy. Applying frailty analysis to patients in the National Surgical Quality Improvement Project, increasing frailty scores correlated with a marked increase risk of 30-day complications in patients undergoing both symptomatic and asymptomatic CEA. Reprinted from J Vasc Surg, 61(3), Melin AA, Schmid KK, Lynch TG, Pipinos II, Kappes S, Longo GM, et al. Preoperative frailty Risk Analysis Index (horizontal axis) to stratify patients undergoing carotid endarterectomy, 683–689, Copyright 2015, with permission from Elsevier

of the aneurysm occurs in a staccato fashion with potential long periods of absence of growth. An aneurysm once identified warrants careful surveillance. Co-morbidities or physical activity, in spite of a common perception, does not cause rupture. Rather the size of the aneurysm is the most predictive factor for rupture of the aneurysm.

Most aneurysms are identified during the time of radiographic scanning either for unrelated reasons or by clinicians following the current USPSTF recommendations for a one time screen using ultrasound of men ages 65–75 who ever smoked [18]. Physical examination of the aorta is very difficult and especially unreliable in those with an elevated BMI.

Abdominal aortic aneurysms can be assessed utilizing multiple diagnostic imaging techniques. From a screening perspective, ultrasound is able to assess the infrarenal aorta diameter with a sensitivity and specificity nearing 100 %. Because ultrasound has no risk and is reliable it should be performed in patients for both a screening study and those suspected of having an aneurysm. Ultrasound is unable to assess the perivisceral, thoracic and iliac vasculature and therefore once an abdominal aortic aneurysm is identified, a CTA is the most commonly obtained study to fully delineate the concomitant arterial circulation and assess its potential for future repair. The use of magnetic resonance imaging can also document the presence of an aneurysm and help define its morphology. However its use is limited both in routine diagnostic and emergent situations due to the typical delay often experienced in obtaining the study as well as the anxiety many patients experience. Once an aneurysm has been identified, it should be followed at regular intervals if it does not meet size criteria for repair. Currently in the USA, aneurysms are routinely repaired once they reach the size of 5–5.5 cm. This recommendation is based upon multiple trials showing acceptable mortality and morbidity at this aneurysm size. If an aneurysm measures 3–4 cm, it is reasonable to

follow this on a yearly or bi-yearly basis with ultrasound. Once the aneurysm reaches 4–4.5 cm, a vascular surgeon will likely reassess the patient at no longer than 1 year intervals, although no definitive recommendations have been established for this surveillance.

Treatment for AAA is specifically aimed at reducing a patient's risk of rupture and once rupture occurs the mortality with or without surgery is very high. Currently no medical treatment exists for an abdominal aortic aneurysm. Propanolol beta blockade has been shown to be ineffective. Current ongoing trials of antibiotics specifically doxycycline are enrolling patients based on matrix metalloproteinase blockade [19]. Thus for now, surgery remains the only form of treatment that will reduce the mortality risk associated with aneurysm rupture. The risk of the operation must be lower than the risk of aortic rupture. Currently, surgery is indicated when the aneurysm reaches 5–5.5 cm for a standard infrarenal AAA. Mortality from rupture at this size is approximately 1–2 % per year and likely to begin to be greater than the operative mortality. Most importantly intervening on small aneurysms has not been shown to be beneficial. Meta-analysis of the four randomized trials of early AAA repair has not shown a survival benefit and there is a definite burden for the patient with operative repair (Fig. 19.2) [20].

Surgical intervention can be open or endovascular. Standard open operations are performed through either a midline laparotomy or retroperitoneal approach with clamping of the aorta and sewing in a bypass graft. This technique has the advantage of eliminating the aneurysm but is associated with hernia formation and potential for postoperative bowel obstructions and aorto-duodenal fistula. More recently endovascular treatment has been popularized with placement of the grafts through the femoral arterial circulation and exclusion of flow into the aortic sac by repairing the aneurysm from within the arterial circulation. This form of treatment typically is associated with a shorter hospital length of stay

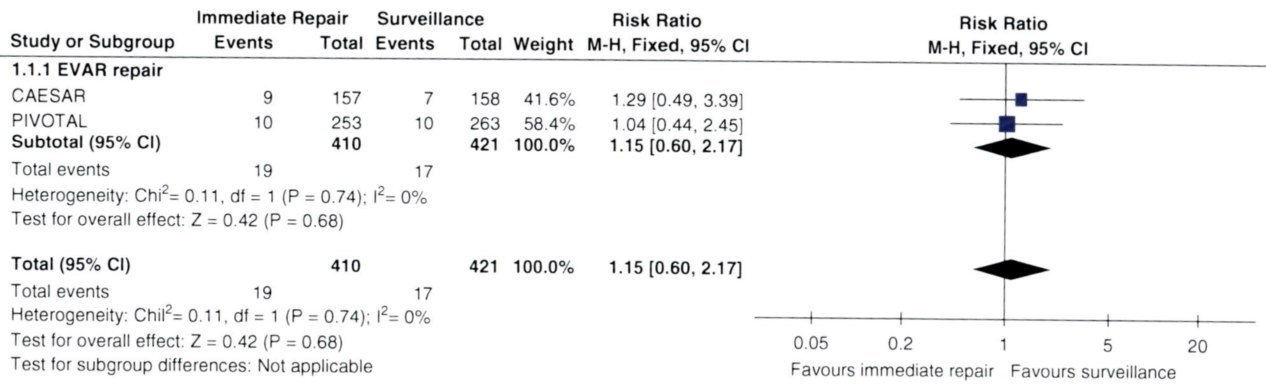

Fig. 19.2 Currently there is no indication for either open or endovascular intervention for patients with aneurysms less than 5 cm based on four well-performed randomized trials demonstrating no benefit to early intervention. From Filardo G, Powell JT, Martinez MA, Ballard DJ. Surgery for small asymptomatic abdominal aortic aneurysms. Cochrane Database Syst Rev. 2015 Feb 8;2:CD001835

Table 19.2 The poor long-term survival of octo- and nonagenarians undergoing endarterectomy in long term follow-up

Time	Cumulative mortality risk %	
	Octogenarian	Nonagenarian
1 year	10.7	16.5
2 year	20	28.3
3 year	27.6	38.3
4 year	35.6	47.3
5 year	43.3	56.2

Data from Lichtman JH, Jones SB, Wang Y, Watanabe E, Allen NB, Fayad P, et al. Postendarterectomy mortality in octogenarians and nonagenarians in the USA from 1993 to 1999. Cerebrovasc Dis. 2010 Jan;29(2):154–161

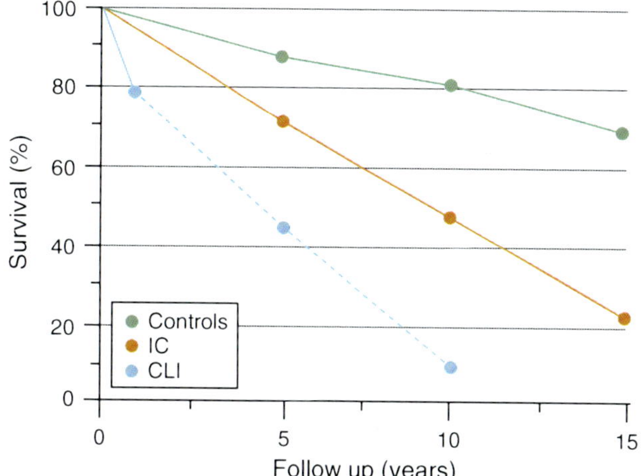

Fig. 19.3 Survival of patients with peripheral arterial disease is markedly decreased in comparison with patients with no evidence of disease. The presence of symptomatic status of a patients PAD markedly worsens long-term survival. Reprinted from Norgren L, Hiatt WR, Dormandy JA, Nehler MR, Harris KA, Fowkes FG, et al. Inter-Society Consensus for the Management of Peripheral Arterial Disease (TASC II). J Vasc Surg. Jan;45 Suppl: S5-67, Copyright 2007, with permission from Elsevier

and recovery time but leaves the aneurysm in situ. Leaving the aneurysm in situ requires close follow-up using CTA with the risk of excessive radiation and inconvenience to the patient resulting from this surveillance. Endovascular repair not uncommonly needs revision because of graft movement and/or re-pressurization of the aortic sac. Nonetheless, with appropriate exclusion of the aneurysm, endovascular repair has been found to have similar mortality rates to open repair over time. In the elderly patient the gain in the immediate perioperative period must be balanced with the burden of repeat imaging to insure a stable aortic repair. Accordingly, the surgeon in discussions with the patient will need to explain carefully the immediate and long-term benefits and burdens of an open or endovascular procedure (Table 19.2).

19.6 Lower Extremity Arterial Disease

Peripheral arterial disease (PAD) is a disease of the elderly. Approximately 20–25 % of patients over age 75 have disease based on an ankle brachial index of less than 0.90. Approximately 50 % of the population with reduced ABIs will be asymptomatic. Of the remaining patients with reduced ABIs, 40 % will present with intermittent claudication and 10 % will present with critical limb ischemia. Regardless of their presentation, the PAD population is most notable for systemic atherosclerotic disease, which predisposes the patient to a high risk of cardiovascular disease and death. Therefore, any patient with a reduced ABI should be counseled regarding risk reduction activities (smoking cessation and exercise) and treated appropriately for cardiac and cerebrovascular disease, if identified. This impact of the systematic nature of asymptomatic disease is emphasized when examining the survival curve of patients with asymptomatic disease compared to normal patients (Fig. 19.3). Once a patient with PVD becomes symptomatic with either intermittent claudication (IC) or critical limb ischemia (CLI) the survival of the patient worsens [21].

When selecting patients for intervention with reduced ABIs, foremost a detailed history focusing on the patient's lower extremity complaints should be obtained. The classic presentation of patients with peripheral arterial disease is that of classical (Rose) claudication which is described as pain or discomfort of calf or buttock muscles with a defined time of exertion and that subsides with 5–10 min of rest. Unfortunately, not all patients present with classic claudication and many remain asymptomatic or have atypical symptoms. Often elderly patients have minimal complaints as their associated co-morbidities limit ambulatory function either due to cardio-pulmonary disease, arthritis or spinal stenosis, for example. The presence of significant coexistent disease in the PAD patient is 50–75 %. Thus it is imperative to assess whether the PAD is the primary cause of complaints. Testing in the form of exercise treadmill or reactive hyperemia is indicated in this situation to determine if vascular disease is truly the cause of the patient's symptoms. In the elderly patient, neurogenic claudication secondary to spinal stenosis and osteoarthritis of the hip or knee must be differentiated from vasculogenic claudication. Osteoarthritis is differentiated from claudication as the pain of osteoarthritis generally localizes to the joint, improves with pain medications, and is commonly brought on with movement of the involved joint. Neurogenic claudication in contrast is more difficult to differentiate from vasculogenic disease. Neurogenic claudication most commonly presents with pain in the calves and posterior thigh and buttocks. In contrast to vasculogenic disease, neurogenic claudication has variable distance to onset and variable recovery time often worsening with repeated episodes of activity. Neurogenic claudication can often be diagnosed through use of assistive devices such as having the patient evaluate the pain walking with a shopping cart and other measures that decompress the spinal canal. It is not unusual for these conditions to co-exist in the elderly patient. Therefore, the surgeon will need to carefully consider the patients most dominate symptoms in order to determine which treatment options to pursue for optimal outcome and the maintenance of ambulation and function. Similar to both carotid and aortic diagnoses, the use of the non-invasive ABIs and ultrasound can document the extent and location of the disease in the majority of patients. Similarly, CTA has proven to be invaluable in providing a roadmap for surgical planning and with modern scanners, angiography is reserved to assessing tibial arteries not clearly seen on CTA and angiography is usually performed with intervention in mind and not simply for diagnostic purposes.

The paradigm for treating the patient with PAD should focus initially on lifestyle issues and medical management. Based on the natural history of PAD many patients remain stable with regard to their disease at presentation or improve regardless of treatment. Institution of medical management with antiplatelet and cholesterol lowering therapy in conjunction with smoking cessation are the mainstays of medical therapy. In addition to medical therapy, an initial trial of exercise therapy should be attempted. Data are robust that exercise therapy will improve maximal walking time and ability. These outcomes are independent of increased ABI. Indeed, typically no significant change is expected in ABI. Importantly when comparing trials of exercise therapy with endovascular intervention, data demonstrate that supervised exercise therapy offers equivalent results over time (usually 1–2 years) with no complication rate and equivalent progression to limb loss. The combination of supervised exercise therapy and endovascular intervention likely offers the best option for the claudication patient in need of treatment. Trials examining dual therapy show a clear improvement in walking distances compared to endovascular intervention alone [22].

If medical management and supervised exercise therapy have failed to give the desired result for the patient and they are willing to undergo intervention, it is reasonable to offer patients with lifestyle limiting claudication options for intervention including stenting of the aorto-iliac and femoral segments or surgical bypass when long segment stenosis or occlusion is present in a patient with an acceptable risk. For the patient with claudication, it should be emphasized that the intervention is for lifestyle improvement and not for limb salvage. This is so despite the occasionally expressed notion that limb salvage is improved. The risk of amputation is quite low for the patient with severe claudication (Fig. 19.4).

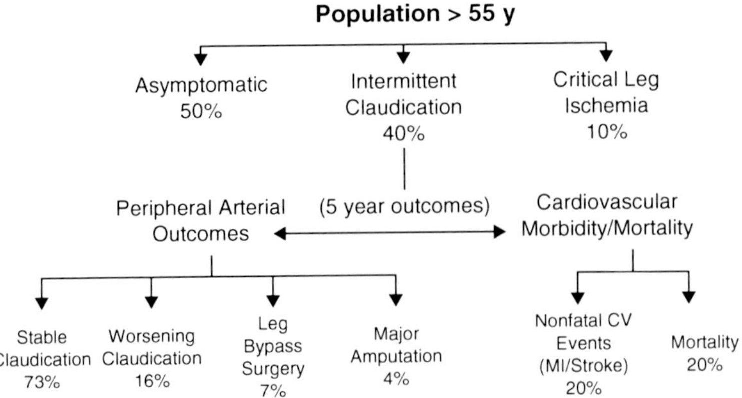

Fig. 19.4 The benign nature of PAD in the lower extremities is noted in the flow chart with 90 % of patients presenting with no or minimal symptoms. Of patients with intermittent claudication, the risk of amputation is approximately 4 %, with less than 10 % of patients needing intervention alluding to the lifestyle nature of intervention for claudication. From Weitz JI, Byrne J, Clagett GP, Farkouh ME, Porter JM, Sackett DL, et al. Diagnosis and treatment of chronic arterial insufficiency of the lower extremities: a critical review. Circulation. 1996 Dec 1;94(11):3026–3049

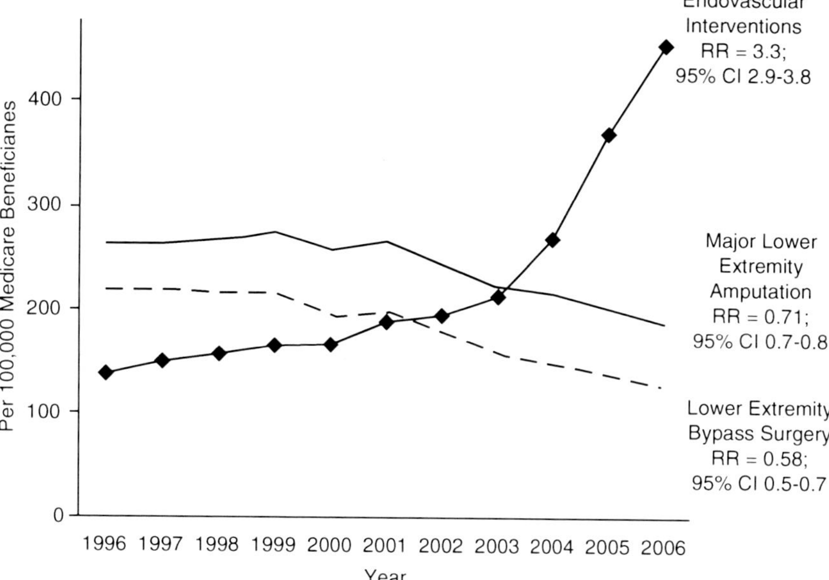

Fig. 19.5 A marked rise in endovascular interventions is noted with a concomitant decrease in open surgical bypass and amputations in the USA. A causal relationship between alterations in revascularization procedures and improvement in amputation rates has yet to be formally determined. Reprinted from J Vasc Surg, Jul;50(1), Goodney PP, Beck AW, Nagle J, Welch HG, Zwolak RM, National trends in lower extremity bypass surgery, endovascular interventions, and major amputations, 54–60, Copyright 2009, with permission from Elsevier

Patients should not be counseled that due to reduced ABIs they are at a high risk of amputation without surgical treatment: that is blatantly false. This is in contrast to patients with critical leg ischemia where all efforts to revascularize lower extremity should proceed promptly due to the high rate of amputation without revascularization. This can be accomplished with either endovascular or open surgical approach. The open surgical approach usually reserved for patients in whom inline endovascular flow cannot be restored or in patients with a significant amount of tissue necrosis. This endovascular first approach is commonly utilized as first line therapy regardless of lesion length given the perceived lack of morbidity and mortality. This concept is based on the BASIL trial where 30-day morbidity and all cause mortality at 6 months was higher in open than endovascular intervention. Yet patients undergoing open surgery had a better amputation free survival and lower all cause mortality at 2 years [23]. Currently the BEST-CLI trial is hoping to answer the surgery vs. endovascular conundrum utilizing an innovative pragmatic randomized design focusing on outcomes of amputation rate, repeat intervention, and mortality [24].

Given the ease of endovascular intervention, the relative lack of complications and the rapid advances in devices to treat peripheral arterial disease, it is not surprising to see the marked rise in this procedure in the USA. The increase in endovascular interventions is related to the need for them to be repeated often in a patient to achieve lasting benefit. This increase in endovascular procedures is associated with a corresponding reduction in surgical bypass and amputations (see Fig. 19.5). The causal relation between alterations in revascularization procedures and improvement in amputation rates has yet to be precisely determined [25]. One must keep in mind that the goal of intervention is to maintain an ambulatory and functional patient. And it has yet to be proven that those patients who are non-ambulatory and dependent prior to intervention will regain functional with an invasive intervention. In fact, when nursing home residents undergo lower extremity revascularization few survive to be alive and ambulatory at 1 year and regain little to no function [26, 27]. Thus in these non-ambulatory patients the choice between limb salvage and palliative amputation must be contemplated considering carefully the patient's goals of care and preferences. The best choice is the least invasive treatment with the lowest morbidity and mortality while achieving the patient's goals.

References

1. O'Rourke MF, Hashimoto J. Mechanical factors in arterial aging: a clinical perspective. J Am Coll Cardiol. 2007;50(1):1–13.
2. Arya S, et al. Frailty increases the risk of 30-day mortality, morbidity, and failure to rescue after elective abdominal aortic aneurysm repair independent of age and comorbidities. J Vasc Surg. 2015; 61(2):324–31.
3. Karam J, et al. Simplified frailty index to predict adverse outcomes and mortality in vascular surgery patients. Ann Vasc Surg. 2013;27(7):904–8.
4. Lee JS, et al. Frailty, core muscle size, and mortality in patients undergoing open abdominal aortic aneurysm repair. J Vasc Surg. 2011;53(4):912–7.
5. Srinivasan A, et al. Premorbid function, comorbidity, and frailty predict outcomes after ruptured abdominal aortic aneurysm repair. J Vasc Surg. 2016;63:603–9.
6. Melin AA, et al. Preoperative frailty risk analysis index to stratify patients undergoing carotid endarterectomy. J Vasc Surg. 2015; 61(3):683–9.
7. Partridge JS, et al. Frailty and poor functional status are common in arterial vascular surgical patients and affect postoperative outcomes. Int J Surg. 2015;18:57–63.

8. Ambler GK, et al. Effect of frailty on short- and mid-term outcomes in vascular surgical patients. Br J Surg. 2015;102(6):638–45.

9. Noorani A, Hippelainen M, Nashef SA. Time until treatment equipoise: a new concept in surgical decision making. JAMA Surg. 2014;149(2):109–11.

10. Chambers BR, Norris JW. Outcome in patients with asymptomatic neck bruits. N Engl J Med. 1986;315(14):860–5.

11. Brott TG, et al. Stenting versus endarterectomy for treatment of carotid-artery stenosis. N Engl J Med. 2010;363(1):11–23.

12. Barnett HJ, et al. Benefit of carotid endarterectomy in patients with symptomatic moderate or severe stenosis. North American Symptomatic Carotid Endarterectomy Trial Collaborators. N Engl J Med. 1998;339(20):1415–25.

13. Schneider JR, et al. A comparison of results with eversion versus conventional carotid endarterectomy from the Vascular Quality Initiative and the Mid-America Vascular Study Group. J Vasc Surg. 2015;61(5):1216–22.

14. Jalbert JJ, et al. Outcomes after carotid artery stenting in Medicare beneficiaries, 2005 to 2009. JAMA Neurol. 2015;72(3):276–86.

15. Lichtman JH, et al. Postendarterectomy mortality in octogenarians and nonagenarians in the USA from 1993 to 1999. Cerebrovasc Dis. 2010;29(2):154–61.

16. LeFevre ML, U.S. Preventive Services Task Force. Screening for asymptomatic carotid artery stenosis: U.S. Preventive Services Task Force recommendation statement. Ann Intern Med. 2014;161(5): 356–62.

17. Wallaert JB, et al. Optimal selection of asymptomatic patients for carotid endarterectomy based on predicted 5-year survival. J Vasc Surg. 2013;58(1):112–8.

18. LeFevre ML, U.S. Preventive Services Task Force. Screening for abdominal aortic aneurysm: U.S. Preventive Services Task Force recommendation statement. Ann Intern Med. 2014;161(4): 281–90.

19. Baxter BT, Terrin MC, Dalman RL. Medical management of small abdominal aortic aneurysms. Circulation. 2008;117(14):1883–9.

20. Filardo G, et al. Surgery for small asymptomatic abdominal aortic aneurysms. Cochrane Database Syst Rev. 2015;2, CD001835.

21. Hirsch AT, et al. Peripheral arterial disease detection, awareness, and treatment in primary care. JAMA. 2001;286(11):1317–24.

22. Frans FA, et al. Systematic review of exercise training or percutaneous transluminal angioplasty for intermittent claudication. Br J Surg. 2012;99(1):16–28.

23. Bradbury AW, et al. Bypass versus angioplasty in severe ischaemia of the leg (BASIL) trial: a survival prediction model to facilitate clinical decision making. J Vasc Surg. 2010;51(5 Suppl): 52S–68.

24. Menard MT, Farber A. The BEST-CLI trial: a multidisciplinary effort to assess whether surgical or endovascular therapy is better for patients with critical limb ischemia. Semin Vasc Surg. 2014;27(1):82–4.

25. Goodney PP, et al. National trends in lower extremity bypass surgery, endovascular interventions, and major amputations. J Vasc Surg. 2009;50(1):54–60.

26. Oresanya L, et al. Functional outcomes after lower extremity revascularization in nursing home residents: a national cohort study. JAMA Inter Med. 2015;175:951–7.

27. Goodney PP, et al. Predicting ambulation status one year after lower extremity bypass. J Vasc Surg. 2009;49(6):1431.9.e1.

Part III

Medical Specialties

Rheumatology

20

Rebecca L. Manno and Jason E. Liebowitz

20.1   Introduction

Many rheumatic diseases disproportionately affect older individuals. Osteoarthritis is almost universally present among octogenarians, and giant cell arteritis, the most common systemic vasculitis in North America, occurs exclusively in individuals over the age of 50 with a mean age of onset between 70 and 80 years. Rheumatoid arthritis has a prevalence of 2 % in the USA among individuals over the age of 60 [1]. In fact, the earliest recorded description of rheumatoid arthritis was among older individuals in the year 1800 when Dr. A.J. Landre-Beauvais described a severe illness with involvement of the joints, female predominance, a chronic course, and precipitous decline in general health among three patients over the age of 70 [2]. Rheumatic, autoimmune, and musculoskeletal diseases may be common among older individuals, but the care of these patients is far from routine.

Rheumatic diseases, and the medications used to treat them, often affect muscles and joints. This has a profound and unique impact on older individuals who are often already dealing with aging-related musculoskeletal issues that are the consequence of multiple co-morbidities, poor functional status, malnutrition, sarcopenia, and cognitive impairment. Fixed incomes and complicated medication regimens with biologic agents that have rarely been studied in older individuals add layers of complexity to management for both patients and providers. Many of these important issues are not being adequately addressed in our current health care system.

The objective of this chapter is to review the current epidemiologic, diagnostic, and therapeutic data for some of the most common rheumatic conditions among older individuals in the realms of arthritis, myositis, vasculitis, and connective tissue disorders. By highlighting some of the important unanswered questions in the multifaceted care of older patients with rheumatic disease we hope to generate future investigation in these areas. Research in geriatric rheumatology has the potential to generate comprehensive, individualized, and data driven management strategies that will improve quality of life and quality of care for older patients suffering with these conditions.

20.2   Arthritis and the Older Patient

20.2.1 Osteoarthritis

20.2.1.1   Epidemiology

Osteoarthritis (OA) is the most prevalent joint disease in the USA with greater than 33 % (12.4 million) of individuals over age 65 affected [3]. Risk factors for OA include female gender, obesity, joint injury, repetitive use of joints, and family history, but the most important risk factor is advanced age. With a predicted 88.5 million Americans reaching the age of 65 or older by 2050, nearly 30 million individuals in the USA will have OA in the future [4].

Studies evaluating the annual health care costs of OA per individual in the USA have provided a wide range of estimates from $989 to 10,313 per year [5, 6]. Although substantial variation exists across studies, it is universally accepted that this is an expensive problem with the cost of knee OA-related health care estimated to account for approximately 10 % of direct medical costs per individual over their lifetime [5]. OA is undoubtedly a prevalent and costly medical condition which targets older individuals.

20.2.1.2   Diagnosis of OA in Older Individuals

Much like everything else when caring for older patients, there can be a unique level of complexity in diagnosis even for the most routine and common medical conditions, such

R.L. Manno, MD, MHS (✉)
Department of Internal Medicine, Division of Rheumatology,
Johns Hopkins University, 5501 Hopkins Bayview Circle,
Room 1B.13, Baltimore, MD 21224, USA
e-mail: rmanno3@jhmi.edu

J.E. Liebowitz, MD
Department of Internal Medicine, Johns Hopkins Bayview,
301 Mason F. Lord Drive, Baltimore, MD 21224, USA

© Springer International Publishing Switzerland 2017
J.R. Burton et al. (eds.), *Geriatrics for Specialists*, DOI 10.1007/978-3-319-31831-8_20

as OA. Classification criteria for knee OA endorsed by the American College of Rheumatology based on clinical features alone (age, stiffness <30 min, crepitus, bony tenderness, bony enlargement, absence of warmth) has a 95% sensitivity but only 69% specificity [7]. Specificity increases to 75% with the addition of laboratory features (negative autoantibodies, normal ESR, synovial fluid consistent with OA) and to up to 86% with confirmatory X-ray data [7].

It is the opinion of these authors that clinical features are generally sufficient to diagnose OA in older patients. However, red flags which should prompt further diagnostic investigation with laboratory studies, imaging, and/or arthrocentesis include: joint warmth, joint effusions or dominate involvement of the metacarpophalangeal (MCP) or metatarsophalangeal joints. Particularly in the multi-morbid older adult, a diagnosis of OA (versus other forms of arthritis) may be challenging because of pain and functional impairment from other sources such as neuropathy, myelopathy, or depression. This is an area where additional research and investigation to develop diagnostic arthritis algorithms, specific for older individuals, would be extremely valuable to streamline joint assessments so that management can begin swiftly.

20.2.1.3 Management of OA in Older Individuals

There are multiple guidelines that have been published by highly reputable professional organizations [American College of Rheumatology (ACR); European League Against Rheumatism (EULAR); Osteoarthritis Research Society International (OARSI); European Society for Clinical and Economic Aspects of Osteoporosis and Osteoarthritis (ESCEO)] with regard to the treatment of OA (specifically knee OA). There is agreement among these guidelines that OA management requires a combination of non-pharmacologic and pharmacologic (oral, topical, intra-articular) treatments [8].

Patient education, weight loss, and exercise programs are universally recommended, although the effects of these interventions on early symptoms and long-term disease modification remain controversial [8]. Even a modest 5% reduction in weight among patients with BMI ≥25 and knee OA has been shown to produce small, but significant, improvements in physical function [9]. Exercise is a critical component of any weight loss program, but often weight loss is not an appropriate goal for older individuals with OA because of co-morbid conditions such as sarcopenia and frailty. Thankfully the benefits of exercise extend well beyond weight loss for OA management.

Exercise is one of the few OA treatments that has consistently demonstrated efficacy in reducing pain, disability and improving joint function. For these reasons, it is universally accepted that it should be an integral part of any OA treatment plan for older adults [8]. A recent systematic review and meta-analysis of 48 exercise trials concluded that the optimal exercise program for individuals with knee OA entails supervised sessions three times per week with fitness goals of improving aerobic capacity, quadriceps strength, and lower extremity performance [10]. However, barriers are often encountered when trying to implement an exercise program for older adults with OA. Advanced, symptomatic OA may prevent moderate to strenuous exercise, and co-morbidities such as heart disease or neuropathy can make conventional exercise programs challenging. In our opinion, the solution is to create a customized and creative OA exercise program based on the individual needs of the older patient. For some older patients, this may include aquatic therapy, tai chi or yoga. All exercise programs should include a resistance exercise component.

Perhaps one of the biggest barriers to implementing an exercise program for older individuals with OA is physicians themselves. In a survey of primary care physicians, geriatricians were among the medical specialties that counseled patients the least (22%) on aerobic exercise [11]. Recommendations for strength training were low among all physician groups, although doctors who exercise are more likely to counsel their patients to exercise [11]. In a balanced factorial experiment among primary care physicians in the USA who were presented with a case of diagnosed knee OA, only 30% made recommendations to the patient for exercise [12]. Physician education on how to prescribe exercise for the management of OA is a large unmet need which should be improved upon to optimize care for older arthritis patients.

The objective of pharmacologic treatment for OA is to manage symptoms, because there is not a single disease modifying OA agent on the market. Acetaminophen (≤3 g per day) remains first line therapy for OA [8, 13]. However, when acetaminophen is not sufficient to control OA symptoms, then nonsteroidal anti-inflammatory drugs (NSAIDs) may be recommended. Topical NSAIDs have minimal systemic side effects and are a very good option for older individuals with OA. Prescribing oral NSAIDs becomes much more complex. Oral NSAIDs have a greater impact on pain, stiffness, and physical function compared to acetaminophen, but worrisome side effects such as gastrointestinal bleeding, renal and cardiovascular toxicity often limit their use in the geriatric population [14]. The long-term use of NSAIDs for a chronic medical condition, such as OA, is generally not recommended for older patients (>75 years) because of these adverse effects [15]. However, if NSAIDs are to be used for the management of OA in an older patient, then using the lowest dose possible for the shortest amount of time possible is prudent. Data from a meta-analysis suggest a two to three-fold increase in relative risk of gastrointestinal complications with daily high dose NSAIDs compared to low or medium doses, except for celecoxib [16]. The use of concomitant gastroprotective agents, such as proton pump inhibitors, may decrease the GI risk but does not negate it. ESCEO recommends cycles of NSAIDs instead of "chronic" use which is a feasible approach for older patients although there are no specific recommendations on duration or dose cutoffs [17]. Some NSAIDs are considered higher risk or less cost-effective than others for older individuals. Indomethacin, in particular, is more likely than other NSAIDs to have adverse CNS effects and should be avoided in elderly patients [15]. Using an Osteoarthritis Policy Model, a recent investigation found naproxen and ibuprofen more cost-effective than opioids or celecoxib for the treatment of OA among multimorbid older adults [18]. Other oral analgesic agents such as opioids, duloxetine and tramadol may have a role for the management of OA in carefully selected older patients, although thoughtful consideration should be given to dosage and side effect monitoring because of the potential for these agents to cause dizziness, lower the seizure threshold, and cause severe constipation [8, 13, 15, 17].

Chondroitin sulfate (CS) and glucosamine sulfate (GS) are natural compounds containing glycosaminoglycans that have demonstrated some symptom amelioration in OA [19]. There is wide heterogeneity in the regulatory status and labeling of commercial forms of these compounds in the USA compared to Europe, which may be why the pooled results from several high quality studies have failed to demonstrate significant effects on pain [20]. The 2012 ACR guidelines do not universally recommend CS or GS for knee OA [21], but the 2003 EULAR guidelines do endorse their use [22]. More research is needed on these compounds before widespread use among older adults with OA can be universally recommended, although the general safety of CS and GS make them an attractive therapeutic option in this high risk population.

Intra-articular injections, either with corticosteroids or hyaluronic acid, may be a therapeutic strategy for older individuals with OA, particularly of the knee. The frequency with which intra-articular steroid injections are administered is generally determined by symptom severity. In an important OA study, patients with knee OA were randomized to receive intra-articular injections every 3 months with either 40 mg triamcinolone or saline [23]. No detrimental effects were observed to the knee structure or joint space at this dosing interval [23]. Further, the group that received intra-articular corticosteroid injections had significant improvements in pain and stiffness compared to saline injections [23]. A dosing interval of every 3–6 months for corticosteroid injections to manage OA is generally considered safe.

The routine use of hyaluronics for OA management is controversial as evidenced by the varied recommendations from key professional societies [8]. In a recent systematic review and meta-analysis of 137 randomized controlled trials of adults with knee OA, all intra-articular therapies (corticosteroid, hyaluronic acid, or placebo) were superior in improving pain, stiffness, and function compared to oral agents (acetaminophen, diclofenac, ibuprofen, naproxen, celecoxib, oral placebo) [24]. Of note, in this evaluation even intra-articular placebo was comparable to oral therapies which raise interesting questions about the placebo-effect in OA trials and perhaps other pain pathways involved in OA [24]. In general, intra-articular therapies are a great therapeutic option for older individuals with OA because of their effectiveness and relative safety, although, for multi-joint OA, this is not a practical approach.

20.2.1.4 Surgical Management of OA

Surgical management for OA becomes an option once medical therapies have been exhausted. As of 2010, the prevalence of total hip replacements and total knee replacements among 80-year-old Americans was 5.26 and 10.38 %, respectively [25]. Treatment with total knee replacement can alleviate pain and improve function. Ninety-five patients with knee OA were randomized to receive total knee replacement (mean age 65.8 ± 8.7 years) or nonsurgical treatment (mean age 67.0 ± 8.7 years) which consisted of five interventions: exercise, education, dietary advice, use of insoles and pain medication. The surgical intervention group demonstrated superior pain relief and functional improvement after 12 months compared to nonsurgical treatment. Interestingly, the nonsurgical intervention group still had significant improvement in pain and function with only 26 % progressing to total knee replacement the following year [26]. As expected, the serious adverse events in the surgical group were higher [26]. The data for arthroscopic debridement of OA affected joints or meniscectomy is more controversial with randomized controlled trials showing similar benefit to sham control or optimized physical and medical therapies [27, 28].

Ultimately, the decision regarding surgery for OA management requires careful consideration of surgical risk versus quality of life and functional benefits. For older individuals who often have multiple joints affected by OA, the implication of post-operative immobility, pain and rehabilitation on other arthritic joints should also be considered. Importantly, OA nonsurgical management should be continued post-operatively in order to maintain the health of all joints affected with OA.

20.2.2 Rheumatoid Arthritis

20.2.2.1 Epidemiology

An estimated 0.5–1 % of the population in the USA has rheumatoid arthritis (RA), and the largest proportion of these patients are older adults [29]. The Rochester Epidemiology Project of Olmsted County suggests there has been an increase in the overall incidence of RA among adult women from 1995 to 2007 compared to the previous 4 decades with a peak annual incidence of RA among individuals aged 65–74 years (89 per 100,000) [30]. Although late-age onset RA remains less common, the estimated annual incidence in the USA among those aged ≥85 years is 54 per 100,000 people is still markedly higher than the youngest age group (18–34 years) with an incidence of 8.7 per 100,000 [30].

20.2.2.2 Clinical Features and Differential Diagnosis in Older Individuals

The hallmark clinical feature of RA is a symmetric inflammatory polyarthritis which involves the small joints of the hands, wrists, and feet. Patients typically recount a history of morning stiffness, joint swelling, and systemic constitutional symptoms. This may occur with an indolent course over several months or with sudden onset. There have been conflicting reports of the elderly or late-age onset RA phenotype in the literature, but it is undisputable that the full spectrum of clinical manifestations of RA can present in older individuals [31–34]. Most importantly, RA can be equally as severe in the old as in the young with erosions, joint destruction, and profound disability occurring within just 3 years after diagnosis [35].

The 2010 ACR/EULAR classification criteria for rheumatoid arthritis apply to all age groups and provide a scoring system to diagnose definite RA based on synovitis, autoantibodies, evidence of systemic inflammation, and duration of symptoms [36]. Importantly, other causes of arthritis must be ruled out before applying these RA classification criteria, and thus the differential diagnosis for polyarthritis in an older individual should be considered carefully. OA and RA often occur concomitantly in older individuals. Bony hypertrophy from Heberden's and Bouchard's nodes can make clinical assessment of synovitis challenging, so evaluation for other features of RA becomes critical. The presence of prolonged morning stiffness, MCP and wrist arthritis, autoantibodies and inflammatory synovial fluid are important clues to the presence of RA even in a patient with multi-joint OA. Crystalline arthropathies (gout, pseudogout) are common RA mimics in older individuals, especially in their more advanced phases when multiple joints are involved. Tophaceous deposits may be mistaken for rheumatoid nodules or Heberden's and Bouchard's nodes. In such cases, joint aspiration and synovial fluid analysis for the presence or absence of monosodium urate and/or calcium pyrophosphate crystals are necessary to make the correct diagnosis. Remitting seronegative symmetrical synovitis with pitting edema syndrome (RS3PE) is a rare inflammatory arthritis which occurs almost exclusively in individuals over the age of 60. RS3PE is an RA mimic that does not progress to joint erosions or deformities. Patients with RS3PE respond very well to therapy with corticosteroids, but the association between RS3PE and malignancy obligates evaluation for an occult cancer [37]. Finally, other autoimmune conditions which have arthritis as a key component and occur with frequency in older individuals, namely dermatomyositis, scleroderma and Sjogren's syndrome, should be considered if additional rheumatic features such as skin rash, sicca, muscle weakness or Raynaud's are also present.

20.2.2.3 Laboratory Features in Older Individuals with RA

RA is a chronic autoimmune condition, and generally laboratory studies will reflect systemic inflammation. An unexplained anemia of chronic disease, thrombocytosis, and hypoalbuminemia in an older individual with articular symptoms should prompt consideration of RA. Rheumatoid factor (RF) is present in 50–90 % of patients with RA. However, it is also one of the most common autoantibodies found in the healthy elderly population without RA. The prevalence of RF in the general older population (≥60 years) ranges from 10 to 48 % [38–40]. RF lacks specificity for RA as it is found in a multitude of other common conditions. When presented with an older patient who has a positive RF and arthralgias, the following conditions should be considered in addition to RA: subacute bacterial endocarditis, paraproteinemias (monoclonal gammopathy of unknown significance, multiple myeloma), hepatitis C infection, cryoglobulinemia, and Sjogren's syndrome [41–43]. Anti-citrullinated peptide antibodies (ACPA), which include anti-cyclic citrullinated antibodies (anti-CCP), are much more specific for RA (up to 98 %) compared to RF [42, 44]. Therefore, ACPA may be more useful diagnostically for older patients. In addition to being specific for RA, ACPA antibodies are prognostic for aggressive erosive disease, even among older individuals [45–47].

In a study using data from the Department of Defense Serum Repository it was found that the preclinical period for RA, defined as the time during which RF and/or ACPA are positive but clinical symptoms are not present, lengthens as the age at RA diagnosis increases [48]. The clinical significance of this is not clear. However, it opens the door to interesting areas for future investigation regarding the interactions between an aging immune system, genetic and environmental exposures on the emergence of a clinical phenotype and autoantibodies in RA.

20.2.2.4 Cardiovascular Disease and RA

Cardiovascular disease (CVD) is common among older individuals, and it is the leading cause of death in RA [49]. Hence, this is an extremely important co-morbidity to be aware of while managing the care of an older RA patient. CVD can be subtle in RA. Individuals with RA are less likely to report angina and more likely to have unrecognized myocardial infarction and sudden cardiac death compared to age-matched individuals without RA [50]. Traditional cardiovascular risk factors should be carefully monitored in older RA patients and medications with associated cardiovascular risk (such as NSAIDs) used with extreme caution. Finally, there is an association between RA disease activity (joint pain severity and systemic inflammation) and CVD risk [51].

20.2.2.5 RA Management for the Older Patient

The treatment of RA has been revolutionized over the past 15 years. Early and appropriate treatment with disease modifying anti-rheumatic drugs (DMARDs) in order to achieve a goal of low disease activity or remission (treat to target) is now the standard of care for RA management. This approach is outlined in the 2015 ACR Guidelines for the Treatment of Rheumatoid Arthritis [52]. In these recent ACR guidelines, DMARDs should be selected based on disease severity, disease activity, and important co-morbidities [52]. There are no absolute contraindications to any DMARDs in older individuals, and the approach to RA management should never be adjusted based on advanced chronologic age alone. Yet older patients are significantly less likely to receive DMARDs compared to their younger counterparts despite data which support comparable disease severity and duration [53–56]. Older individuals (≥65 years) with RA who are not seen by a rheumatologist are more likely to be treated with glucocorticoids alone and not prescribed DMARDs [57].

The observation of decreased use of DMARDs in the elderly has multiple etiologies; however, lack of DMARD efficacy in older RA patients is not among them. In a recent study of 151 methotrexate naïve older RA patients (mean age 75 years) in whom an aggressive treat to target approach using methotrexate, TNFα-inhibitors (TNFi), and/or tocilizumab was utilized, there was a high treatment adherence rate (76%) and 50% achieved structural remission (change in van der Hejde-modified total Sharp score ≤0.5), 63% achieved functional remission (HAQ-DI ≤0.5), and 51% achieved low disease activity (DAS28-ESR ≤3.2) over 52 weeks [58]. The most common serious adverse events were infections which occurred in 13% of patients and required discontinuation of RA therapy in only three patients [58]. Modern day RA therapeutics can be effective in the elderly and remission can be achieved in this age group. This study is commendable in that it begins to explore the application of current treatment paradigms to older RA patients with co-morbidities. It opens the door for future studies to examine intensive (or less intensive) treatment regimens specific to older RA patients.

Co-morbidities, risk of infection, and drug interactions are all important considerations in DMARD selection for older RA patients. In addition, we propose the following medication precautions. Methotrexate remains the first line DMARD for all patients with RA regardless of age. Potential methotrexate hepatotoxicity can be worsened by concomitant medications (such as statins) or fatty infiltration of the liver, issues not uncommon among older individuals.

Methotrexate is renally excreted, and creatinine should be calculated for all older patients in whom it is being considered and doses adjusted as appropriate [59]. Of particular importance in older individuals are methotrexate-induced CNS side effects such as headache, altered mood, or memory impairment [60]. This rare complication has been described primarily among older RA patients (>60 years) and should be monitored for closely in this population.

Leflunomide shares many of the same adverse effects as methotrexate in terms of hepatotoxicity and cytopenias. However, the gastrointestinal side effects of leflunomide can be severe and indolent in older individuals. Anorexia, nausea, and diarrhea may occur with drug initiation or in a subtle manner in the weeks following even small dose escalations. Weight loss in the absence of gastrointestinal symptoms has been attributed to leflunomide and often prompts fruitless, but expensive and exhaustive, evaluations for malignancy and infections [61]. The mechanism for leflunomide-associated weight loss is not known, but it seems to occur predominately in older individuals. Awareness of these leflunomide toxicities in older RA patients can prevent extensive and invasive workups.

Glucocorticoids are often used in the treatment of RA, typically as a bridge to DMARD therapy. The use of low-dose glucocorticoids chronically (defined as ≤10 mg/day prednisone equivalent), usually in combination with synthetic (non-biologic) DMARD therapy, is controversial. There are data which suggest improvements in structural outcomes and symptom severity with low-dose steroid use [62]. The risks with corticosteroids are well established in older patients and include infection osteoporosis, hyperglycemia, hypertension, and cataracts. However, many glucocorticoid side effects correspond with high doses [63]. The risk benefit ratio of low-dose glucocorticoids, specifically for older RA patients, has not been assessed. We propose that the risk assessment for the use of low-dose prednisone in older individuals with RA may be unique. In elderly RA patients, co-morbidities, infection risk, and specific DMARD toxicities may limit the use of synthetic and biologic DMARDs in select older patients. Therefore, in very specific cases, low-dose prednisone may be a reasonable option. Future research regarding the utility of low-dose glucocorticoid therapy and algorithms for its use (or not) in older RA patients will be important to guide future recommendations.

Biologic DMARDs have revolutionized the treatment of RA. TNFi have demonstrated equal efficacy among older and younger RA patients with a comparable safety profile regardless of age [64, 65]. Risk of infection is always a concern when treating older RA patients with TNFi. Whether or not infection risk with TNFi is influenced by age alone remains a matter of debate. A large retrospective cohort study of older Canadian RA patients (>66 years) in a nested case–control analyses demonstrated an increased risk of infection associated with TNFi, although the greatest infectious risk was attributed to prednisone with an associated dose response [66]. In a study using data from the US Medicare and Medicaid population, the rate of serious infections among older RA patients on TNFi was found to occur at a constant rate (~1–4 infections per 100 person years) above the rate predicted by age, co-morbidity, and other factors that contribute to infections independent of exposure to biologics [67]. These data support the observation that the increased risk of infection with TNFi is constant across age groups, although the background risk of infection is higher among older individuals in general. In summary, older RA patients should be educated about infections and closely monitored for infections while on treatment with TNFi, but this general risk alone should not be a reason to withhold TNFi therapy from the elderly.

Rituximab is an attractive biologic option for older individuals with RA because of the ease of administration. In a study of 1709 RA patients treated with rituximab from a French multicenter prospective cohort, patients in the 65–75 year age group had the highest percentage of responders at 12 months [68]. Patients in the >75 year age group had the lowest response rates. The incidence of severe infections was highest in the oldest age group (26.5%) and decreased accordingly (19.5% age 65–74 years; 6.8% 50–64 years; 5% <50 years) in the younger strata [68]. It cannot be established if the increased number of infections was attributable to rituximab or aging alone from these data.

Tocilizumab, an IL-6 inhibitor, demonstrated a good short-term safety profile among a retrospective cohort of older (≥65 years) French RA patients; however, after 6 months of treatment older RA patients were less likely to have a high EULAR response category (representing low disease activity) compared to their younger counterparts [69]. Tofacitinib, a janus kinase inhibitor, is the first oral biologic agent. There are no data specifically regarding the use of tofacitinib in older RA patients, but the very high rates of zoster infection with this biologic agent are worthy of consideration in an elderly population [70, 71]. There are no data specifically for the use of abatacept or anakinra among older RA patients.

Screening for latent tuberculosis (TB) risk is always advised before starting any biologic therapy. Among older RA patients, a positive TB screen (PPD or quantiferonTB gold testing) will raise important clinical management issues regarding treatment with isoniazid (INH), which carries considerable risk of hepatitis among older individuals [72]. Data using a Markov decision analytic model examining the risk of INH versus the risk of TB reactivation found that withholding prophylaxis prior to TNFi may be an appropriate option in low-risk elderly RA patients [73]. These decisions need to be considered carefully and discussed with the patient and family members.

In summary, while risks associated with traditional and biologic DMARD treatment in older RA patients are real, these are generally manageable and preventable with careful patient selection, education, and close monitoring. The risk of undertreating older adults with RA is significant and may lead to CVD, precipitous functional decline, and poor quality of life.

20.2.2.6 Special Considerations in Older Patients with RA

Older RA patients have a higher prevalence of age related syndromes (cognitive impairment, depression, falls, urinary incontinence, malnutrition) compared to younger RA patients [74]. Risk factors for the presence of geriatric syndromes among elderly RA patients include high RA disease activity, long disease duration, and functional impairment as measured by the Health Assessment Questionnaire (HAQ) [74]. Functional impairment, as measured by HAQ, increases with age among the general population and is highest among female RA patients over age 70 [75, 76]. Evaluation for geriatric syndromes is not routine practice for rheumatologists. Further, it is not included as a component of instruments frequently used to measure RA disease activity, such as the CDAI or DAS28. Such instruments focus primarily on the number of tender and swollen joints, ESR/CRP values and general disease activity impressions alone. These authors propose that consideration of geriatric syndromes in the routine assessment of older individuals with RA by rheumatologists when evaluating disease activity could have important benefits. For example, when making a decision about the treatment regimen for an 87-year-old RA patient, if cognitive impairment is recognized then complicated RA regimens, such as triple therapy with methotrexate, sulfasalazine, and hydroxychloroquine would be quickly ruled out. However, if cognition is not considered in the evaluation of an older RA patient with mild-moderate cognitive impairment, then this issue may be easily overlooked. Geriatric syndromes are intimately tied to RA because of the synergistic effects on functional status, nutrition, and co-morbidities. There is great opportunity for research in care models and care delivery systems which incorporate co-management of RA and geriatric syndromes to optimize the health of this vulnerable population. See Chap. 8, for additional information on detection of geriatric syndromes suitable for research and clinical care.

Work disability can be a serious problem for individuals with RA. In a study using data from the National Data Bank for Rheumatic Diseases, a longitudinal study of RA outcomes, a sample of approximately 2500 patients with RA age 55–64 years demonstrated significantly higher rates of premature work cessation and lower employment rates compared to age-matched controls [77]. As expected, early workforce withdrawal had a significant impact on the financial security of these patients in their retirement years [77].

In a subsequent study (from the same data source) using a nested case–control design, older age was the most prominent predictor of work disability among individuals with RA [78]. These findings demonstrate the effect of this chronic disease on finances, work satisfaction, quality of life, and retirement planning for individuals aging with RA as they transition into the seventh and eighth decades of life. Health care providers should recognize these issues that are unique to older RA patients in order to formulate comprehensive, yet feasible, treatment plans for their geriatric patients.

20.3 Myositis and Myopathy in Older Individuals

20.3.1 Idiopathic Inflammatory Myopathies

20.3.1.1 Epidemiology

Muscular weakness is a common complaint among older individuals. The differential diagnosis for weakness is broad and includes nutritional deficiencies, poor conditioning, frailty, and metabolic derangements such as thyroid dysfunction or anemia. However, objective findings such as rash, fever, dyspnea, dysphagia, elevation in creatine kinase (CK), and measurable impairments in muscular strength should raise red flags for a systemic autoimmune myopathic process.

The idiopathic inflammatory myopathies (IIM), which include dermatomyositis, polymyositis, and immune-mediated necrotizing myopathies, are relatively rare with an estimated incidence of 1.16–19/million/year and prevalence of 2.4–33.8 per 100,000 individuals [79]. The incidence of IIM increases with age and peaks in 35–44 and 55–64 year old age groups [80–82]. Age is an important predictor of mortality in IIM and may convey a poorer prognosis overall with regard to treatment response [83–85].

20.3.1.2 Clinical Features of IIM in Older Adults

Few studies have investigated the clinical presentation and phenotype of IIM among older individuals. A retrospective study of 23 older (median age 69 years) patients with IIM compared to younger (age <65 years) adults found similar frequencies of myalgias, muscle weakness, skin manifestations, and interstitial lung disease [84]. Older patients had more esophageal dysfunction [84]. A case–control study of 21 older IIM patients (mean age 69.9 years) compared to 21 younger (mean age 46.4 years) patients yielded similar findings with the exception of lower CK at diagnosis among the older group [86].

The association between IIM and cancer is well established with advanced age being a key risk factor. Individuals with cancer-associated myositis are generally older, have a dermatomyositis phenotype and shorter survival [84, 86–88]. In a retrospective study of 139 patients with a new diagnosis of

dermatomyositis, 8.6% were diagnosed with cancer within 12 months. Age at dermatomyositis onset was significantly older (by more than 15 years) among those who developed a malignancy compared to those who did not [89]. The risk of malignancy with IMM is thought to be greatest within the first year of diagnosis and does not normalize to the general population even after 5 years [90]. Therefore, a careful and thorough search for cancer should be performed in older individuals who develop a new IIM, particularly dermatomyositis.

20.3.2 Statins and Myopathy

At least 60–80% of Medicare beneficiaries with coronary heart disease are currently on statin therapy [91]. Overall, statin-induced myopathy is rare with a spectrum of myotoxicities that range from mild myalgias without CK elevation to rhabdomyolysis [92, 93]. Genetic variants and undiagnosed metabolic myopathies can predispose individuals to statin-associated myopathy [94–96]. Additional risk factors for the development of high CK levels while on treatment with a statin include older age (>65 years), diabetes, and male gender [97]. Several medications frequently prescribed for older patients such as verapamil, macrolide antibiotics, and amiodarone may also increase the risk of statin myotoxicity [98].

The National Lipid Association Statin Safety Assessment Task Force recommends obtaining baseline CK levels in adults at high risk for developing a statin-related myotoxicity [99]. Older adults, particularly those with polypharmacy or on medications which may increase myotoxicity risk when given concomitantly with a statin, fall into this category. Repeat CK measurements are not necessary unless the patient develops muscle symptoms. The presence of intolerable muscle symptoms, with or without CK elevation, should prompt discontinuation of the drug. In most instances, this should be sufficient to resolve the statin myopathy within a relatively short period of time (<2 months). Then if the symptoms resolve, a thoughtful discussion with the patient, the generalist, and cardiologist about the long-term benefit and burden of reinstituting a statin must occur so the patient's goals of care can be honored.

In cases of persistent muscle symptoms, despite termination of statin therapy, the patient may be suffering from an autoimmune process that is a distinct clinical entity from self-limited statin-associated myopathy and can be further evaluated with serologic testing. Specifically, patients should be tested for antibodies to 3-hydroxy-3-methylglutaryl-coenzyme A reductase (anti-HMGCR). The presence of these antibodies is highly suggestive of an immune-mediated necrotizing myopathy that may have been "unmasked" in the presence of statin therapy. Individuals with anti-HMGCR myopathy have proximal muscle weakness, very high CK levels (mean 10,000 IU/L) and a necrotizing myopathy on muscle biopsy [100, 101]. Additionally, despite its name, anti-HMGCR antibodies are frequently, but not always, associated with statin-triggered autoimmune myopathy. In fact, studies have shown that 33–56 % of anti-HMGCR-positive patients had no prior exposure to statins [101, 102]. It is not yet known what triggers the IIM in these non-statin exposed individuals. Although there is no established age association with anti-HMGCR at this time, it is clear that the prevalence of statin exposure increases with age, thereby placing older individuals at disproportionate risk.

20.3.3 Inclusion Body Myositis

Inclusion body myositis (IBM) is a common mimic of inflammatory myositis in older adults. It rarely occurs among individuals less than age 50, and it has a male predominance [103]. Slow, progressive, asymmetric muscular weakness is common and can initially appear very similar to polymyositis. However, IBM has key clinical features which distinguish it from the inflammatory myopathies, such as distal weakness in the wrist and deep finger flexors with sparing of wrist and finger extensors. Facial weakness and dysphagia may also be present [103–105]. A diagnosis of IBM can be made on the basis of clinical features, muscle pathology and new biomarkers with relatively high specificity but varying sensitivity, according to current diagnostic categories [106]. Distinguishing IBM from IIM is extremely important because immunosuppressive and immunomodulatory agents, which are highly effective in treating IIM, have not shown efficacy in IBM and may be detrimental [104]. Resistance exercise and orthoses are the primary treatment modalities for IBM [107].

20.3.4 An Approach to Diagnosis and Management of Older Patients with Myopathy

When faced with an older patient who has symptoms of weakness, we propose a systematic approach to diagnosis and management. Diagnostic precision is key because without an accurate diagnosis the wrong or unnecessary treatment may be prescribed to an elderly frail individual which could be devastating. Although diagnostic testing in this evaluation may be extensive and include imaging and invasive procedures, such as muscle biopsy and EMG/NCS, the acquisition of data will be valuable when teasing out the source of this vague common complaint in older patients.

On physical exam the pattern of *objective* weakness (proximal vs distal) can narrow the differential diagnosis if it is consistent with IIM, IBM, or spinal cord pathology (myelopathy). The presence of a new rash, Raynaud's phenomenon,

inflammatory arthritis with synovitis or cuticular abnormalities (abnormal nailfold capillary microscopy) in an older individual with muscular complaints suggests an immune-mediated process. A thorough review of a patient's medication and supplement lists, particularly the presence (or absence) of statin therapy, may reveal a single myotoxic agent or medications which when used together predispose to myopathy. Laboratory data, namely myositis-specific autoantibodies, thyroid studies, and CK measurements, are incredibly useful although these need to be interpreted in the context of the clinical picture. Normal or very minor CK elevations in older patients with sarcopenia, low BMI, and weakness may be highly significant. Similarly, elevated CK (above the upper limit of normal) in a very physically active older individual with high muscle mass, normal strength and who engages in resistance training may be a normal finding.

Therapeutic interventions for myopathy in older adults are targeted at the disease process. For IIM (including anti-HMGCR immune-mediated necrotizing myopathy), immunosuppression with corticosteroids, methotrexate, intravenous immunoglobulins, and other agents is standard of care. Adverse events which may be seen more frequently in older individuals include volume overload, infection (typical and opportunistic), cognitive impairment, and anorexia. Regular surveillance for these complications should be conducted routinely.

Resistance exercise should be a part of the treatment plan for every patient with IIM or IBM. Multiple studies, including randomized controlled trials, have demonstrated safety and efficacy of resistance exercise in IIM and IBM [108, 109]. Little is known specifically about how to tailor resistance training programs to the needs of older adults with myopathy, and this is an important area for future investigation. We propose that a resistance exercise program with a focus on large muscle groups (legs, back, chest) in order to improve functional mobility and increase muscular strength should be prescribed routinely for older individuals with myopathy as a standard part of their treatment plan.

20.4 Vasculitis in Older Individuals

20.4.1 Giant Cell Arteritis and Polymyalgia Rheumatica

Giant cell arteritis (GCA) is a systemic inflammatory disease that occurs almost exclusively in the elderly. It is the most common form of systemic vasculitis in older persons in North America with an annual incidence which is highest among those over age 70 [110, 111]. Common symptoms of cranial GCA are headache, jaw claudication, and diplopia with the latter two symptoms having the highest positive predictive value for a positive temporal artery biopsy [112]. Jaw claudication is a red flag in older patients, because it is associated with a high likelihood of visual symptoms in GCA [113]. Large-vessel GCA may occur with cranial GCA or independently. Large-vessel GCA can present with indolent non-specific symptoms such as arthralgias, myalgias, fever, and/or limb claudication. GCA should always be considered in the evaluation of an older patient with fever of unknown origin or unexplained laboratory evidence of inflammation (high ESR/CRP, hypoalbuminemia, anemia of chronic inflammation) and systemic symptoms [114]. An accurate diagnosis of GCA is important in order to avoid unnecessarily treating older patients with high dose corticosteroids. Temporal artery biopsies (bilateral, >1 cm length) and imaging of the aorta can provide important data for diagnostic certainty [115–118]. MRI, CT angiography, or PET-CT can be useful to demonstrate aortitis in a patient in whom GCA is suspected but the temporal artery biopsy is negative or in a patient presenting with signs and symptoms of large-vessel GCA alone.

The association between GCA and varicella-zoster (VZV) infection has been an area of great interest as of recent. Exciting studies have demonstrated VZV antigen in temporal artery biopsies of patients with confirmed GCA and among those with biopsy-negative GCA [119–121]. At this time, routine treatment with anti-viral agents is not part of standard of care management for GCA nor are temporal artery biopsies routinely assessed for VZV antigens. As this story unfolds it could have important ramifications for diagnosis and management of GCA in the future.

Corticosteroids, starting at a dose of 1 mg/kg, are still first line treatment for GCA [122]. Yet more than half of patients with GCA experience two or more adverse steroid-associated events with the majority being bone fractures [123]. The well-established morbidity of corticosteroids in older individuals makes the recent advances in steroid-sparing therapies for GCA encouraging. There are data that support the use of methotrexate in GCA. However, the overall effect size of methotrexate for GCA is modest, and the use of methotrexate has not translated into fewer steroid-associated side effects [124]. The same caveats apply to the use of methotrexate in older patients with GCA as for older individuals with RA. Tociliziumab has shown great promise as a steroid-sparing agent for GCA and large-vessel vasculitis [125–127]. Transaminitis, neutropenia, and infections have been observed during treatment with tocilizumab for GCA [125, 127].

In a systemic disease which generates robust inflammation and primarily utilizes a therapy that is fraught with complications in older individuals, it is not surprising that additional co-morbidities are common. Patients with GCA are at increased risk (compared to non-GCA age-matched individuals) for infections, particularly in the first 6 months after diagnosis [128]. GCA patients are also more likely to be hospitalized for pneumonia, hip fracture, and stroke than those without GCA [127]. During hospitalization, GCA patients are more likely to have inpatient complications, namely delirium, adrenal insufficiency, deep vein thrombosis, and pulmonary embolism [127]. The mechanism for increased risk of venous thromboembolism in GCA is not known, but the phenomenon appears to be a real trend [129]. Small, retrospective studies have suggested the low-dose aspirin may be beneficial in GCA as its use was associated with decreased risk of vision loss and stroke [130]. However, there have not been any randomized controlled trials to establish the safety and efficacy of aspirin as adjuvant therapy in GCA [131].

GCA is a disease of older individuals and when managing elderly GCA patients (>70 years) it is our opinion that the following issues are considered. In the context of high dose steroids, close monitoring and frequent follow-up can be helpful to regularly assess for complications which may occur suddenly, namely infections, delirium, changes in blood pressure, and hyperglycemia. Appropriate initiation of bone protective strategies and counseling on fall risk should be addressed at every visit. Due to the increased thromboembolic risk associated with GCA, patients and their family members should be advised and educated about this risk. If an older GCA patient is hospitalized, appropriate prophylaxis for thromboembolic disease should be utilized. We recommend that a prescription for physical therapy and/or an exercise program is provided to older patients at the time of GCA diagnosis in order to combat steroid myopathy, fat gain, and muscle loss associated with corticosteroids. There has been little research on how to prevent musculoskeletal complications from corticosteroids among older GCA patients, and this is an area of research which is desperately needed.

Polymyalgia rheumatica (PMR) is a systemic inflammatory condition which presents with disabling pain and stiffness in the shoulder and hip girdle regions. It occurs almost exclusively in individuals over the age of 50 with an incidence that increases with age (mean age onset 73 years) [132, 133]. There is a relationship between PMR and GCA. Approximately 40–60 % of patients with GCA have PMR, and 16–21 % of patients with PMR have GCA [134].

The diagnosis of PMR in an older individual can be challenging because there are many mimics such as malignancy, chronic infections, and other inflammatory musculoskeletal conditions. The new 2012 Provisional Classification Criteria developed by ACR/EULAR include the key components of PMR: age (≥50 years), abnormal ESR and/or CRP, morning stiffness, and bilateral shoulder symptoms [135]. However, it is well recognized that early in the disease course, late-age onset RA can look clinically just like PMR. Therefore, the absence of ACPA, RF, and other joint symptoms (i.e., inflammatory arthritis of the small joints of the hands and feet) increase the likelihood of a PMR diagnosis by the 2012 ACR/EULAR criteria [135]. ACPA, in particular, have shown value in distinguishing late-age onset RA from PMR. In a study of 57 late-age onset RA patients, 49 PMR patients, and 24 aged healthy controls it was found that 65 % of late-age onset RA patients were positive for ACPA while none of the PMR or healthy controls were [136]. Therefore, serologic testing for ACPA is an important part of the evaluation for PMR in older individuals.

Low-dose corticosteroids remain the mainstay of treatment for PMR. The 2015 ACR/EULAR recommendations for the management of PMR acknowledge the morbidity of corticosteroids in older individuals and endorse some key geriatric practices and principles to minimize toxicity [137]. For example, comprehensive assessment of co-morbidities and frequent physician visits with direct and easy access to providers are strategies advised by these recommendations [137]. In that regard, Chap. 8, describes basic elements for evaluating and tracking the common problems likely to be encountered in this population.

20.4.2 ANCA-Associated Vasculitis

The ANCA-associated vasculitides (AAV) include granulomatosis with polyangiitis (GPA, Wegener's), microscopic polyangiitis, and eosinophilic granulomatosis with polyangiitis (Churg–Strauss syndrome). Although AAV is rare in the general population, there is an increased incidence in older age groups [138]. The spectrum of organ involvement is similar among older and younger individuals with AAV [139]. GCA is often on the differential diagnosis of an older patient presenting with fever, headache, myalgias, and systemic inflammatory symptoms. In a descriptive study of 22 patients with newly diagnosed AAV after age 75, 18 % had undergone TA biopsy prior to AAV diagnosis [139]. However, in retrospect there were clues to the diagnosis of AAV in these older individuals, namely hematuria, neuropathy, and otolaryngologic manifestations of GPA [139]. ANCA testing can be very helpful in the evaluation of an older patient with systemic inflammatory signs and symptoms.

The treatment paradigm for AAV is the same for older and younger individuals. Life and organ threatening manifestation of vasculitis are managed with induction therapy (cyclophosphamide or rituximab) followed by long-term immunosuppressive maintenance therapy. Older individuals are particularly susceptible to cyclophosphamide toxicities such as leukopenia and infection [140]. A recent randomized controlled trial of older patients (≥65 years) with systemic necrotizing vasculitis (93 % AAV) demonstrated that an induction protocol using <u>lower</u> doses of cyclophosphamide and corticosteroids than conventional protocols was comparable in terms of efficacy [141]. Importantly, there were fewer serious adverse events in the low-dose cyclophosphamide group [141]. Rituximab as an induction agent for AAV

in an older individual is an attractive option because of the lower risk of cytopenias and less frequent monitoring that is required compared to cyclophosphamide. There are data which support the use of rituximab in older individuals with AAV, although more studies are needed in order to confirm dosing regimens and intervals for maintenance [142]. The decision to treat an older patient with severe renal failure from AAV and requiring dialysis can be challenging. Renal recovery is a realistic expectation even for older patients with AAV if appropriate treatment is initiated [143]. See Chap. 25 for discussion of the special considerations around dialysis decisions in older patients.

20.5 Connective Tissue Disease and Raynaud's in Older Individuals

20.5.1 Raynaud's Phenomenon in Older Individuals

Cold hands and feet are common complaints among older individuals. However, a careful history and physical exam will distinguish between cold hands and Raynaud's phenomenon (RP). RP is characterized by recurrent vasospasm of the fingers and toes in response to stress or cold exposure. Primary RP is a benign process, usually among young women (<40 years of age), and it is characterized by symmetric bilateral RP, normal laboratory studies (negative autoantibodies), and normal physical exam (no evidence of ischemia, normal nailfold capillaroscopy) [144]. Often primary RP will diminish with time and age.

The new onset of RP in individuals over age 40 years should prompt investigation for a systemic inflammatory condition, because late-age onset RP is strongly associated with the development of such [145–147]. When presented with an older patient with RP, a careful history can determine the age of onset. Physical exam should focus on evaluation for features of connective tissues disease (scleroderma, lupus, myositis, etc.) and mimics of RP (atherosclerosis, hyperviscosity syndromes, malignancy, medication effects) with close attention to the vascular exam and nailfold capillaries [148]. Evaluation of autoantibodies may be a helpful guide to longitudinal monitoring for the development of systemic autoimmune disease, such as scleroderma, in older patients with new RP [149].

20.5.2 Late-Age Onset Scleroderma

Scleroderma or systemic sclerosis (SSc) is a relatively rare condition across all age groups with a prevalence of 240 patients per 1 million US adults, and a peak age of onset between 40 and 50 years old [150, 151]. However, incident disease after age 60 is not uncommon with at least one study demonstrating a peak incidence in Caucasian women occurring between the ages of 65–74 years [150, 151]. Older patients with late-age onset SSc (≥65 years of age) are at increased risk for pulmonary hypertension, cardiac disease, muscle weakness, and renal impairment compared to those with onset of disease at younger ages [152]. Pulmonary hypertension, in particular, should be screened for regularly in the older SSc population. A relationship between SSc and malignancy has been clearly identified, particularly among individuals with antibodies against RNA polymerase III [153]. Given the increased overall prevalence of malignancy in the elderly, the new onset of SSc features in an older individual should prompt a comprehensive cancer evaluation as well [154].

20.5.3 Late-Age Onset Systemic Lupus Erythematosus

The incidence of systemic lupus erythematosus (SLE) after age 50 is estimated to be between 3 and 18 % [155–157]. Although SLE is predominately seen in women, advanced age decreases this gender gap [158]. The phenotype of late-age onset SLE is heterogenous and most manifestations in younger patients have also been described in older individuals [158, 159]. When considering a diagnosis of late-age onset SLE it is particularly important to exclude drug-induced lupus. Many of the medications implicated in drug-induced lupus are commonly used in older individuals such as procainamide, hydralazine, carbamazepine, methyldopa, minocycline, interferon-alpha, TNFi agents and rarely beta-blockers [160]. There are no age-specific recommendations regarding management of SLE. Hydroxychloroquine (HCQ) is a cornerstone of therapy for SLE. Careful attention should be paid to HCQ dosage in older SLE patients, as this should be based on weight (not exceeding 6.5 mg/kg/day) and creatinine clearance to minimize risk of retinal toxicity [161, 162]. The risk of HCQ retinopathy may not be associated with age, but it clearly increases with duration of therapy [163]. Therefore, it is important to considering total cumulative exposure of HCQ when determining screening intervals for older SLE patients.

20.5.4 Primary Sjogren's Syndrome

Primary Sjogren's syndrome (SS) is a systemic inflammatory condition that affects the salivary and lacrimal glands. The hallmark feature is sicca or dryness of the eyes and mouth. The overall prevalence of SS is about 0.5–1 %, and estimates in older populations are higher [164, 165]. Dry mouth is very common in the geriatric population. Older individuals (without SS) have less salivary secretion and higher rates of xerostomia then younger individuals [166, 167]. This is due to a combination of factors including age related decreases in acinar cells and medications (anti-histamines, SSRIs, diuretics, etc.) [166, 167]. Since sicca symptoms alone lack specificity for SS, it becomes particularly important to obtain objective evidence of an immune-mediated process when considering a diagnosis of SS for an older patient. The proposed new classification criteria for SS emphasize objective evidence of inflammation and/or autoimmunity with the presence of autoantibodies (anti-SSA, anti-SSB, RF, ANA), focal lymphocytic sialadenitis (labial salivary gland biopsy), or high ocular staining score demonstrating keratoconjunctivitis sicca [168]. Cancer, namely lymphoma, is a concern in SS regardless of age. Red flags which should prompt a more thorough investigation for an occult lymphoproliferative process in an older patient with SS include low C4 levels, new development of vasculitis, monoclonal gammopathy, and cryoglobulinemia [169]. Treatment of SS in elderly patients does not differ from management in younger adults, and in both cases the goals are to manage glandular and extra-glandular manifestations, prevent organ damage, and decrease morbidity and mortality [170].

References

1. Rasch EK, Hirsch R, Paulose-Ram R, Hochberg MC. Prevalence of rheumatoid arthritis in persons 60 years of age and older in the United States: effect of different methods of case classification. Arthritis Rheum. 2003;48(4):917–26.
2. Landre-Beauvais AJ. The first description of rheumatoid arthritis. Unabridged text of the doctoral dissertation presented in 1800. Joint Bone Spine. 2001;68(2):130–43.
3. Lawrence RC, Felson DT, Helmick CG, Arnold LM, Choi H, Deyo RA, et al. Estimates of the prevalence of arthritis and other rheumatic conditions in the United States. Part II. Arthritis Rheum. 2008;58(1):26–35.
4. Vincent GK, Velkoff VA. The next four decades: the older population in the United States: 2010 to 2050. Washington: U.S. Dept. of Commerce, Economics and Statistics Administration, U.S. Census Bureau; 2010.
5. Losina E, Paltiel AD, Weinstein AM, Yelin E, Hunter DJ, Chen SP, et al. Lifetime medical costs of knee osteoarthritis management in the United States: impact of extending indications for total knee arthroplasty. Arthritis Care Res (Hoboken). 2015;67(2):203–15.
6. Xie F, Thumboo J, Li SC. True difference or something else? Problems in cost of osteoarthritis studies. Semin Arthritis Rheum. 2007;37(2):127–32.
7. Altman R, Asch E, Bloch D, Bole G, Borenstein D, Brandt K, et al. Development of criteria for the classification and reporting of osteoarthritis. Classification of osteoarthritis of the knee. Diagnostic and Therapeutic Criteria Committee of the American Rheumatism Association. Arthritis Rheum. 1986;29(8):1039–49.
8. Cutolo M, Berenbaum F, Hochberg M, Punzi L, Reginster JY. Commentary on recent therapeutic guidelines for osteoarthritis. Semin Arthritis Rheum. 2015;44(6):611–7.
9. Christensen R, Bartels EM, Astrup A, Bliddal H. Effect of weight reduction in obese patients diagnosed with knee osteoarthritis: a systematic review and meta-analysis. Ann Rheum Dis. 2007;66(4): 433–9.

10. Juhl C, Christensen R, Roos EM, Zhang W, Lund H. Impact of exercise type and dose on pain and disability in knee osteoarthritis: a systematic review and meta-regression analysis of randomized controlled trials. Arthritis Rheumatol. 2014;66(3):622–36.

11. Abramson S, Stein J, Schaufele M, Frates E, Rogan S. Personal exercise habits and counseling practices of primary care physicians: a national survey. Clin J Sport Med. 2000;10(1):40–8.

12. Maserejian NN, Fischer MA, Trachtenberg FL, Yu J, Marceau LD, McKinlay JB, et al. Variations among primary care physicians in exercise advice, imaging, and analgesics for musculoskeletal pain: results from a factorial experiment. Arthritis Care Res (Hoboken). 2014;66(1):147–56.

13. Makris UE, Abrams RC, Gurland B, Reid MC. Management of persistent pain in the older patient: a clinical review. JAMA. 2014;312(8):825–36.

14. Zhang W, Jones A, Doherty M. Does paracetamol (acetaminophen) reduce the pain of osteoarthritis? A meta-analysis of randomised controlled trials. Ann Rheum Dis. 2004;63(8):901–7.

15. By the American Geriatrics Society 2015 Beers Criteria Update Expert Panel. American Geriatrics Society 2015 Updated Beers Criteria for potentially inappropriate medication use in older adults. J Am Geriatr Soc. 2015;63(11):2227–46.

16. Castellsague J, Riera-Guardia N, Calingaert B, Varas-Lorenzo C, Fourrier-Reglat A, Nicotra F, et al. Individual NSAIDs and upper gastrointestinal complications: a systematic review and meta-analysis of observational studies (the SOS project). Drug Saf. 2012;35(12):1127–46.

17. Bruyere O, Cooper C, Pelletier JP, Branco J, Luisa Brandi M, Guillemin F, et al. An algorithm recommendation for the management of knee osteoarthritis in Europe and internationally: a report from a task force of the European Society for Clinical and Economic Aspects of Osteoporosis and Osteoarthritis (ESCEO). Semin Arthritis Rheum. 2014;44(3):253–63.

18. Katz JN, Smith SR, Collins JE, Solomon DH, Jordan JM, Hunter DJ, et al. Cost-effectiveness of nonsteroidal anti-inflammatory drugs and opioids in the treatment of knee osteoarthritis in older patients with multiple comorbidities. Osteoarthritis Cartilage. 2016;24:409–18.

19. Henrotin Y, Marty M, Mobasheri A. What is the current status of chondroitin sulfate and glucosamine for the treatment of knee osteoarthritis? Maturitas. 2014;78(3):184–7.

20. Towheed TE, Maxwell L, Anastassiades TP, Shea B, Houpt J, Robinson V, et al. Glucosamine therapy for treating osteoarthritis. Cochrane Database Syst Rev. 2005;(2):CD002946.

21. Hochberg MC, Altman RD, April KT, Benkhalti M, Guyatt G, McGowan J, et al. American College of Rheumatology 2012 recommendations for the use of nonpharmacologic and pharmacologic therapies in osteoarthritis of the hand, hip, and knee. Arthritis Care Res (Hoboken). 2012;64(4):465–74.

22. Jordan KM, Arden NK, Doherty M, Bannwarth B, Bijlsma JW, Dieppe P, et al. EULAR Recommendations 2003: an evidence based approach to the management of knee osteoarthritis: Report of a Task Force of the Standing Committee for International Clinical Studies Including Therapeutic Trials (ESCISIT). Ann Rheum Dis. 2003;62(12):1145–55.

23. Raynauld JP, Buckland-Wright C, Ward R, Choquette D, Haraoui B, Martel-Pelletier J, et al. Safety and efficacy of long-term intraarticular steroid injections in osteoarthritis of the knee: a randomized, double-blind, placebo-controlled trial. Arthritis Rheum. 2003;48(2):370–7.

24. Bannuru RR, Schmid CH, Kent DM, Vaysbrot EE, Wong JB, McAlindon TE. Comparative effectiveness of pharmacologic interventions for knee osteoarthritis: a systematic review and network meta-analysis. Ann Intern Med. 2015;162(1):46–54.

25. Maradit Kremers H, Larson DR, Crowson CS, Kremers WK, Washington RE, Steiner CA, et al. Prevalence of total hip and knee replacement in the United States. J Bone Joint Surg Am. 2015;97(17):1386–97.

26. Skou ST, Roos EM, Laursen MB, Rathleff MS, Arendt-Nielsen L, Simonsen O, et al. A randomized, controlled trial of total knee replacement. N Engl J Med. 2015;373(17):1597–606.

27. Kirkley A, Birmingham TB, Litchfield RB, Giffin JR, Willits KR, Wong CJ, et al. A randomized trial of arthroscopic surgery for osteoarthritis of the knee. N Engl J Med. 2008;359(11):1097–107.

28. Moseley JB, O'Malley K, Petersen NJ, Menke TJ, Brody BA, Kuykendall DH, et al. A controlled trial of arthroscopic surgery for osteoarthritis of the knee. N Engl J Med. 2002;347(2):81–8.

29. Helmick CG, Felson DT, Lawrence RC, Gabriel S, Hirsch R, Kwoh CK, et al. Estimates of the prevalence of arthritis and other rheumatic conditions in the United States. Part I. Arthritis Rheum. 2008;58(1):15–25.

30. Myasoedova E, Crowson CS, Kremers HM, Therneau TM, Gabriel SE. Is the incidence of rheumatoid arthritis rising? Results from Olmsted County, Minnesota, 1955–2007. Arthritis Rheum. 2010;62(6):1576–82.

31. van Schaardenburg D, Breedveld FC. Elderly-onset rheumatoid arthritis. Semin Arthritis Rheum. 1994;23(6):367–78.

32. van der Heijde DM, van Riel PL, van Leeuwen MA, van't Hof MA, van Rijswijk MH, van de Putte LB. Older versus younger onset rheumatoid arthritis: results at onset and after 2 years of a prospective followup study of early rheumatoid arthritis. J Rheumatol. 1991;18(9):1285–9.

33. Kavanaugh AF. Rheumatoid arthritis in the elderly: is it a different disease? Am J Med. 1997;103(6A):40S–8.

34. Glennas A, Kvien TK, Andrup O, Karstensen B, Munthe E. Recent onset arthritis in the elderly: a 5 year longitudinal observational study. J Rheumatol. 2000;27(1):101–8.

35. Pease CT, Bhakta BB, Devlin J, Emery P. Does the age of onset of rheumatoid arthritis influence phenotype? A prospective study of outcome and prognostic factors. Rheumatology (Oxford). 1999;38(3):228–34.

36. Aletaha D, Neogi T, Silman AJ, Funovits J, Felson DT, Bingham 3rd CO, et al. 2010 Rheumatoid arthritis classification criteria: an American College of Rheumatology/European League Against Rheumatism collaborative initiative. Arthritis Rheum. 2010;62(9):2569–81.

37. McCarty DJ, O'Duffy JD, Pearson L, Hunter JB. Remitting seronegative symmetrical synovitis with pitting edema. RS3PE syndrome. JAMA. 1985;254(19):2763–7.

38. Juby AG, Davis P. Prevalence and disease associations of certain autoantibodies in elderly patients. Clin Invest Med. 1998;21(1):4–11.

39. Manoussakis MN, Stavropoulos ED, Germanidis GS, Papasteriades CA, Garalea KL, Dontas AS, et al. Soluble interleukin-2 receptors and autoantibodies in the serum of healthy elderly individuals. Autoimmunity. 1990;7(2–3):129–37.

40. Ramos-Casals M, Garcia-Carrasco M, Brito MP, Lopez-Soto A, Font J. Autoimmunity and geriatrics: clinical significance of autoimmune manifestations in the elderly. Lupus. 2003;12(5):341–55.

41. Araujo IR, Ferrari TC, Teixeira-Carvalho A, Campi-Azevedo AC, Rodrigues LV, Guimaraes Junior MH, et al. Cytokine signature in infective endocarditis. PLoS One. 2015;10(7), e0133631.

42. Palosuo T, Tilvis R, Strandberg T, Aho K. Filaggrin related antibodies among the aged. Ann Rheum Dis. 2003;62(3):261–3.

43. van Schaardenburg D, Lagaay AM, Otten HG, Breedveld FC. The relation between class-specific serum rheumatoid factors and age in the general population. Br J Rheumatol. 1993;32(7):546–9.

44. Schellekens GA, Visser H, de Jong BA, van den Hoogen FH, Hazes JM, Breedveld FC, et al. The diagnostic properties of

rheumatoid arthritis antibodies recognizing a cyclic citrullinated peptide. Arthritis Rheum. 2000;43(1):155–63.

45. Meyer O, Labarre C, Dougados M, Goupille P, Cantagrel A, Dubois A, et al. Anticitrullinated protein/peptide antibody assays in early rheumatoid arthritis for predicting five year radiographic damage. Ann Rheum Dis. 2003;62(2):120–6.

46. Kroot EJ, de Jong BA, van Leeuwen MA, Swinkels H, van den Hoogen FH, van't Hof M, et al. The prognostic value of anti-cyclic citrullinated peptide antibody in patients with recent-onset rheumatoid arthritis. Arthritis Rheum. 2000;43(8):1831–5.

47. Forslind K, Ahlmen M, Eberhardt K, Hafstrom I, Svensson B, BARFOT Study Group. Prediction of radiological outcome in early rheumatoid arthritis in clinical practice: role of antibodies to citrullinated peptides (anti-CCP). Ann Rheum Dis. 2004;63(9): 1090–5.

48. Majka DS, Deane KD, Parrish LA, Lazar AA, Baron AE, Walker CW, et al. Duration of preclinical rheumatoid arthritis-related autoantibody positivity increases in subjects with older age at time of disease diagnosis. Ann Rheum Dis. 2008;67(6):801–7.

49. del Rincon ID, Williams K, Stern MP, Freeman GL, Escalante A. High incidence of cardiovascular events in a rheumatoid arthritis cohort not explained by traditional cardiac risk factors. Arthritis Rheum. 2001;44(12):2737–45.

50. Maradit-Kremers H, Crowson CS, Nicola PJ, Ballman KV, Roger VL, Jacobsen SJ, et al. Increased unrecognized coronary heart disease and sudden deaths in rheumatoid arthritis: a population-based cohort study. Arthritis Rheum. 2005;52(2):402–11.

51. Mackey RH, Kuller LH, Deane KD, Walitt BT, Chang YF, Holers VM, et al. Rheumatoid arthritis, anti-cyclic citrullinated peptide positivity, and cardiovascular disease risk in the women's health initiative. Arthritis Rheumatol. 2015;67(9):2311–22.

52. Singh JA, Saag KG, Bridges Jr SL, Akl EA, Bannuru RR, Sullivan MC, et al. 2015 American College of Rheumatology guideline for the treatment of rheumatoid arthritis. Arthritis Rheumatol. 2016;68(1):1–26.

53. Tutuncu Z, Reed G, Kremer J, Kavanaugh A. Do patients with older-onset rheumatoid arthritis receive less aggressive treatment? Ann Rheum Dis. 2006;65(9):1226–9.

54. Schmajuk G, Schneeweiss S, Katz JN, Weinblatt ME, Setoguchi S, Avorn J, et al. Treatment of older adult patients diagnosed with rheumatoid arthritis: improved but not optimal. Arthritis Rheum. 2007;57(6):928–34.

55. Ogasawara M, Tamura N, Onuma S, Kusaoi M, Sekiya F, Matsudaira R, et al. Observational cross-sectional study revealing less aggressive treatment in Japanese elderly than nonelderly patients with rheumatoid arthritis. J Clin Rheumatol. 2010;16(8):370–4.

56. DeWitt EM, Lin L, Glick HA, Anstrom KJ, Schulman KA, Reed SD. Pattern and predictors of the initiation of biologic agents for the treatment of rheumatoid arthritis in the United States: an analysis using a large observational data bank. Clin Ther. 2009;31(8):1871–80. discussion 1858.

57. Yazdany J, Tonner C, Schmajuk G, Lin GA, Trivedi AN. Receipt of glucocorticoid monotherapy among Medicare beneficiaries with rheumatoid arthritis. Arthritis Care Res (Hoboken). 2014;66(10):1447–55.

58. Sugihara T, Ishizaki T, Hosoya T, Iga S, Yokoyama W, Hirano F, et al. Structural and functional outcomes of a therapeutic strategy targeting low disease activity in patients with elderly-onset rheumatoid arthritis: a prospective cohort study (CRANE). Rheumatology (Oxford). 2015;54(5):798–807.

59. Bressolle F, Bologna C, Kinowski JM, Sany J, Combe B. Effects of moderate renal insufficiency on pharmacokinetics of methotrexate in rheumatoid arthritis patients. Ann Rheum Dis. 1998;57(2):110–3.

60. Wernick R, Smith DL. Central nervous system toxicity associated with weekly low-dose methotrexate treatment. Arthritis Rheum. 1989;32(6):770–5.

61. Coblyn JS, Shadick N, Helfgott S. Leflunomide-associated weight loss in rheumatoid arthritis. Arthritis Rheum. 2001;44(5):1048–51.

62. Kavanaugh A, Wells AF. Benefits and risks of low-dose glucocorticoid treatment in the patient with rheumatoid arthritis. Rheumatology (Oxford). 2014;53(10):1742–51.

63. Da Silva JA, Jacobs JW, Kirwan JR, Boers M, Saag KG, Ines LB, et al. Safety of low dose glucocorticoid treatment in rheumatoid arthritis: published evidence and prospective trial data. Ann Rheum Dis. 2006;65(3):285–93.

64. Fleischmann RM, Baumgartner SW, Tindall EA, Weaver AL, Moreland LW, Schiff MH, et al. Response to etanercept (Enbrel) in elderly patients with rheumatoid arthritis: a retrospective analysis of clinical trial results. J Rheumatol. 2003;30(4):691–6.

65. Fleischmann R, Baumgartner SW, Weisman MH, Liu T, White B, Peloso P. Long term safety of etanercept in elderly subjects with rheumatic diseases. Ann Rheum Dis. 2006;65(3):379–84.

66. Widdifield J, Bernatsky S, Paterson JM, Gunraj N, Thorne JC, Pope J, et al. Serious infections in a population-based cohort of 86,039 seniors with rheumatoid arthritis. Arthritis Care Res (Hoboken). 2013;65(3):353–61.

67. Curtis JR, Xie F, Chen L, Muntner P, Grijalva CG, Spettell C, et al. Use of a disease risk score to compare serious infections associated with anti-tumor necrosis factor therapy among high-versus lower-risk rheumatoid arthritis patients. Arthritis Care Res (Hoboken). 2012;64(10):1480–9.

68. Payet S, Soubrier M, Perrodeau E, Bardin T, Cantagrel A, Combe B, et al. Efficacy and safety of rituximab in elderly patients with rheumatoid arthritis enrolled in a French Society of Rheumatology registry. Arthritis Care Res (Hoboken). 2014;66(9):1289–95.

69. Pers YM, Schaub R, Constant E, Lambert J, Godfrin-Valnet M, Fortunet C, et al. Efficacy and safety of tocilizumab in elderly patients with rheumatoid arthritis. Joint Bone Spine. 2015;82(1): 25–30.

70. Winthrop KL, Yamanaka H, Valdez H, Mortensen E, Chew R, Krishnaswami S, et al. Herpes zoster and tofacitinib therapy in patients with rheumatoid arthritis. Arthritis Rheumatol. 2014;66(10):2675–84.

71. Lee EB, Fleischmann R, Hall S, Wilkinson B, Bradley JD, Gruben D, et al. Tofacitinib versus methotrexate in rheumatoid arthritis. N Engl J Med. 2014;370(25):2377–86.

72. Nolan CM, Goldberg SV, Buskin SE. Hepatotoxicity associated with isoniazid preventive therapy: a 7-year survey from a public health tuberculosis clinic. JAMA. 1999;281(11):1014–8.

73. Hazlewood GS, Naimark D, Gardam M, Bykerk V, Bombardier C. Prophylaxis for latent tuberculosis infection prior to anti-tumor necrosis factor therapy in low-risk elderly patients with rheumatoid arthritis: a decision analysis. Arthritis Care Res (Hoboken). 2013;65(11):1722–31.

74. Chen YM, Chen LK, Lan JL, Chen DY. Geriatric syndromes in elderly patients with rheumatoid arthritis. Rheumatology (Oxford). 2009;48(10):1261–4.

75. Krishnan E, Sokka T, Hakkinen A, Hubert H, Hannonen P. Normative values for the Health Assessment Questionnaire disability index: benchmarking disability in the general population. Arthritis Rheum. 2004;50(3):953–60.

76. Sokka T, Kautiainen H, Hannonen P, Pincus T. Changes in Health Assessment Questionnaire disability scores over five years in patients with rheumatoid arthritis compared with the general population. Arthritis Rheum. 2006;54(10):3113–8.

77. Allaire S, Wolfe F, Niu J, Lavalley M, Michaud K. Work disability and its economic effect on 55–64-year-old adults with rheumatoid arthritis. Arthritis Rheum. 2005;53(4):603–8.

78. Allaire S, Wolfe F, Niu J, LaValley MP, Zhang B, Reisine S. Current risk factors for work disability associated with rheumatoid arthritis: recent data from a US national cohort. Arthritis Rheum. 2009;61(3):321–8.

79. Meyer A, Meyer N, Schaeffer M, Gottenberg JE, Geny B, Sibilia J. Incidence and prevalence of inflammatory myopathies: a systematic review. Rheumatology (Oxford). 2015;54(1):50–63.

80. Christopher-Stine L, Plotz PH. Adult inflammatory myopathies. Best Pract Res Clin Rheumatol. 2004;18(3):331–44.

81. Medsger Jr TA, Dawson Jr WN, Masi AT. The epidemiology of polymyositis. Am J Med. 1970;48(6):715–23.

82. Oddis CV, Conte CG, Steen VD, Medsger Jr TA. Incidence of polymyositis-dermatomyositis: a 20-year study of hospital diagnosed cases in Allegheny County, PA 1963–1982. J Rheumatol. 1990;17(10):1329–34.

83. Koh ET, Seow A, Ong B, Ratnagopal P, Tjia H, Chng HH. Adult onset polymyositis/dermatomyositis: clinical and laboratory features and treatment response in 75 patients. Ann Rheum Dis. 1993;52(12):857–61.

84. Marie I, Hatron PY, Levesque H, Hachulla E, Hellot MF, Michon-Pasturel U, et al. Influence of age on characteristics of polymyositis and dermatomyositis in adults. Medicine (Baltimore). 1999;78(3):139–47.

85. Hochberg MC, Lopez-Acuna D, Gittelsohn AM. Mortality from polymyositis and dermatomyositis in the United States, 1968–1978. Arthritis Rheum. 1983;26(12):1465–71.

86. Pautas E, Cherin P, Piette JC, Pelletier S, Wechsler B, Cabane J, et al. Features of polymyositis and dermatomyositis in the elderly: a case-control study. Clin Exp Rheumatol. 2000;18(2):241–4.

87. Danko K, Ponyi A, Constantin T, Borgulya G, Szegedi G. Long-term survival of patients with idiopathic inflammatory myopathies according to clinical features: a longitudinal study of 162 cases. Medicine (Baltimore). 2004;83(1):35–42.

88. Marie I, Hachulla E, Hatron PY, Hellot MF, Levesque H, Devulder B, et al. Polymyositis and dermatomyositis: short term and long-term outcome, and predictive factors of prognosis. J Rheumatol. 2001;28(10):2230–7.

89. de Souza FH, Shinjo SK. Newly diagnosed dermatomyositis in the elderly as predictor of malignancy. Rev Bras Reumatol. 2012;52(5):713–21.

90. Hill CL, Zhang Y, Sigurgeirsson B, Pukkala E, Mellemkjaer L, Airio A, et al. Frequency of specific cancer types in dermatomyositis and polymyositis: a population-based study. Lancet. 2001;357(9250):96–100.

91. Yun H, Safford MM, Brown TM, Farkouh ME, Kent S, Sharma P, et al. Statin use following hospitalization among Medicare beneficiaries with a secondary discharge diagnosis of acute myocardial infarction. J Am Heart Assoc. 2015;4(2), e001208. doi:10.1161/JAHA.114.001208.

92. Gaist D, Rodriguez LA, Huerta C, Hallas J, Sindrup SH. Lipid-lowering drugs and risk of myopathy: a population-based follow-up study. Epidemiology. 2001;12(5):565–9.

93. Antons KA, Williams CD, Baker SK, Phillips PS. Clinical perspectives of statin-induced rhabdomyolysis. Am J Med. 2006;119(5):400–9.

94. SEARCH Collaborative Group, Link E, Parish S, Armitage J, Bowman L, Heath S, et al. SLCO1B1 variants and statin-induced myopathy—a genomewide study. N Engl J Med. 2008;359(8):789–99.

95. Patel J, Superko HR, Martin SS, Blumenthal RS, Christopher-Stine L. Genetic and immunologic susceptibility to statin-related myopathy. Atherosclerosis. 2015;240(1):260–71.

96. Vladutiu GD, Simmons Z, Isackson PJ, Tarnopolsky M, Peltier WL, Barboi AC, et al. Genetic risk factors associated with lipid-lowering drug-induced myopathies. Muscle Nerve. 2006;34(2):153–62.

97. Chan J, Hui RL, Levin E. Differential association between statin exposure and elevated levels of creatine kinase. Ann Pharmacother. 2005;39(10):1611–6.

98. Christopher-Stine L. Statin myopathy: an update. Curr Opin Rheumatol. 2006;18(6):647–53.

99. McKenney JM, Davidson MH, Jacobson TA, Guyton JR, National Lipid Association Statin Safety Assessment Task Force. Final conclusions and recommendations of the National Lipid Association Statin Safety Assessment Task Force. Am J Cardiol. 2006;97(8A):89C–94.

100. Christopher-Stine L, Casciola-Rosen LA, Hong G, Chung T, Corse AM, Mammen AL. A novel autoantibody recognizing 200-kd and 100-kd proteins is associated with an immune-mediated necrotizing myopathy. Arthritis Rheum. 2010;62(9):2757–66.

101. Mammen AL, Chung T, Christopher-Stine L, Rosen P, Rosen A, Doering KR, et al. Autoantibodies against 3-hydroxy-3-methylglutaryl-coenzyme A reductase in patients with statin-associated autoimmune myopathy. Arthritis Rheum. 2011;63(3):713–21.

102. Allenbach Y, Drouot L, Rigolet A, Charuel JL, Jouen F, Romero NB, et al. Anti-HMGCR autoantibodies in European patients with autoimmune necrotizing myopathies: inconstant exposure to statin. Medicine (Baltimore). 2014;93(3):150–7.

103. Paltiel AD, Ingvarsson E, Lee DK, Leff RL, Nowak RJ, Petschke KD, et al. Demographic and clinical features of inclusion body myositis in North America. Muscle Nerve. 2015;52(4):527–33.

104. Benveniste O, Guiguet M, Freebody J, Dubourg O, Squier W, Maisonobe T, et al. Long-term observational study of sporadic inclusion body myositis. Brain. 2011;134(Pt 11):3176–84.

105. Michelle EH, Mammen AL. Myositis mimics. Curr Rheumatol Rep. 2015;17(10):63.

106. Lloyd TE, Mammen AL, Amato AA, Weiss MD, Needham M, Greenberg SA. Evaluation and construction of diagnostic criteria for inclusion body myositis. Neurology. 2014;83(5):426–33.

107. Alfano LN, Lowes LP. Emerging therapeutic options for sporadic inclusion body myositis. Ther Clin Risk Manag. 2015;11:1459–67.

108. Alexanderson H, Munters LA, Dastmalchi M, Loell I, Heimburger M, Opava CH, et al. Resistive home exercise in patients with recent-onset polymyositis and dermatomyositis – a randomized controlled single-blinded study with a 2-year followup. J Rheumatol. 2014;41(6):1124–32.

109. Alemo Munters L, Alexanderson H, Crofford LJ, Lundberg IE. New insights into the benefits of exercise for muscle health in patients with idiopathic inflammatory myositis. Curr Rheumatol Rep. 2014;16(7):429.

110. Hochberg MC, Silman AJ, Smolen JS, Weinblatt ME, Weisman MH, editors. Rheumatology. 4th ed. Spain: Elsevier Limited; 2008.

111. Chandran AK, Udayakumar PD, Crowson CS, Warrington KJ, Matteson EL. The incidence of giant cell arteritis in Olmsted County, Minnesota, over a 60-year period 1950–2009. Scand J Rheumatol. 2015;44(3):215–8.

112. Smetana GW, Shmerling RH. Does this patient have temporal arteritis? JAMA. 2002;287(1):92–101.

113. Singh AG, Kermani TA, Crowson CS, Weyand CM, Matteson EL, Warrington KJ. Visual manifestations in giant cell arteritis: trend over 5 decades in a population-based cohort. J Rheumatol. 2015;42(2):309–15.

114. Knockaert DC, Vanneste LJ, Bobbaers HJ. Fever of unknown origin in elderly patients. J Am Geriatr Soc. 1993;41(11):1187–92.

115. Breuer GS, Nesher R, Nesher G. Effect of biopsy length on the rate of positive temporal artery biopsies. Clin Exp Rheumatol. 2009;27(1 Suppl 52):S10–3.

116. Breuer GS, Nesher G, Nesher R. Rate of discordant findings in bilateral temporal artery biopsy to diagnose giant cell arteritis. J Rheumatol. 2009;36(4):794–6.

117. Khan A, Dasgupta B. Imaging in giant cell arteritis. Curr Rheumatol Rep. 2015;17(8):52.

118. Grossman C, Barshack I, Bornstein G, Ben-Zvi I. Is temporal artery biopsy essential in all cases of suspected giant cell arteritis? Clin Exp Rheumatol. 2015;33(2 Suppl 89):S-84-9.

119. Lavi E, Gilden D, Nagel M, White T, Grose C. Prevalence and distribution of VZV in temporal arteries of patients with giant cell arteritis. Neurology. 2015;85(21):1914–5.

120. Gilden D, White T, Khmeleva N, Heintzman A, Choe A, Boyer PJ, et al. Prevalence and distribution of VZV in temporal arteries of patients with giant cell arteritis. Neurology. 2015;84(19):1948–55.

121. Nagel MA, White T, Khmeleva N, Rempel A, Boyer PJ, Bennett JL, et al. Analysis of varicella-zoster virus in temporal arteries biopsy positive and negative for giant cell arteritis. JAMA Neurol. 2015;72(11):1281–7.

122. Weyand CM, Goronzy JJ. Clinical practice. Giant-cell arteritis and polymyalgia rheumatica. N Engl J Med. 2014;371(1):50–7.

123. Proven A, Gabriel SE, Orces C, O'Fallon WM, Hunder GG. Glucocorticoid therapy in giant cell arteritis: duration and adverse outcomes. Arthritis Rheum. 2003;49(5):703–8.

124. Mahr AD, Jover JA, Spiera RF, Hernandez-Garcia C, Fernandez-Gutierrez B, Lavalley MP, et al. Adjunctive methotrexate for treatment of giant cell arteritis: an individual patient data meta-analysis. Arthritis Rheum. 2007;56(8):2789–97.

125. Loricera J, Blanco R, Hernandez JL, Castaneda S, Mera A, Perez-Pampin E, et al. Tocilizumab in giant cell arteritis: multicenter open-label study of 22 patients. Semin Arthritis Rheum. 2015;44(6):717–23.

126. Loricera J, Blanco R, Castaneda S, Humbria A, Ortego-Centeno N, Narvaez J, et al. Tocilizumab in refractory aortitis: study on 16 patients and literature review. Clin Exp Rheumatol. 2014;32(3 Suppl 82):S79–89.

127. Unizony S, Arias-Urdaneta L, Miloslavsky E, Arvikar S, Khosroshahi A, Keroack B, et al. Tocilizumab for the treatment of large-vessel vasculitis (giant cell arteritis, Takayasu arteritis) and polymyalgia rheumatica. Arthritis Care Res (Hoboken). 2012; 64(11):1720–9.

128. Durand M, Thomas SL. Incidence of infections in patients with giant cell arteritis: a cohort study. Arthritis Care Res (Hoboken). 2012;64(4):581–8.

129. Avina-Zubieta JA, Bhole VM, Amiri N, Sayre EC, Choi HK. The risk of deep venous thrombosis and pulmonary embolism in giant cell arteritis: a general population-based study. Ann Rheum Dis. 2016;75(1):148–54.

130. Nesher G, Berkun Y, Mates M, Baras M, Rubinow A, Sonnenblick M. Low-dose aspirin and prevention of cranial ischemic complications in giant cell arteritis. Arthritis Rheum. 2004;50(4):1332–7.

131. Mollan SP, Sharrack N, Burdon MA, Denniston AK. Aspirin as adjunctive treatment for giant cell arteritis. Cochrane Database Syst Rev. 2014;8, CD010453.

132. Doran MF, Crowson CS, O'Fallon WM, Hunder GG, Gabriel SE. Trends in the incidence of polymyalgia rheumatica over a 30 year period in Olmsted County, Minnesota, USA. J Rheumatol. 2002;29(8):1694–7.

133. Gonzalez-Gay MA, Vazquez-Rodriguez TR, Lopez-Diaz MJ, Miranda-Filloy JA, Gonzalez-Juanatey C, Martin J, et al. Epidemiology of giant cell arteritis and polymyalgia rheumatica. Arthritis Rheum. 2009;61(10):1454–61.

134. Salvarani C, Cantini F, Hunder GG. Polymyalgia rheumatica and giant-cell arteritis. Lancet. 2008;372(9634):234–45.

135. Dasgupta B, Cimmino MA, Maradit-Kremers H, Schmidt WA, Schirmer M, Salvarani C, et al. 2012 provisional classification criteria for polymyalgia rheumatica: a European League Against Rheumatism/American College of Rheumatology collaborative initiative. Ann Rheum Dis. 2012;71(4):484–92.

136. Lopez-Hoyos M, Ruiz de Alegria C, Blanco R, Crespo J, Pena M, Rodriguez-Valverde V, et al. Clinical utility of anti-CCP antibodies in the differential diagnosis of elderly-onset rheumatoid arthritis and polymyalgia rheumatica. Rheumatology (Oxford). 2004;43(5): 655–7.

137. Dejaco C, Singh YP, Perel P, Hutchings A, Camellino D, Mackie S, et al. 2015 recommendations for the management of polymyalgia rheumatica: a European League Against Rheumatism/American College of Rheumatology collaborative initiative. Arthritis Rheumatol. 2015;67(10):2569–80.

138. Watts RA, Lane SE, Bentham G, Scott DG. Epidemiology of systemic vasculitis: a ten-year study in the United Kingdom. Arthritis Rheum. 2000;43(2):414–9.

139. Hoganson DD, From AM, Michet CJ. ANCA vasculitis in the elderly. J Clin Rheumatol. 2008;14(2):78–81.

140. Mouthon L, Le Toumelin P, Andre MH, Gayraud M, Casassus P, Guillevin L. Polyarteritis nodosa and Churg-Strauss angiitis: characteristics and outcome in 38 patients over 65 years. Medicine (Baltimore). 2002;81(1):27–40.

141. Pagnoux C, Quemeneur T, Ninet J, Diot E, Kyndt X, de Wazieres B, et al. Treatment of systemic necrotizing vasculitides in patients aged sixty-five years or older: results of a multicenter, open-label, randomized controlled trial of corticosteroid and cyclophosphamide-based induction therapy. Arthritis Rheumatol. 2015;67(4):1117–27.

142. Timlin H, Lee SM, Manno RL, Seo P, Geetha D. Rituximab for remission induction in elderly patients with ANCA-associated vasculitis. Semin Arthritis Rheum. 2015;45(1):67–9.

143. Manno RL, Seo P, Geetha D. Older patients with ANCA-associated vasculitis and dialysis dependent renal failure: a retrospective study. BMC Nephrol. 2015;16:88.

144. Koenig M, Joyal F, Fritzler MJ, Roussin A, Abrahamowicz M, Boire G, et al. Autoantibodies and microvascular damage are independent predictive factors for the progression of Raynaud's phenomenon to systemic sclerosis: a twenty-year prospective study of 586 patients, with validation of proposed criteria for early systemic sclerosis. Arthritis Rheum. 2008;58(12):3902–12.

145. Planchon B, Pistorius MA, Beurrier P, De Faucal P. Primary Raynaud's phenomenon. Age of onset and pathogenesis in a prospective study of 424 patients. Angiology. 1994;45(8):677–86.

146. Friedman EI, Taylor Jr LM, Porter JM. Late-onset Raynaud's syndrome: diagnostic and therapeutic considerations. Geriatrics. 1988;43(12):59–63. 67–70.

147. Pavlov-Dolijanovic S, Damjanov NS, Vujasinovic Stupar NZ, Radunovic GL, Stojanovic RM, Babic D. Late appearance and exacerbation of primary Raynaud's phenomenon attacks can predict future development of connective tissue disease: a retrospective chart review of 3,035 patients. Rheumatol Int. 2013;33(4): 921–6.

148. Ling SM, Wigley FM. Raynaud's phenomenon in older adults: diagnostic considerations and management. Drugs Aging. 1999;15(3):183–95.

149. Pavlov-Dolijanovic SR, Damjanov NS, Vujasinovic Stupar NZ, Baltic S, Babic DD. The value of pattern capillary changes and antibodies to predict the development of systemic sclerosis in patients with primary Raynaud's phenomenon. Rheumatol Int. 2013;33(12):2967–73.

150. Mayes MD, Lacey Jr JV, Beebe-Dimmer J, Gillespie BW, Cooper B, Laing TJ, et al. Prevalence, incidence, survival, and disease characteristics of systemic sclerosis in a large US population. Arthritis Rheum. 2003;48(8):2246–55.

151. Steen VD, Medsger Jr TA. Epidemiology and natural history of systemic sclerosis. Rheum Dis Clin North Am. 1990;16(1):1–10.

152. Manno RL, Wigley FM, Gelber AC, Hummers LK. Late-age onset systemic sclerosis. J Rheumatol. 2011;38(7):1317–25.

153. Shah AA, Hummers LK, Casciola-Rosen L, Visvanathan K, Rosen A, Wigley FM. Examination of autoantibody status and clinical features associated with cancer risk and cancer-associated scleroderma. Arthritis Rheumatol. 2015;67(4):1053–61.

154. Joseph CG, Darrah E, Shah AA, Skora AD, Casciola-Rosen LA, Wigley FM, et al. Association of the autoimmune disease scleroderma with an immunologic response to cancer. Science. 2014;343(6167):152–7.

155. Arnaud L, Mathian A, Boddaert J, Amoura Z. Late-onset systemic lupus erythematosus: epidemiology, diagnosis and treatment. Drugs Aging. 2012;29(3):181–9.

156. Font J, Pallares L, Cervera R, Lopez-Soto A, Navarro M, Bosch X, et al. Systemic lupus erythematosus in the elderly: clinical and immunological characteristics. Ann Rheum Dis. 1991;50(10):702–5.

157. Cervera R, Khamashta MA, Font J, Sebastiani GD, Gil A, Lavilla P, et al. Systemic lupus erythematosus: clinical and immunologic patterns of disease expression in a cohort of 1,000 patients. The European Working Party on Systemic Lupus Erythematosus. Medicine (Baltimore). 1993;72(2):113–24.

158. Boddaert J, Huong DL, Amoura Z, Wechsler B, Godeau P, Piette JC. Late-onset systemic lupus erythematosus: a personal series of 47 patients and pooled analysis of 714 cases in the literature. Medicine (Baltimore). 2004;83(6):348–59.

159. Padovan M, Govoni M, Castellino G, Rizzo N, Fotinidi M, Trotta F. Late onset systemic lupus erythematosus: no substantial differences using different cut-off ages. Rheumatol Int. 2007;27(8):735–41.

160. Katz U, Zandman-Goddard G. Drug-induced lupus: an update. Autoimmun Rev. 2010;10(1):46–50.

161. Durcan L, Clarke WA, Magder LS, Petri M. Hydroxychloroquine blood levels in systemic lupus erythematosus: clarifying dosing controversies and improving adherence. J Rheumatol. 2015;42(11):2092–7.

162. Jallouli M, Galicier L, Zahr N, Aumaitre O, Frances C, Le Guern V, et al. Determinants of hydroxychloroquine blood concentration variations in systemic lupus erythematosus. Arthritis Rheumatol. 2015;67(8):2176–84.

163. Wolfe F, Marmor MF. Rates and predictors of hydroxychloroquine retinal toxicity in patients with rheumatoid arthritis and systemic lupus erythematosus. Arthritis Care Res (Hoboken). 2010;62(6):775–84.

164. Botsios C, Furlan A, Ostuni P, Sfriso P, Andretta M, Ometto F, et al. Elderly onset of primary Sjogren's syndrome: clinical manifestations, serological features and oral/ocular diagnostic tests. Comparison with adult and young onset of the disease in a cohort of 336 Italian patients. Joint Bone Spine. 2011;78(2):171–4.

165. Haugen AJ, Peen E, Hulten B, Johannessen AC, Brun JG, Halse AK, et al. Estimation of the prevalence of primary Sjogren's syndrome in two age-different community-based populations using two sets of classification criteria: the Hordaland Health Study. Scand J Rheumatol. 2008;37(1):30–4.

166. Nagler RM, Hershkovich O. Relationships between age, drugs, oral sensorial complaints and salivary profile. Arch Oral Biol. 2005;50(1):7–16.

167. Nagler RM, Hershkovich O. Age-related changes in unstimulated salivary function and composition and its relations to medications and oral sensorial complaints. Aging Clin Exp Res. 2005;17(5):358–66.

168. Shiboski SC, Shiboski CH, Criswell L, Baer A, Challacombe S, Lanfranchi H, et al. American College of Rheumatology classification criteria for Sjogren's syndrome: a data-driven, expert consensus approach in the Sjogren's International Collaborative Clinical Alliance cohort. Arthritis Care Res (Hoboken). 2012;64(4):475–87.

169. Tzioufas AG, Boumba DS, Skopouli FN, Moutsopoulos HM. Mixed monoclonal cryoglobulinemia and monoclonal rheumatoid factor cross-reactive idiotypes as predictive factors for the development of lymphoma in primary Sjogren's syndrome. Arthritis Rheum. 1996;39(5):767–72.

170. Moerman RV, Bootsma H, Kroese FG, Vissink A. Sjogren's syndrome in older patients: aetiology, diagnosis and management. Drugs Aging. 2013;30(3):137–53.

Susan P. Bell and Michael W. Rich

21.1 Introduction

The number and proportion of adults over the age of 65 worldwide is increasing at a rapid rate due to improved sanitation, nutrition, access to health care, and medical advances in prevention, diagnosis, and treatment for both communicable and non-communicable diseases [1]. In the USA, 13 % of the current population is over the age of 65 and it is estimated that the proportion will increase to 19 % by the year 2030, including 19 million people aged 85 and older [2].

In parallel, the global burden of cardiovascular disease (CVD) has increased exponentially over the last 25 years despite remarkable advances in CVD prevention and treatment [1]. In the USA, approximately 40 million adults over the age of 65 report one or more cardiovascular (CV) disorders and CVD is the leading cause of major morbidity and mortality in that population [3]. Notably, although advancing age is the most potent predictor of CVD, it is a non-modifiable risk factor. Nonetheless, biological aging and the effects of aging on the CV system vary considerably from individual to individual, and there is evidence that behavioral factors, including diet, physical activity, and smoking, modulate the aging process and the incidence of age-related disease. It is therefore essential that cardiovascular providers understand the marked interactions between aging and CVD, the impact of co-existing disease processes, limitations of currently available evidence, and the inherent complexities involved in providing patient-centered care aligned with individual

patient preferences. This chapter examines the principal effects of aging on the CV system, geriatric factors that modulate CVD in older adults, and differences in the management of CVD in older compared to younger individuals.

21.2 Aging and the Heart

Biological aging has a fundamental effect on the development and progression of CVD through two different but synergistic mechanisms. Age-associated vascular changes do not independently cause vascular disease, but alterations in cellular and molecular mechanisms, especially those responsible for regeneration and response to stress, greatly increase the vulnerability of the heart and vasculature to the development of CVD [4, 5]. In addition, the longitudinal nature of aging allows for the accumulation of genetic risk factors, acquired risk factors (e.g., hypertension), lifestyle choices, and environmental factors, which taken together, greatly increase the likelihood of developing CVD with increasing age. Cardiovascular changes associated with aging are widespread and include alterations in both structure and function. Table 21.1 lists major changes in the heart, vasculature, hemodynamics, and response to exercise that impact the clinical presentation of CVD in older adults.

21.3 Traditional Cardiovascular Risk Factors

21.3.1 Hypertension

Age-associated increased central arterial stiffness, increased peripheral resistance, and impaired vascular reactivity contributed to hypertension being the most prevalent risk factor for CVD in older adults [6]. By age 75, approximately 80 % of women and 70 % of men in the USA are classified as hypertensive, yet they have the lowest rates of optimal control [7, 8]. With vascular aging, the systolic blood pressure

S.P. Bell, MBBS, MSCI (✉)
Division of Cardiovascular and Geriatric Medicine, Department of Medicine, Vanderbilt University School of Medicine, Center for Quality Aging, 2525 West End Avenue, Suite 350, Nashville, TN 37203, USA
e-mail: susan.p.bell@vanderbilt.edu

M.W. Rich, MD
Department of Medicine, Division of Cardiology, Washington University School of Medicine, 660 S. Euclid Ave., Campus Box 8086, St. Louis, MO 63110, USA

© Springer International Publishing Switzerland 2017
J.R. Burton et al. (eds.), *Geriatrics for Specialists*, DOI 10.1007/978-3-319-31831-8_21

Table 21.1 Cardiovascular changes associated with aging

Arterial structure and function
  Increased lumen size
  Increased wall thickness (intimal-media thickening)
  Increased calcification
  Increased tortuosity of large vessels
  Increased collagen cross-linking
  Degeneration and fragmentation of elastin
  Decreased endothelial function
  Increased stiffness of large and medium-sized arteries
  (decreased distensibility)

Cardiac anatomy
  Increased atrial size (LA>RA)
  Increased LV wall mass and thickness
  Increased LV stiffness (decreased compliance)
  LV fibrosis and collagen accumulation
  Degeneration (calcific) of valve leaflets and annulus
  Decreased LV cavity size and longitudinal shortening
  Fibrosis, calcification, and degeneration of conducting system
  Decline in number of sinoatrial node pacemaker cells

Hemodynamics
  Increase in systolic blood pressure
  Increase in pulse wave velocity
  Earlier reflection of pulse wave and augmentation of blood
  pressure in late systole
  Decrease in aortic peak flow velocity
  Reduction in peak LV filling rate
  Decreased ratio of early LV filling (E) to atrial filling (A)

Changes during exercise
  Decrease in maximum heart rate (220-age)
  Decline in heart rate variability
  Increase in atrial and ventricular ectopy
  Reduced cardiac output reserve
  Reduction in end systolic volume reserve
  Reduction in VO_2 Max
  Impaired peripheral vasodilation

LA left atrium, *RA* right atrium, *LV left ventricular*/ventricle, *A-V* atrioventricular, *VO2 Max* maximal oxygen consumption

Table 21.2 Clinical trials of hypertension in older adults

Trials	Risk reduction %					
	N	Age	CVA	CAD	CHF	All CVD
Australian [152]	582	60–69	33%	18%	NR	31%
EWPHE [153]	840	>60	36%	20%	22%	29%
Coope [154]	884	60–79	42%	−3%	32%	24%
STOP_HTN [155]	1627	70–84	47%	13%	51%	40%
MRC [156]	4396	65–74	25%	19%	NR	17%
HDFP [157]	2374	60–69	44%	15%	NR	16%
SHEP [158]	4736	≥60	33%	27%	55%	32%
SYST-Eur [159]	4695	≥60	42%	26%	36%	31%
STONE [160]	1632	60–79	57%	6%	68%	60%
Syst-China [161]	2394	≥60	38%	33%	38%	37%
HYVET [10]	3845	≥80	30%	28%	64%	34%
SPRINT [11]	9361	≥50	11%	12%	33%	25%

CAD coronary artery disease, *CHF* congestive heart failure, *CVA* cerebrovascular accident, *CVD* cardiovascular disease, *EWPHE* European Working Party on High Blood Pressure in the Elderly, *HDFP* Hypertension Detection and Followup Program, *MRC* Medical Research Council, *NR* not reported, *SHEP* Systolic Hypertension in the Elderly Program, *STONE* Shanghai Trial of Nifedipine in the Elderly, *STOP-HTN* Swedish Trial in Old Patients with Hypertension, *Syst-China* Systolic Hypertension in China, *Syst-Eur* Systolic Hypertension in Europe

increases progressively, whereas the diastolic blood pressure peaks at approximately age 50 and then plateaus before declining after 60 years of age in both men and women. As a result, isolated systolic hypertension (ISH, defined as systolic blood pressure over 140 mmHg and diastolic blood pressure below 90 mmHg) is the dominant form of hypertension in older adults. In turn, ISH is strongly associated with an increased risk for stroke, end-stage renal disease, myocardial infarction (MI), heart failure, and CV and all-cause mortality. While the treatment of hypertension at any age (including the very elderly), reduces CV and cerebrovascular events (Table 21.2), optimal treatment thresholds and target blood pressures have not been clearly defined [9, 10].

In the Hypertension in the Very Elderly Trial (HYVET), 3845 patients 80 years of age or older (mean 83.6 years, 60.5% women) with systolic blood pressure ≥160 mmHg were randomized to the diuretic indapamide 1.5 mg or matching placebo [10]. Perindopril or placebo was added as needed to achieve a target blood pressure <150/80 mmHg. The primary outcome was fatal or nonfatal stroke. After a mean follow-up of 1.8 years, active treatment was associated with a 30% reduction in the primary outcome, and reductions in secondary outcomes of incident heart failure and all-cause mortality. The results of HYVET led to a recommendation by several hypertension guideline committees to aim for a goal of <150 mmHg when treating systolic hypertension in patients ≥80 years of age.

More recently, the Systolic Blood Pressure Intervention Trial (SPRINT) randomized 9361 patients ≥50 years of age (28.2% ≥75 years of age) at increased cardiovascular risk (as defined by subclinical or clinical CVD, chronic kidney disease, 10-year risk of CVD ≥15% based on the Framingham Risk Score, and/or age ≥75 years) and with baseline systolic blood pressure 130–180 mmHg to intensive treatment (target blood pressure <120 mmHg) or standard treatment (target blood pressure <140 mmHg) [11]. Patients with diabetes mellitus, symptomatic heart failure in the preceding 6 months, recent acute coronary syndrome (ACS), prior stroke, orthostatic systolic blood pressure <110 mmHg, unintentional weight loss (a component of frailty), or residence in a nursing home or assisted living facility were excluded. Women and patients with multimorbidity were also under-represented. The primary outcome was a composite of myocardial infarction (MI), other ACS, stroke, heart failure, or cardiovascular death. The study was stopped prematurely at a median follow-up of 3.26 years due to a significant benefit of intensive treatment on the primary outcome (2.19% per year with standard treatment vs. 1.65% per year with intensive treatment, hazard ratio 0.75, 95% CI 0.69–0.89, $p < 0.001$). Outcomes were similar in patients ≥75 years of age compared to those <75 years but the absolute benefit was numerically greater in the older subgroup. All-cause mortality, CV mortality, and incident heart failure were significantly reduced with intensive treatment, but there was no effect on MI, ACS, or stroke. The number needed to treat for 1 year to prevent one primary outcome event was 185. The mean number of blood pressure medications was 1.8 in the standard treatment group and 2.8 in the intensive treatment group. Serious adverse events, including acute kidney injury, electrolyte abnormalities, hypotension, and syncope (but not injurious falls) were all significantly more frequent in the intensive therapy group. Annual rates of serious adverse events attributed to anti-hypertensive treatment were 1.44 % in the intensive therapy group and 0.77 % in the standard therapy group (number needed to harm 149). The incidence of adverse events was similar among patients older or younger than age 75. The effects of intensive treatment on quality of life and cognitive function have not yet been reported.

The implications of SPRINT for treatment of older adults with hypertension are uncertain, as the modest absolute benefit with respect to major CV events and death must be balanced against the potential for adverse events, increased burden of medications, and unknown impact on quality of life, functional status, and cognition. In addition, a substantial proportion of older adults would not have met the SPRINT inclusion/exclusion criteria, and the applicability of the findings to these individuals is unknown. Based on the results of HYVET and current guidelines, it is reasonable to treat individuals ≥75 years of age who are suitable candidates for anti-hypertensive drug therapy to a target systolic blood pressure of <140 mmHg (age 75–79 years) or <150 mmHg (age ≥80 years). More aggressive treatment should be individualized based on the clinical profile and patient preferences.

Management of hypertension in older adults is often complicated by orthostatic or post-prandial hypotension [12], which may be associated with light-headedness and increased risk for falls and syncope. In addition, "white coat" hypertension is common in older adults (i.e., office blood pressure higher than home blood pressure), and older individuals with stiff arteries may exhibit pseudohypertension (blood pressure measured by sphygmomanometer higher than central aortic pressure) [13, 14]. For these reasons, it is important to measure blood pressure in the sitting and standing positions and, when feasible, to obtain blood pressure readings in the home environment [12]. In some cases, 24-hour ambulatory blood pressure monitoring may be helpful in determining the presence and severity of hypertension, as well as the variability in blood pressure readings [15]. In patients with significant orthostatic hypotension (decline in systolic blood pressure ≥20 mmHg on standing), titration of anti-hypertensive therapy should be very gradual and should include periodic assessments of orthostatic blood pressure changes and evaluation for symptoms attributable to orthostasis.

21.3.2 Hyperlipidemia

Dyslipidemia remains an important risk factor for CVD in older adults up to age 85; after age 85, the association of lipid levels with CVD is less clear [16–18]. In addition, the strength of association between cholesterol levels and CVD declines with age, such that total cholesterol and LDL cholesterol become less predictive of CV events at older age. Factors affecting the relationship between cholesterol and CVD risk at increased age include survival bias among individuals with low CVD risk despite increased cholesterol levels, and the impact of co-existing diseases (e.g., malignancy, chronic inflammatory disorders) and malnutrition (a common condition in older adults). Statins are highly efficacious for the treatment of dyslipidemia, and numerous trials have documented the benefits of statins on CVD outcomes [19–22]. However, few patients over age 80 have been enrolled in these trials, and patients with complex comorbidity have been excluded. In addition, statin side effects, such as myalgias, may be more common in older adults, and there is weak evidence that statins may be associated with cognitive impairment in some individuals. Recognizing the paucity of evidence on statins in older patients, current guidelines recommend that treatment decisions consider anticipated benefits and adverse effects (including their time horizon), life expectancy, comorbidities, and individual treatment priorities [23]. In addition, the guidelines advise caution in using high intensity statin therapy in individuals over 75 years of age.

21.3.3 Diabetes Mellitus

Diabetes mellitus (DM) is a powerful and independent predictor of the development and progression of CVD in older adults, imparting an increase in relative risk of CAD of 1.4 in men and 2.1 in women 65 and older with a significant sex interaction (i.e., stronger association in women) [24]. Although the relative risk in individuals over the age of 65 is lower than in younger individuals with DM, the high prevalence of DM in older adults results in greater excess risk [25].

Management of CV risk in patients with DM should focus on treating co-existing CVD risk factors, including hypertension and dyslipidemia, which are present in 71 and 65 % of older diabetics, respectively [21]. Additionally, utilization of an angiotensin-converting enzyme inhibitor (ACE-I) in older adults with diabetes is effective for reducing CV mortality [26]. Regular physical activity and maintaining a healthy body weight should be encouraged. Additional recommendations for managing DM in older adults are provided in Chap. 23.

21.3.4 Smoking

Smoking accounts for 30% of the attributable risk of all strokes and 36% of first acute coronary events [27]. In older adults the prevalence of smoking decreases but it still remains a significant risk factor. Although the relative risk for MI or death as a result of smoking in an individual over the age of 70 is twice that of an individual age 55–60, older patients are less likely to receive smoking cessation counselling or interventions [28].

Individuals who smoke should be advised of the risks associated with smoking and given guidance on cessation strategies. Elderly individuals may be resistant to changing life-long habits, but the negative effects of continued smoking irrespective of age demand continued efforts to promote smoking cessation.

21.4 Geriatric Syndromes and Cardiovascular Disease

21.4.1 Multimorbidity

Multimorbidity, defined as the presence of 2 or more chronic conditions, increases exponentially with age and is present in over 70% of individuals 75 years or older [29]. By the age of 65, more than 60% of individuals have 2 or more chronic conditions, >25% have 4 or more chronic conditions, and nearly 10% have 6 or more conditions; by age 85, >50% of individuals have 4 or more chronic conditions and 25% have 6 or more conditions. The accumulation of chronic conditions culminates in a vastly heterogeneous population of older adults for whom balancing the management of multiple medical problems becomes paramount.

Among Medicare beneficiaries with CVD, the burden of multimorbidity is substantial; for example, over 50% of individuals with a diagnosis of heart failure or stroke have 5 or more co-existing chronic medical conditions [29]. In older adults with CVD, the most common concomitant non-CVD conditions are arthritis, anemia, and diabetes mellitus, with prevalence rates ranging from 40 to 50%. Other common conditions include chronic kidney disease, cognitive impairment, chronic obstructive lung disease, and depression, each of which much be considered when developing individual treatment strategies for the management of CVD [30].

21.4.2 Polypharmacy and Drug Interactions

Older adults with multimorbidity are frequently seen by numerous general and specialist providers which can result in competing management strategies and numerous prescriptions for medications. Polypharmacy, often defined as concomitant use of five or more medications, is associated with markedly increased risk for drug–drug interactions, drug–disease interactions, and therapeutic competition (the recommended treatment for one condition may adversely affect and/or compete with another co-existing condition) [31]. Approximately 50% of older adults are taking at least one medication with no active indication, and many of these drugs are initiated during hospitalization, such as stress ulcer prophylaxis and antipsychotics for delirium [32]. Careful medication reconciliation including prescribed medicines, over the counter pharmaceuticals, and herbal therapies should be performed at each provider interaction. Adverse consequences of polypharmacy including poor adherence, adverse drug events, hospitalization, and mortality are related not only to the number of medications but also to the regimen complexity, so attention should be given to limiting the number of medications as well as simplifying the dosing schedule [32–34].

Non-steroidal anti-inflammatory drugs (NSAIDs) are frequently taken by older adults to relieve burdensome pain or for treatment of arthritis. However, NSAIDs, including the cyclo-oxygenase 2 (COX-2) inhibitors, increase the risk of atherothrombotic vascular events and incident heart failure [35]. In addition, NSAIDs have adverse interactions with many CV medications, including diuretics, other anti-hypertensive agents, and antithrombotic drugs. NSAIDs have also been associated with worsening renal function and increased risk for gastrointestinal bleeding. For these reasons, the FDA and the American Heart Association suggest minimizing the use of NSAIDs when feasible, and using the lowest possible doses for the shortest period of time [36]. Polypharmacy and medication management are discussed in greater detail in Chap. 5.

21.4.3 Cognitive Impairment

Approximately 13% of community dwelling adults over the age of 65 have a diagnosis of dementia. However, the total burden of disease is likely to be much higher due to under-recognition of dementia by patients, families, and health care providers, particularly in the early stages [37, 38]. In people over the age of 80, the prevalence of dementia increases to 40%, and in advanced heart failure patients, 30–60% have comorbid dementia [39, 40]. Older individuals with CVD also have a high prevalence of mild cognitive impairment (the prodromal phase of dementia) as compared to individuals without CVD, and patients with cognitive impairment and CVD have worse outcomes than those with CVD alone. Older adults with heart failure have a twofold increased risk of impaired cognition, including deficits in attention, executive function, and episodic memory, and these impairments tend to be more pronounced during episodes of decompensation [41]. Executive dysfunction, in particular, can reduce the ability to adhere to recommended therapies and participate in disease management programs [42]. In part for these reasons, the presence of cognitive impairment increases cost, management complexity, and mortality rates in older adults with CVD. Diagnosis and management of dementia are discussed in Chap. 4.

21.4.4 Frailty

Frailty is a geriatric syndrome that represents an accelerated path of biological decline across multiple interrelated organ systems and a loss of homeostatic reserve in response to stressors [43]. Although different criteria for frailty have been proposed, the frailty phenotype originally described in the Cardiovascular Health Study comprises unintentional weight loss, exhaustion, weakness, slowness, and low physical activity (pre-frail: 1–2 criteria; frail: ≥3 criteria) [43]. More recently, cognitive impairment has emerged as an additional component of frailty [44]. The estimated prevalence of frailty in community cohorts is 7 % but increases to 20 % in individuals over age 80. In older patients hospitalized with CVD, especially heart failure, it is estimated that frailty rates approach 50 % [45]. Frailty is associated with an increased risk of adverse outcomes including falls, functional decline, disability, institutionalization, and death [43, 46, 47]. A bidirectional relationship exists between frailty and CVD such that frailty is an independent predictor of the development and progression of a wide range of CV disorders [48]. Conversely, the presence of CVD increases the risk of frailty, and older adults with concomitant frailty and CVD have significantly worse outcomes than those with CVD alone (hazard ratios ranges from 2 to 4 depending on the specific disease). Chapter 1 provides a comprehensive discussion of the recognition and management of frailty.

21.4.5 Comprehensive Geriatric Evaluation

Although disease-focused evaluation of symptoms may facilitate assessment of the primary CV diagnosis, it does not allow for a more comprehensive evaluation of the multitude of factors that may impact optimal management. Implementing a more patient-centered approach to prioritizing goals of care within the context of co-existing multimorbidity, geriatric syndromes, cognitive impairment, and social and psychological factors can result in a management strategy better aligned with patient preferences. Table 21.3 provides an overview of commonly used tools for assessment of geriatric patients. The reader is also referred to Chap. 8 for practical guidance on office based geriatric assessment.

Table 21.3 Screening tools for common geriatric conditions

Geriatric condition	Assessment tool
Frailty	Fried frailty scale: grip strength, gait speed, exhaustion, weight loss, and physical activity questionnaire [43] Short physical performance battery [162] Rockwood frailty index
Functional status	Katz activities of daily living [163] Lawton instrumental activities of daily living [164] Timed up and go [165] Functional reach [166]
Cognition	Montreal cognitive assessment (www.mocatest.org) Mini-Cog [167] Mini mental state examination (MMSE)
Weight loss/ Sarcopenia	Grip strength Body mass index or weight change, 3–5 % decline [43, 168, 169] annually
Depression	Geriatric depression scale [170] Patient health questionnaire-9 [171]

21.5 Cardiovascular Diseases Common in Older Adults

21.5.1 Coronary Artery Disease

While chest pain or discomfort is the most common presenting symptom in patients of all ages with coronary artery disease (CAD), dyspnea is frequently the presenting symptom in older adults and women, particularly in the presence of multimorbidity. Atypical or non-specific symptoms are also common in older adults with CAD and may include weakness, confusion, decline in functional status, reduced physical activity, nausea, and loss of appetite. For these reasons, a high clinical suspicion for CAD in older adults should be maintained (especially the very elderly). Older adults may also be less likely to recognize or report symptoms of CAD due to reduced physical activity or cognitive impairment. Further, older adults may minimize symptoms owing to fear of possible interventions, hospitalization, and loss of independence.

21.5.2 Acute Myocardial Infarction

Ischemic heart disease is the leading cause of mortality in both men and women in the USA, with nearly 85 % of deaths occurring in individuals 65 years and older and over 50 % in those 75 and older [49, 50]. The high prevalence of ischemic heart disease in older adults contributes to the increased number of deaths, but greater in-hospital and 6-month mortality rates are also a significant factor.

A critical step in optimum management of older adults with acute myocardial infarction (AMI) is prompt diagnosis and re-vascularization, if appropriate, but such treatment is contingent upon recognition of symptoms and the presence of diagnostic electrocardiographic (ECG) changes. In the Global Registry of Acute Coronary Events (GRACE), almost 50 % of participants >85 years with an ACS presented with dyspnea rather than chest pain [51]. In the Framingham cohort, silent or unrecognized infarcts accounted for almost 60 % of all MIs in individuals over age 85 [52]. Current practice guidelines recommend that an ECG should be obtained and reviewed within 10 min of presentation in individuals with symptoms consistent with ACS. In older adults, particularly women, the time to first ECG is considerably longer than in younger patients and it is more likely to be non-diagnostic [52]. The higher prevalence of non-specific symptoms, pre-existing ECG abnormalities, and non-ST segment elevation MI (NSTEMI) in elderly patients can further delay treatment initiation.

Reperfusion therapy in the form of fibrinolysis or more commonly primary percutaneous coronary intervention (PCI) in ST-elevation MI (STEMI) is associated with reduced in-hospital mortality, subsequent heart failure, and long-term morbidity and mortality [53, 54]. Despite a greater incremental benefit obtained by elderly patients, they are less likely to receive reperfusion therapy [55]. In the Myocardial Infarction National Audit Project (MINAP), only 55 % of patients ≥85 presenting with STEMI received reperfusion therapy as compared to 84 % of patients age 65 or younger. Primary PCI is the treatment of choice if performed within 90 min of arrival to the hospital and within 12 h of onset of symptoms. [56] Increased actual and perceived risks in older adults undergoing PCI likely contribute to lower utilization rates.

21.5.2.1 Antiplatelet Therapy

In the second International Study of Infarct Survival-2 (ISIS-2) [57], early aspirin therapy in patients with STEMI reduced 35-day mortality by 23 % overall with corresponding effects in individuals over the age of 70. Chronic aspirin therapy following MI also decreases recurrent MI, stroke, and all-cause mortality irrespective of age. Clopidogrel in addition to aspirin reduces recurrent MI and death in the 12 months following hospital admission for ACS, whether or not PCI is performed [58, 59]. Table 21.4 summarizes clinical trials of antiplatelet agents in the treatment of ACS, including outcomes and caveats for older adults. Older adults are at increased risk for bleeding complications associated with all antiplatelet agents, including aspirin, and the use of dual antiplatelet therapy (e.g., aspirin with clopidogrel) and especially triple therapy (2 antiplatelet agents and an anticoagulant) further increases risk. Compared to clopidogrel, prasugrel is associated with increased risk of intracranial hemorrhage in patients ≥75 years of age and is not recommended for use in that age group except in patients at high

risk for stent thrombosis [60]. Similarly, vorapaxar is associated with significantly higher risk of bleeding in patients over age 75 [61].

21.5.2.2 Antithrombotic Therapy

Activation of thrombin plays an important role in the pathway of ACS and blockade of thrombin by heparin is a recommended therapy. Unfractionated heparin is associated with higher rates of bleeding in older adults as a result of low protein binding and impaired renal function [62]. If appropriate, low molecular weight heparin (LMWH) provides a more reliable therapeutic effect and has been shown to reduce recurrent angina, MI, and death [63]. However, LMWH should be used with caution in patients with stage IV-V chronic kidney disease (est. creatinine clearance <30 cc/min).

Following a large anterior MI, the risk of apical LV thrombosis warrants treatment with warfarin for at least 3 months to reduce thromboembolic events [64]. As noted above, the risk of bleeding on triple antithrombotic therapy is increased in older adults, and this factor should be carefully considered in therapeutic decision-making [65]. As a general principle, intensive antithrombotic therapy should be continued for as short a duration as clinically warranted, especially in patients at high risk for bleeding complications.

21.5.2.3 Secondary Prevention

In addition to aspirin, oral beta-blockers reduce recurrent events and mortality irrespective of age in both the acute phase and during long-term follow-up after ACS [66–68]. Risk factors for drug–disease interactions with beta-blockers (i.e., bradycardia, hypotension, exacerbation of acute heart failure) are more common in older adults but should not preclude administration of these medications; close observation and careful titration are recommended [69].

Angiotensin-converting enzyme inhibitors (ACE-I) are beneficial in older adults following AMI, particularly in the setting of LV dysfunction and heart failure. ACE-I therapy initiated in the hospital and continuing after discharge reduces mortality, hospitalizations, and the progression of LV dysfunction [70, 71]. Angiotensin receptor blockers (ARBs), including losartan and valsartan, have comparable effects to ACE-I and are appropriate second line agents when ACE-I are not tolerated due to cough [72, 73]. Combination treatment with an ACE-I and ARB does not reduce mortality but increases risk of adverse drug events.

21.5.3 Stable Coronary Artery Disease

The management of chronic CAD with or without antecedent MI focuses on optimum risk factor modification and symptom control. As a result of vascular aging and

Table 21.4 Antiplatelet therapy for use in acute coronary syndromes or coronary artery disease

	Trial[a] (sample size)	Intervention vs control	Outcomes	Age (years)	Bleeding risk	Precautions/Geriatric considerations (per Lexicomp®)
Irreversible cyclo-oxygenase inhibitors						
Aspirin	ISIS-2 [57] $N = 17,187$	Aspirin (162.5 mg) Versus Placebo	35 day CV mortality: • 9.4 % in aspirin group versus 11.8 % in Placebo group • 23 % reduction in odds of primary outcome in the aspirin group compared with placebo • Outcome % by age: <60 years: 4.5 % in aspirin group versus 5.5 % in Placebo group 60–69 years: 10.9 % in aspirin group versus 14.0 % in Placebo group ≥70 years: 17.6 % in aspirin group versus 22.3 % in Placebo group	<60 = 45 % 60–69 = 35 % ≥70 = 20 % (Aspirin group)	Major bleeding: • 0.4 % in Both groups	• Risk for peptic ulcers and/or hemorrhage • CNS adverse effects in elderly even with low doses • >325 mg Potentially inappropriate according to BEERS criteria
	M-HEART II [172] $N = 752$	Aspirin 325 daily Versus Sulotroban 800 mg four times daily Versus Placebo 6 h before planned percutaneous transluminal coronary angioplasty	Death, myocardial infarction, or clinically important restenosis at 6 months: • 30 % in Aspirin group versus 41 % in Placebo group • OR 0.63 ($p = 0.05$) compared to placebo	Mean in Aspirin group = 58 (±10)		
Adenosine diphosphate (ADP P2Y12) receptor inhibitors						
Clopidogrel	CURE [59] $N = 12,562$	Clopidogrel 300 mg loading dose + 75 mg daily Versus Placebo (In addition to Aspirin in both groups)	Composite of death from CV causes, nonfatal MI or stroke: • 9.3 % in Clopidogrel group versus 11.4 % in Placebo group • RR 0.8 ($p < 0.001$) • Outcome % by age: ≤65 years: 5.4 % in Clopidogrel group versus 7.6 % in Placebo group +>65 years: 13.3 % in Clopidogrel group versus 15.3 % in Placebo group	Mean in Clopidogrel group = 64.2 (±11.3)	Major bleeding: • 3.7 % in Clopidogrel group versus 2.7 % in Placebo group • RR 1.38 ($p = 0.001$)	• Plasma concentrations of the main metabolite were significantly higher in the elderly (≥75 years) • Use with caution in hepatic or renal impairment
	PCI CURE [58] $N = 2658$	Clopidogrel 300 mg loading dose Versus Placebo (In both groups Aspirin 75–325 mg and PCI after randomization)	Composite of CV death, MI, or urgent target-vessel revascularization within 30 days of PCI: • 8.8 % in clopidogrel group versus 12.6 % in Placebo group • RR 0.69 (95 %CI 0.54–0.87) • Outcome % and RR by age: ≥65 years: 13.4 % in Aspirin group versus 16.9 % in Placebo group And RR 0.79 (95 % CI 0.57–1.08) <65 years: 5.9 % in Aspirin group versus 9.8 % in Placebo group And RR 0.59 (95 % CI 0.41–0.84)	Mean in Clopidogrel group = 61.6 (±11.2)	Major bleeding: PCI to 30days- • 1.6 % in Clopidogrel group versus 1.4 % in Placebo group • RR 1.13 ($p = 0.69$) PCItofollowup(8months)- • 2.7 % in Clopidogrel group versus 2.5 % in Placebo group • RR 1.12 ($p = 0.64$)	
	CHARISMA [173] $N = 9478$	Clopidogrel 75 mg + Aspirin (75–162 mg) daily Versus Placebo + Aspirin (75–162 mg) daily	CV death (including hemorrhagic death), MI, or stroke (from any cause): • 7.3 % in Clopidogrel group versus 8.8 % in Placebo group • HR 0.83 ($p = 0.010$)	Median = 64 IQR = 56–71	Severe bleeding: • 1.7 % in Clopidogrel group versus 1.5 % in Placebo group • HR 1.1 ($p = 0.51$)	

(continued)

Table 21.4 (continued)

	Trial[a] (sample size)	Intervention vs control	Outcomes	Age (years)	Bleeding risk	Precautions/Geriatric considerations (per Lexicomp®)
Prasugrel	TRITON-TIMI-38 [60] $N = 13,608$	Prasugrel 60 mg loading dose Versus Clopidogrel 300 mg loading dose	Composite rate of CV mortality, nonfatal MI, or nonfatal stroke: • 9.9 % in Prasugrel group versus 12.1 % in Clopidogrel group • 0.81 HR $p < 0.001$	Median = 61 IQR = 53–69	Major bleeding: • 2.4 % in Prasugrel group versus 1.8 % in Clopidogrel group • HR 1.32 ($p = 0.03$)	• Not recommended for use in elderly ≥75 years unless high cardiac risk due to risk of fatal intracranial bleeding and lack of certain benefit in this age group • AUC of the active metabolite was 19 % higher in ≥75 years of age
Tricagrelor (Brilinta)	PLATO [61] $N = 18,624$	Tricagrelor 180 mg loading dose, 90 mg twice daily Versus Clopidogrel 300 mg loading dose with 75 mg daily	Composite of CV mortality, MI, or stroke at 12 months: • 9.8 % in Ticagrelor group versus 11.7 % in Clopidogrel group • 0.84 HR p <0.001	Median = 62 43 % of the participants were ≥65 years and 15 % were ≥75 years of age	Bleeding: • 11.6 % in Ticagrelor group versus 11.2 % in Clopidogrel group ($p = 0.43$)	• Avoid use in severe hepatic impairment • Caution in renal impairment, hyperuricemia, or gouty arthritis
Protease-activated receptor-1 (PAR-1) antagonists						
Vorapaxar	TRACER [174] $N = 12,944$	Vorapaxar 40 mg loading dose 2.5 mg daily Versus Placebo with stratification (intention to use a glycoprotein IIb/IIIa inhibitor (vs. none) and parenteral direct thrombin inhibitor (vs. other antithrombinagents)	Composite of CV mortality, MI, stroke, recurrent ischemia with rehospitalization, or urgent coronary revascularization at 2 years: • 18.5 % in Voraxapar group versus 19.9 % in Placebo group • HR 0.92 ($p = 0.07$)	Median =64 IQR = 58–72 ≥75 = 16.9 %	Moderate and severe BLEEDING (GUSTO) 2 years: • 7.2 % in Voraxapar group versus 5.2 % in Placebo group • HR 1.35 ($p < 0.001$)	• Moderate/severe bleeding was much higher for vorapaxar in the ≥74 year quintile at 13 % vs 8.4 % with placebo
Glycoprotein IIB/IIIA inhibitors (IV use only)						
Abciximab	GUSTO IV-ACS [175] $N = 7800$	Abciximab 24 h or 48 h (0.25 mg/kg bolus followed by a 0.125 µg/kg per min maxi of 10 µg/min Versus Placebo (all receive aspirin)	30-day death from any cause or MI 24 h: • 8.2 % in Abciximab group with OR 1 (95 % CI 0·83–1·24) 48 h: • 9.1 % in Abciximab group with OR 1.1 (95 % CI 0·94–1·39) Versus 8 % in Placebo group	Mean = 65 (±11)	Major bleeding requiring blood transfusion: 24 h: Abciximab — 2 % 48 h: Abciximab — 3 % ($p < 0.05$) Versus 2 % in placebo	• Use with caution in patients >65 years and <75 kg = due to increased risk of bleeding
Eptifibatide	PURSUIT [176] $N = 10,948$	Eptifibatide Bolus dose of 180 µg/kg + infusion of 1.3 µg/kg/min, or bolus dose of 180 µg/kg + infusion of 2 µg/kg/min Versus Placebo	30-day death from any cause or MI: • 14.2 % in Eptifibatide versus 15.7 % in Placebo • 1.5 % absolute reduction ($p = 0.04$) • Odds ratio closer to null for more than 65 year olds	Median = 64 IQR = 55–71	Major (TIMI): • 10.6 % in Eptifibatide versus 9.1 % in Placebo ($p = 0.02$)	• Dose reduction for renal impairment (CrCl <50 ml/min) Increased bleeding risk in older patients and <70 kg
Tirofiban	RESTORE [177] $N = 2139$	Tirofiban Bolus 10 µg/kg Versus Placebo over a 3-minute period	Composite end point (mortality, MI, CABG recurrent surgical or interventional revascularization of target vessel or ischemia) at 30 days: • 10.3 % in Tirofiban group versus 12.2 % in Placebo group • 16 % relative reduction ($p = 0.160$)	Mean = 59.2	Major bleeding: • 5.3 % in Tirofiban group versus 3.7 % in Placebo group ($p = 0.096$)	• Elderly patients receiving tirofiban with heparin or heparin alone had a higher incidence of bleeding

CV cardiovascular, *MI* myocardial infarction, *HR* hazard ratio, *OR* odds ratio, *RR* relative risk, *IQR* interquartile range

[a]Trial acronyms: *ISIS-2* The Second International Study of Infarct Survival, *M-HEART II* Multi Hospital Eastern Atlantic Restenosis Trial; *CURE* Clopidogrel in Unstable angina to prevent Recurrent Events; *PCI CURE* Percutaneous Coronary Intervention Clopidogrel in Unstable angina to prevent Recurrent Events, *CHARISMA* Clopidogrel for High Atherothrombotic Risk and Ischemic Stabilization, Management, and Avoidance; *TRITON-TIMI* Trial to Assess Improvement in Therapeutic Outcomes by Optimizing Platelet Inhibition with Prasugrel–Thrombolysis in Myocardial Infarction, *PLATO* The Study of Platelet Inhibition and Patient Outcomes, *TACER* Thrombin Receptor Antagonist for Clinical Event Reduction in Acute Coronary Syndrome, *GUSTO-IV ACS* glycoprotein IIb/IIIa receptor blocker abciximab on outcome in patients with acute coronary syndromes, *PURSUIT* Platelet Glycoprotein IIb/IIIa in Unstable Angina: Receptor Suppression Using Integrilin Therapy; *RESTORE* Randomized Efficacy Study of Tirofiban for Outcomes and REstenosis

accumulation of risk factors, CAD in older adults tends to affect multiple arteries and to be more diffuse and more severe than in younger adults. Diagnostic stress testing is indicated in older adults to investigate suspected CAD but baseline ECG abnormalities warrant concomitant imaging (echo, magnetic resonance imaging, or nuclear perfusion) to improve accuracy. Physical limitations may restrict the use of exercise stress testing but pharmacological stress testing (e.g., adenosine, regadenoson or dobutamine) provides a suitable alternative. Coronary computed tomographic angiography (CTA) is an alternative to stress imaging in selected cases; a limitation of this technique is the need for intravenous contrast administration and potential risk for acute kidney injury. Coronary angiography is appropriate in selected older patients with markedly abnormal stress test findings and/or limiting symptoms that do not respond adequately to medical therapy.

Management of stable CAD is designed to alleviate symptoms, improve quality of life, and reduce the risk of adverse ischemic events. First line anti-anginal therapy should include a beta-blocker if tolerated. Alternative medications include calcium channel blockers, nitrates and ranolazine. Side effects from beta-blockers and calcium channel blockers are more common in older adults and may include fatigue, weakness, and loss of energy, constipation, dizziness, low blood pressure, lower extremity swelling, and depressive symptoms.

Elective PCI for the management of stable angina symptoms is an alternative treatment strategy and may be beneficial in individuals intolerant of optimal medical therapy or in those who remain symptomatic despite medications. Although PCI is effective in reducing symptoms, data from the COURAGE trial indicate that routine PCI in patients with chronic stable CAD does not reduce mortality or risk of MI compared to optimal medical therapy alone (including aggressive CV risk reduction) [74]. The findings of COURAGE were similar in patients younger or older than 65 years.

In appropriately selected patients, coronary artery-bypass grafting (CABG) reduces symptoms and improves quality of life. In high risk individuals, CABG also confers a mortality benefit [75]. Older patients undergoing CABG are more likely than younger patients to have multimorbidity, cognitive impairment, reduced functional status, and more advanced and diffuse CAD [76]. As a result, perioperative morbidity and mortality are higher, with higher rates of respiratory failure, bleeding, acute kidney injury, atrial fibrillation, heart failure, and delirium. In addition, postoperative cognitive impairment is more common in elderly individuals. For additional information on cardiothoracic surgery, see Chap. 10.

21.5.4 Heart Failure

Heart failure is primarily a disorder of older adults in part because CV aging, especially increased vascular and myocardial stiffness, increases vulnerability for developing heart failure [77]. In addition, heart failure is the "final common pathway" for nearly all CV disorders afflicting older adults. Heart failure affects 5.7 million Americans with approximately 870,000 new cases annually in individuals ≥55 years. It is the most common cause of hospital admission in individuals >65 years of age and is responsible for an estimated 1 million hospital discharges as primary diagnosis each year at a cost of approximately \$30 billion in 2012 [78]. Heart failure contributes to more than 250,000 deaths annually in the USA, of which >85 % are in individuals over the age of 65. Mortality rates in advanced heart failure approach those of metastatic lung cancer; however, these poor outcomes are infrequently communicated to and comprehended by patients and families. Not only does heart failure account for significant adverse health outcomes, it has a major impact on quality of life, disability, and independence in elderly patients. See Chap. 6 for further discussion of palliative and end-of-life care in advanced heart failure.

Dyspnea on exertion, reduced exercise tolerance, orthopnea, lower extremity and abdominal swelling, and general fatigue are characteristic symptoms in both young and older adults with heart failure. Reduced baseline physical activity in older adults due to disability or sedentary life style can mask exertional symptoms. In contrast, non-specific symptoms including confusion, reductions in physical activity and functional status, nausea and loss of appetite are more common expressions of heart failure in elderly patients.

The goals of heart failure management in older adults should focus on reduction of symptom severity, improving quality of life, maintenance of functional status and independence, avoidance of hospitalization and institutionalization, and extending life in alignment with patient-centered goals. An interprofessional team approach to care is critical and should incorporate cardiovascular, non-cardiovascular, and social factors. Studies have shown that team care reduces readmissions and improves quality of life in older patients with heart failure. However, recent data indicate that up to two-thirds of readmissions are due to causes other than heart failure, which underscores the need to individualize care and to address prevalent comorbidities [79].

21.5.4.1 Medical Therapy

The mainstay of treatment for heart failure with reduced ejection fraction (HFrEF) includes beta-blockers, ACE-I or ARBs, diuretics, and mineralocorticoid antagonists. In addition, digoxin and vasodilators can be beneficial in selected cases. During long-term use beta-blockers improve LV systolic function and reduce hospital admissions and mortality [80, 81]. These effects are evident for all stages of heart failure and across all age groups, including beneficial effects in the elderly. Beta-blockers shown to be effective in clinical trials and approved for use in the USA for treatment of heart failure include metoprolol succinate and carvedilol. Bisoprolol and nebivolol have also demonstrated improved outcomes in heart failure patients but are not FDA approved for that indication [82, 83]. As with use in coronary artery disease, side effects and adverse events are more common in older adults; hence, it is appropriate to start with low doses, titrate gradually, and monitor closely.

ACE-I have favorable effects on left ventricular remodeling and are beneficial in patients with HFrEF irrespective of symptoms [84–86]. However, since most landmark ACE-I trials included low numbers of elderly patients, the benefits of these agents in patients over 75–80 years of age are less well established. Nonetheless, ACE-I for HFrEF carry a class I indication regardless of age [42]. ARBs are a suitable alternative in the setting of ACE-I intolerance and benefits of ARBs have been shown in both young and older adults [87, 88]. ACE-I and ARBs are generally well tolerated but should be started at lower doses in older adults and titrated slowly while monitoring closely for hypotension, renal dysfunction, and electrolyte abnormalities (especially hyperkalemia).

Mineralocorticoid receptor antagonists (aldosterone receptor antagonists), including spironolactone and eplerenone, reduce mortality in patients with New York Heart Association (NYHA) class II-IV HFrEF and are recommended in these patients unless contraindicated [89, 90]. Patients with NYHA class II heart failure should have a history of prior CV hospitalization or elevated plasma natriuretic peptide levels to be considered for mineralocorticoid receptor antagonists [42]. Mineralocorticoid receptor antagonists are not recommended if the estimated glomerular filtration rate (eGFR) is <30 mL/min/M^2 or if the serum potassium level is >5 meq/L. Adverse effects include hyperkalemia, especially in the setting of chronic kidney disease, but with close observation severe hyperkalemia is uncommon.

Diuretics, in combination with sodium restriction, are essential for treating acute decompensation and for maintaining euvolemia in the outpatient setting. In elderly patients, management of fluid and sodium balance must be considered in the context of social support, as well as functional and physical limitations. Titrating diuretic therapy according to daily weights and close monitoring of daily sodium and fluid intake may not be feasible in older adults with limited social support or significant functional, physical, or cognitive impairments.

Digoxin reduces heart failure symptoms and heart failure admissions in patients with HFrEF [91]. However, digoxin has no effect on mortality and it has a low therapeutic index with relatively high potential for serious adverse events, especially in older patients with reduced renal function. In older adults with preserved renal function (est. GFR ≥60 cc/min) digoxin may be useful as an adjunctive agent in patients who remain symptomatic despite standard therapy [92]. In such cases, low doses (e.g., 0.125 mg daily or every other day) should be utilized and levels should be monitored periodically, targeting a therapeutic range of 0.5–0.9 ng/ml [93].

The vasodilators hydralazine and isosorbide dinitrate are indicated in African American patients with moderate to severe heart failure symptoms, and they may also be useful in patients who are unable to take ACE-I or ARBs due to renal insufficiency or side effects [94, 95]. Limitations of these medications in older adults include the relatively high side effect profile and thrice daily dosing, which impacts the complexity of the regimen and may reduce medication adherence.

21.5.4.2 Implantable Cardioverter-Defibrillators and Cardiac Resynchronization Therapy

Despite optimal medical therapy, patients with HFrEF are at an increased risk for sudden cardiac death due to ventricular arrhythmias. Implantable cardioverter-defibrillators (ICDs) reduce CV and all-cause mortality in selected patients and are recommended for individuals with irreversible heart failure (ischemic or non-ischemic), an LV ejection fraction ≤35 %, NYHA class II-III heart failure symptoms, and a life expectancy of at least 1 year [96, 97]. In the USA, >40 % of ICDs are implanted in patients over age 70 and 10–12 % are implanted in individuals over the age of 80. However, the majority of trials for primary and secondary prevention of sudden cardiac death with ICDs did not enroll patients over the age of 80 [98], and data from clinical trials and observational studies indicate that the mortality benefit of ICDs declines with age, primarily due to competing risks of death. For these reasons, the decision to implant an ICD in an older adult must be considered carefully and should include an estimation of the individual's likely benefit in the context of other medical problems. In addition, shared decision-making to ensure alignment with the patients' preferences and goals is essential. For example, frail individuals with recurrent hospital admissions are unlikely to benefit from an ICD. On the other hand, older adults who are otherwise suitable candidates should not be denied an ICD based solely on age. However, prior to implanting a device there should be a discussion about the potential for recurrent shock therapies and associated post-traumatic stress and anxiety, as well as options and preferences for disabling the device in the setting of terminal illness.

Cardiac resynchronization therapy (CRT) aims to improve hemodynamic parameters associated with impaired left ventricular function resulting from dyssynchronous LV contraction. In patients with HFrEF, a prolonged QRS duration ($\geq$120 ms), and class II-IV symptoms, CRT has demonstrated improvements in symptoms, quality of life, and survival [99, 100]. Patients with left bundle branch block and QRS duration $\geq$150 ms are most likely to benefit, and there is evidence that women derive greater benefit than men. Although patients over the age of 80 were excluded from most of the randomized CRT trials, observational studies suggest that appropriately selected older adults often experience improved symptoms and quality of life. Therefore, CRT should be offered as an option in the management of advanced heart failure in older adults who are suitable candidates for the device.

21.5.4.3 Heart Transplant and Advanced Heart Failure Devices

Although there is no widely accepted upper age limit for heart transplantation, most transplant centers use a cut-off of either 70 or 75 years. Among patients 65–74 undergoing orthotopic heart transplantation, outcomes are comparable to those in younger individuals [101]. However, due to low availability of donor hearts, few individuals are selected for transplantation and they generally have low rates of co-existing diseases. To address this disparity, some centers are performing the procedure using hearts from older donors for an increasing number of older adults who previously would have been declined for transplantation.

Left ventricular assist devices (LVADs) for destination therapy (DT) are increasingly used in patients with advanced heart failure with reduced left ventricular ejection fraction who are ineligible for heart transplantation [102, 103]. As a result, many DT-LVAD candidates are older and have greater comorbidity than younger device candidates. LVAD implantation is associated with substantial morbidity and mortality despite improvements in device technology and operative skills. Currently, 2-year survival rates following LVAD implantation are less than 60%, the overall stroke rates is 11% [102], and 5-year costs are >$350,000 [104]. For these reasons optimal patient selection for DT-LVAD implantation is critical.

The prevalence of frailty in patients with advanced heart failure approaches 50% as a result of reduced cardiac output, deconditioning, cognitive impairment, and muscle cachexia [105]. Additionally, hallmark symptoms of advanced heart failure, including exhaustion, reduction in physical activity, and weakness are also fundamental components of frailty. The presence of frailty and/or cognitive impairment negatively impacts short- and long-term outcomes. Whether elements of frailty can be reversed with restoration of adequate cardiac output has not been determined. The concept of "LVAD responsive" and "LVAD un-responsive" frailty has been proposed in an effort to optimize patient selection for DT-LVAD implantation, but additional studies are needed.

21.5.4.4 Heart Failure with Preserved Ejection Fraction

Up to 50% of patients with heart failure have normal or near normal LV ejection fractions [i.e., heart failure with preserved ejection fraction (HFpEF)]. The majority of patients with HFpEF have antecedent hypertension (60–80%), and HFpEF prevalence is substantially higher in women than in men. Multimorbidity is common and often includes other CV disorders, such as CAD, atrial fibrillation, and valvular heart disease. Although prognosis is somewhat better for HFpEF than for HFrEF, symptoms, quality of life, and hospitalization rates are similar between the two forms of heart failure. However, unlike HFrEF, for which numerous therapies have been shown to improve symptoms and clinical outcomes, to date no pharmacological or device-based interventions have demonstrated efficacy in HFpEF (Table 21.5). For this reason, current management of HFpEF focuses on optimizing blood pressure control (see above Sect. 23.3.1), treating ischemia in patients with concomitant CAD, controlling heart rate in patients with atrial fibrillation, and avoiding excess dietary salt and fluid intake. Diuretics are indicated to maintain euvolemia and minimize symptoms of shortness of breath and edema, but must be used judiciously to avoid over-diuresis, which may lead to reduced organ perfusion and pre-renal azotemia.

Cardiac amyloidosis is an increasingly recognized cause of HFpEF in older adults. Myocardial amyloid deposition may be due to a chronic systemic illness (e.g., multiple myeloma), systemic amyloidosis, or as a primary cardiac condition [106]. Senile systemic amyloidosis is a disease preferentially affecting older adults, especially men, and is present in approximately 25% of individuals over the age of 80 [107]. This form of amyloidosis is derived from an inherited wild-type transthyretin (TTR), an amino acid transporter protein of thyroxine and retinol produced by the liver, and can involve the atria, conduction system and on occasion the entire heart [108]. A subset of TTR amyloidosis associated with specific mutations of the TTR gene has recently been identified. A common mutation (Val12Ile) is predominantly found in African Americans with an estimated carrier prevalence of 3–4% [109].

The clinical presentation of cardiac amyloid is highly variable, ranging from asymptomatic disease that runs a relatively benign course to severe restrictive cardiomyopathy associated with heart failure, atrial fibrillation, conduction abnormalities, and poor prognosis. Echocardiography, magnetic resonance imaging, and nuclear scintigraphy are useful for evaluating suspected cardiac amyloid, but tissue biopsy is needed to confirm the diagnosis. Until recently, treatment was primarily supportive, but several novel agents currently under investigation show promise for slowing the rate of disease progression.

Table 21.5 Clinical trials in heart failure with preserved ejection fraction

Trial[a]	Patients	Treatment	LVEF	Age	Outcomes compared to placebo[b]
PEP-CHF [178]	850	Periondopril	65 (56–66)	75 (72–79)	Death/hospitalization by 1 year—HR 0.69 (0.47–1.01, $p=0.055$). HF hospitalization by 1 year—HR 0.63 (0.41–0.97, $p=0.033$)
CHARM-Preserved [179]	3023	Candesartan	54±9	67±11	CV death/HF admission—HR 0.89 (0.77–1.03, $p=0.118$). HF admission—HR 0.85 (0.72–1.01, $p=0.072$)
I-PRESERVE [180]	4128	Irbesartan	60±9	72±7	Death/hospitalization—HR 0.95 (0.86–1.05, $p=0.35$)
SENIORS (EF>35 % subgroup) [181]	643	Nebivolol	49±10	76±5	All cause death/CV hospitalization—HR 0.81 (0.63–1.04)
TOPCAT [182]	3445	Spironolactone	56 (51–62)	69 (61–76)	CV death/HF hospitalization/aborted SCD—HR 0.89 (0.77–1.04, $p=0.14$) HF hospitalization—HR 0.83 (0.69–0.99, $p=0.04$)
Aldo-DHF [183]	422	Spironolactone	67±8	67±8	Reduced E/e' avg 1.5 ($p<0.001$)
RELAX [184]	216	Sildenafil	60 (56–65)	69 (62–77)	No difference Δ VO2 peak at 24 weeks
ESS-DHF [185]	192	Sitaxsentan	61±12	65±10	Median 43 s relative increase in Naughton treadmill time ($p=0.03$)
DIG Ancillary [186]	988	Digoxin	55±8	67±10	HF hospitalization—HR 0.79 (0.59–1.04, $p=0.09$). Hospitalization for unstable angina—HR 1.37 (0.99–1.91, $p=0.06$)

Age (in years) and LVEF (%) presented as mean ± SD or median (IQR)

CV cardiovascular. *E/e' avg* echocardiographic mitral inflow velocity/tissue Doppler velocity ratio. *HR* hazard ratio with (95 % confidence interval). *LVEF* left ventricular ejection fraction, *SCD* sudden cardiac death

[a]Trial acronyms: *PEP-CHF* Perindopril in Elderly People with Chronic Heart Failure, *CHARM-Preserved* Candesartan in Heart failure: Assessment of Reduction in Mortality and morbidity—Preserved LVEF, *I-PRESERVE* Irbesartan in Heart Failure with Preserved Ejection Fraction Study, *SENIORS* Study of the Effects of Nebivolol Intervention on Outcomes and Rehospitalisation in Seniors with Heart Failure, *TOPCAT* Treatment of Preserved Cardiac Function Heart Failure with an Aldosterone Antagonist, *Aldo-DHF* Aldosterone Receptor Blockade in Diastolic Heart Failure, *RELAX* Phosphodiesterase-5 Inhibition to Improve Clinical Status and Exercise Capacity in Heart Failure with Preserved Ejection Fraction, *ESS-DHF* Effectiveness of Sitaxsentan Sodium in Patients With Diastolic Heart Failure, *DIG* Ancillary Digitalis Investigation Group Ancillary Trial

[b]All-cause mortality was not significantly reduced in *any* trial

21.6 Valvular Heart Disease

21.6.1 Aortic Valve

Aortic stenosis (AS) is the most common valvular heart disease requiring intervention in older adults [110], with an estimated prevalence of severe AS of approximately 8 % by 85 years of age [111, 112]. Risk factors for developing AS include age, male sex, smoking, hypertension, and increased LDL cholesterol levels. Classical symptoms of AS include angina, syncope (and pre-syncope), and shortness of breath, which occur as a result of severe obstruction to left ventricular ejection. This culminates in increased LV systolic and diastolic pressures and prolonged emptying time of the LV. Pathological responses include increased myocardial mass and ischemia due to increased myocardial oxygen consumption in the face of decreased oxygen supply.

Surgical aortic valve replacement (SAVR) is the gold standard and definitive treatment for severe symptomatic AS. However, the decision to perform SAVR in elderly patients is challenging due to increasing comorbidities and the associated increase in operative mortality. Despite improved survival with SAVR compared to conservative medical therapy, 30–40 % of patients are denied or refuse surgery due to real or perceived increased perioperative risk [113].

Since 2002, transcatheter aortic valve replacement (TAVR) has emerged as a successful alternative therapy for patients at prohibitive or high operative risk [114, 115]. Initial studies demonstrated TAVR to be non-inferior to SAVR in patients with severe AS at high operative risk [116]. Additionally, in patients unable to undergo surgery due to prohibitively high risk, TAVR conferred a 20 % absolute reduction in all-cause mortality compared to medical therapy [117]. However, 1-year mortality following TAVR was 30 % and an additional 20 % had no significant improvement in quality of life or functional status. Similar results were also observed with a self-expanding bioprosthesis; i.e., non-inferiority to SAVR in high risk patients but with 26 % 1-year mortality. Even though procedural complications have decreased with increased operator experience, 1-year mortality rates have remained in excess of 20 %. While there is growing interest in TAVR, there is paucity of data on optimal patient selection for successful procedural and long-term outcomes. The ability to distinguish which patients will achieve significant improvements in quality and quantity of life from those for whom the procedure may be futile is critical for aligning patient-centered goals with available therapeutic options [118]. Importantly, incorporating frailty indicators into risk assessment models shows promise for identifying patients likely to have a favorable or unfavorable outcome following TAVR [119]. See also Chap. 10 for further discussion of TAVR.

Aortic regurgitation in older adults occurs as a result of valve leaflet degeneration (e.g., rheumatic or calcific aortic valve disease, endocarditis) or dilatation of the ascending aorta and aortic root (e.g., long standing central aortic hypertension, atherosclerosis, and other disorders affecting the aortic root). Chronic moderate or severe aortic regurgitation leads to chronic LV volume overload and increased stroke volume. Over time increased LV dilatation and an imbalance between myocardial oxygen consumption and supply results in myocardial ischemia and LV dysfunction, ultimately leading to LV failure. Symptoms related to aortic regurgitation can manifest late in the disease process and may include shortness of breath, exercise intolerance, and angina. Treatment of aortic regurgitation in older adults is similar to that in younger individuals. Medical therapies aimed at reducing LV afterload, such as ACE-I or nifedipine, can provide symptomatic benefit [120, 121]. In patients with severe aortic regurgitation, valve replacement should be performed prior to the development of irreversible LV dysfunction (if feasible) [122].

21.6.2 Mitral Valve

The prevalence of mitral valve regurgitation increases with age as a consequence of ischemic heart disease, degenerative valve disease, or mitral valve annulus enlargement from LV dilatation in the setting of HFrEF. Chronic moderate or severe mitral regurgitation leads to LV volume overload with increasing left atrial and left ventricular pressures, pulmonary venous hypertension, and pulmonary arterial hypertension. As with aortic regurgitation, mitral regurgitation may not cause symptoms until LV dysfunction is evident. For those with mild to moderate disease, medical management with afterload reduction is appropriate [122]. In patients with severe mitral regurgitation, surgical mitral valve repair is the treatment of choice when feasible and is preferred to mitral valve replacement due to more salutary outcomes [123, 124]. Older adults with severe mitral regurgitation may be high risk surgical candidates or ineligible for surgery due to co-existing conditions such as chronic kidney disease, neurological disease, and pulmonary disease, and outcomes are less favorable in individuals with impaired LV systolic function. In addition, decision-making should consider patient preferences with respect to quality of life versus length of life, as well as functional, cognitive, and geriatric factors central to surgical outcomes regardless of type of procedure (also see Chap. 10).

For older adults at high or prohibitive surgical risk percutaneous transcatheter techniques to repair the mitral valve have emerged [125]. The EVEREST II trail randomized individuals with degenerative mitral valve regurgitation to mitral valve surgery or percutaneous repair using the MitraClip device [126]. Mortality at 4 years was similar between groups, although a small number of individuals who received the MitraClip required subsequent surgical intervention. In addition, the MitraClip was less efficacious in reducing the severity of mitral regurgitation. Although EVEREST II enrolled primarily low-risk surgical candidates, registry data have demonstrated that transcatheter mitral valve repair is safe and associated with advantageous clinical outcomes in older individuals with significant or prohibitive surgical risk. Nonetheless, additional studies are needed to better define the role of this technology in the management of older patients with moderate or severe mitral regurgitation.

The leading cause of mitral stenosis globally is rheumatic heart disease. In developed countries, however, the prevalence of mitral stenosis has declined, and in older adults mitral valve obstruction due to mitral annular calcification has become the most common cause of mitral stenosis [127]. Additional risk factors include systemic hypertension, genetic connective tissue disorders, and DM. Clinical features of rheumatic mitral stenosis tend to develop over several decades; as a result, the condition occasionally presents in older adults. Predominant symptoms include shortness of breath, fatigue, and weakness. Medical therapy includes sodium restriction, diuretics, and anticoagulation with warfarin in the presence of atrial fibrillation (AF). Rates of thromboembolic events in individuals with AF and mitral stenosis are high, ranging from 7 to 15 % annually [128]. Newer oral anticoagulants have not been studied in this setting and are not approved for AF attributable to valvular heart disease. Isolated rheumatic mitral stenosis (without significant mitral regurgitation) with favorable valve characteristics may be suitable for percutaneous mitral valvuloplasty, which often results in prompt improvement in symptoms and hemodynamics. In addition, 60–70 % of patients with successful valvuloplasty are free of recurrent stenosis at 10-year follow-up [129, 130]. Older adults often have unfavorable characteristics of the mitral valve and annulus, such as calcification, leaflet immobility, disease involving the subvalvular apparatus, and significant mitral regurgitation, which, taken together, may make them poor candidates for valvuloplasty. In addition, the presence of left atrial thrombus prior to the procedure is a contraindication. Surgical mitral valve replacement is an alternative for very symptomatic older adults who are not candidates for valvulopasty, but perioperative mortality rates are 5–15 % and recovery can be slow, especially in patients with diminished pre-operative functional status [131].

21.7 Arrhythmias

Age-related changes in the cardiac conduction system, including degeneration, fibrosis, and calcification (Table 21.1), lead to increasing prevalence of cardiac arrhythmias with age [132]. Aging is associated with a decrease in the number of cardiac myocytes and an increase in collagen content throughout the heart and conduction system. In addition, there is an increase in fat deposition adjacent to the sinoatrial node and progressive fibrosis of the node itself resulting in a gradual loss of sinoatrial pacemaker cells such that by age 75 only 10 % of these cells remain functional. The diversity of symptoms related to cardiac arrhythmias tends to be greater in older as compared to younger adults, and may include falls, weakness, fatigue, confusion, and exacerbations of other co-existing diseases. As a result, cardiac arrhythmias should be considered in the differential diagnosis of a broad spectrum of presenting symptoms.

21.7.1 Bradyarrhythmias

Individuals over the age of 65 account for more than 80 % of pacemakers placed in the USA, and approximately half of these pacemakers are for treatment of sick sinus syndrome [133]. Although bradyarrhythmias are the hallmark of sinus sick syndromes, the condition is frequently accompanied by tachyarrhythmias and atrial-ventricular conduction abnormalities. In particular, treatment of a supraventricular tachycardia can precipitate or exacerbate symptomatic bradyarrhythmias. Bradyarrhythmias commonly associated with sick sinus syndrome include chronic and inappropriate sinus bradycardia (i.e., too slow to maintain resting cardiac output and an inadequate response to stress), sinus pauses, and sinus arrest. Symptomatic bradycardia not attributable to a reversible cause (e.g., beta-blocker, donepezil, hypothyroidism) is a class I indication for pacemaker placement, and in the setting of sinus rhythm, a dual chamber device is appropriate. For individuals with symptomatic bradycardia due to medication, indications for that therapy should be reviewed, and only if compelling (e.g., beta-blocker for heart failure) should a pacemaker be considered; otherwise, an alternative medication should be used.

21.7.2 Supraventricular Tachycardias

Atrial fibrillation (AF) affects between 2.7 and 6 million individuals in the US and is the most common sustained cardiac arrhythmia with an estimated prevalence of 9 % in adults 65 and older [134]. AF is predominantly a disorder of older adults, with approximately 50 % of cases occurring in individuals 75 years of age or older. In addition, with the aging of the population it is projected that the median age for patients with AF will approach 80 years by mid-century. Although AF is more common in men than women, increasing prevalence of heart disease in women with aging and their longer life expectancy results in more women with AF at older age. In older adults, AF is nearly always associated with underlying CVD with hypertensive heart disease, ischemic heart disease, and valvular heart disease making up the overwhelming majority. AF can present with varied symptoms; a large proportion of older adults with AF experience mild or no symptoms, whereas others report fatigue, weakness, lightheadedness, decreased activity tolerance, chest discomfort, or shortness of breath. Palpitations, fluttering, and racing heartbeat are also commonly reported. In addition to symptoms caused by AF, the risk of stroke attributable to AF is substantial. In the Framingham Study, AF was associated with a two to threefold increased risk of stroke, and 23.5 % of strokes were attributed to AF in those over age 80 [135].

The management of AF should include (1) identification of underlying cause and potential reversibility, (2) control of symptoms through a rhythm or rate-control strategy, and (3) stroke prevention [136]. Reversible causes include hyperthyroidism, obstructive sleep apnea, alcohol, excess caffeine, drugs (prescribed, illicit, and herbal/OTC medications), and electrolyte imbalance. Additionally, optimum treatment of underlying CVD, such as controlling blood pressure, can reduce the burden of AF and help maintain sinus rhythm.

The balance between rhythm control (aiming to maintain sinus rhythm) and rate control (aiming to reduce ventricular response rate) strategies is complicated and controversial. The AFFIRM trial randomized older adults with AF to rate control or rhythm control and demonstrated a non-significant increase in mortality in individuals in the rhythm control group, as well as a significant increase in hospitalizations [137]. A key observation was that most strokes occurred in patients either not taking warfarin or with sub-therapeutic international normalized ratios (INR). This has contributed to the strong recommendation to maintain older adults with AF on anticoagulation whether or not they are in sinus rhythm. Medications commonly used as first line agents for rate control include beta-blockers and non-dihydropyridine calcium channel blockers (diltiazem, verapamil). Digoxin is relatively ineffective as a single agent but may be a useful adjunct in patients with inadequate rate control despite maximally tolerated doses of beta-blockers and/or calcium channel blockers.

A strategy of maintaining sinus rhythm is appropriate in patients with moderate or severe symptoms related to AF that do not respond to rate control interventions. In addition, rhythm control may be associated with improved quality of life and exercise tolerance, and there is preliminary evidence that cognitive outcomes may be better in patients with AF who are maintained in sinus rhythm [138]. Rhythm control usually includes a trial of antiarrhythmic drug therapy; however, available agents have relatively low efficacy rates and side effects are common. Catheter ablation of AF foci in the left atrium is an alternative to antiarrhythmic drugs for maintaining sinus rhythm. Success rates range from about 65–85 % but tend to be lower in older adults, who are also less often suitable candidates for the procedure due to an enlarged left atrium or other factors. The surgical Maze procedure is effective in maintaining sinus rhythm in up to 90 % of patients with AF, but is usually reserved for severely symptomatic patients or those undergoing cardiac surgery for another reason (e.g., CABG) [136].

Anticoagulation markedly reduces the risk of stroke in older patients with either paroxysmal or chronic AF, and since increasing age is associated with increasing stroke risk, the oldest patients derive the greatest absolute benefit from anticoagulation. Conversely, the oldest patients are also at increased risk for bleeding complications. As a result of this tension, decisions regarding anticoagulation in older adults with AF are often challenging. In general, if there are no significant contraindications or high risk co-existing conditions, older adults with AF should receive systemic anticoagulation. In other cases, risk assessment tools such as $CHADS_2$, CHA_2DS_2-VASc, ATRIA, and HAS-BLED can be useful for assessing benefits and risks of anticoagulation (see Table 21.6) [139–142]. In the past few years, new options for anticoagulation have become available; Table 21.7

Table 21.6 Risk prediction tools for anticoagulation use in atrial fibrillation

Prediction tool	Variables included (points)	Reported risk	
$CHADS_2$ [139]	C congestive heart failure (1) H hypertension (1) A age >75 years (1) D diabetes mellitus (1) S_2 prior stroke, TIA or thromboembolism (2)	$CHADS_2$ score	Annual stroke risk %
		0	1.9
		1	2.8
		2	4.0
		3	5.9
		4	8.5
		5	12.5
		6	18.2
CHA_2DS_2-VASc [140]	C congestive heart failure (1) H hypertension (1) A_2 age >75 years (2) D diabetes mellitus (1) S_2 prior Stroke, TIA or thromboembolism (2) V vascular disease (1)* A age 65–74 YEARS (1) Sc female sex (1)	CHA_2DS_2VASc Score	Annual stroke risk %
		0	0
		1	1.3
		2	2.2
		3	3.2
		4	4.0
		5	6.7
		6	9.8
		7	9.6
		8	6.7
		9	15.2
HAS-BLED [141]	H hypertension (1) A abnormal renal/liver function (1)** S prior stroke (1) B bleeding (1) L Labile INRs (1)*** E elderly >65 years (1) D drugs or alcohol (1)****	Score of ≥3 indicates increased 1 year bleeding risk on anticoagulation Risk is for bleeding requiring hospitalization or hemoglobin decrease >2 g/L or transfusion required	
ATRIA [142]	Anemia (3) Severe renal disease (3) Age ≥75 years (2) Prior bleeding (1) Hypertension (1)	ATRIA score	Major hemorrhage (% per year)
		0	0.4
		1	0.6
		2	1.0
		3	1.0
		4	2.6
		5	5.7
		6	5.0
		7	5.2
		8	9.6
		9	12.4
		10	17.3

ATRIA = Anticoagulation and Risk Factors in Atrial Fibrillation

Table 21.7 Anticoagulants—for use in patients with non-valvular atrial fibrillation (NVAF)

	Trial[a] (sample size)	Intervention vs control	Outcomes	Age	Bleeding risk	Precautions/geriatric considerations (per Lexicomp®)
Warfarin/ Vitamin K inhibitors	SPAF [187] $N=627$	Group 1 (Anticoagulation) Warfarin Versus Placebo	Ischemic stroke and primary embolism: • 2.3%/year in Warfarin group versus 7.4%/year in Placebo group • Risk reduction in warfarin group was 67% ($p=0.01$)	Mean = 65 in Warfarin group Only 4% above 75	Major bleeding: • 1.5%/year in Warfarin group versus 1.6%/year in Placebo group	Risk for bleeding complications secondary to falls, drug interactions, living situation, and cognitive status
	BAFTA [188]	Warfarin (target international normalized ratio 2–3) Versus Aspirin 75 mg daily	Fatal or disabling stroke, intracranial hemorrhage, or clinically significant arterial embolism: • 1.8%/year in Warfarin group vs 3.8%.year in Aspirin group • RR 0.48, 95% CI 0.28–0.80, $p=0.003$ • Outcomes by Age: 75–79 years: 2%/year in Warfarin group vs 2.8%.year in Aspirin group And 0.71 (95% CI 0.29–1.65) $p=0.57$ 80–84 years: 1.1%/year in Warfarin group vs 3.8%.year in Aspirin group And RR 0.30 (95% CI 0.10–0.77) $p=0.45$ ≥85 years: 2.8%/year in Warfarin group vs 5.6%.year in Aspirin group And RR 0.50 (95% CI 0.17–1.31) $p=$n/a	Inclusion criteria was >75 year olds Mean = 81.5 (±4.2)		

Direct thrombin inhibitors

	Trial (sample size)	Intervention vs control	Outcomes	Age	Bleeding risk	Precautions/geriatric considerations
Dabigatran	RE-LY [189] $N=18, 113$	Dabigatran 110 mg or 150 mg twice daily Versus Warfarin	Stroke or systemic embolism: 1.53%/year in 110 mg Dabigatran RR 0.91 ($p<0.001$) *and* 1.11%/year in 150 mg Dabigatran RR 0.66 ($p<0.001$) Versus 1.69% in Warfarin group	≥75 years or 65–74 years with DM, HTN, CAD 110 mg: Mean = 71.4(±8.6) years 150 mg: Mean = 71.5(±8.8) years	Major bleeding: 2.71%/year in 110 mg Dabigatran RR 0.8 ($p=0.003$) *and* 3.11%/year in 150 mg Dabigatran RR 0.93 ($p=031$) Versus 3.36% in Warfarin group	80% excreted renally; dose adjustment for patients with kidney disease: 75 mg BID for eGFR 15–30 cc/min; not recommended for eGFR <15 cc/min Increase in bleeding risk with age

Xa inhibitors

Drug	Trial	Dosing	Stroke or systemic embolism	Age	Bleeding	Comments
Rivaroxaban	ROCKET AF [190] $N = 14,264$	Rivaroxaban 20 mg or 15 mg daily (CrCl 30–49 ml/min) Versus Warfarin	Stroke or systemic embolism: • 1.7 %/year in Rivaroxaban group versus 2.4 %/year in Warfarin group • HR 0.79 ($p < 0.001$)	Median = 74 IQR = 65–78	Major and Minor bleeding : • 14.9 %/year in Rivaroxaban group versus 14.5 %/year in Warfarin group • HR 1.03 ($p = 0.44$) • *Subgroup analysis by age* ($p = 0.118$) <65 years = 14.6 %/year in Rivaroxaban group versus 15.3 %/year and HR 0.93 (95 % CI 0.78–1.11) 65–75 years = 19.48 %/year in Rivaroxaban group versus 19.99 % in Warfarin group and HR 0.98 (95 % CI 0.87–1.1) >75 years = 25.78 %/year in Rivaroxaban group versus 23.48 % in Warfarin group and HR 1.12 (95 % CI 1–1.25)	The mean AUC was 41 % greater in persons >75 years of age. Rivaroxaban's half-life in older adults was 11–13 h Dose reduction to 15 mg daily in patients with NVAF and creatinine clearance 15–50 cc/min; avoid in patients with creatinine clearance <15 cc/min Avoid in: – Moderate to severe hepatic impairment (Child-Pugh classes B and C) – Patients with any hepatic disease associated with coagulopathy
Apixaban	ARISTOTLE [191] $N = 18,201$	Apixaban 5 mg twice daily Versus Warfarin 2.5 mg twice daily in patients with ≥ 2 risk factors: age ≥ 80 years, weight ≤ 60 kg, creatinine ≥ 1.5 mg/dL	Stroke or systemic embolism: • 1.27 %/year in Apixaban group versus 1.6 %/year in Warfarin group • HR 0.79 ($p < 0.001$) • *Outcomes by age ($p = 0.12$)* <65 years = 1 %/year in Apixaban group versus 0.9 %/year in Warfarin group 65–74 years = 1.3 %/year in Apixaban group versus 1.7 %/year in Warfarin group ≥75 years = 1.6 %/year in Apixaban group versus 2.2 %/year in Warfarin group	Median = 70 IQR = 63–76	Major or clinically relevant non-major bleeding: • 4.07/year in Apixaban group versus 6.01 % in Warfarin group • HR 0.68 ($p < 0.001$)	Not recommended in: – Severe hepatic impairment (Child-Pugh class C) – Significant renal impairment (CrCl <30 mL/min) (not included in trials) – Systemic exposure increases with worsening renal function. Bleeding risk may be increased in severe renal impairment (CrCl <30 mL/min) – Patients with ESRD with or without hemodialysis have not been studied – Dosage reduction for patients with ≥2 risk factors: serum creatinine ≥1.5 mg/dL, ≥80 years of age, ≤60 kg
Edoxaban	ENGAGE AF-TIMI [192] $N = 21,105$	Edoxaban 30 or 60 mg daily Versus Warfarin	Stroke or systemic embolism: • 1.61 %/year in 30 mg Edoxaban group HR 1.07 $p = 0.005$ *and* 1.18 %/year in 60 mg Edoxaban group HR 0.79 p <0.001 Versus 1.5 %/year in Warfarin group	Median = 72 IQR = 64–78	Major bleeding: • 2.75 %/year in 30 mg Edoxaban group and HR 0.8 ($p < 0.001$) *and* 1.61 %/year in 60 mg Edoxaban group HR 0.47 (p <0.001) Versus 3.43 %/year in Warfarin Group	Do not administer to patients with CrCl >95 mL/min Reduce dose to 30 mg/day in patients with CrCl of 15 to 50 mL/min or venous thromboembolism (DVT and/or PE) and body weight ≤60 kg Not recommended in patients with moderate or severe hepatic impairment (Child-Pugh class B and C) or patients with CrCl <15 mL/min

HR hazard ratio, *OR* odds ratio, *RR* relative risk, *IQR* interquartile range, *CrCl* creatinine clearance, *DM* diabetes mellitus, *CAD* coronary artery disease, *HTN* hypertension; *CNS* central nervous system

[a]Trial acronyms: *SPAF* Stroke Prevention in Atrial Fibrillation, *BAFTA* Birmingham Atrial Fibrillation Treatment of the Aged Study, *RE-LY* Randomized Evaluation of Long-Term Anticoagulation Therapy, *ROCKETAF* Rivaroxaban Once Daily Oral Direct Factor Xa Inhibition Compared with Vitamin K Antagonism for Prevention of Stroke and Embolism Trial in Atrial Fibrillation, ARISTOTLE = Apixaban for Reduction in Stroke and Other Thromboembolic Events in Atrial Fibrillation, ENGAGE-TIMI = Effective Anticoagulation with Factor Xa Next Generation

summarizes some of the major AF trials and provides caveats for treating older adults. In general, the new oral anticoagulants (NOACs) are at least as effective as warfarin for stroke prevention in patients with non-valvular AF, including those ≥75 years of age. NOACs are also associated with lower risk for intracranial hemorrhage than warfarin, while the incidence of other major bleeding complications varies across agents. Among patients age 75 or older, gastrointestinal bleeding is more common with dabigatran and rivaroxaban than with warfarin, and this observation should be considered when selecting an anticoagulant in older patients [143]. In addition, as noted previously, bleeding risks are increased for individuals on triple antithrombotic therapy. While optimal management of patients with indications for both antiplatelet therapy and anticoagulation remains an area of active investigation, recent data suggest that clopidogrel in combination with warfarin is as effective as triple therapy (i.e., including aspirin) and associated with lower bleeding risk, and that it may be safe to shorten the duration of triple therapy in selected patients following PCI (Table 21.8) [65, 144].

In patients at high risk for stroke who are also poor candidates for anticoagulation, device therapy, such as the WATCHMAN device or LARIAT procedure, may be considered, although experience with these interventions in older adults is very limited [145]. The WATCHMAN left atrial appendage occlusion device is inserted via percutaneous catheterization, while the LARIAT procedure involves percutaneous closure of the left atrial appendage using a specialized suture delivery system; both have been approved by the FDA as alternative therapies for stroke prevention in selected patients with non-valvular atrial fibrillation.

21.7.3 Ventricular Arrhythmias

Ventricular arrhythmias, including isolated ventricular premature depolarizations, couplets, and runs of non-sustained ventricular tachycardia, increase in prevalence with age. Management of ventricular arrhythmias focuses on symptom severity and the risk of sudden cardiac death. In the absence of disturbing symptoms or very high frequency, ventricular premature depolarizations do not require treatment in the majority of patients. Non-sustained and sustained ventricular tachycardia (VT) in older adults are usually associated with structural heart disease, and treatment is predicated on the severity of symptoms and the underlying heart condition. In most cases, short runs of non-sustained VT do not require specific therapy. Patients with symptomatic sustained VT should be referred to an electrophysiologist for further evaluation and management. Patients with reduced LV ejection fraction (≤35 %) are at risk for sudden cardiac death, whether or not ventricular arrhythmias are manifest, and should be considered for an ICD (see above).

Table 21.8 Triple therapy for use in individuals on chronic oral anticoagulants (OAC)

Trial[a] z(sample size)	Intervention vs control	Outcomes	Age	Bleeding risk	Precautions/ geriatric considerations (per Lexicomp®)
WOEST [65] $N=573$	OAC+Clopidogrel (75 mg for 5 days, 300 mg 24 h or Loading dose of 600 mg before PCI +75 mg daily)+Aspirin (80–100 mg daily) (Triple) Versus OAC+Clopidogrel (Double)	Bleeding episode: • 44.4 % in Triple group versus 19.4 % in Double group ($p<0.001$) Composite secondary endpoint of death, myocardial infarction, stroke, target-vessel revascularization, and stent thrombosis: • 17.6 % in Triple group versus 11.1 % in Double group ($p<0.025$)	Mean=70.3 (±7)	See outcomes	Bleeding risk is very high compared to double therapy
ISAR-TRIPLE [144] $N=614$	OAC+Aspirin+Clopidogrel 75 mg for 6 weeks Versus OAC+Aspirin+Clopidogrel 75 mg for 6 months	Composite of death, myocardial infarction (MI), definite stent thrombosis, stroke, or TIMI major bleeding at 9 months: • 9.8 % in 6-week group versus 8.8 % in 6-month group • HR 1.14 ($p=0.63$) • Consistent across age	Mean=73.9 (±7.7) In 6-week group	TIMI Major Bleeding at 9 months: • 5.3 % in 6-week group versus 5 % in 6-month group • HR 1.35 ($p=0.44$)	6-week therapy not superior to 6-month therapy

OAC oral anticoagulant, *HR* hazard ratio
ISAR-TRIPLE Triple therapy in patients on oral anticoagulation after drug eluting stent implantation
[a]Trial acronyms: *WOEST* What is the Optimal antiplatElet and anticoagulant therapy in patients with oral anticoagulation and coronary StenTing

21.8 Cardiac Rehabilitation and Exercise

Regular physical activity, including structured cardiac rehabilitation, provides substantial benefits for older adults through multiple mechanisms [146, 147]. Physical activity improves physical strength and function, cardiovascular indices, social and psychological factors, and cognitive function. Despite these benefits, older adults are less likely to be active and tend towards a sedentary life due to reduced motivation, social barriers, and physical limitations. Older adults are also less likely to initiate and maintain participation in cardiac rehabilitation, even when recommended by their physicians [148]. Reasons for this are multifactorial and relate to both patients and providers. Compared to younger adults, referral rates to cardiac rehabilitation are lower following a qualifying event. There is also poor communication to and understanding by patients and their families of the benefits of cardiac rehabilitation. In addition, there may be significant social, financial, and psychological barriers to participation, including transportation issues, costs, and fears about ability to exercise.

Physical activity beneficial to cardiovascular health can also be achieved outside of the structure of a cardiac rehabilitation program, and indeed for many diagnoses (e.g., HFpEF, AF), formal cardiac rehabilitation is not covered by Medicare [149]. Individuals who remain physically active have a lower incidence of CVD as well as lower rates of frailty, disability, and cognitive decline. Currently, there are numerous activity programs, some of which may be covered by Medicare Advantage plans that specifically focus on older adults. Importantly, exercise programs for older adults must be able to accommodate and adapt to multimorbidity and physical limitations; nonetheless, the value of exercise even in the very elderly is substantial. Good communication between providers, physical therapists, patients, families, and trainers increases the feasibility and safety of exercise for older adults at any age and regardless of functional status (see also Chap. 17).

21.9 Advanced Care Planning and End-of Life

CVD is the leading cause of major morbidity and mortality in older adults and in the advanced stages often results in disabling symptoms that greatly diminish quality of life. Whereas evidence-based care often focuses on the primary goal of increasing longevity, symptom severity, complexity of care, and multimorbidity can undermine the perceived value of prolonging life. In addition, aggressive therapies expose patients to increasing risk of harm. For some elderly patients, living as long as possible may be the primary health care goal, but for others, achieving an acceptable quality of life, maintaining independence, avoiding hospitalization, or dying at home may be more important. Since these preferences are highly personal, conversations regarding goals of care and healthcare choices need to occur prior to life-threatening events [150].

The prognosis for an older adult with advanced heart failure is similar to that of advanced lung cancer; however, this information is infrequently communicated to patients and families. Even when eligible for advanced treatment options (DT-LVAD or rarely heart transplantation), the associated morbidity and mortality rates are high. This obliges providers to discuss patient preferences, short- and long-term goals, and views on life-prolonging therapies.

Palliative care and hospice services improve symptoms, patient and family quality of life, and in some cases may even prolong life [151]. In one non-randomized study of individuals with end-stage heart failure, those that received hospice care survived 81 days longer on average than those not in hospice programs. Patients enrolled in home hospice programs are far more likely to die in their own homes in alignment with their expressed wishes. In addition, there are fewer hospital admissions and doctor visits, as well as reduced overall expenditures. For some older adults, palliative care and hospice provide an acceptable patient-centered alternative to standard disease-focused care. For further information on palliative and end-of-life care, see Chap. 6.

21.10 Summary

Aging is associated with substantial changes in cardiovascular structure and function, as well as alterations in other organ systems that significantly impact the incidence, clinical features, response to therapy, and prognosis of virtually all cardiovascular disorders. In addition, the increasing prevalence of geriatric-specific conditions, including multimorbidity, polypharmacy, frailty, and physical and cognitive impairments, greatly increases the complexity of managing older adults with CVD. Although additional research is needed, optimal care of older adults with CVD requires an individualized multidisciplinary approach that is patient-centered rather than disease-centered, and which incorporates patient preferences and goals of care into the decision-making process.

Disclosures SBP funded by K12HD043483-11 from NIH/NICHD, NIA-K award K23AG048347 and by the Eisenstein Women's Heart Fund. ARISTOTLE = Apixaban for Reduction in Stroke and Other Thromboembolic Events in Atrial Fibrillation ENGAGE = Effective Anticoagulation with Factor Xa Next Generation

References

1. Roth GA, Forouzanfar MH, Moran AE, et al. Demographic and epidemiologic drivers of global cardiovascular mortality. N Engl J Med. 2015;372:1333–41.

2. Vincent GK, Velkoff VA. The next four decades: the older population in the United States: 2010 to 2050. US Department of Commerce, Economics and Statistics Administration, US Census Bureau; 2010.

3. Go AS, Mozaffarian D, Roger VL, et al. Heart disease and stroke statistics—2013 update: a report from the American Heart Association. Circulation. 2013;127, e6.

4. Lakatta EG. Arterial and cardiac aging: major shareholders in cardiovascular disease enterprises: Part I: aging arteries: a "set up" for vascular disease. Circulation. 2003;107:139–46.

5. Lakatta EG. Arterial and cardiac aging: major shareholders in cardiovascular disease enterprises: Part II: the aging heart in health: links to heart disease. Circulation. 2003;107:346–54.

6. Lewington S, Clarke R, Qizilbash N, Peto R, Collins R, Prospective Studies Collaboration. Age-specific relevance of usual blood pressure to vascular mortality: a meta-analysis of individual data for one million adults in 61 prospective studies. Lancet. 2002;360:1903–13.

7. Hyman DJ, Pavlik VN. Characteristics of patients with uncontrolled hypertension in the United States. N Engl J Med. 2001;345:479–86.

8. Chobanian AV. Clinical practice. Isolated systolic hypertension in the elderly. N Engl J Med. 2007;357:789–96.

9. Staessen JA, Gasowski J, Wang JG, et al. Risks of untreated and treated isolated systolic hypertension in the elderly: meta-analysis of outcome trials. Lancet. 2000;355:865–72.

10. Beckett NS, Peters R, Fletcher AE, et al. Treatment of hypertension in patients 80 years of age or older. N Engl J Med. 2008;358:1887–98.

11. Group SR, Wright Jr JT, Williamson JD, et al. A randomized trial of intensive versus standard blood-pressure control. N Engl J Med. 2015;373:2103–16.

12. Gupta V, Lipsitz LA. Orthostatic hypotension in the elderly: diagnosis and treatment. Am J Med. 2007;120:841–7.

13. Spence JD, Sibbald WJ, Cape RD. Direct, indirect and mean blood pressures in hypertensive patients: the problem of cuff artefact due to arterial wall stiffness, and a partial solution. Clin Invest Med. 1979;2:165–73.

14. Franklin SS, Wilkinson IB, McEniery CM. Unusual hypertensive phenotypes: what is their significance? Hypertension. 2012;59:173–8.

15. Staessen JA, Thijs L, Fagard R, et al. Predicting cardiovascular risk using conventional vs ambulatory blood pressure in older patients with systolic hypertension. Systolic hypertension in Europe trial investigators. JAMA. 1999;282:539–46.

16. Manolio TA, Pearson TA, Wenger NK, Barrett-Connor E, Payne GH, Harlan WR. Cholesterol and heart disease in older persons and women. Review of an NHLBI workshop. Ann Epidemiol. 1992;2:161–76.

17. Schatz IJ, Masaki K, Yano K, Chen R, Rodriguez BL, Curb JD. Cholesterol and all-cause mortality in elderly people from the Honolulu Heart Program: a cohort study. Lancet. 2001;358:351–5.

18. Liu HH, Li JJ. Aging and dyslipidemia: a review of potential mechanisms. Ageing Res Rev. 2015;19:43–52.

19. Heart Protection Study Collaborative Group. MRC/BHF Heart Protection Study of cholesterol lowering with simvastatin in 20,536 high-risk individuals: a randomised placebo-controlled trial. Lancet. 2002;360:7–22.

20. Miettinen TA, Pyorala K, Olsson AG, et al. Cholesterol-lowering therapy in women and elderly patients with myocardial infarction or angina pectoris: findings from the Scandinavian Simvastatin Survival Study (4S). Circulation. 1997;96:4211–8.

21. Sacks FM, Pfeffer MA, Moye LA, et al. The effect of pravastatin on coronary events after myocardial infarction in patients with average cholesterol levels. Cholesterol and recurrent events trial investigators. N Engl J Med. 1996;335:1001–9.

22. Shepherd J, Blauw GJ, Murphy MB, et al. Pravastatin in elderly individuals at risk of vascular disease (PROSPER): a randomised controlled trial. Lancet. 2002;360:1623–30.

23. Stone NJ, Robinson JG, Lichtenstein AH, et al. 2013 ACC/AHA guideline on the treatment of blood cholesterol to reduce atherosclerotic cardiovascular risk in adults: a report of the American College of Cardiology/American Heart Association Task Force on Practice Guidelines. Circulation. 2014;129:S1–45.

24. Selvin E, Marinopoulos S, Berkenblit G, et al. Meta-analysis: glycosylated hemoglobin and cardiovascular disease in diabetes mellitus. Ann Intern Med. 2004;141:421–31.

25. American Diabetes Association. Statistics about diabetes. Available at: http://www.diabetes.org/diabetes-basics/statistics/. Accessed 10 Dec 2015.

26. Yusuf S, Sleight P, Pogue J, Bosch J, Davies R, Dagenais G. Effects of an angiotensin-converting-enzyme inhibitor, ramipril, on cardiovascular events in high-risk patients. The Heart Outcomes Prevention Evaluation Study Investigators. N Engl J Med. 2000;342:145–53.

27. Cheng S, Claggett B, Correia AW, et al. Temporal trends in the population attributable risk for cardiovascular disease: the Atherosclerosis Risk in Communities Study. Circulation. 2014;130:820–8.

28. Hermanson B, Omenn GS, Kronmal RA, Gersh BJ. Beneficial six-year outcome of smoking cessation in older men and women with coronary artery disease. Results from the CASS registry. N Engl J Med. 1988;319:1365–9.

29. Centers for Medicare & Medicaid Services. Chronic conditions overview. Available at: https://www.cms.gov/Research-Statistics-Data-and-Systems/Statistics-Trends-and-Reports/Chronic-Conditions/CC_Main.html. Accessed 25 Nov 2015.

30. Arnett DK, Goodman RA, Halperin JL, Anderson JL, Parekh AK, Zoghbi WA. AHA/ACC/HHS strategies to enhance application of clinical practice guidelines in patients with cardiovascular disease and comorbid conditions: from the American Heart Association, American College of Cardiology, and US Department of Health and Human Services. J Am Coll Cardiol. 2014;64:1851–6.

31. Lorgunpai SJ, Grammas M, Lee D, McAvay G, Charpentier P, Tinetti ME. Potential therapeutic competition in community-living older adults in the US: use of medications that may adversely affect a coexisting condition. PLoS One. 2014;9, e89447.

32. Morandi A, Vasilevskis E, Pandharipande PP, et al. Inappropriate medication prescriptions in elderly adults surviving an intensive care unit hospitalization. J Am Geriatr Soc. 2013;61:1128–34.

33. Lau DT, Kasper JD, Potter D, Lyles A, Bennett RG. Hospitalization and death associated with potentially inappropriate medication prescriptions among elderly nursing home residents. Arch Intern Med. 2005;165:68–74.

34. Claxton AJ, Cramer J, Pierce C. A systematic review of the associations between dose regimens and medication compliance. Clin Ther. 2001;23:1296–310.

35. Solomon SD, McMurray JJ, Pfeffer MA, et al. Cardiovascular risk associated with celecoxib in a clinical trial for colorectal adenoma prevention. N Engl J Med. 2005;352:1071–80.

36. Coxib, traditional NTC, Bhala N, et al. Vascular and upper gastrointestinal effects of non-steroidal anti-inflammatory drugs: meta-analyses of individual participant data from randomised trials. Lancet. 2013;382:769–79.

37. Rocca WA, Petersen RC, Knopman DS, et al. Trends in the incidence and prevalence of Alzheimer's disease, dementia, and cognitive impairment in the United States. Alzheimers Dement. 2011;7:80–93.

38. Alzheimer's Association. Alzheimer's disease facts and figures. Available at: http://www.alz.org/facts/ (2015). Accessed 10 Dec 2015.

39. Harkness K, Demers C, Heckman GA, McKelvie RS. Screening for cognitive deficits using the Montreal cognitive assessment tool in outpatients >/=65 years of age with heart failure. Am J Cardiol. 2011;107:1203–7.

40. Vogels RL, Scheltens P, Schroeder-Tanka JM, Weinstein HC. Cognitive impairment in heart failure: a systematic review of the literature. Eur J Heart Fail. 2007;9:440–9.

41. Zuccala G, Cattel C, Manes-Gravina E, Di Niro MG, Cocchi A, Bernabei R. Left ventricular dysfunction: a clue to cognitive impairment in older patients with heart failure. J Neurol Neurosurg Psychiatry. 1997;63:509–12.

42. Hunt SA, Abraham WT, Chin MH, et al. 2009 focused update incorporated into the ACC/AHA 2005 guidelines for the diagnosis and management of heart failure in adults: a report of the American College of Cardiology Foundation/American Heart Association Task Force on Practice Guidelines: developed in collaboration with the International Society for Heart and Lung Transplantation. Circulation. 2009;119:e391–479.

43. Fried LP, Tangen CM, Walston J, et al. Frailty in older adults: evidence for a phenotype. J Gerontol A Biol Sci Med Sci. 2001;56:M146–56.

44. Boyle PA, Buchman AS, Wilson RS, Leurgans SE, Bennett DA. Physical frailty is associated with incident mild cognitive impairment in community-based older persons. J Am Geriatr Soc. 2010;58:248–55.

45. Afilalo J, Karunananthan S, Eisenberg MJ, Alexander KP, Bergman H. Role of frailty in patients with cardiovascular disease. Am J Cardiol. 2009;103:1616–21.

46. Woods NF, LaCroix AZ, Gray SL, et al. Frailty: emergence and consequences in women aged 65 and older in the Women's Health Initiative Observational Study. J Am Geriatr Soc. 2005;53:1321–30.

47. Fried LP, Walston JD, Ferrucci L. Chapter 52. Frailty. In: Halter JB, Ouslander JG, Tinetti ME, Studenski S, High KP, Asthana S, editors. Hazzard's geriatric medicine and gerontology. 6th ed. New York: McGraw-Hill; 2009. http://accessmedicine.mhmedical.com/content.aspx?bookid=371&Sectionid=41587664. Accessed 10 Dec 2015.

48. Afilalo J, Alexander KP, Mack MJ, et al. Frailty assessment in the cardiovascular care of older adults. J Am Coll Cardiol. 2014;63:747–62.

49. Maggioni AP, Maseri A, Fresco C, et al. Age-related increase in mortality among patients with first myocardial infarctions treated with thrombolysis. The Investigators of the Gruppo Italiano per lo Studio della Sopravvivenza nell'Infarto Miocardico (GISSI-2). N Engl J Med. 1993;329:1442–8.

50. White HD, Barbash GI, Califf RM, et al. Age and outcome with contemporary thrombolytic therapy. Results from the GUSTO-I trial. Global utilization of streptokinase and TPA for occluded coronary arteries trial. Circulation. 1996;94:1826–33.

51. Steg PG, Goldberg RJ, Gore JM, et al. Baseline characteristics, management practices, and in-hospital outcomes of patients hospitalized with acute coronary syndromes in the Global Registry of Acute Coronary Events (GRACE). Am J Cardiol. 2002;90:358–63.

52. Alexander KP, Newby LK, Cannon CP, et al. Acute coronary care in the elderly, part I: non-ST-segment-elevation acute coronary syndromes: a scientific statement for healthcare professionals from the American Heart Association Council on Clinical Cardiology: in collaboration with the Society of Geriatric Cardiology. Circulation. 2007;115:2549–69.

53. An international randomized trial comparing four thrombolytic strategies for acute myocardial infarction. The GUSTO investigators. N Engl J Med. 1993;329:673–82.

54. A clinical trial comparing primary coronary angioplasty with tissue plasminogen activator for acute myocardial infarction. The Global Use of Strategies to Open Occluded Coronary Arteries in Acute Coronary Syndromes (GUSTO IIb) Angioplasty Substudy Investigators. N Engl J Med. 1997;336:1621–8.

55. Zaman MJ, Stirling S, Shepstone L, et al. The association between older age and receipt of care and outcomes in patients with acute coronary syndromes: a cohort study of the Myocardial Ischaemia National Audit Project (MINAP). Eur Heart J. 2014;35:1551–8.

56. Kolte D, Khera S, Palaniswamy C, et al. Early invasive versus initial conservative treatment strategies in octogenarians with UA/NSTEMI. Am J Med. 2013;126:1076–83. e1.

57. Randomised trial of intravenous streptokinase, oral aspirin, both, or neither among 17,187 cases of suspected acute myocardial infarction: ISIS-2. ISIS-2 (Second International Study of Infarct Survival) Collaborative Group. Lancet. 1988;2:349–60.

58. Mehta SR, Yusuf S, Peters RJG, et al. Effects of pretreatment with clopidogrel and aspirin followed by long-term therapy in patients undergoing percutaneous coronary intervention: the PCI-CURE study. Lancet. 2001;358:527–33.

59. Yusuf S, Zhao F, Mehta SR, et al. Effects of clopidogrel in addition to aspirin in patients with acute coronary syndromes without ST-segment elevation. N Engl J Med. 2001;345:494–502.

60. Wiviott SD, Braunwald E, McCabe CH, et al. Prasugrel versus clopidogrel in patients with acute coronary syndromes. N Engl J Med. 2007;357:2001–15.

61. Wallentin L, Becker RC, Budaj A, et al. Ticagrelor versus clopidogrel in patients with acute coronary syndromes. N Engl J Med. 2009;361:1045–57.

62. Krumholz HM, Hennen J, Ridker PM, et al. Use and effectiveness of intravenous heparin therapy for treatment of acute myocardial infarction in the elderly. J Am Coll Cardiol. 1998;31:973–9.

63. Cohen M, Demers C, Gurfinkel EP, et al. A comparison of low-molecular-weight heparin with unfractionated heparin for unstable coronary artery disease. Efficacy and Safety of Subcutaneous Enoxaparin in Non-Q-Wave Coronary Events Study Group. N Engl J Med. 1997;337:447–52.

64. Hurlen M, Abdelnoor M, Smith P, Erikssen J, Arnesen H. Warfarin, aspirin, or both after myocardial infarction. N Engl J Med. 2002;347:969–74.

65. Dewilde WJM, Oirbans T, Verheugt FWA, et al. Use of clopidogrel with or without aspirin in patients taking oral anticoagulant therapy and undergoing percutaneous coronary intervention: an open-label, randomised, controlled trial. Lancet. 2013;381:1107–15.

66. Antman EM, Anbe DT, Armstrong PW, et al. ACC/AHA guidelines for the management of patients with ST-elevation myocardial infarction--executive summary: a report of the American College of Cardiology/American Heart Association Task Force on Practice Guidelines (Writing Committee to Revise the 1999 Guidelines for the Management of Patients With Acute Myocardial Infarction). Circulation. 2004;110:588–636.

67. Krumholz HM, Radford MJ, Wang Y, Chen J, Heiat A, Marciniak TA. National use and effectiveness of beta-blockers for the treatment of elderly patients after acute myocardial infarction: National Cooperative Cardiovascular Project. JAMA. 1998;280:623–9.

68. Fleg JL, Forman DE, Berra K, et al. Secondary prevention of atherosclerotic cardiovascular disease in older adults: a scientific statement from the American Heart Association. Circulation. 2013;128:2422–46.

69. Alexander KP, Newby LK, Armstrong PW, et al. Acute coronary care in the elderly, part II: ST-segment-elevation myocardial infarction: a scientific statement for healthcare professionals from the American Heart Association Council on Clinical Cardiology: in collaboration with the Society of Geriatric Cardiology. Circulation. 2007;115:2570–89.

70. GISSI-3: effects of lisinopril and transdermal glyceryl trinitrate singly and together on 6-week mortality and ventricular function after acute myocardial infarction. Gruppo Italiano per lo Studio della Sopravvivenza nell'infarto Miocardico. Lancet. 1994;343:1115–22.

71. Ambrosioni E, Borghi C, Magnani B. The effect of the angiotensin-converting-enzyme inhibitor zofenopril on mortality and morbidity after anterior myocardial infarction. The Survival of Myocardial Infarction Long-Term Evaluation (SMILE) Study Investigators. N Engl J Med. 1995;332:80–5.

72. Hamon M, Filippi-Codaccioni E. The OPTIMAAL trial: losartan or captopril after acute myocardial infarction. Lancet. 2002;360: 1886–7.

73. Pfeffer MA, McMurray JJ, Velazquez EJ, et al. Valsartan, captopril, or both in myocardial infarction complicated by heart failure, left ventricular dysfunction, or both. N Engl J Med. 2003;349:1893–906.

74. Boden WE, O'Rourke RA, Teo KK, et al. Optimal medical therapy with or without PCI for stable coronary disease. N Engl J Med. 2007;356:1503–16.

75. McKellar SH, Brown ML, Frye RL, Schaff HV, Sundt 3rd TM. Comparison of coronary revascularization procedures in octogenarians: a systematic review and meta-analysis. Nat Clin Pract Cardiovasc Med. 2008;5:738–46.

76. Selnes OA, Gottesman RF, Grega MA, Baumgartner WA, Zeger SL, McKhann GM. Cognitive and neurologic outcomes after coronary-artery bypass surgery. N Engl J Med. 2012;366:250–7.

77. Rich MW. Epidemiology, pathophysiology, and etiology of congestive heart failure in older adults. J Am Geriatr Soc. 1997;45:968–74.

78. Centers for Disease Control and Prevention. Heart failure fact sheet. Available at: http://www.cdc.gov/dhdsp/data_statistics/fact_sheets/fs_heart_failure.htm. Accessed 10 Dec 2015.

79. Dharmarajan K, Hsieh AF, Lin Z, et al. Diagnoses and timing of 30-day readmissions after hospitalization for heart failure, acute myocardial infarction, or pneumonia. JAMA. 2013;309:355–63.

80. Effect of metoprolol CR/XL in chronic heart failure: Metoprolol CR/XL Randomised Intervention Trial in-Congestive Heart Failure (MERIT-HF). Lancet. 1999;353:2001–7.

81. Packer M, Coats AJ, Fowler MB, et al. Effect of carvedilol on survival in severe chronic heart failure. N Engl J Med. 2001;344:1651–8.

82. A randomized trial of beta-blockade in heart failure. The Cardiac Insufficiency Bisoprolol Study (CIBIS). CIBIS Investigators and Committees. Circulation. 1994;90:1765–73.

83. Flather MD, Shibata MC, Coats AJ, et al. Randomized trial to determine the effect of nebivolol on mortality and cardiovascular hospital admission in elderly patients with heart failure (SENIORS). Eur Heart J. 2005;26:215–25.

84. Effect of enalapril on survival in patients with reduced left ventricular ejection fractions and congestive heart failure. The SOLVD Investigators. N Engl J Med. 1991;325:293–302.

85. Effect of enalapril on mortality and the development of heart failure in asymptomatic patients with reduced left ventricular ejection fractions. The SOLVD Investigators. N Engl J Med. 1992;327: 685–91.

86. Effects of enalapril on mortality in severe congestive heart failure. Results of the Cooperative North Scandinavian Enalapril Survival Study (CONSENSUS). The CONSENSUS Trial Study Group. N Engl J Med. 1987;316:1429–35.

87. Maggioni AP, Anand I, Gottlieb SO, et al. Effects of valsartan on morbidity and mortality in patients with heart failure not receiving angiotensin-converting enzyme inhibitors. J Am Coll Cardiol. 2002;40:1414–21.

88. Granger CB, McMurray JJ, Yusuf S, et al. Effects of candesartan in patients with chronic heart failure and reduced left-ventricular systolic function intolerant to angiotensin-converting-enzyme inhibitors: the CHARM-Alternative trial. Lancet. 2003;362: 772–6.

89. Pitt B, Zannad F, Remme WJ, et al. The effect of spironolactone on morbidity and mortality in patients with severe heart failure. Randomized Aldactone Evaluation Study Investigators. N Engl J Med. 1999;341:709–17.

90. Pitt B, Remme W, Zannad F, et al. Eplerenone, a selective aldosterone blocker, in patients with left ventricular dysfunction after myocardial infarction. N Engl J Med. 2003;348:1309–21.

91. Digitalis Investigation Group. The effect of digoxin on mortality and morbidity in patients with heart failure. N Engl J Med. 1997;336:525–33.

92. Rich MW, McSherry F, Williford WO, Yusuf S, Digitalis Investigation Group. Effect of age on mortality, hospitalizations and response to digoxin in patients with heart failure: the DIG study. J Am Coll Cardiol. 2001;38:806–13.

93. Ahmed A, Rich MW, Love TE, et al. Digoxin and reduction in mortality and hospitalization in heart failure: a comprehensive post hoc analysis of the DIG trial. Eur Heart J. 2006;27:178–86.

94. Cohn JN, Archibald DG, Ziesche S, et al. Effect of vasodilator therapy on mortality in chronic congestive heart failure. Results of a Veterans Administration Cooperative Study. N Engl J Med. 1986;314:1547–52.

95. Cohn JN, Johnson G, Ziesche S, et al. A comparison of enalapril with hydralazine-isosorbide dinitrate in the treatment of chronic congestive heart failure. N Engl J Med. 1991;325:303–10.

96. Moss AJ, Zareba W, Hall WJ, et al. Prophylactic implantation of a defibrillator in patients with myocardial infarction and reduced ejection fraction. N Engl J Med. 2002;346:877–83.

97. Bardy GH, Lee KL, Mark DB, et al. Amiodarone or an implantable cardioverter-defibrillator for congestive heart failure. N Engl J Med. 2005;352:225–37.

98. Santangeli P, Di Biase L, Dello Russo A, et al. Meta-analysis: age and effectiveness of prophylactic implantable cardioverter-defibrillators. Ann Intern Med. 2010;153:592–9.

99. Bristow MR, Saxon LA, Boehmer J, et al. Cardiac-resynchronization therapy with or without an implantable defibrillator in advanced chronic heart failure. N Engl J Med. 2004;350:2140–50.

100. Cleland JG, Daubert JC, Erdmann E, et al. The effect of cardiac resynchronization on morbidity and mortality in heart failure. N Engl J Med. 2005;352:1539–49.

101. Daneshvar DA, Czer LS, Phan A, Trento A, Schwarz ER. Heart transplantation in the elderly: why cardiac transplantation does not need to be limited to younger patients but can be safely performed in patients above 65 years of age. Ann Transplant. 2010;15:110–9.

102. Slaughter MS, Rogers JG, Milano CA, et al. Advanced heart failure treated with continuous-flow left ventricular assist device. N Engl J Med. 2009;361:2241–51.

103. Kirklin JK, Naftel DC, Kormos RL, et al. Third INTERMACS Annual Report: the evolution of destination therapy in the United States. J Heart Lung Transplant. 2011;30:115–23.

104. Rogers JG, Bostic RR, Tong KB, Adamson R, Russo M, Slaughter MS. Cost-effectiveness analysis of continuous-flow left ventricular assist devices as destination therapy. Circ Heart Fail. 2012;5:10–6.

105. Flint KM, Matlock DD, Lindenfeld J, Allen LA. Frailty and the selection of patients for destination therapy left ventricular assist device. Circ Heart Fail. 2012;5:286–93.

106. Cohen FE, Kelly JW. Therapeutic approaches to protein-misfolding diseases. Nature. 2003;426:905–9.

107. Westermark P, Sletten K, Johansson B, Cornwell 3rd GG. Fibril in senile systemic amyloidosis is derived from normal transthyretin. Proc Natl Acad Sci U S A. 1990;87:2843–5.

108. Rapezzi C, Quarta CC, Riva L, et al. Transthyretin-related amyloidoses and the heart: a clinical overview. Nat Rev Cardiol. 2010;7:398–408.

109. Jacobson DR, Pastore RD, Yaghoubian R, et al. Variant-sequence transthyretin (isoleucine 122) in late-onset cardiac amyloidosis in black Americans. N Engl J Med. 1997;336:466–73.

110. Martinez-Selles M, Gomez Doblas JJ, Carro Hevia A, et al. Prospective registry of symptomatic severe aortic stenosis in octogenarians: a need for intervention. J Intern Med. 2014;275:608–20.

111. Ungar A, Ceccofiglio A. Prospective registry of symptomatic severe aortic stenosis in octogenarians: a need for intervention. J Intern Med. 2014;275:605–7.

112. Lindroos M, Kupari M, Heikkila J, Tilvis R. Prevalence of aortic valve abnormalities in the elderly: an echocardiographic study of a random population sample. J Am Coll Cardiol. 1993;21:1220–5.

113. Pierard S, Seldrum S, de Meester C, et al. Incidence, determinants, and prognostic impact of operative refusal or denial in octogenarians with severe aortic stenosis. Ann Thorac Surg. 2011;91:1107–12.

114. Shroyer AL, Coombs LP, Peterson ED, et al. The Society of Thoracic Surgeons: 30-day operative mortality and morbidity risk models. Ann Thorac Surg. 2003;75:1856–64. discussion 64–5.

115. Roques F, Nashef SA, Michel P, et al. Risk factors and outcome in European cardiac surgery: analysis of the EuroSCORE multinational database of 19030 patients. Eur J Cardiothorac Surg. 1999;15:816–22. discussion 22–3.

116. Adams DH, Popma JJ, Reardon MJ, et al. Transcatheter aortic-valve replacement with a self-expanding prosthesis. N Engl J Med. 2014;370:1790–8.

117. Smith CR, Leon MB, Mack MJ, et al. Transcatheter versus surgical aortic-valve replacement in high-risk patients. N Engl J Med. 2011;364:2187–98.

118. Lindman BR, Alexander KP, O'Gara PT, Afilalo J. Futility, benefit, and transcatheter aortic valve replacement. JACC Cardiovasc Interv. 2014;7:707–16.

119. Green P, Woglom AE, Genereux P, et al. The impact of frailty status on survival after transcatheter aortic valve replacement in older adults with severe aortic stenosis: a single-center experience. JACC Cardiovasc Interv. 2012;5:974–81.

120. Scognamiglio R, Rahimtoola SH, Fasoli G, Nistri S, Dalla Volta S. Nifedipine in asymptomatic patients with severe aortic regurgitation and normal left ventricular function. N Engl J Med. 1994;331:689–94.

121. Evangelista A, Tornos P, Sambola A, Permanyer-Miralda G, Soler-Soler J. Long-term vasodilator therapy in patients with severe aortic regurgitation. N Engl J Med. 2005;353:1342–9.

122. Nishimura RA, Otto CM, Bonow RO, et al. 2014 AHA/ACC guideline for the management of patients with valvular heart disease: a report of the American College of Cardiology/American Heart Association Task Force on Practice Guidelines. J Am Coll Cardiol. 2014;63:e57–185.

123. Detaint D, Sundt TM, Nkomo VT, et al. Surgical correction of mitral regurgitation in the elderly: outcomes and recent improvements. Circulation. 2006;114:265–72.

124. Gaur P, Kaneko T, McGurk S, Rawn JD, Maloney A, Cohn LH. Mitral valve repair versus replacement in the elderly: short-term and long-term outcomes. J Thorac Cardiovasc Surg. 2014;148:1400–6.

125. Feldman T, Foster E, Glower DD, et al. Percutaneous repair or surgery for mitral regurgitation. N Engl J Med. 2011;364:1395–406.

126. Glower D, Ailawadi G, Argenziano M, et al. EVEREST II randomized clinical trial: predictors of mitral valve replacement in de novo surgery or after the MitraClip procedure. J Thorac Cardiovasc Surg. 2012;143:S60–3.

127. Carabello BA. Modern management of mitral stenosis. Circulation. 2005;112:432–7.

128. Perez-Gomez F, Salvador A, Zumalde J, et al. Effect of antithrombotic therapy in patients with mitral stenosis and atrial fibrillation: a sub-analysis of NASPEAF randomized trial. Eur Heart J. 2006;27:960–7.

129. Reyes VP, Raju BS, Wynne J, et al. Percutaneous balloon valvuloplasty compared with open surgical commissurotomy for mitral stenosis. N Engl J Med. 1994;331:961–7.

130. Ben Farhat M, Ayari M, Maatouk F, et al. Percutaneous balloon versus surgical closed and open mitral commissurotomy: seven-year follow-up results of a randomized trial. Circulation. 1998;97:245–50.

131. Jamieson WR, Edwards FH, Schwartz M, Bero JW, Clark RE, Grover FL. Risk stratification for cardiac valve replacement. National Cardiac Surgery Database. Database Committee of The Society of Thoracic Surgeons. Ann Thorac Surg. 1999;67:943–51.

132. Baine WB, Yu W, Weis KA. Trends and outcomes in the hospitalization of older Americans for cardiac conduction disorders or arrhythmias, 1991–1998. J Am Geriatr Soc. 2001;49:763–70.

133. Lamas GA, Lee KL, Sweeney MO, et al. Ventricular pacing or dual-chamber pacing for sinus-node dysfunction. N Engl J Med. 2002;346:1854–62.

134. Go AS, Hylek EM, Phillips KA, et al. Prevalence of diagnosed atrial fibrillation in adults: national implications for rhythm management and stroke prevention: the AnTicoagulation and Risk Factors in Atrial Fibrillation (ATRIA) Study. JAMA. 2001;285:2370–5.

135. Wolf PA, Abbott RD, Kannel WB. Atrial fibrillation as an independent risk factor for stroke: the Framingham Study. Stroke. 1991;22:983–8.

136. January CT, Wann LS, Alpert JS, et al. 2014 AHA/ACC/HRS guideline for the management of patients with atrial fibrillation: a report of the American College of Cardiology/American Heart Association Task Force on Practice Guidelines and the Heart Rhythm Society. J Am Coll Cardiol. 2014;64:e1–76.

137. Jenkins LS, Brodsky M, Schron E, et al. Quality of life in atrial fibrillation: the Atrial Fibrillation Follow-up Investigation of Rhythm Management (AFFIRM) study. Am Heart J. 2005;149:112–20.

138. Hui DS, Morley JE, Mikolajczak PC, Lee R. Atrial fibrillation: a major risk factor for cognitive decline. Am Heart J. 2015;169:448–56.

139. Gage BF, Waterman AD, Shannon W, Boechler M, Rich MW, Radford MJ. Validation of clinical classification schemes for predicting stroke: results from the National Registry of Atrial Fibrillation. JAMA. 2001;285:2864–70.

140. Lip GY, Nieuwlaat R, Pisters R, Lane DA, Crijns HJ. Refining clinical risk stratification for predicting stroke and thromboembolism in atrial fibrillation using a novel risk factor-based approach: the euro heart survey on atrial fibrillation. Chest. 2010;137:263–72.

141. Pisters R, Lane DA, Nieuwlaat R, de Vos CB, Crijns HJ, Lip GY. A novel user-friendly score (HAS-BLED) to assess 1-year risk of major bleeding in patients with atrial fibrillation: the Euro Heart Survey. Chest. 2010;138:1093–100.

142. Fang MC, Go AS, Chang Y, et al. A new risk scheme to predict warfarin-associated hemorrhage: the ATRIA (Anticoagulation and Risk Factors in Atrial Fibrillation) study. J Am Coll Cardiol. 2011;58:395–401.

143. Abraham NS, Singh S, Alexander GC, et al. Comparative risk of gastrointestinal bleeding with dabigatran, rivaroxaban, and warfarin: population based cohort study. BMJ. 2015;350:h1857.

144. Fiedler KA, Maeng M, Mehilli J, et al. Duration of triple therapy in patients requiring oral anticoagulation after drug-eluting stent implantation: the ISAR-TRIPLE Trial. J Am Coll Cardiol. 2015;65:1619–29.

145. Reddy VY, Doshi SK, Sievert H, et al. Percutaneous left atrial appendage closure for stroke prophylaxis in patients with atrial fibrillation: 2.3-Year Follow-up of the PROTECT AF (Watchman

Left Atrial Appendage System for Embolic Protection in Patients with Atrial Fibrillation) Trial. Circulation. 2013;127:720–9.

146. Laurin D, Verreault R, Lindsay J, MacPherson K, Rockwood K. Physical activity and risk of cognitive impairment and dementia in elderly persons. Arch Neurol. 2001;58:498–504.

147. Taylor RS, Brown A, Ebrahim S, et al. Exercise-based rehabilitation for patients with coronary heart disease: systematic review and meta-analysis of randomized controlled trials. Am J Med. 2004;116:682–92.

148. Balady GJ, Ades PA, Bittner VA, et al. Referral, enrollment, and delivery of cardiac rehabilitation/secondary prevention programs at clinical centers and beyond: a presidential advisory from the American Heart Association. Circulation. 2011;124:2951–60.

149. Vogel T, Brechat PH, Lepretre PM, Kaltenbach G, Berthel M, Lonsdorfer J. Health benefits of physical activity in older patients: a review. Int J Clin Pract. 2009;63:303–20.

150. Hofmann JC, Wenger NS, Davis RB, et al. Patient preferences for communication with physicians about end-of-life decisions. SUPPORT Investigators. Study to understand prognoses and preference for outcomes and risks of treatment. Ann Intern Med. 1997;127:1–12.

151. Goodlin SJ. Palliative care in congestive heart failure. J Am Coll Cardiol. 2009;54:386–96.

152. Treatment of mild hypertension in the elderly. A study initiated and administered by the National Heart Foundation of Australia. Med J Aust. 1981;2:398–402.

153. Amery A, Birkenhager W, Brixko P, et al. Mortality and morbidity results from the European Working Party on high blood pressure in the elderly trial. Lancet. 1985;1:1349–54.

154. Coope J, Warrender TS. Randomised trial of treatment of hypertension in elderly patients in primary care. Br Med J (Clin Res Ed). 1986;293:1145–51.

155. Dahlof B, Lindholm LH, Hansson L, Schersten B, Ekbom T, Wester PO. Morbidity and mortality in the Swedish trial in old patients with hypertension (STOP-Hypertension). Lancet. 1991;338:1281–5.

156. Medical Research Council trial of treatment of hypertension in older adults: principal results. MRC Working Party. BMJ. 1992;304:405–12.

157. Five-year findings of the hypertension detection and follow-up program. I. Reduction in mortality of persons with high blood pressure, including mild hypertension. Hypertension Detection and Follow-up Program Cooperative Group. JAMA. 1979;242: 2562–71.

158. Prevention of stroke by antihypertensive drug treatment in older persons with isolated systolic hypertension. Final results of the Systolic Hypertension in the Elderly Program (SHEP). SHEP Cooperative Research Group. JAMA. 1991;265:3255–64.

159. Staessen JA, Fagard R, Thijs L, et al. Randomised double-blind comparison of placebo and active treatment for older patients with isolated systolic hypertension. The Systolic Hypertension in Europe (Syst-Eur) Trial Investigators. Lancet. 1997;350:757–64.

160. Gong L, Zhang W, Zhu Y, et al. Shanghai trial of nifedipine in the elderly (STONE). J Hypertens. 1996;14:1237–45.

161. Liu L, Wang JG, Gong L, Liu G, Staessen JA. Comparison of active treatment and placebo in older Chinese patients with isolated systolic hypertension. Systolic Hypertension in China (Syst-China) Collaborative Group. J Hypertens. 1998;16:1823–9.

162. Volpato S, Cavalieri M, Guerra G, et al. Performance-based functional assessment in older hospitalized patients: feasibility and clinical correlates. J Gerontol A Biol Sci Med Sci. 2008;63:1393–8.

163. Katz S, Downs TD, Cash HR, Grotz RC. Progress in development of the index of ADL. The Gerontologist. 1970;10:20–30.

164. Lawton MP, Brody EM. Assessment of older people: self-maintaining and instrumental activities of daily living. The Gerontologist. 1969;9:179–86.

165. Podsiadlo D, Richardson S. The timed "Up & Go": a test of basic functional mobility for frail elderly persons. J Am Geriatr Soc. 1991;39:142–8.

166. Duncan PW, Weiner DK, Chandler J, Studenski S. Functional reach: a new clinical measure of balance. J Gerontol. 1990;45: M192–7.

167. Borson S, Scanlan J, Brush M, Vitaliano P, Dokmak A. The mini-cog: a cognitive 'vital signs' measure for dementia screening in multi-lingual elderly. Int J Geriatr Psychiatry. 2000;15:1021–7.

168. Tully CL, Snowdon DA. Weight change and physical function in older women: findings from the Nun Study. J Am Geriatr Soc. 1995;43:1394–7.

169. Wallace JI, Schwartz RS, LaCroix AZ, Uhlmann RF, Pearlman RA. Involuntary weight loss in older outpatients: incidence and clinical significance. J Am Geriatr Soc. 1995;43:329–37.

170. Hoyl MT, Alessi CA, Harker JO, et al. Development and testing of a five-item version of the geriatric depression scale. J Am Geriatr Soc. 1999;47:873–8.

171. Kroenke K, Spitzer RL, Williams JB, Lowe B. The patient health questionnaire somatic, anxiety, and depressive symptom scales: a systematic review. Gen Hosp Psychiatry. 2010;32:345–59.

172. Savage MP, Goldberg S, Bove AA, et al. Effect of thromboxane A2 blockade on clinical outcome and restenosis after successful coronary angioplasty: Multi-Hospital Eastern Atlantic Restenosis Trial (M-HEART II). Circulation. 1995;92:3194–200.

173. Bhatt DL, Topol EJ, Clopidogrel for High Atherothrombotic Risk and Ischemic Stabilization, Management, Avoidance Executive Committee. Clopidogrel added to aspirin versus aspirin alone in secondary prevention and high-risk primary prevention: rationale and design of the Clopidogrel for High Atherothrombotic Risk and Ischemic Stabilization, Management, and Avoidance (CHARISMA) trial. Am Heart J. 2004;148: 263–8.

174. Tricoci P, Huang Z, Held C, et al. Thrombin-receptor antagonist vorapaxar in acute coronary syndromes. N Engl J Med. 2012;366:20–33.

175. Effect of glycoprotein IIb/IIIa receptor blocker abciximab on outcome in patients with acute coronary syndromes without early coronary revascularisation: the GUSTO IV-ACS randomised trial. Lancet. 2001;357:1915–24.

176. Inhibition of platelet glycoprotein IIb/IIIa with eptifibatide in patients with acute coronary syndromes. The PURSUIT Trial Investigators. Platelet glycoprotein IIb/IIIa in unstable angina: receptor suppression using integrilin therapy. N Engl J Med. 1998;339:436–43.

177. Effects of platelet glycoprotein IIb/IIIa blockade with tirofiban on adverse cardiac events in patients with unstable angina or acute myocardial infarction undergoing coronary angioplasty. The RESTORE Investigators. Randomized Efficacy Study of Tirofiban for Outcomes and REstenosis. Circulation. 1997;96: 1445–53.

178. Cleland JG, Tendera M, Adamus J, et al. The perindopril in elderly people with chronic heart failure (PEP-CHF) study. Eur Heart J. 2006;27:2338–45.

179. Yusuf S, Pfeffer MA, Swedberg K, et al. Effects of candesartan in patients with chronic heart failure and preserved left-ventricular ejection fraction: the CHARM-Preserved Trial. Lancet. 2003;362:777–81.

180. Massie BM, Carson PE, McMurray JJ, et al. Irbesartan in patients with heart failure and preserved ejection fraction. N Engl J Med. 2008;359:2456–67.

181. van Veldhuisen DJ, Cohen-Solal A, Bohm M, et al. Beta-blockade with nebivolol in elderly heart failure patients with impaired and preserved left ventricular ejection fraction: data from SENIORS (Study of Effects of Nebivolol Intervention on Outcomes and Rehospitalization in Seniors with Heart Failure). J Am Coll Cardiol. 2009;53:2150–8.

182. Pitt B, Pfeffer MA, Assmann SF, et al. Spironolactone for heart failure with preserved ejection fraction. N Engl J Med. 2014;370:1383–92.
183. Edelmann F, Wachter R, Schmidt AG, et al. Effect of spironolactone on diastolic function and exercise capacity in patients with heart failure with preserved ejection fraction: the Aldo-DHF randomized controlled trial. JAMA. 2013;309:781–91.
184. Redfield MM, Chen HH, Borlaug BA, et al. Effect of phosphodiesterase-5 inhibition on exercise capacity and clinical status in heart failure with preserved ejection fraction: a randomized clinical trial. JAMA. 2013;309:1268–77.
185. Zile MR, Bourge RC, Redfield MM, Zhou D, Baicu CF, Little WC. Randomized, double-blind, placebo-controlled study of sitaxsentan to improve impaired exercise tolerance in patients with heart failure and a preserved ejection fraction. JACC Heart Fail. 2014;2:123–30.
186. Ahmed A, Rich MW, Fleg JL, et al. Effects of digoxin on morbidity and mortality in diastolic heart failure: the ancillary digitalis investigation group trial. Circulation. 2006;114:397–403.
187. Stroke Prevention in Atrial Fibrillation Study. Final results. Circulation. 1991;84:527–39.
188. Mant J, Hobbs FDR, Fletcher K, et al. Warfarin versus aspirin for stroke prevention in an elderly community population with atrial fibrillation (the Birmingham Atrial Fibrillation Treatment of the Aged Study, BAFTA): a randomised controlled trial. Lancet. 2007;370:493–503.
189. Connolly SJ, Ezekowitz MD, Yusuf S, et al. Dabigatran versus warfarin in patients with atrial fibrillation. N Engl J Med. 2009;361:1139–51.
190. Patel MR, Mahaffey KW, Garg J, et al. Rivaroxaban versus warfarin in nonvalvular atrial fibrillation. N Engl J Med. 2011;365:883–91.
191. Granger CB, Alexander JH, McMurray JJ, et al. Apixaban versus warfarin in patients with atrial fibrillation. N Engl J Med. 2011;365:981–92.
192. Giugliano RP, Ruff CT, Braunwald E, et al. Edoxaban versus warfarin in patients with atrial fibrillation. N Engl J Med. 2013;369:2093–104.

Endocrinology

22

Willy Marcos Valencia and Hermes Florez

This chapter focuses on frequent endocrinology problems in older adults looking through a "geriatrician prism." The following learning-cases facilitate discussion of pertinent topics:

22.1 Case 1

Mr. F. is a 78-year-old white non-Hispanic patient without any known major chronic disease. His body mass index (BMI) is 29 kg/m^2. He exercises daily, between home and a supervised exercise group program. He remains active at home and volunteers in a local hospital. He reports good memory and enjoys a happy life with his wife. Both his parents survived into their 90s.

22.2 Case 2

Mrs. O. is a 67-year-old Hispanic patient with recently diagnosed type 2 diabetes. She does not have micro- or macrovascular complications but is concerned about being at-risk for them. Her BMI has increased over the past few years, despite her efforts, and currently is 33 kg/m^2. She has tried to be physically active but reports limitations as she takes care of her 7-year-old grandson while her daughter goes to school and work. Her functional status is preserved, but she now manifests features of mild cognitive impairment.

W.M. Valencia, MD, MSc (✉) • H. Florez, MD, MPH, PhD
Division of Epidemiology & Population Health,
Department of Public Health Sciences, Miami VA Medical Center,
Geriatrics Research, Education and Clinical Center (GRECC),
University of Miami, 1201 NW 16St., 11 GRC CLC 207 A2,
Miami, FL 33125, USA
e-mail: wvalenciarodrigo@med.miami.edu

22.3 Case 3

Mr. P. is a 66-year-old African American patient with long-standing type 2 diabetes and metastatic prostate cancer, treated with bilateral orchiectomy 4 years ago. Since then he has been receiving androgen-suppression therapy. His medical history includes controlled coronary heart disease, diastolic heart failure, and embolic stroke, without residual neurological deficits. He complains of weight gain, depression, lack of energy, and has recently become more forgetful. His family (wife, children, and brothers) are supportive, and they usually take turns to come to the appointments.

22.4 Case 4

Mrs. B is a 72-year-old white non-Hispanic patient with type 2 diabetes and coronary heart disease who was recently discharged home from a skilled-nursing facility after completing rehabilitation following hip fracture and replacement. Her BMI is 26 kg/m^2 and she has tolerated her new regimen of medications for diabetes and osteoporosis. She is now at home, where she lives alone, but reports having a number of neighbors who look after her.

The chapter will be presented in four sections addressing the most common endocrinologic problems in the elderly: diabetes (including prediabetes and obesity), osteoporosis (and hypercalcemia), thyroid diseases, and male hypogonadism.

22.5 Diabetes in Older Adults

More than 11.2 million or 26% of those age 65 years and older have diabetes in the USA [1]. The annual incidence in those ages 65–9 years is 10.5 per 1000 people [2]. Based on Hemoglobin HbA1c (HbA1c) data, the Centers for Disease Prevention and Control (CDC) reported that about 37% of

© Springer International Publishing Switzerland 2017
J.R. Burton et al. (eds.), *Geriatrics for Specialists*, DOI 10.1007/978-3-319-31831-8_22

US adults adult population has prediabetes, and more than half of them were age 65 years and older [3]. There is growing concern since 1 out of 4 people with diabetes remained unaware of the diagnosis [4]. Similarly, prediabetes has been widely unrecognized, and more than 60% of those at-high risk for prediabetes are 65 years and older.

Understanding the challenges associated with the diabetes epidemic in this age group is paramount for both endocrinologists and geriatricians. Older patients with diabetes have significant clinical and functional heterogeneity that should impact the choice of pharmacological agents and management targets [5–7]. Most providers recognize the importance of a patient-centered approach considering specific features such as diabetes duration, life-expectancy, comorbidities, complications, attitudes, resources, and support systems [8].

There is variability in the development of diabetes-related complications. Using the clinical vignettes, Mr. F. (Case 1) is at risk of developing diabetes due to his age and high BMI, but has no comorbidities, while Mr. P. (Case 3) has long-standing diabetic macro-vascular complications, metastatic prostate cancer and is experiencing a decline in physical function and depression. These very different patients warrant very different approaches to prevention and treatment. In addition, Mr. P's. clinical presentation is typical of older adults with diabetes that often includes several comorbid conditions that impact functional status, life-expectancy, and increase the risk for side effects and adverse reactions from diabetes interventions [9].

Life-expectancy varies significantly depending on the number and severity of diabetic complications and co-morbidities, functional reserve, physical and cognitive function, social support and environment, as well as genetic background (i.e., parental longevity vs. those with family history of premature death). Diabetes duration and advancing age independently predict diabetes morbidity and mortality rates [10]; while an accurate determination of life-expectancy is not possible, an estimation of short, intermediate, and long-term life-expectancy can facilitate establishing goals and the management intensity needed to reach them.

Since there is limited data from clinical trials focusing on older adults with diabetes, it is challenging to implement evidence-based care for diabetes in this age group [11]. Decisions should be individualized using data available from clinical studies, recommendations from clinical guidelines and the clinical experience of the providers.

Most endocrinologists implement a comprehensive approach for diabetes management [12], and include coordination of care and specialized services (ophthalmology, podiatry, nephrology, cardiology, neurologist, home health care, etc.), while involving the patient's family and any other support available. Additional geriatric assessment could improve care, particularly considering the association of diabetes with dementia, dysmobility, and falls. Therefore endocrinologists and other practitioners should consider incorporating cognitive and physical function assessments in their evaluation of older patients [13].

22.5.1 Diabetes and Clinical Inertia

There is growing concern about clinical inertia in older patients with diabetes [14], which may result in either under or over treatment. These can be described with the three different scenarios: (1) resistance to implement early intensive preventive therapies for weight and glucose control in healthy older adults with newly diagnosed diabetes or prediabetes; (2) lack of adoption of current recommendations for the management of older adults with diabetes that tailor targets according to health status, multimorbidity, cognition, and life-expectancy; and (3) lack of awareness of patient's preferences and circumstances related to their functional, mental, and social domains.

The first inertia scenario may occur among primary care providers related to concerns about overtreatment, underestimation of life-expectancy, and low confidence in the ability of older adults to respond to life-style interventions. For example, Mr. F. (Case 1) is at risk for developing diabetes due to his BMI of 29 kg/m². He should be screened with a HbA1c, and if in a prediabetic range he would be an ideal candidate for the Diabetes Prevention Program (DPP) [15]. While most clinicians are aware of the efficacy of these programs in younger adults, the benefits from lifestyle improvements are even greater for older individuals [16]. If despite DPP interventions Mr. F develops diabetes at age 78, the recommended HbA1c target would be <7.5% [5], and lower HbA1c values would be appropriate only if this is accomplished without hypoglycemia and done in consideration of the patient's preferences, access, and support [8]. Using targets similar to the general adult population (HbA1c <6.5%) [17] may be reasonable for some healthy older adults with short diabetes duration, but may not apply in the patient described here who is approaching age 80. Individualized targets [5–8] require further assessment of physical and cognitive function, life-expectancy, and patient's preferences, and avoids hypoglycemic events.

The second inertia scenario may occur when older patients with diabetes are not treated according to recommendations from the American Geriatrics Society and American Diabetes Association guidelines for this age group [6], which recommend less intensive glycemic control in older adults with diabetes. Even these guidelines were based on major studies that recruited "young" old adults (62.2±6.8 years in ACCORD [18], 66±6 years in ADVANCE [19], and 60.4±8.7 in VADT [20]). For adults in their late 70s and 80s, even great caution and clinical judgment must guide therapeutic targets and interventions, since there are no clinical trials in those age groups.

Finally the third inertia scenario occurs when there is failure to recognize that geriatric syndromes are more common in older people with diabetes. These syndromes (impaired mobility, dementia, depression, etc.) impact the patient's ability for self-monitoring, and others (falls syndrome, osteoporosis, frailty syndrome, poor dentition, malnutrition, etc.) increase the risk for negative outcomes from hypoglycemia or hyperglycemia. Thus, tight glycemic control in the older adult and particularly in the oldest old can be difficult and potentially detrimental.

Table 22.1 illustrates the evolving targets for an older individual whose diabetes progresses, when diabetic complications occur and when there is a decline in physical and cognitive function or when geriatric syndromes develop.

22.5.2 Diabetes and Renal Disease

Progressive loss of renal function is associated with aging although the degree of loss is highly variable. Chronic kidney disease (CKD) is a complication of diabetes or can be associated with hypertension (HTN), another common age-related disease. In addition, older adults may be treated with pharmacologic agents that could lead to kidney damage. Since several anti-hyperglycemic medications (Table 22.2) are renally excreted, the management of older adults with diabetes and kidney disease is challenging, particularly in those with advanced CKD.

The reader is also referred to Chap. 25, Nephrology.

22.5.3 Geriatric Syndromes and Diabetes

Geriatric syndromes are prevalent in older adults, associated with aging and comorbidities, and often lead to poor quality of life, loss of independence, and admission to long-term care facilities [23]. These syndromes include cognitive decline, depression, persistent pain, polypharmacy, urinary incontinence, and reduced mobility and falls. Some of these may impair diabetes self-management, lead to poor glycemic control, and increase the risk for hypoglycemia especially those described below [24].

Table 22.1 Evolving glycemic targets and changes in geriatric domains during diabetes disease progression in the older patient

Clinical Scenario	HbA1c goals ADA and AGS[a]	Comments
Mrs. O. (Case 2) 67-year-old Hispanic patient **Medical** recently diagnosed T2D. **Functional** preserved functional status **Mental:** mild cognitive impairment (MCI). **Social:** lives at home, independent, has family support	<7.5% Or 6.5–7.5% As long as no hypoglycemic events	There is potential harm in lowering HbA1c <6.5% in older adults [19]. Implement lifestyle changes towards modest intentional weight loss. Start low, go slow, with pharmacologic interventions, and monitor; follow up and titrate to reach the target
Two years later, Mrs. O. presents with one or several of the following scenarios: **Medical (1):** a myocardial infarction, and heart failure **Medical (2):** Parkinson's disease, chronic kidney disease stage 3, and emphysema. **Medical (3):** newly diagnosed colon cancer. **Functional**: requires assistance with ADLs (bathing and dressing) **Mental:** MCI has progressed to dementia **Social:** lives in an Assisted Living Facility which cannot administer insulin four times per day	<8.0% Or 7.0–8.0% As long as no hypoglycemic events	Studies support avoiding intensive glycemic control in individuals with macrovascular complications. Similar approach applies in multimorbidity (more than three chronic diseases), cancer, or mild to moderate cognitive impairment, and with two or more Instrumental ADL impairments
Six years later, Mrs. O. presents with one or several of the following scenarios: **Medical (1):** has a massive stroke with major neurological and functional sequel **Medical (2):** develops severe liver damage due to acetaminophen toxicity, and now presents end-stage liver disease **Medical (3):** develops rapidly progressive chronic kidney disease, and requires hemodialysis **Functional:** loss of physical function, bedridden, dependent for most activities of daily living **Mental:** advanced dementia **Social:** admitted to a nursing home Her family requests a focus on quality of life and avoidance of polypharmacy	<8.5% Or 8.0–8.5% And up to 9% in cases unlikely to benefit from lower values, due to limited life expectancy	Higher targets relate to lack of benefit from more aggressive interventions and the need to avoid hypoglycemia. Still aims to avoid severe hyperglycemia and glycosuria, which may be associated with impaired wound healing, infection, and urinary incontinence, volume depletion, hypernatremia, delirium, falls, as well as hyperosmolar hyperglycemic nonketotic syndrome or diabetic ketoacidosis

Goals must be achievable without recurrent or severe hypoglycemia or undue treatment burden. For cases experiencing those, reducing antihyperglycemic medications and allowing higher HbA1c values is appropriate. This recommendation increases in relevance as the clinical scenarios progress to situations with end-organ failure, long-term care, and end-of-life care

Note: HbA1c might not be reliable in severe illness or disease, and targets may be based on measured glucose values

[a]Recommendations based on the American Diabetes Association and the American Geriatrics Society, including individualization of targets and patient-centered characteristics [5, 6, 8, 21]

Table 22.2 Pharmacotherapy for diabetes in the older adult

HbA1c Target based on clinical scenarios In Table 22.1	Management	
	First line	Second line ([a])
<7.5% Or 6.5–7.5% As long as no hypoglycemic events	Maximize lifestyle interventions. Avoid medications associated with weight gain **Metformin** • May help with weight loss • Start 500 mg PO with largest meal, monitor tolerance, increase slowly, towards target of 1000 mg PO BID • Monitor renal function, counsel patients when to hold medication in settings where renal function may be impaired (procedures using iodinated contrast)	**Glucagon like peptide-1 receptor agonists (GLP-1 RA)** • Reduces appetite, useful if the patient has concomitant obesity • Requires injection (check manual dexterity, vision) **Dipeptidyl peptidase inhibitors (DPP)-4 inhibitors** • Weight neutral • May be preferred if the patient has limitations in vision, or prefers an oral agent • Dose adjust based on renal function; except linagliptin **SGLT-2 inhibitors** • Risk of urinary tract infections and ketoacidosis • Reduces glucose resorption from kidney; caution in patients with urinary incontinence (UI); may cause or contribute to UI. If UI identified, refer to primary care or geriatrics for further evaluation and management **Second generation sulfonylureas** • May cause hypoglycemia and weight gain, start with low dose glipizide or glimepiride, monitor and titrate • Useful when drug cost is important (generics available) • Do not use glyburide [22] which is long acting and has numerous drug interactions • Evolving concern on cardiovascular safety **Basal insulin** for patients who are not eligible or amenable to any of the above options • Start 0.2 units/kg/day, monitor and titrate [16] • Older patients with new onset diabetes and HbA1c above 10%; patients may not fully respond to oral agents. Start basal insulin and preprandial short-acting insulin
<8.0% Or 7.0–8.0% As long as no hypoglycemic events	**Metformin**	**DPP-4 inh** (same as above) **GLP-1 RA** (same as above) **SGLT-2 inh** (same as above) **Insulin**: as above
<8.5% Or 8.0–8.5% And up to 9% in selected cases unlikely to benefit from lower values, due to limited life expectancy	Most non-insulin antihyperglycemic agents will require to be stopped due to limitations in renal excretion and disease status **Begin** • Insulin basal bolus and preprandial • Daily home skilled nursing services not feasible long term • Basal insulin plus oral agents, as long as glycemic target can be achieved **Other considerations** • Use alternatives to insulin if the patient/caregiver cannot check glucose or inject insulin 4 times/day • Most patients with advanced chronic kidney or liver disease require insulin, due to risks, lack of evidence, unpredictability, or contraindications to non-insulin options. • Insulin can be challenging, if caloric intake fluctuates, for procedures, e.g. hemodialysis, etc.	**DPP-4 inhibitor alone** (reduces HbA1c by 0.7%) consider when this may be sufficient to reach target **DPP-4 inhibitor plus Alpha glucosidase inhibitor (if tolerated)** **Long-acting GLP-1 RA** (weekly), if effective and safe, may be convenient in certain settings, especially when the patient requires assistance with medications **Other considerations** • Avoid glucose values above 220 mg/dl, since this can be associated with glycosuria (dehydration and UI). • Not only avoid glucose values close to 100 mg/dl, but if a trend towards these values is detected, a decrease in the intensity of regimen may be required, before a hypoglycemic event occurs. • Avoid weight loss, which will be mostly be from muscle and bone mass, due to low physical activity levels in many of these patients

[a]With proper monitoring, titrate up as needed to accomplish the desired target

22.5.3.1 Polypharmacy

In prescribing for an older person with diabetes, it is important to recognize that older people may carry chronic diseases from earlier life, as well as develop new diseases, and that multimorbidity leads to being prescribed a great number of medications, with higher risk for drug–drug or drug–disease interactions. In addition, adherence to medications declines as the number of medications and the frequency of dosing increases. Polypharmacy in older people with diabetes has also been driven by pay-for-performance and the use of HbA1c as a quality outcome measure [25]. Often when providers follow guidelines for a series of conditions, the result is polypharmacy. Guidelines are not based on studies of patients with multimorbidity. The recent shift toward quality outcomes that include reduction of polypharmacy by incorporating age- and patient-specific factors to assess quality and performance should lessen medication burden [26].

The American Geriatrics Society published the "Beers criteria," a list of medications that should be avoided or used with caution in older patients [22]. Among them, Glyburide is listed as a drug to avoid, as it is associated with a high risk for hypoglycemia due to its long half-life. While sulfonylureas may have decreased due to new alternative agents, it these agents are still sometimes useful. While glyburide ought to be avoided other sulfonylureas (like glipizide or glimepiride) are acceptable. Similarly the routine use of regular insulin sliding scale is discouraged by the Beers Criteria in older adults with diabetes. Table 22.2 presents an overview of pharmacologic options, and considerations in the geriatric population.

22.5.3.2 Cognitive Impairment

There is epidemiological evidence that diabetes increases risk for cognitive impairment [27, 28]. Long-standing diabetes may contribute to the development of dementia, however there are insufficient longitudinal studies to address the impact of patient attrition (i.e., patients with diabetes may not live long enough to develop dementia). The Atherosclerosis Risk in Communities study showed the association between diabetes in midlife and long-term cognitive decline [29], suggesting that diabetes prevention and control in midlife may protect against cognitive decline later in life.

Poor glycemic control with recurrent especially severe hypoglycemic events is independently associated with accelerated late-life cognitive decline [30], and there is no evidence that more intensive glycemic control will slow progression towards dementia.

The Memory in Diabetes study (ACCORD MIND) evaluated patients with type 2 diabetes with a mean age 62.5 years, and showed no benefit from intensive glycemic or blood pressure interventions on cognitive testing [31]. Similarly, an ancillary analysis from the Look AHEAD study showed no benefit in cognitive function after 8 years of intensive lifestyle intervention in adults with obesity and type 2 diabetes [32]. Studies in older adults at high-risk or with newly diagnosed type 2 diabetes may provide better understanding on the potential benefits of earlier interventions to reduce the risk of cognitive decline and preserve function in these patients.

Hypoglycemia in older adults with type 2 diabetes is associated with increased risk for cognitive decline and dementia [33]. Conversely, a post-hoc analysis in the ACCORD study showed that poor cognitive function may increase the risk of severe hypoglycemia [34]. These points

emphasize the importance of incorporating cognitive assessment as pertinent to refine a treatment plan and to avoid hypoglycemia in the older adult with diabetes.

The reader is referred to Chap. 8, Office Tools for Assessment for recommendations on screening for cognitive impairment.

22.5.4 Challenges with Insulin Use

Due to the progressive natural history of type 2 diabetes, most patients will eventually require insulin. However, the dexterity and ability needed to implement an insulin regimen could be affected by neuropathy, arthritis, cognitive impairment, and other comorbidities. If self-management skills are limited, then providers should assess the availability of informal (i.e., family or friends) or formal (e.g., home health nursing) support to implement and monitor an insulin regimen. In addition, documenting in the patient's record the presence of these chronic conditions and comorbidities will help providers reach the level of complexity needed for appropriate clinical reimbursement and facilitate coordination of care for older adults with diabetes on insulin.

22.5.5 Challenges with Obesity Management

The prevalence of obesity and its comorbidities increase with age [35]. Obesity could impact the medical (e.g., type 2 diabetes, cardiovascular disease, and cancer), mental (e.g., depression and dementia), social (e.g., stigmatization and isolation), and functional domains (e.g., impaired mobility) in the geriatric population [36–39]. However, the assessment and management of obesity in older adults with diabetes may not be common practice among providers. One contributing factor may be the limited evidence on potential benefits associated with weight loss medications and bariatric surgery in older adults. However, modest intentional weight loss through lifestyle (healthy nutrition and increased physical activity) could reduce the burden of obesity-related comorbidities and improve the quality of life of otherwise healthy obese older adults [36].

The "obesity paradox" is a term used to describe the fact that better outcomes are seen in older people at higher BMIs compared to younger people [40–42]. Epidemiological studies have described better survival in overweight older adults with heart failure, hypertension, stroke, and end-organ damage. However, better outcomes are also seen in each BMI category, when better fitness was also present [41, 43, 44] suggesting that fitness and not simply fatness is important. Therefore, it is important that cardiovascular and physical conditioning with modest weight management should be a part of the plan of care in older patients with diabetes. In

Case 1, Mr. F. who has a BMI of 29 kg/m² would benefit from the lifestyle interventions consisting of exercise, and modest intentional weight loss. He may lose 10 lb in 1 year, and lower his BMI to 28 kg/m². While remaining in the overweight group, he has likely improved his clinical, metabolic, and functional profiles.

22.6 Osteoporosis and Bone Metabolism

Osteoporosis increases with age but there are potential gender differences in its consequences. Osteoporosis-related fractures are more common in older women, probably related to accelerated bone loss in the postmenopausal period, but mortality is greater in older men within the first year after a hip or femoral fracture [45, 46]. In addition, the prevalence of osteoporosis increases in the oldest old (age 80 and older), in whom the average T-score is lower than −2.5 SD. Furthermore, more than 50% of patients admitted to a hospital with hip fracture belong to this age group [47, 48].

Among non-communicable chronic diseases, osteoporosis is fifth in disability burden behind coronary heart disease, lung disease, osteoarthritis and Alzheimer's dementia [49]. Therefore, timely assessment and appropriate therapy could reduce the growing burden associated with osteoporosis.

22.6.1 Osteoporosis Screening

Current guidelines provide recommendations for osteoporosis screening for both women (age 65 and older with or without risk factors) [50, 51] and men (age 70 and older with risk factors) [52, 53]. Approximately 50% of women and 20% of men are at risk for an osteoporosis-related fracture during their lifetime. Osteoporotic fractures accelerate functional decline in older adults and have major economic impact [54, 55]. The annual costs of incident fractures are estimated at $ 17 billion with men accounting for 29% of fractures and 25% of costs. An economic model incorporating the growth of the older adult population projected that by 2025 the annual fractures and costs will increase by 50% [54]. Forty percent of people who break their hip do not fully recover to their functional level before the fracture and 20% have such major functional decline that independence is lost and long-term care placement may result [55].

Prevalence studies find nearly half of all women age 80 and older have a vertebral fracture [56]. Additionally, older adults with vertebral fractures present with progressive height loss, pain, loss of mobility and independence, psychological distress, decreased quality of life, and increased risk of disability [57–59]. Furthermore, patients with vertebral fractures also have increased risk for non-vertebral fractures.

22.6.2 Osteoporosis Risk Assessment

In addition to age-related decline in bone, the loss of gonadal function in both women and men, and conditions associated with inflammation may contribute to increased risk of fracture [60–62]. In the World Health Organization (WHO) Fracture Risk Algorithm (FRAX®, available at https://www.shef.ac.uk/FRAX/), increasing age is one of the strongest predictors for fracture risk, only second to personal history or family history of previous fragility fracture. Of interest, there is a remarkable variation in the age-specific risk for fracture worldwide. In the 45 countries studied, there was greater heterogeneity between countries than between gender differences within a country [63]. A revision of FRAX (3.0) uses updated epidemiological information in the USA and shows the predictive value for hip fracture even in men and women age 70 and older [64].

Data from the Osteoporotic Fractures in Men Study (MrOS), suggests that pharmacologic treatment would be needed in one-third of USA; white men aged 65 years and older and one-half of those aged 75 years and older [65]. A practical approach to screening for men is to address height loss, especially if ~1.5–2 in., as potentially associated with asymptomatic vertebral fractures [17]. Additional clinical risk factors that should prompt earlier screening include low body weight, history of prior fragility fracture, family history of osteoporosis, smoking, excessive alcohol intake, and long-term use of high-risk medications (e.g., glucocorticoids at doses >5 mg/d of prednisone, or its equivalent) [66].

22.6.3 Special Considerations in Older Adults

Falls, sarcopenia, and frailty are not included in FRAX, but they are associated with increased fracture risk in older adults [67–74]. In addition, more than 50% of people hospitalized due to hip fracture are older than 80, and many of those will sustain another fracture [47, 75–78] For patients with spine and hip fractures, there is a broad body of literature supporting the reduction of fracture risk from pharmacological treatment [50]. In general, these medications are safe in the older population as long as pertinent precautions are followed. For instance, in older adults with CKD stages 4 and 5 bisphosphonates are contraindicated, and proper monitoring is required to avoid adynamic bone disease [79, 80] (see also Chap. 25, for a discussion of metabolic bone disease.) However, the alternative antiresorptive monoclonal antibody denosumab could be considered.

Before starting either type of antresorptive therapy, examination of the oral cavity by a dental professional is indicated. This is especially important in the older people who are at greater risk for oral disease (poor dentition requiring dentoalveolar surgery, tooth extraction, dental fractures) and poor oral health (including periodontal disease, caries, infections) [81]. Oral disease increases risk of osteonecrosis of the jaw. While most cases have been reported after IV formulation in frail older adults with multimorbidity and/or history of malignancy, it is recommended to treatment dental diseases prior to beginning antiresorptives [82].

In addition, calcium and vitamin D supplementation and exercise (see below) are important in prevention and management of osteoporosis [83, 84]. The recommended calcium intake for older adults is 1200 mg per day, ideally from dietary sources [50, 52, 84, 85]. The National Institutes of Health offer a fact sheet for calcium supplementation, with detailed information on dietary sources of calcium (available at https://ods.od.nih.gov/factsheets/Calcium-HealthProfessional/#h3). However, the dietary intake of calcium in older adults is usually insufficient (about 600 mg per day), thus prescription supplementation is often required to reach the target (additional 500–600 mg per day). Furthermore, older adults have an increased prevalence of chronic or atrophic gastritis, with achlorhydria, leading to malabsorption of calcium [86]. Therefore, some experts suggest calcium citrate over calcium carbonate [87]. Constipation may develop with either, and it is important to advise proper hydration and measures to avoid this geriatric syndrome. Concomitant intake and maintenance of proper vitamin D is required to ensure calcium absorption. However, older adults commonly have low levels of 25 hydroxyvitamin D (25OHD) and, in spite of reports of measurement inconsistencies [88, 89], this should be measured. Vitamin D supplementation is recommended when levels are below 30 ng/ml, aiming to maintain levels above 35 ng/dl using D3 (cholecalciferol) [90, 91]. Toxicity is rare, as vitamin D has a wide therapeutic range. Additional potential benefits of vitamin D repletion include reduction of falls and improvement of physical function [51, 89, 91].

There is evidence of the effectiveness of exercise to preserve or improve bone mass and also to reduce falls [92–94]. Falls are reduced particularly with the combination of aerobic, flexibility, resistance and balance training. Exercise recommendations must be tailored, especially for those with severe osteoporosis, who should avoid forward flexion exercises, using heavy weights, or side-bending exercises, because pushing, pulling, lifting, and bending exert compressive forces on the spine that may lead to fracture. These patients may benefit from specific recommendations provided by a physical therapist [50]. For the majority of older patients, at risk for or with osteoporosis, resources include the National Institute on Aging Go4Life program, which offers free education materials (available at https://go4life.nia.nih.gov) [95] and the National Council on Aging, which lists a number of evidence-based programs (available at https://www.ncoa.org/center-for-healthy-aging/physical-activity/physical-activity-programs-for-older-adults/) [96].

For primary prevention of fractures, a patient with known osteoporosis should have an assessment of gait and balance, especially if there is a history of falls. For details see Chap. 8 on Office Based Assessment. While not specific to osteoporosis, the practice guidelines from the American Geriatrics Society and the British Geriatrics Society [97] outline recommendations for older adults who present with the falls syndrome. Patients with osteoporosis may benefit greatly from a multifactorial risk assessment for falls if they present with more than 2 falls per year, or if a fall leads to an injury or is the chief complaint in the clinical visit. The endocrinologist should ask about falls, and refer the patient to a geriatrician or to a falls clinic. Prevention of falls plays a major role in the prevention of morbidity in patients with osteoporosis. The CDC Stopping Elderly Accidents, Deaths & Injuries (STEADI) program offers tools for assessment and prevention of falls (available at http://www.cdc.gov/steadi/) [98]. Furthermore, for patients at high risk for falls, home safety assessment and modification in those with a previous fall can reduce the rate of falls and risk for falling [99].

Regarding secondary prevention, it is important to recognize patient characteristics that are associated with greater risk for a subsequent fall. A recent systematic review and meta-analysis found that female, institutionalization, decreased vision, dizziness, dementia, cardiac and respiratory diseases, in addition to osteoporosis, increased the risk for a second contralateral hip fracture [100]. Special attention ought to be placed for secondary prevention in those cases.

22.6.4 Problems with Calcium Metabolism

The incidence and prevalence of primary hyperparathyroidism (PHP) is greater with aging. Similarly, the prevalence of cancer associated with non-parathyroid hormone dependent hypercalcemia also increases with aging. For PHP, advanced age is not a contraindication for parathyroidectomy; however, assessments of function, cognition, life-expectancy, and other age-related conditions are needed to complete the assessment and recommendation towards surgery, or chronic medical management with a calcimimetic (Cinacalcet) [101], as well as the pertinent interventions for diagnosis and management of secondary osteoporosis, falls and fracture prevention.

Older adults are a heterogeneous population with a range of comorbidities that influence treatment in all illnesses including calcium disorders. If 10 years passes and PHP is found in Mr. F. (Case 1) who is now 88 years old, with well-controlled diabetes, and preserved physical and cognitive function, parathyroidectomy will be the procedure of choice. However, for Mrs. B. (Case 4), now 82 years old, with cardiovascular disease, severe heart failure, advanced dementia and poor physical function, parathyroidectomy may not be applicable, and medical management may be the first option to discuss with her family.

22.7 Thyroid Disorders

Thyroid disorders are common in older adults with clinical presentations that include both long-standing and new-onset illnesses. Clinical and subclinical hypothyroidism and hyperthyroidism are common as thyroid nodular disease and differentiated thyroid cancer (DTC).

22.7.1 Hypothyroidism

The incidence of hypothyroidism (defined as high TSH and low T-4) increases with age as a result of long-standing hypothyroid disease, resulting from the treatment for hyperthyroidism and differentiated thyroid cancer (DTC), or as a side effect of amiodarone therapy. Diagnosis of hypothyroidism can be delayed by comorbidities, including depression and cognitive decline, thus proper screening must be implemented.

Thyroid hormone replacement with levothyroxine (LT4) is usually based on lean body mass (~1.6 mcg per kg-weight) for healthy middle age patients [99]; age-related loss of lean body mass [103] often means dose adjustments are needed with increasing age. In addition, lower starting dosages (25–50 mcg per day) is recommended for healthy older adults, lower (12.5–25 mcg per day) for those with known or possible cardiovascular disease. Replacement therapy must strive to avoid overtreatment, with careful monitoring every 4–6 weeks, and dose adjustments of 12.5 mcg, until TSH target is reached. A start and go slow approach may also provide more stable TSH values over time [102, 104, 105].

For a patient with a clinical presentation similar to Mr. F. (Case 1), who is otherwise healthy and recently developed primary hypothyroidism, LT4 therapy could reach a full dose replacement similar to a younger person. In contrast, for a patient similar to Mrs. B. (Case 4), a more careful approach is required, given concerns for bone and cardiovascular risk.

Guidelines recommend TSH targets between 1 and 2.5 mIU/L, but normal age-specific TSH values are higher in older adults when compared with younger people [106]. The NHANES study has shown that the 97.5 centiles for TSH in the 20- to 29-year and the 80-year and older groups were 3.56 and 7.49 mIU/L, respectively and 70 % of older patients with TSH greater than 4.5 mIU/L were within their age-specific reference range. In addition, some suggest that higher TSH values in healthy older individuals might be associated with better cognitive and physical function [107, 108].

While there are no randomized controlled trials, we recommend caution when treating hypothyroidism in older adults, especially in the oldest old. A TSH closer to 2.5 mIU/L, and perhaps higher (within the normal range) may be more appropriate, whereas reaching TSH of 1 mIU/L may be potentially harmful.

In addition, for older adults with hypothyroidism related to Hashimoto's thyroiditis, it is important to be aware of the risk of autoimmune atrophic gastritis [109], given potential clinical implications for nutrition and pharmacologic therapies.

22.7.2 Subclinical Hypothyroidism

This condition is defined as a high TSH and normal T-4. The European Thyroid Association provides guidelines for subclinical hypothyroidism management [110] with two potential scenarios: the first one with TSH values range between the upper limit of normal and 10 mIU/L, and the second when TSH is greater than 10 mIU/L. About 90 % of cases fall in the first scenario [111] and have milder clinical consequences [112, 113].

Guidelines recommend careful monitoring and a watchful waiting in the oldest old [9], avoiding a rush to diagnosis based on one value and rather rechecking TSH at 3–6 months intervals.

A recent systematic-review assessed the risk of stroke in those with subclinical hypothyroidism [114]. Compared to those with normal thyroid function, no increased risks were found in individuals with subclinical hypothyroidism in those aged 65 and older. A subsequent analysis from this research group suggested a pattern of increased risk for fatal stroke in younger individuals with higher TSH concentrations [115].

Increased risk for depression has been reported in subjects older than 60 years with untreated subclinical hypothyroidism [116], while a more recent prospective study in adults age 70–82 [117] did not show an association of subclinical hypothyroidism with increased depressive symptoms among those at high cardiovascular risk.

Regarding cognitive decline, a recently published meta-analysis [118] found no association between subclinical hypothyroidism and cognitive performance (impaired mini-mental state examination, executive function, and memory).

Regarding quality of life, a small randomized trial compared the impact of thyroid hormone replacement versus placebo in adults who screened positive for hypothyroidism and those with subclinical hypothyroidism. They found improved quality of life (less tiredness) for the hypothyroid [119] but not those with subclinical hypothyroidism. Therefore, clinical judgment is crucial in the management of subclinical hypothyroidism in older adults. Caution with over-screening leading to overtreatment has been raised, particularly if age-adjusted normal limits of TSH are not used [120]. Decisions should include a specific evaluation of the pre-existent cardiovascular risk, degree of TSH elevation, comorbidity, and frailty [107].

22.7.3 Hyperthyroidism

Excess thyroid hormone may have major impact on bone and cardiovascular health in older adults [121]. Graves' disease is the most common cause of hyperthyroidism, while toxic multinodular goiter and toxic adenoma are more prevalent in iodine deficiency regions [122], and have a faster progression to hypothyroidism post-treatment [123].

Any abnormality in thyroid function can present with non-specific symptoms. For example, apathetic hyperthyroidism in seniors classically has none of the typical symptoms of younger onset hyperthyroidism such as heat intolerance, tremor, nervousness, tachycardia, and others [124], and rather presents with cardiovascular features (atrial fibrillation), depression, lethargy, weakness, weight loss, and without goiter or ocular manifestations [125]. In general, anorexia and atrial fibrillation are more frequent in older than in younger patients [126]. Furthermore, the greater prevalence of HTN and cardiovascular disease in this age group may lead to chronic use of beta-blockers, which mask hyperadrenergic symptoms [124].

Radioactive iodine (RAI) is the preferred therapeutic approach, based on better success rate and safety profile with lesser risk for recurrence. Thionamides become second line alternative therapy, and consideration should be given to the risk-benefit, due to potential adverse reactions, medication interaction, and the greater prevalence of liver and bone marrow diseases in this age group.

22.7.4 Subclinical Hyperthyroidism

Regarding subclinical hyperthyroidism, two scenarios have been described: the first one with TSH between 0.1 mIU/L and the lower limit of normal (grade 1), and the second with TSH below 0.1 mIU/L (grade 2). There is greater concern in grade 2 for cardiovascular risk (heart dysfunction, coronary heart disease, and atrial fibrillation), osteoporosis, and progression to overt hyperthyroidism. Therefore, both American and European guidelines recommend treatment for grade 2 subclinical hyperthyroidism [121, 127]. Nonetheless, persistently suppressed TSH in the grade 1 range may need treatment in older adults given the increased risk for atrial fibrillation and heart failure.

A recent analysis from the Rotterdam Study examined the association between increased thyroid hormone levels and risks for atrial fibrillation [128]. Among subjects with normal free T4 (FT4) levels, higher risks for atrial fibrillation were found in those with FT4 levels in the highest quartile when compared to those in the lowest quartile. The absolute 10-year risk was greater in subjects older than 65 compared to younger subjects.

22.7.5 Differentiated Thyroid Cancer

Late-onset DTC typically presents in older patients and has unique recurrence features, an atypical TNM model, different responses to total thyroidectomy, and a different survival [129]. The older the age the greater the risk for more advanced stage at presentation and the greater the risk for recurrence.

Older adults undergoing TSH suppression with thyroid hormone replacement, post-thyroidectomy for DTC, may be at greater risk of adverse events (e.g., atrial fibrillation and osteoporosis) compared to younger individuals [130, 131]. Potential benefits with beta blockers for prophylaxis have been suggested but more research is needed [132]. Current management guidelines also suggest therapy for osteoporosis [125] and recommendations to preserve bone health such as exercise and supplementation with calcium and vitamin D.

22.8 Hypogonadism

The endocrine evaluation of older men should include evaluation of their gonadal function. Most symptoms associated with gonadal dysfunction are non-specific but may impact quality of life and wellbeing.

22.8.1 Clinical Diagnosis

There is significant heterogeneity in the way older men with hypogonadism present clinically. For men with early-onset hypogonadism due primary to testicular failure or secondary to pituitary tumor resection, long-term monitoring and management is required. Many of the symptoms of testosterone deficiency of late onset (i.e., erectile dysfunction, depression, decreased energy, weakness) may also occur in age-related comorbidities (diabetes, cardiovascular disease, depression, frailty syndrome) and will not improve with testosterone replacement alone. Thus, counseling about expectations from evaluation and treatment for hypogonadism is advised [133, 134].

Since the diagnosis of late-onset hypogonadism often is challenging, a European study evaluated the clinical and hormonal profile in middle-age and older men [129]. Sexual symptoms (poor morning erection, low sexual desire, and erectile dysfunction) were significantly related to low testosterone levels. Less specific symptoms such as depression and fatigue were more typically related to co-existing conditions and had greater impact in quality of life and ability for self-care [136–138]. This fact makes the clinical monitoring of patients on replacement testosterone difficult.

22.8.2 Laboratory Assessment

It is important to recognize that chronic diseases may impact hormonal values [139]. Obesity was associated with lower testosterone values in the Massachusetts Male Aging Study and the European Male Aging Study [140, 141]. Diabetes and heart failure have also been associated with hypogonadism [142, 143]. These diseases are associated with fatigue, poor sleep, insomnia, and other non-specific symptom, which may lead to impaired metabolism, obesity, and impaired gonadal function. In addition, older patients may require medications (opioids, glucocorticoids, and spironolactone) which decrease testosterone levels [144]. Thus, after thorough discussion with patients, laboratory screening for hypogonadism can be considered in older adults with symptoms of hypogonadism [133, 134].

There are changes in the circadian rhythm for testosterone, so blood sample collection is recommended early in the morning after a good night's rest and tested using reliable assays; low levels should be confirmed with a second morning sample. An older person with insomnia or sleep disorders may have inaccurate levels. Consider assessment of free testosterone in the setting of abnormal sex hormone binding globulin, especially in older men with total testosterone concentrations near the lower limit of the normal range and in whom alterations of sex-hormone binding globulin are suspected [134].

Late-onset hypogonadism develops in a relative small percentage of all older men (2.1 % in the European Male Aging Study) [145]. Those with testosterone levels well below the lower limit of 300 ng/dl, i.e. values below 150 ng/dl [146] ought to be reassed (diagnosis requires confirmation in separate occassions). Then, further informed discussion for treatment should follow if results are consistently low in the setting of syndromal presentation (low values alone do not justify treatment). Moreover, it is important to consider potential risks affecting those in whom therapy may be clinically indicated.

22.8.3 Adverse Effects of Testosterone Replacement Therapy

There is growing concern with the increase in testosterone prescriptions and potential health consequences [147]. The American Association of Clinical Endocrinologists recently addressed potential cardiovascular risk [148] and concluded that there is no compelling evidence that testosterone therapy either increases or decreases cardiovascular risk but stated that treatment in older adults should be extra cautious.

Controversy related to cardiovascular safety of testosterone supplementation continues among experts. Several authors have stated the need for adequate randomized trials, powered to assess the impact of testosterone on cardiovascular health and outcomes in the older population [149]. Until then, the decision to treat hypogonadism in older adults must be based on a clinical approach considering the patient's health status, physical and cognitive function, and incorporating the patients' goals, risks, and any special considerations [150].

For those cases in whom testosterone treatment clearly offer greater benefits than risks, recommended monitoring includes surveillance for erythrocytosis, hypertension, prostate disease, and liver abnormalities [151].

22.8.4 Testosterone Replacement Therapy

When treatment is warranted, replacement should aim for testosterone levels in the mid-normal range [146, 151], with suggested target around 400 ng/dl for older men, which is less than in younger individuals.

Building on the clinical scenarios of the learning cases:

If an otherwise healthy older adult, like Mr. F. (Case 1), returns to the clinic for a yearly follow-up, and reports decreased libido, and erectile dysfunction, his symptoms may be due to hypogonadism, and require evaluation. Assuming the laboratory assessments confirm low testosterone values, e.g. 180, and 140 ng/dL, with corresponding increased gonadotropins, the diagnosis of testicular hypogonadism is established and it will be appropriate to discuss testosterone replacement. For this relatively healthy older man, with preserved physical function, cognition and good social support, treatment can improve symptoms and his quality of life.

However, there will be more complex scenarios. For example, a 70-year-old man who has diabetes, coronary artery disease, and a known family history of prostate cancer, presents with complaints of fatigue, depression, and inability to perform vigorous activity. Laboratory assessment shows borderline low testosterone values of 290 and 280 ng/dL. Given the family history of prostate cancer and the potential concerns about cardiovascular safety, testosterone therapy may not be initially recommended. These non-specific symptoms could be explained by stress, poor sleep, and impaired physical function. Furthermore, the risk benefit ratio of testosterone replacement is not clearly favorable. On the other hand, a healthy, functional, and cognitively intact

68-year-old man with hypertension and family history (cousin) of prostate cancer is found to have osteoporosis, and unequivocally low testosterone values (e.g., 150 and 140 ng/dL), and a normal prostate specific antigen. In this case, testosterone replacement will improve bone health, quality of life, function, and future outcomes, since a fracture could be devastating to him.

References

1. American Diabetes Association. Fast facts data and statistics about diabetes. March, 2015. Available at http://professional.diabetes.org/admin/UserFiles/0%20-%20Sean/14_fast_facts_june2014_final3.pdf. Accessed 8 Oct 2015.
2. Centers for Disease Prevention and Control. Incidence of diagnosed diabetes per 1,000 population aged 18-79 years, by age, United States, 1980-2014. Available at http://www.cdc.gov/diabetes/statistics/incidence/fig3.htm. Accessed 8 Oct 2015.
3. Centers for Disease Control and Prevention. National Diabetes Statistics Report, 2014. Available at http://www.cdc.gov/diabetes/pubs/statsreport14/national-diabetes-report-web.pdf. Accessed 8 Oct 2015.
4. Centers for Disease Control and Prevention. National Diabetes Statistics Report: estimates of diabetes and its burden in the United States, 2014. Atlanta, GA: US Department of Health and Human Services; 2014. Available at http://www.cdc.gov/diabetes/pubs/statsreport14/national-diabetes-report-web.pdf. Accessed 8 Oct 2015.
5. Kirkman SM, Briscoe VJ, Clark N, et al. Diabetes in older adults. Diabetes Care. 2012;35:2650–64.
6. American Diabetes Association. Older adults. Sec 10. In standards of Medical care in Diabetes – 2015. Diabetes Care 2015;38(Suppl 1):S67–S9.
7. Valencia WM, Florez H. Pharmacological treatment of diabetes in older people. Diabetes Obes Metab. 2014;16(12):1192–203.
8. Inzucchi SE, Bergenstal RM, Buse JB, et al. Management of hyperglycemia in type 2 diabetes, 2015: a patient-centered approach. Update to a Position Statement of the American Diabetes Association and the European Association for the Study of Diabetes. Diabetes Care. 2015;38:140–9.
9. American Geriatrics Society. Guiding principles for the care of older adults with multimorbidity: an approach for clinicians. American Geriatrics Society Expert Panel on the care of older adults with multimorbidity. J Am Geriatr Soc. 2012;60(10):E1–E25.
10. Huang ES, Laiteerapong N, Liu JY, et al. Rates of complications and mortality in older patients with diabetes mellitus. The diabetes and aging study. JAMA Inter Med. 2014;174(2):251–8.
11. Strotmeyer ES. Diabetes and aging. Clin Geriatr Med 2015;31(1):xiii–xvi.
12. American Diabetes Association. Initial evaluation and diabetes management planning. Sec 3. In standards of Medical care in Diabetes – 2015. Diabetes Care 2015;38(Suppl 1):S17–S9.
13. Sinclair A, Morley JE, Rodriguez-Manas L, et al. Diabetes mellitus in older people: position statement on behalf of the International Association of Gerontology and Geriatrics (IAGG), the European Diabetes Working Party for older people (EDWPOP), and the International Task Force of Experts in Diabetes. J Am Med Dir Assoc. 2012;13:497–502.
14. Lin J, Zhou S, Wei W, Pan C, Lingohr-Smith M, Levin P. Does clinical inertia vary by personalized A1c goal? A study of predictors and prevalence of clinical inertia in a US managed care setting. Endocr Pract. 2015. [Epub ahead of print].
15. Diabetes Prevention Program Research Group. Reduction in the incidence of type 2 diabetes with lifestyle intervention or metformin. N Engl J Med. 2002;346(6):393–403.
16. Diabetes Prevention Program Research Group, Crandall J, Schade D, et al. The influence of age on the effects of lifestyle modification and metformin in prevention of diabetes. J Gerontol A Biol Sci Med Sci. 2006;61(1):1075–81.
17. Garber AJ, Abrahamson MJ, Barzilay JI, et al. AACE/ACE comprehensive diabetes management algorithm 2015. Endocr Pract. 2015;21(4):438–47.
18. The Action to Control Cardiovascular Risk in Diabetes Study Group. Effects of intensive glucose lowering in type 2 diabetes. N Engl J Med. 2008;368(24):2545–59.
19. The ADVANCE Collaborative Group. Intensive blood glucose control and vascular outcomes in patients with type 2 diabetes. N Engl J Med. 2008;358:2560–72.
20. Duckworth WC, Abraira C, Moritz T, et al. Glucose control and vascular complications in Veterans with type 2 diabetes. N Eng J Med. 2009;360:129–39.
21. American Geriatrics Society Expert Panel on the Care of Older Adults with Diabetes Mellitus. Guidelines abstracted from the American Geriatrics Society guidelines for improving the care of older adults with diabetes mellitus: 2013 Update. J Am Geriatr Soc. 2013;61:2020–26
22. The American Geriatrics Society 2015 Beers Criteria Update Expert Panel. American Geriatrics Society 2015 updated Beers Criteria for potentially inappropriate medication use in older adults. J Am Geriatr Soc. 2015;63:2227–46.
23. Inouye SK, Studenski S, Tinetti ME, Kuchel GA. Geriatric syndromes: clinical, research and policy implications of a core geriatric concept. J Am Geriatr Soc. 2007;55(5):780–91.
24. Munshi M. Managing the "geriatric syndrome" in patients with type 2 diabetes. Consult Pharm. 2008;23(Suppl B):12–6.
25. Boyd CM, Darer J, Boult C, et al. Clinical practice guidelines and quality of care for older patients with multiple comorbid diseases: implications for pay for performance. JAMA. 2005;294(60):716–24.
26. Peron EP, Ogbonna KC, Donohoe KL. Antidiabetic medications and polypharmacy. Clin Geriatr Med. 2015;31:17–27.
27. Wu Q, Tchetgen Tchetgen EJ, Qsypuk T, et al. Estimating the cognitive effects of prevalent diabetes, recent onset diabetes, and the duration of diabetes among older adults. Dement Geriatr Cogn Disord. 2015;39:239–49.
28. Bangen KJ, Gu Y, Gross AL, et al. Relationship between type 2 diabetes mellitus and cognitive change in a multiethnic elderly cohort. J Am Geriatr Soc. 2015;63:1075–83.
29. Rawlings AM, Sharrett AR, Schneider ALC, et al. Diabetes in midlife and cognitive change over 20 years. A cohort study. Ann Intern Med. 2014;161:785–93.
30. Feinkohl I, Aung PP, Keller M, et al. Severe hypoglycemia and cognitive decline in older people with type 2 diabetes: the Edinburg type 2 diabetes study. Diabetes Care. 2014;37:507–15.
31. Launer LJ, Miller ME, Williamson JD, et al. Effects of intensive glucose lowering on brain structure and function in people with type 2 diabetes (ACCORD MIND): a randomized open-label substudy. Lancet Neurol. 2011;10:969–77.
32. Espeland MA, Rapp SR, Bray GA, et al. Long-term impact of behavioral weight loss intervention on cognitive function. J Gerontol A Biol Sci Med Sci. 2014;69(9):1101–8.
33. Whitmer RA, Karter AJ, Yaffe K, Quesenberry CPJ, Selby JV. Hypoglycemic episodes and risk of dementia in older patients with type 2 diabetes. JAMA. 2009;301:1565–72.
34. Punthakee Z, Miller ME, Launer LE, et al. Poor cognitive function and risk of severe hypoglycemia in type 2 diabetes. Diabetes Care. 2012;35:787–93.

35. CDC overweight and obesity facts. Centers for Disease Control and Prevention. 2014. Available at. http://www.cdc.gov/obesity/data/adult.html. Accessed 8 Oct 2015.

36. Valencia WM, Stoutenberg M, Florez H. Weight loss and physical activity for disease prevention in obese older adults: an important role for lifestyle management. Curr Diab Rep. 2014;14:539–48.

37. Loef M, Walach H. Midlife obesity and dementia: meta-analysis and adjusted forecast of dementia prevalence in the United States and China. Obesity. 2013;21:E51–5.

38. WHO Global strategy on diet, physical activity and health. Obesity and overweight facts. World Health Organization. 2003. Available at http://www.who.int/dietphysicalactivity/media/en/gsfs_obesity.pdf. Accessed 8 Oct 2015.

39. The Obesity Society. Obesity, bias and stigmatization. Available at http://www.obesity.org/resources/facts-about-obesity/bias-stigmatization. Accessed 8 Oct 2015.

40. Carnethon MR, De Chavez PJD, Biggs ML, et al. Association of weight status with mortality in adults with incident diabetes. JAMA. 2012;308:581–90.

41. Lavie CJ, McAuley PA, Church TS, Milani RV, Blair SN. Obesity and cardiovascular diseases: implications regarding fitness, fatness, and severity in the obesity paradox. J Am Coll Cardiol. 2014;63:1345–54.

42. Hainer V, Aldhoon-Hainerová I. Obesity paradox does exist. Diabetes Care. 2013;36 Suppl 2:S276–81.

43. McAuley PA, Beavers KM. Contribution of cardiorespiratory fitness to the obesity paradox. Prog Cardiovasc Dis. 2014;56:434–40.

44. Barry VW, Baruth M, Beets MW, Durstine JL, Liu J, Blair SN. Fitness vs fatness on all-cause mortality: a meta-analysis. Prog Cardiovasc Dis. 2014;56:382–90.

45. Center JR, Nguyen TV, Schneider D, Sambrook PN, Eisman JA. Mortality after all major types of osteoporotic fracture in men and women: an observational study. Lancet. 1999;353(9156):878–82.

46. Kannegaard PN, van derMark S, Eiken P, Abrahamsen B. Excess mortality in men compared with women following a hip fracture. National analysis of comedications, comorbidity and survival. Age Ageing. 2010;39(2):203–9.

47. Rizzoli R, Branco J, Brandi ML, et al. Management of osteoporosis in the oldest old. Osteoporos Int. 2014;25:2507–29.

48. Chevalley T, Guilley E, Hermann FR, Hoffmeyer P, Rapin CH, Rizzoli R. Incidence of hip fracture over a 10-year period (1991-2000): reversal of a secular trend. Bone. 2007;40:1284–9.

49. Johnell O, Kanis JA. An estimate of the worldwide prevalence and disability associated with osteoporotic fractures. Osteoporos Int. 2006;17:1726–33.

50. Watts NB, Bilezikian JP, Camacho PM, et al. American Association of Clinical Endocrinologists medical guidelines for clinical practice for the diagnosis and treatment of postmenopausal osteoporosis. Endocr Pract. 2010;16 Suppl 3:1–37.

51. U.S. Preventive Services Task Force. Screening for osteoporosis: U.S. Preventive Services Task Force Recommendation Statement. Ann Intern Med. 2011;154:356–64.

52. Watts NB, Adler RA, Bilezikian JP, et al. Osteoporosis in men: an endocrine society clinical practice guideline. J Clin Endocrinol Metab. 2012;97(6):1802–22.

53. Cosman F, de Beur SJ, LeBoff MS, et al. Clinician's guide to prevention and treatment of osteoporosis. Osteoporos Int. 2014;25:2359–81.

54. Burge R, Dawson-Hughes B, Solomon DH, Wong JB, King A, Tosteson A. Incidence and economic burden of osteoporosis-related fractures in the United States, 2005-2025. J Bone Miner Res. 2007;22:465–75.

55. Office of the Surgeon General. Rockville (MD). Bone health and osteoporosis: a report of the surgeon general. Available on line at http://www.ncbi.nlm.nih.gov/books/NBK45502/#ch5.s8; 2004.

56. Bouxsein ML, Genant HK, International Osteoporosis Foundation. The breaking spine. Available at http://www.iofbonehealth.org/sites/default/files/PDFs/WOD%20Reports/2010_the_breaking_spine_en.pdf. Accessed 16 Nov 2015.

57. Goldstein CL, Chutkan NB, Choma TJ, Orr RD. Management of the elderly with vertebral compression fractures. Neurosurgery. 2015;77:533–45.

58. International Osteoporosis Foundation (IOF). Impact of osteoporosis. Available online at http://www.iofbonehealth.org/impact-osteoporosis. Accessed 23 Oct 2015.

59. Darba J, Kaskens L, Perez-Alvarez N, Palacios S, Neyro JL, Rejas J. Disability-adjusted-life-years losses in postmenopausal women with osteoporosis: a burden of illness study. BMC Public Health. 2015;15:234–43.

60. Stenderup K, Justesen J, Clausen C, Kassem M. Aging is associated with decreased maximal life span and accelerated senescence of bone marrow stromal cells. Bone. 2003;33:919–26.

61. Zhou S, Greenberger JS, Epperly MW, et al. Age-related intrinsic changes in human bone-marrow-derived mesenchymal stem cells and their differentiation to osteoblasts. Aging Cell. 2008;7:335–43.

62. D'Amelio P, Roato I, D'Amico L, et al. Bone and bone marrow pro-osteoclastogenic cytokines are upregulated in osteoporosis fragility fractures. Osteoporos Int. 2011;22:2869–77.

63. Kanis JA, Oden A, McCloskey EV, Johansson H, Wahl DA, Cooper C, on behalf of the IOF Working Group on Epidemiology and Quality of Life. A systematic review of hip fracture incidence and probability of fracture worldwide. Osteoporos Int. 2012;23:2239–56.

64. Kanis JA, Johansson H, Oden A, Dawson-Hughes B, Melton 3rd LJ, McCloskey EV. The effects of a FRAX revision for the USA. Osteoporos Int. 2010;21(1):35–40.

65. Donaldson MG, Cawton PM, Lui LY, et al. Estimates of the proportion of older white men who would be recommended for pharmacologic treatment by the new US National Osteoporosis Foundation guidelines. J Bone Miner Res. 2010;25:1506–11.

66. Watts NB. Osteoporosis in men. Endocr Pract. 2013;19:834–8.

67. Laurent M, Gielen E, Claessens F, Boonen S, Vanderschueren D. Osteoporosis in older men: recent advances in pathophysiology and treatment. Best Pract Res Clin Endocrinol Metab. 2013;27(4):527–39.

68. Sayer AA, Robinson SM, Patel HP, Shavlakadze T, Cooper C, Grounds MD. New horizons in the pathogenesis, diagnosis and management of sarcopenia. Age Ageing. 2013;42:145–50.

69. Di Monaco M, Castiglione C, Vallero F, Di Monaco R, Tappero R. Sarcopenia is more prevalent in men than in women after hip fracture: a cross-sectional study of 591 inpatients. Arch Gerontol Geriatr. 2012;55:e48–52.

70. Bijlsma AY, Meskers CG, Westendorp RG, Maier AB. Chronology of age-related disease definitions: osteoporosis and sarcopenia. Ageing Res Rev. 2012;11(2):320–4.

71. Gibson MJ, Andres RO, Isaacs B, Radebaugh T, Worm-Petersen J. The prevention of falls in later life. A report of the Kellogg International Work Group on the prevention of falls by the elderly. Dan Med Bull. 1987;34 Suppl 4:1–24.

72. Centers for Disease Control and Prevention. Important facts about falls. Available at http://www.cdc.gov/homeandrecreational-safety/falls/adultfalls.html. Accessed 16 Nov 2016.

73. Hayes WC, Myers ER, Morris JN, Gerhart TN, Yett HS, Lipsitz LA. Impact near the hip dominates fracture risk in elderly nursing home residents who fall. Calcif Tissue Int. 1993;52:192–8.

74. Fried LP, Tangen CM, Walston J, et al. Frailty in older adults: evidence for a phenotype. J Gerontol A Biol Sci Med Sci. 2001;56(3):M146–56.

75. Klotzbuecher CM, Ross PD, Landsman PB, et al. Patients with prior fractures have an increased risk of future fractures: a sum-

mary of the literature and statistical synthesis. J Bone Miner Res. 2000;15:721–39.

76. Lonnroos E, Kautiainen H, Karppi P, et al. Incidence of second hip fractures. A population-based study. Osteoporos Int. 2007;18:1279–85.

77. Berry SD, Samelson EJ, Hannan MT, et al. Second hip fracture in older men and women: the Framingham Study. Arch Intern Med. 2007;167:1971–6.

78. Shen S-H, Huang K-C, Tsai Y-H, et al. Risk analysis for second hip fracture in patients after hip fracture surgery: a nationwide population-based study. J Am Med Dir Assoc. 2014;2015:725–31.

79. Toussaint ND, Elder GJ, Kerr PG. Bisphosphonates in chronic kidney disease; balancing potential benefits and adverse effects on bone and soft tissue. Clin J Am Soc Nephrol. 2009;4(1):221–33.

80. Miller PD. The kidney and bisphosphonates. Bone. 2011;49(1):77–81.

81. Batchelor P. The changing epidemiology of oral diseases in the elderly, their growing importance for care and how they can be managed. Age Aging. 2015;44:1064–70.

82. Spanou A, Lyritis GP, Chronopoulos E, Tournis S. Management of bisphosphonate-related osteonecrosis of the jaw: a literature review. Oral Dis. 2015;21(8):927–36.

83. Body JJ, Bergmann P, Boonen S, et al. Non-pharmacological management of osteoporosis: a consensus of the Belgian Bone Club. Osteoporos Int. 2011;22:2769–88.

84. Diab DL, Watts NB. Diagnosis and treatment of osteoporosis in older adults. Endocrinol Metab Clin N Am. 2013;42:305–17.

85. Verbrugge FH, Gielen E, Milisen K, Boonen S. Who should receive calcium and vitamin D supplementation? Age Ageing. 2012;41:576–80.

86. Sipponen P, Maaross HI. Chronic gastritis. Scand J Gastroenterol. 2015;50(6):657–67.

87. Mayo Clinic. Healthy Lifestyle. Nutrition and healthy aging. Available at http://www.mayoclinic.org/healthy-lifestyle/nutrition-and-healthy-eating/in-depth/calcium-supplements/art-20047097?pg=2. Accessed 31 Dec 2015.

88. Black LJ, Anderson D, Clarke MW, Ponsonby A-L, Lucas RM, Ausimmune Investigator Group. Analytical bias in the measurement of serum 25-hydroxyvitamin D concentrations impairs assessment of vitamin D status in clinical and research settings. PLoS One. 2015;10:1–14.

89. Gallagher JC. Vitamin D, and aging. Endocrinol Metab Clin N Am. 2013;42:319–32.

90. Armas LA, Hollis BW, Heaney RP. Vitamin D2 is much less effective than vitamin D3 in humans. J Clin Endocrinol Metab. 2004;89(11):5387–91.

91. Bjelakovic G, Gluud LL. Nikolova, et al. Vitamin D supplementation for prevention of mortality in adults. Cochrane Database Syst Rev. 2014;10(1), CD007470.

92. Sherrington C, Whitney JC, Lord SR, Herbert RD, Cumming RG, Close JC. Effective exercise for the prevention of falls: a systematic review and meta-analysis. J Am Geriatr Soc. 2008;56(12):2234–43.

93. Choi M, Hector M. Effectiveness of intervention programs in preventing falls: a systematic review of recent 10 years and meta-analysis. J Am Med Dir Assoc. 2012;13(2):188.e13–188.e21

94. Lee MS, Pittler MH, Shin BC, Ernst E. Tai Chi for osteoporosis: a systematic review. Osteoporos Int. 2008;19:139–46.

95. Go4Life from the National Institute on Aging at NIH. Available at https://go4life.nia.nih.gov/. Accessed 14 Dec 2015.

96. National Council on Aging. Exercise programs that promote senior fitness. Available at https://www.ncoa.org/center-for-healthy-aging/physical-activity/physical-activity-programs-for-older-adults/. Accessed 14 Dec 2015.

97. American Geriatrics Society and British Geriatrics Society. Summary of the updated American Geriatrics Society/British Geriatrics Society clinical practice guideline for prevention of falls in older persons. J Am Geriatr Soc. 2011;59:148–57.

98. Centers for Disease Control and Prevention. STEADI stopping elderly accidents, deaths and injuries. Available at http://www.cdc.gov/steadi/. Accessed 14 Dec 2015.

99. Gillispie LD, Robertson MC, Gillispie WJ, et al. Interventions for preventing falls in older people living in the community. Cochrane Database Syst Rev. 2012;12(9), CD007146.

100. Liu S, Zhu Y, Chen W, Sun T, Cheng J, Zhang Y. Risk factors for the second contralateral hip fracture in elderly patients: a systematic review and meta-analysis. Clin Rehabil. 2015;29(3):285–94.

101. Marcocci C, Bollerslev J, Khan AA, Shoback DM. Medical management of primary hyperparathyroidism: proceedings of the fourth International Workshop on the Management of Asymptomatic Primary Hyperparathyroidism. J Clin Endocrinol Metab. 2014;99(10):3607–18.

102. Jonklaas J, Bianco AC, Bauer AJ, et al. Guidelines for the treatment of hypothyroidism: prepared by the American Thyroid Association task force on thyroid hormone replacement. Thyroid. 2014;24(12):1670–751.

103. Cunningham JJ, Barzel US. Lean body mass is a predictor of the daily requirement for thyroid hormone in older men and women. J Am Geriatr Soc. 1984;32:204–7.

104. Kabadi UM. Variability of L-thyroxine replacement dose in elderly patients with primary hypothyroidism. J Fam Pract. 1987;24:473–7.

105. Pecina J, Garrison GM, Bernard M. Levothyroxine dosage is associated with stability of TSH values. Am J Med. 2014;127:240–5.

106. Surks MI, Hollowell JG. Age-specific distribution of serum thyrotropin and antithyroid antibodies in the US population: implications for the prevalence of subclinical hypothyroidism. J Clin Endocrinol Metab. 2007;92:4575–82.

107. Gussekloo J, van Exel E, de Craen AJ, Meinders AE, Frolich M, Westendorp RG. Thyroid status, disability and cognitive function, and survival in old age. JAMA. 2004;292:2591–9.

108. Simonsick EM, Newman AB, Ferrucci L, et al. Subclinical hypothyroidism and functional mobility in older adults. Arch Intern Med. 2009;169:2011–7.

109. Centanni M, Marignani M, Gargano L, et al. Atrophic body gastritis in patients with autoimmune thyroid disease: an underdiagnosed association. Arch Intern Med. 1999;159:1726–30.

110. Pearce SHS, Brabant G, Duntas LH, et al. 2013 ETA guideline: management of subclinical hypothyroidism. Eur Thyroid J. 2013;2:215–28.

111. Hollowell JG, Staehling NW, Flanders WD, et al. Serum TSH, T4, and thyroid antibodies in the United States population (1988 to 1994): National Health and Nutrition Examination Survey (NHANES III). J Clin Endocrinol Metab. 2002;87:489–99.

112. Surks MI, Ortiz E, Daniels GH, et al. Subclinical thyroid disease: scientific review and guidelines for diagnosis and management. JAMA. 2004;29:228–38.

113. Canaris GJ, Manowitz NR, Mayor G, Ridgway EC. The Colorado thyroid disease prevalence study. Arch Intern Med. 2000;160:526–34.

114. Chaker L, Baumgartner C, Ikram MA, et al. Subclinical thyroid dysfunction and the risk of stroke: a systematic review and meta-analysis. Eur J Epidemiol. 2014;29:791–800.

115. Chaker L, Baumgartner C, den Elzen WPJ, et al. Subclinical hypothyroidism and the risk of stroke events and fatal stroke: an individual participant data analysis. J Clin Endocrinol Metab. 2015;100:2181–91.

116. Chueire VB, Romaldini JH, Ward LS. Subclinical hypothyroidism increases the risk for depression in the elderly. Arch Gerontol Geriatr. 2007;44(1):21–8.

117. Blum MR, Bauer DC, Collet T-H, et al. Subclinical thyroid dysfunction and fracture risk. A meta-analysis. JAMA. 2015;313(20): 2055–65.

118. Akintola AA, Jansen SW, van Bodegom D, et al. Subclinical hypothyroidism and cognitive function in people over 60 years: a systematic review and meta-analysis. Front Aging Neurosci. 2015;7(150):1–10.

119. Abu-Helalah M, Law MR, Bestwick JP, Monson JP, Wald NJ. A randomized double-blind crossover trial to investigate the efficacy of screening for adult hypothyroidism. J Med Screen. 2010;17: 164–9.

120. Hennessey JV, Espaillat R. Diagnosis and management of subclinical hypothyroidism in elderly adults: a review of the literature. J Am Geriatr Soc. 2015;63:1663–73.

121. Bahn RS, Burch HB, Cooper DS, et al. American Thyroid Association/American Association of Clinical Endocrinologists. Hyperthyroidism and other causes of thyrotoxicosis: management guidelines of the American Thyroid Association and American Association of Clinical Endocrinologists. Thyroid. 2011;21(6): 593–687.

122. Laurberg P, Pedersen KM, Vestergaard H, Sigurdsson G. High incidence of multinodular toxic goitre in the elderly population in a low iodine intake area vs. high incidence of Graves' disease in the young in a high iodine intake area: comparative surveys of thyrotoxicosis epidemiology in East-Jutland Denmark and Iceland. J Intern Med. 1991;229:415–20.

123. Ceccarelli C, Bencivelli W, Vitti P, Grasso L, Pinchera A. Outcome of radioiodine-131 therapy in hyperfunctioning thyroid nodules: a 20 years' retrospective study. Clin Endocrinol (Oxf). 2005;62:331–5.

124. Mitrou P, Raptis SA, Dmitriadis G. Thyroid disease in older people. Maturitas. 2011;70:5–9.

125. Wu W, Sun Z, Yu J, et al. A clinical retrospective analysis of factors associated with apathetic hyperthyroidism. Pathobiology. 2010;77:46–51.

126. Trivalle C, Doucet J, Chassagne P, et al. Differences in the signs and symptoms of hyperthyroidism in older and younger patients. J Am Geriatr Soc. 1996;46:50–3.

127. Biondi B, Bartalena L, Cooper D, Hegedus L, Laurberg P, Kahaly G. The 2015 European Thyroid Association Guidelines on diagnosis and treatment of endogenous subclinical hyperthyroidism. Eur Thyroid J. 2015;4:149–63.

128. Chaker L, Heeringa J, Dehghan A, et al. Normal thyroid function and the risk of atrial fibrillation: the Rotterdam study. J Clin Endocrinol Metab. 2015;100:3718–24.

129. Alexander EK, Bible KC, Doherty GM, et al. 2015 American Thyroid Association management guidelines for adult patients with thyroid nodules and differentiated thyroid cancer. Thyroid. 2016;26:1–133.

130. Sawin CT, Geller A, Wolf PA, et al. Low serum thyrotropin concentrations as a risk factor for atrial fibrillation in older persons. N Engl J Med. 1994;331:1249–52.

131. Flynn RW, Bonellie SR, Jung RT, MacDonald TM, Morris AD, Leese GP. Serum thyroid-stimulating hormone concentration and morbidity from cardiovascular disease and fractures in patients on long-term thyroxine therapy. J Clin Endocrinol Metab. 2010;95:186–93.

132. Taillard V, Sardinoux M, Oudot C, et al. Early detection of isolated left ventricular diastolic dysfunction in highrisk differentiated thyroid carcinoma patients on TSH-suppressive therapy. Clin Endocrinol (Oxf). 2011;75:709–14.

133. Petak SM, Nankin HR, Spark RF, Swerdloff RS, Rodriguez-Riqau LJ. American Association of Clinical Endocrinologists medical guidelines for clinical practice for the evaluation and treatment of hypogonadism in adult male patients – 2002 update. Endocr Pract. 2002;8:440–59.

134. Bhasin S, Cunningham GR, Hayes FJ, et al. Testosterone therapy in men with androgen deficiency syndromes: an Endocrine Society clinical practice guideline. J Clin Endocrinol Metab. 2010;95:2536–59.

135. Wu FC, Tajar A, Beynon JM, et al. Identification of late-onset hypogonadism in middle-aged and elderly men. N Engl J Med. 2010;363:123–35.

136. Gielissen MF, Knoop H, Servaes P, et al. Differences in the experience of fatigue in patients and healthy controls: patients' descriptions. Health Qual Life Outcomes. 2007;5:36–42.

137. Park M, Reynolds III CF. Depression among older adults with diabetes. Clin Geriatr Med. 2015;31:117–37.

138. Ginsberg TB. Male sexuality. Clin Geriatr Med. 2010;26: 185–95.

139. Travison TG, Araujo AB, Kupelian V, et al. The relative contributions of aging, health, and lifestyle factors to serum testosterone decline in men. J Clin Endocrinol Metab. 2007;92:549–55.

140. Mohr BA, Bhasin S, Link CL, O'Donnell AB, McKinlay JB. The effect of changes in adiposity on testosterone levels in older men: longitudinal results from the Massachusetts Male Aging Study. Eur J Endocrinol. 2006;155:443–52.

141. Wu FC, Tajar A, Pye SR, et al. Hypothalamic-pituitary-testicular axis dysruptions in older men are differentially linked to age and modifiable risk factors: the European male aging study. J Clin Endocrinol Metab. 2008;93:2737–45.

142. Dandona P, Dhindsa S. Hypogonadotropic hypogonadism in type 2 diabetes and obesity. J Clin Endocrinol Metab. 2011;96: 2643–51.

143. Jankowska EA, Biel B, Majda J, et al. Anabolic deficiency in men with chronic heart failure: prevalence and detrimental impact on survival. Circulation. 2006;114:1829–37.

144. Basaria S. Reproductive aging in men. Endocrinol Metab Clin N Am. 2013;42:255–70.

145. Tajar A, Huhtaniemi IT, O'Neil TW, et al. Characteristics of androgen deficiency in late-onset hypogonadism: results from the European Male Aging Study (EMAS). J Clin Endocrinol Metab. 2012;97:1508–16.

146. Feldman HA, Loncope C, Derby CA, et al. Age trends in the level of serum testosterone and other hormones in middle-aged men: longitudinal results from the Massachusetts male aging study. J Clin Endocrinol Metab. 2002;87:589–98.

147. Gan EH, Pattman S, Pearce S, Quinton R. Many men are receiving unnecessary testosterone prescriptions. BMJ. 2012;345, e5469.

148. Goodman N, Guay A, Dandona P, et al. American Association of Clinical Endocrinologists and American College of Endocrinology position statement on the association of testosterone and cardiovascular risk. Endocr Pract. 2015;21:1066–73.

149. Gencer B, Mach F. Testosterone: a hormone preventing cardiovascular disease or a therapy increasing cardiovascular events? Eur Heart J. 2015; pii: ehv439. [Epub ahead of print].

150. Matsumoto AM. Testosterone administration in older men. Endocrinol Metab Clin N Am. 2013;43:271–86.

151. Bhattacharya RK, Bhattacharya SB. Late-onset hypogonadism and testosterone replacement in older men. Clin Geriatr Med. 2015;31:631–44.

Gastroenterology

23

Marc S. Piper and Karen E. Hall

23.1 The Extent of the Problem

Gastrointestinal symptoms are common in patients aged 65 and older and can range from mild self-limited episodes of constipation or acid reflux to life-threatening episodes of infectious colitis or bowel ischemia. This chapter highlights common GI problems in older patients that may affect care by specialists.

23.2 Gastroesophageal Reflux Disease

Gastroesophageal reflux disease (GERD) is one of the more common GI disorders affecting the elderly [1]. Population studies indicate that more than 20 % of adults over age 65 have heartburn at least weekly. This may actually underestimate the true prevalence of GERD because symptoms appear to decrease in intensity with age, and the severity of reflux and complications increase. The use of proton pump inhibitors (PPIs) has probably resulted in treatment of unsuspected GERD. GERD is straightforward to diagnose if it presents with the classic symptoms of pyrosis (substernal burning with radiation to the mouth and throat) and sour regurgitation, however geriatric patients may present with more subtle symptoms, such as a chronic cough, difficult-to-control asthma, laryngitis, recurrent chest pain, or may be asymptomatic and present with anemia or dysphagia due to dysmotility or stricture. Complications associated with GERD such as esophagitis, esophageal ulceration, bleeding, strictures, Barrett's esophagus, and esophageal adenocarcinoma are more common in patients over 65 years of age [2]. Upper endoscopy (EGD) should be performed in all patients with new-onset GERD over age 50, persistent symptoms of reflux despite medical therapy, patients with a history of acid reflux longer than 5 years, and those with possible complications from acid reflux, as these groups have an increased risk of malignancy. EGD is safe even in the very elderly frail patient—the main contraindication is end-stage chronic obstructive pulmonary disease (COPD) or when sedation is contraindicated. Other testing, such as 24-h pH monitoring or esophageal manometry, is reserved for patients who do not respond to therapy or who have atypical symptoms. Treatment of GERD in the elderly is essentially the same as that in younger patients with a notable exception. While the "step-up" approach of lifestyle changes followed by acid-reducing drugs may work for mild GERD, immediate initiation of a PPI along with lifestyle modifications usually results in fewer office visits, a reduction in procedures, improved patient satisfaction, and reduced overall costs (Table 23.1).

Histamine 2 receptor antagonists (H2RAs) are effective for mild symptoms, and avoid the side effects of PPIs such as fracture and Clostridium difficile infection. Cimetidine and ranitidine are not recommended in older patients because of drug interactions and greater anticholinergic effects compared with other H_2RAs. While effective, chronic PPI use is associated with an increased relative risk of osteoporosis of 1.97 (>7 years) [3]. There have been reports of other concerns, such as decreased efficacy of clopidogrel against coronary stent occlusion when used in conjunction with PPIs, and increased risk of pneumonia in ventilated ICU patients, and Clostridium difficile infection [4]. Re-evaluate the need for PPIs in patients who have been taking them for longer than 6 months or who had PPIs started for ulcer prophylaxis during hospitalization. Antireflux surgery is reserved for patients with severe refractory GERD with complications. Results from high-volume centers indicate that mortality and morbidity are not increased in patients over 70 years who are at low surgical risk for complications. However, while only 10–15 % of patients have symptoms immediately post-surgery, 5–15 years later 60 % of patients are taking acid suppressive medications.

M.S. Piper, MD • K.E. Hall, MD, PhD (✉)
Division of Gastroenterology, Department of Internal Medicine, University of Michigan Healthcare System, 3912 Taubman Center 1500 E. Medical Center Dr, Ann Arbor, MI 48109-5362, USA
e-mail: kehall@med.umich.edu

© Springer International Publishing Switzerland 2017
J.R. Burton et al. (eds.), *Geriatrics for Specialists*, DOI 10.1007/978-3-319-31831-8_23

Table 23.1 Treatment of GERD in older patients

Step 1
Lifestyle modifications
Smaller, more frequent meals
Avoid chocolate, peppermint, acidic foods, or foods that stimulate acid production (caffeine-containing foods)
Stop eating 3–4 h before going to bed
Minimize fats, alcohol, caffeine, and nicotine, especially at night
Sleep with head of bed elevated 6 in
Proton pump inhibitors (re-evaluate after 8–12 weeks)
Esomeprazole (Nexium; 20–40 mg qd)
Lansoprazole (Prevacid; 15–30 mg qd)
Omeprazole (Prilosec; 20–40 mg qd) — available OTC as Prilosec 20 mg
Pantoprazole (Protonix; 40 mg qd)
Rabeprazole (Aciphex; 20 mg qd)
Step 2
Add antacid liquids or tablets for occasional breakthrough
Mylanta, Maalox, Gaviscon, Tums, Rolaids
*Add H2 receptor antagonists (H2RAs) at night*a
Cimetidine (Tagamet; not recommended in older patients because of drug interactions and delirium risk)
Famotidine (Pepcid; 20 mg qd or bid)
Nizatidine (Axid; 150 mg qd or bid)
Ranitidine (Zantac not recommended in older patients because of increased risk of delirium; 150 mg qd or bid)
Step 3
Surgery
Laparoscopic fundoplication
Nissen fundoplication

aThis entire class of medications appears on the Beers List of Potentially Inappropriate Medications. All agents have some anticholinergic activity and have been implicated in delirium; all require dose adjustment for creatinine clearance <50 ml/min

Table 23.2 Causes of odynophagia

1. Medications
Tetracycline
Quinidine
Doxycycline
Alendronate
Iron
NSAIDs
ASA
Vitamin C
Potassium chloride
2. Infections
Viral (HSV, CMV, HIV, VZV)
Bacterial (*Mycobacteria*)
Fungal (*Candida, Asperigillus*)
3. Acid reflux disease
4. Malignancy
Squamous cell carcinoma
Adenocarcinoma
5. Miscellaneous
Ischemia
Chemotherapy
Radiation
Crohn's disease
Sarcoid

NSAIDs nonsteroidal anti-inflammatory drugs, *ASA* acetylsalicylic acid, *HSV* herpes simplex virus, *CMV* cytomegalovirus, *V2V* varicella zoster virus

23.3 Dysphagia

Dysphagia is prevalent in the elderly (20 % compared to 5–9 % in the general population). It is a cause of difficulty eating in 40–60 % of the institutionalized elderly. The incidence of dysphagia increases with increasing obesity [5], as obesity increases the risk of GERD. In a review of patients presenting with dysphagia in a primary care setting, the most common etiologies were GERD (44 %), benign strictures (36 %), esophageal motility disorder (11 %), neoplasm (6 %), infectious esophagitis (2 %), and achalasia (1 %) [6]. Eosinophilic esophagitis (EoE), while rare (18.6 per 100,000 people), can present with difficulty swallowing and food impactions in older patients rather than the atopic symptoms routinely found in the pediatric population [7].

Patients over 65 have multiple changes with aging that predispose to oropharyngeal dysphagia, such as painful or diseased teeth, xerostomia, poorly fitting dentures, slow muscle function resulting in impaired transfer of food into the pharynx, and delayed relaxation of the upper esophageal sphincter (UES). Barium cinefluroscopic studies of normal adults over age 85 demonstrate that approximately 10 % have silent aspiration of food or fluids. Comorbidities that increase the risk of dysphagia still further include cerebrovascular disease, Parkinson's disease, multiple sclerosis, Alzheimer's disease, upper motor neuron diseases, myasthenia gravis, polymyositis, amyloidosis, and a history of surgery or radiation to the oral cavity or neck. In the latter group, recurrence of cancer should be in the differential diagnosis.

Patients with oropharyngeal dysphagia typically cough, gag, choke, or aspirate their food during the initiation of a swallow. Patients may also complain of odynophagia, painful swallowing. Those with esophageal dysphagia often complain of solid foods or liquids "sticking," "catching," or "hanging up" in their chest, and may point to their substernal area as the location. This does not always indicate the true location of the problem, as patients with distal esophageal obstruction may have sensations referred higher up in the chest. Dysphagia only to solids often reflects mechanical obstruction, whereas dysphagia to both liquids and solids starting simultaneously suggests a neuromuscular motility disorder. Causes of odynophagia are listed in Table 23.2.

Review of a patient's medication list may suggest pill-induced esophagitis. Elderly patients are at an increased risk for this due to: more medications, decreased saliva production, and anatomical abnormalities compressing the esophagus such as strictures, webs, rings, and vascular anomalies (i.e., enlarged left atrium and dilated aortic arch). History of smoking or heavy alcohol use is associated with increased risk of squamous cell esophageal cancer. Physicians should inquire about these, and look for anemia and unintentional weight loss. Finally, symptoms of GERD should be elicited, as it can cause peptic strictures, Barrett's esophagus, and adenocarcinoma [2].

A speech-language pathologist can coordinate a cinefluroscopic swallowing study using thin, thick, and solid food materials for patients suspected of having oropharyngeal dysphagia. Patients can be taught proper swallowing techniques and how to modify their posture to improve their swallowing.

In addition to a barium esophagogram, an EGD should be performed to check for malignancy and take biopsies [8]. The diagnostic yield of EGD is around 55 % in the initial evaluation of patients >40 years old who present with heartburn, odynophagia, and weight loss [9]. If upper endoscopy is normal and complaints of dysphagia persist, then esophageal manometry should be performed. Treatment is directed toward the underlying disorder in addition to ensuring adequate nutrition and preventing aspiration. Patients with dysphagia due to decreased esophageal contractility and increased lower esophageal sphincter (LES) pressure (achalasia) may benefit from lower esophageal sphincter (LES) dilation or botulinum toxin injection. In addition to being diagnostic, EGD also offers therapeutic interventions such as dilation, which can be accomplished safely in the elderly (Table 23.3).

Drugs that decrease smooth muscle contractions (anticholinergics, calcium antagonists, nitrates) may treat diffuse esophageal spasm. Laparoscopic Heller myotomy to open the LES has been performed in older patients with achalasia with reasonable safety and efficacy. If aspiration occurs or the nutritional status of the patient suffers, a feeding jejunostomy or gastrostomy can be considered, but ideally the patient should participate in the decision to proceed with a feeding tube. Current recommendations are to avoid placing G tubes in demented patients, as those have not been shown to improve quality of life. Table 23.4 provides practice tips for dysphagia.

23.4 Peptic Ulcer Disease

Peptic ulcer disease (PUD) refers to both gastric (GUs) and duodenal ulcers (DUs), with the two most common causes being NSAIDs and *H. pylori* [10]. Approximately 5 million cases of PUD will occur this year in the USA, and the demographics are shifting towards older age of presentation.

Table 23.3 Dysphagia: Conditions for which EGD may provide therapeutic interventions

Benign conditions
1. Peptic strictures
2. Schatzki rings
3. Esophageal web
4. Eosinophilic Esophagitis
5. Caustic injury
6. Radiation injury
7. Anastomotic stricture
8. Pill-induced stricture
9. Cricopharyngeal bar
Malignant conditions
1. Esophageal adenocarcinoma
2. Esophageal squamous cell carcinoma
3. Pseudoachalasia
Motility Disorders
1. Achalasia

Modified from *Gastrointestinal Endoscopy*, 79(2), Pasha S, Acosta R, Chandrasekhara V et al., The role of endoscopy in the evaluation and management of dysphagia, p. 191–201, Copyright 2014, with permission from Elsevier

EGD cannot provide therapeutic intervention in extrinsic compression, diffuse esophageal spasms and hypomotility disorders secondary to connective tissue disorder

EGD endoscopic gastroduodenoscopy

Table 23.4 Practice Tips for Dysphagia in the Elderly Patient

- Dysphagia in the elderly is common and should always be investigated
- Dysphagia is associated with aspiration, weight loss, and poor quality of life
- Dysphagia may be oropharyngeal (mostly caused by neurological disorders) or esophageal; the causes of esophageal dysphagia are often indicated by history
- Common causes of dysphagia include neuromuscular, mechanical, motility, neoplastic and inflammatory conditions
- Check history of smoking, alcohol use, review medications, do neurologic exam
- EGD can be diagnostic and therapeutic
- Patients considered for a feeding tube should be able to participate in the decision
- Esophageal cancer usually presents in an advanced stage in the elderly, with symptoms of progressive dysphagia and weight loss
- Surveillance of Barrett's esophagus should be performed at 1–3 year intervals to detect early adenocarcinoma

EGD esophageal gastroduodenoscopy

Older people are more likely to suffer complications of PUD, including hospitalization, need for blood transfusions, emergency surgery, and death. Patients may present with overt bleeding with hematemesis or coffee-ground emesis, or occult bleeding with anemia. Older patients are less likely to have epigastric pain than younger patients, due to decreased visceral sensitivity. About half of patients have minimal pain, and complications such as perforation are more common in

Table 23.5 Practice tips for peptic ulcer disease in the elderly

- Peptic ulcer disease is usually caused by NSAIDs or *Helicobacter pylori*
- Complications of peptic ulcer disease are more common in the elderly and morbidity and mortality are higher in this age group
- PUD in the elderly may present without pain, particularly with NSAID use, and hemorrhage or perforation may be the first sign of an ulcer
- Dyspepsia is a common complaint in the elderly and requires endoscopy to rule out ulcer or cancer
- Consider depression as a cause of dyspepsia in an older patient with a negative workup and other symptoms of depression
- A CT scan of the abdomen may be helpful to diagnose abdominal pain, as elderly patients often present with atypical symptoms of diseases such as cholecystitis, appendicitis, and renal stones
- Mesenteric ischemia is a diagnosis often missed in older adults: consider it if pain occurs after meals and is progressively worse with time

NSAIDs nonsteroidal anti-inflammatory drugs

this age group [11]. Patients should be asked about a history of PUD; use of aspirin, NSAIDs, and oral anticoagulants; and previous diagnostic studies (upper GI series, testing for *H. pylori*). Upper endoscopy should be performed in patients suspected of having PUD to identify the lesion, perform a biopsy for *H. pylori*, rule out a malignancy, and initiate endoscopic therapy if necessary [12]. Morbidity and mortality of GI bleeding is higher in patients over 70 due to a higher risk of continued hemorrhage causing hypotension and cardiac ischemia. If an ulcer is found, therapy should be initiated with a PPI for at least 8 weeks. NSAIDs and aspirin (including 81 mg ASA) should be stopped [13]. If the patient is found to be *H. pylori* positive, therapy with antibiotics and a PPI should be started. In the case of a GU, a follow-up EGD should be performed 8–12 weeks later to confirm healing and rule out malignancy. Patients with a prior history of PUD who did not have a significant bleed, and who require chronic NSAID or aspirin use should be treated concurrently with a PPI or misoprostol. Both agents reduce the risk of PUD in chronic NSAID users, although the PPIs are generally better tolerated. Older patients with hemorrhage or perforation should avoid NSAIDs and ASA, as risk of bleeding even with prophylaxis is high and outweighs potential benefit (Table 23.5).

23.5 Dyspepsia

Dyspepsia is defined as chronic or recurrent pain or discomfort in the upper abdomen with or without nausea, bloating, early satiety, or reflux and affects 20–30 % of older adults. Dyspeptic pain lasts for hours, distinguishing it from spasmodic pain of colonic contractions or renal stones. There is overlap with the symptoms of cholecystitis and patients often

are evaluated for gallbladder disease. It is important to distinguish patients with structural problems such as ulcers from those with "functional" or non-ulcer dyspepsia. Patients should be asked about unintentional weight loss, odynophagia, dysphagia, prior PUD, pancreatitis, biliary tract disease, bleeding, prior trauma, a family history of GI tract cancer, and evidence of blood loss or jaundice. *H. pylori* infection accounts for a significant number of cases of dyspepsia in patients aged <60. Older patients are more likely to be infected but most are asymptomatic. Non-invasive tests for *H. pylori* infection that can be done in the outpatient setting include *H. pylori serum* antibody, urease breath testing, and *H. pylori* stool antigen.

If prevalence in community is below <20 %, then a *H. pylori* antibody test (iGG) will have a low positive predictive value, as a positive result is more likely to be a false positive than a true indication of infection. A negative test has a high negative predictive value (>95 %). Both the urease breath test and stool antigen test for active infection can be used before and after treatment. Both have an excellent positive predictive value and negative predictive value of over 90 % regardless of prevalence [14]. If urease breath testing is performed, bismuth and antibiotics need to be stopped for at least 28 days, and PPIs discontinued for at least a week prior to testing due to suppression of active infection by these agents. Stool antigen detection in the setting of use of PPIs or antibiotics may also be affected for the same reason.

In addition to other non-invasive tests for abdominal pathology (complete blood count (CBC), erythrocyte sedimentation rate (ESR), liver function tests (LFTs), electrolytes, amylase, and lipase), consider performing upper endoscopy in *H. pylori*+ older patients to rule out ulcer and cancer before initiating triple therapy. If *H. pylori* testing is negative, endoscopy is normal and symptoms persist, then it is reasonable to check for cholecystitis and gastroparesis. In older patients with persistent symptoms, workup should include a CT scan of the abdomen with both oral and intravenous contrast if renal function does not preclude use of IV contrast. If no organic cause is found, patients are categorized as having non-ulcer dyspepsia. There is little data to support routine use of antacids, antimuscarinics, or sucralfate. Routine treatment with H_2RAs is of slight benefit, but better results are obtained with once-or twice-daily PPIs in patients with burning pain or pain relieved by food. This suggests that these patients have GERD or some effect of acid on gastroesophageal motility.

Non-ulcer dyspepsia may be the presenting symptom for depression with somatization. Data from the Rome III classification of GI motility disorders supports a relationship between chronic abdominal pain and depression based on evidence that patients with chronic abdominal pain (without irritable-bowel-type relief with defecation) respond better to antidepressants than GI-directed medications [15]. Somatic manifestations of depression (chest pain, abdominal pain, nausea, and early satiety) are more common in the elderly. While there are no controlled studies of selective serotonin reuptake inhibitors in treatment of dyspepsia in older patients, if there other symptoms and signs of depression, a trial of antidepressants may be warranted. Choice should be guided by the side effect profile, as some antidepressants (e.g., tricyclics, mirtazapine) may worsen other common conditions such as constipation.

23.6 Gastric Cancer

In 2002, the number of new cases of gastric cancer reached 900,000; most were in patients older than 60 [16]. Gastric cancer is increasing in the elderly worldwide, while it is decreasing in younger cohorts. The overall 5-year survival rate is estimated at 16 %. Nearly 95 % of gastric cancers are adenocarcinomas, followed by lymphoma at 4 %. Stromal tumors (GISTs), carcinoids, and sarcomas make up 1 %. Risk factors for gastric cancer include chronic atrophic gastritis, *H. pylori*, pernicious anemia, family history of gastric cancer, partial gastrectomy, tobacco use, alcohol use, and consumption of large quantities of salted or smoked foods containing nitrites and nitrates. Presenting symptoms are often nonspecific (nausea, early satiety, epigastric fullness, intermitted vomiting, weight loss, and abdominal pain). Physical examination may reveal a mass, a succussion splash from gastric outlet obstruction, or peripheral lymphadenopathy. By the time symptoms or physical examination findings are apparent, patients usually have advanced disease. There are no specific chemical tests for gastric cancer, although CEA is often elevated, which can be used to monitor treatment. Gastric cancer is best detected by upper endoscopy. CT scanning with contrast, or MRI can assess depth of tumor invasion and lymphadenopathy. Endoscopic ultrasonography and positron emission tomography scans are increasingly used to improve tumor staging, as patients undergoing EUS are 1.26× more likely to have >15 lymph nodes examined and undergo both pre-and post-operative chemotherapy (Table 23.6) [17]. The general approach to the older patient with cancer is discussed in Chap. 26, Geriatric Oncology.

Table 23.6 Practice tips for gastric cancer

• Symptoms of gastric cancer are nonspecific, and diagnosis is often delayed
• Gastric cancer is most common in China, Japan, Korean, and Eastern Europe, therefore consider this diagnosis in patients from those areas
• MALT lymphoma, while uncommon, has a relatively good prognosis and appears to be sequelae of chronic *H. pylori* infection
• Patients need continued endoscopic and EUS surveillance for at least 5 years after surgical resection of gastric cancer

MALT mucosal-associated lymphoid tissue

Mucosal-associated lymphoid tissue (MALT lymphoma), which is confined to the gastric mucosa, has the best prognosis of all gastric cancers. There appears to be an association between this tumor and infection with *H. pylori*, and treatment of *H. pylori* (if present) is first line treatment of low-grade MALT lymphoma. Surgery offers the only cure for non-MALT gastric cancer; however, the overall 5-year survival is poor (20–40 %) and operative mortality high (15–25 %). Patients undergoing surgery should have EGD and EUS surveillance at least yearly for at least 5 years. Endoscopic resection of large masses, laser therapy, and stent placement may provide palliation for patients with obstructive symptoms and inoperable disease. Neo-adjuvant chemotherapy may improve survival by a few months. Palliative chemotherapy may prolong survival and preserve quality of life. Both chemotherapy and radiation are used for treatment of high-grade MALT lymphoma.

23.7 Diarrhea

Patients with diarrhea most often complain of frequent stools (>3/day) or loose stools; however, the term *diarrhea* is also used to describe fecal incontinence or fecal urgency. Most cases of acute diarrhea (lasting <2 weeks) in the elderly are related to viral or bacterial infections, but medications, medication interactions, or dietary supplements should also be considered. *Clostridium difficile* colitis is more prevalent in the elderly because of colonization during hospitalizations, antibiotic use, and care in institutional settings. *C. difficile* colonization in long-term-care facilities is estimated to be at least 50 % in the USA. Lactase deficiency can develop acutely after an episode of diarrhea due to other causes such as viral gastroenteritis. This usually resolves, but may take weeks or months.

Causes of chronic diarrhea, lasting >2 weeks, include: fecal impaction, medications, irritable bowel, microscopic or lymphocytic colitis, inflammatory bowel disease, obstruction from colon cancer, malabsorption, small bowel bacterial overgrowth, thyrotoxicosis, and lymphoma. Patients with neuromuscular disease such as Parkinson's disease who use anticholinergic medications that decrease GI transit are at risk of small bowel bacterial overgrowth and may present with diarrhea.

Celiac disease is an increasingly recognized cause of diarrhea and bloating in older adults. It is not clear whether this develops de novo in later life or reflects chronic undiagnosed gluten intolerance. Uncommon causes of diarrhea in older patients include Whipple's disease, jejunal diverticulosis, bowel ischemia, amyloidosis, lymphoma, and scleroderma with bacterial overgrowth. An appropriate history and physical examination, including a rectal examination should be performed. Medication history may reveal the cause. A history of weight loss raises concern for malignancy, inflammatory bowel disease (IBD), microscopic colitis, malabsorption, or thyrotoxicosis. Fluid status with orthostatic blood pressure measurement should be assessed in all elderly patients with diarrhea. Stool cultures should be obtained to exclude infection in patients with acute diarrhea accompanied by fever, abdominal pain, or blood in the stool. Routine stool cultures usually give a specific diagnosis in only 20–30 % of cases [18]. This is likely due to the fact that most infectious diarrheas are due to viruses such as rotavirus and Norwalk agent. For chronic diarrhea, qualitative or quantitative stool fat should be checked for steatorrhea, and a TSH for thyroid disease. *C. difficile* toxin assay of the stool should be obtained if there is recent antibiotic use. Colonoscopy should be performed in patients with a history of weight loss, bloody diarrhea, and diarrhea lasting >4 weeks. Even if the colonoscopy appears normal, biopsies should be taken for microscopic colitis. X-rays and oral and IV contrast CT scan may demonstrate bowel wall thickening with severe enteritis or colitis; they are also useful if complications such as perforation or abscess are suspected. In patients with possible small bowel bacterial overgrowth due to a variety of risk factors such as motility disorders or structural changes in the GI tract that cause slow GI transit, prior use of antibiotics or immune deficiencies [19], a positive breath hydrogen/methane test confirms fermentation of ingested sugars in the small bowel. Serum antibodies to tissue transglutamidase (tTG) are often positive in celiac disease. Diagnosis is confirmed by villous damage and atrophy in small bowel biopsies.

Treatment of diarrhea focuses on the underlying cause if one is found. In patients without sepsis who are C. difficile negative and have no blood in the stool, loperamide (≤8 tablets/day) can be effective in treating symptoms. Diphenoxylate/atropine (Lomotil®) may cause CNS toxicity, and should be avoided, as should anti-spasmodics such as dicylcomine. Bismuth subsalicylate, which has bactericidal action on common bacterial pathogens, can also be used. *C. difficile* should be treated with oral metronidazole for mild infections, and oral vancomycin for moderate to severe colitis. Elderly patients have a decreased response to metronidazole compared to younger patients (85 % vs. 95 %), and relapse of *C. difficile* diarrhea is more common in older patients. Antidiarrheal agents should be avoided in *C. difficile* colitis due to the risk of toxic megacolon. In microscopic colitis, antidiarrheal agents such as loperamide and bismuth subsalicylate can be tried; however, budesonide is the most effective treatment [20]. If small bowel overgrowth is present, bismuth-containing medications may be helpful in mild cases. For severe cases, treatment with 14–21 days of antibiotics eradicates the offending bacteria. If the cause of slow transit is not addressed or is not treatable, then overgrowth is likely to recur. Elimination of gluten is the treatment for celiac disease and improvement in diarrhea usually occurs within 4 weeks, although healing of the small bowel mucosa can take several months. Medication review is helpful in

Table 23.7 Practice tips for diarrhea in the elderly

• Acute diarrhea is usually self-limited and caused by infections. Chronic diarrhea has many causes, and an extensive workup may be needed.
– Consider early hospitalization or admission to an observation unit for older patients with diarrhea: increased risk of dehydration, falls, and inability to perform activities of daily living
• Avoid diphenoxylate/atropine (Lomotil®) due to risk of confusion and ileus from atropine
• Avoid antidiarrheals until bleeding and C. difficile ruled out
• Chronic diarrhea—check for:
– metabolic causes (thyroid disease)
– microscopic colitis
– medications
– malabsorbtion
– small bowel overgrowth (slow transit)
– celiac disease
• IBS (FODMAP diet)

FODMAP fermentable oligo-di-monosaccharides and polyols

patients with refractory celiac disease, as medications are an unsuspected source of gluten. For those with irritable bowel syndrome (IBS), a focus on stress and depression reduction, and referral to a nutritionist to discuss a low Fermentable Oligo-Di-Monosaccharides and Polyols (FODMAP) diet may help (Table 23.7).

23.8 Diverticular Disease

Diverticular disease is common in industrialized nations and increases with age; >60 % of those older than 70 and nearly 80 % of those older than 80 have diverticular out-pouchings of the colonic mucosa and submucosa. Diverticuli are most common in the sigmoid colon probably due to increased colonic luminal pressures, with constipation and straining. Approximately 15–20 % of older adults with diverticulosis will have a complication such as diverticular bleeding or diverticulitis.

23.8.1 Diverticular Bleeding

While bleeding from the GI tract can have many origins (Table 23.8), diverticular bleeding is a disease of old age. Forty-five percent of all diverticular bleeding occurs in patients over age 80 [21]. It can present with sudden onset of painless hematochezia. Although most diverticula are on the left side of the colon, 70 % of diverticular bleeding comes from right-sided diverticulae [12]. Eighty percent of diverticular bleeding episodes stop spontaneously, however patients should be hospitalized if bleeding persists, if they are hemodynamically unstable, or if blood loss compromises other organ systems. Older patients are at higher risk for poor

Table 23.8 Causes of GI bleeding in older patients

UGI bleeding	LGI bleeding
Gastric, duodenal, or esophageal ulcer	Colonic diverticuli
Gastritis, duodenitis, or esophagitis	Ischemic bowel disease
Esophageal varices	Inflammatory bowel disease
Mallory–Weiss tear	Angiodysplasia
Neoplasm	Infectious diarrhea
Telangiectasias	Radiation proctitis
Angiodysplasia	Postpolypectomy
	Hemorrhoids
	Stercoral ulcers

GI gastrointestinal, *UGI* upper GI, *LGI* lower GI

outcomes with bleeding, and the threshold for hospitalization should be lower than in younger patients. Evaluation of lower GI bleeding usually involves colonoscopy to exclude sources of bleeding such as arteriovenous malformations (AVMs), ischemia, IBD, and cancer. Diverticular bleeding is a diagnosis of exclusion in patients with diverticuli. If significant bleeding persists, angiography may show the site. In refractory cases, surgical resection of the bleeding area may be required.

23.8.2 Diverticulitis

In uncomplicated diverticulitis, patients have lower abdominal pain, fever, and an elevated white blood cell count [22]. They may have diarrhea or may have decreased bowel movements from spasm in the inflamed colon. On physical examination they may have mild tenderness on palpation over the inflamed site, however there are usually no palpable masses or peritoneal signs such as rebound tenderness or rigidity of the abdominal wall (guarding). An abdominal radiograph should be performed to look for pneumoperitoneum. If there is no evidence of perforation or sepsis, treatment can be initiated in the outpatient setting with clear liquids for 2–3 days and oral antibiotics to cover anaerobes and gram-negative organisms. The physician should call the patient within 24 h to assess the situation and a follow-up visit in 48–72 h is important. If no improvement occurs, the patient should be hospitalized and a CT scan of the abdomen performed, preferable with IV and oral contrast if renal function allows use of IV contrast. Complications of diverticulitis include abscess, stricture, large volume bleeding, or fistula. In addition to presenting with tachycardia or hypotension, older patients may present with delirium. Abdominal examination may reveal a mass in the left lower quadrant, with or without signs of peritonitis; significant blood in the stool; or a fistula to the bladder, uterus, or skin. Patients with complicated diverticulitis require hospitalization. Older patients with an episode of diverticulitis have a 35 % chance of a second episode within the next 5 years. Patients with more than two episodes

of diverticulitis in the same segment of colon, particularly with complications, should be referred for consideration of segmental resection. Older patients tolerate elective resection with primary anastomosis well. Emergency colon resection has a higher morbidity and mortality in patients over 70 compared to younger patients, and diverting colostomy may be a better alternative.

23.9 Inflammatory Bowel Disease

While most patients with IBD are under age 65, approximately 10–15 % of newly diagnosed cases of Crohn's disease and ulcerative colitis occur in patients over age 65 [23]. Older patients with Crohn's disease may have less abdominal pain or cramps, possibly due to reduced visceral sensation or use of medications that suppress pain or decrease intestinal motility. Patients typically have non-bloody diarrhea, unintentional weight loss, and fatigue. They may have anemia causing pallor, shortness of breath, reduced exercise tolerance. Extra-intestinal manifestations of Crohn's disease are common including: joint effusions, oral ulcers, painful nodular lesions on the extremities (erythema nodosum), uveitis, and back pain from sacroileitis. Although Crohn's disease develops anywhere from the mouth to the anus, in older patients it is less likely to involve large portions of the GI tract. Diagnosis is often delayed in older patients because symptoms of Crohn's disease mimic other diseases, including malignancy, infectious diarrhea, ischemic colitis, lactose intolerance, irritable bowel disease, medication-induced diarrhea, diverticulitis, celiac disease, microscopic colitis, or bacterial overgrowth. Serologic antibody panels detecting autoantibodies in IBD can help in distinguishing between ulcerative colitis and Crohn's disease when patients present with indeterminate colitis. These tests are expensive and their use should be deferred to specialists in IBD.

Ulcerative colitis (UC) usually presents with tenesmus and frequent bloody stools, without the weight loss associated with Crohn's disease. Extra-intestinal manifestations of UC include dermatological manifestations such as pyoderma gangrenosum (round or oval lesions on the shins and forearms). Older patients are more likely to have limited left-sided disease or proctitis compared with younger patients. The first attack in an older patient is generally more severe and more likely to require steroids than in a younger patients. Approximately 15 % of older patients with UC will eventually require surgery. The diagnosis of either UC or Crohn's is made on physical examination and history supplemented by laboratory studies and imaging. Patients require endoscopy for definitive diagnosis; however, this is undertaken with caution in patients with severe colitis due to risk of perforation. CT enterography (a CT scan that uses special contrast and image reconstruction to evaluate the small bowel wall more accurately) is used to detect small bowel involvement in Crohn's disease. Patients should be followed by an IBD specialist. There is limited data on IBD treatment in patients over age 70, as few older patients have been included in clinical trials.

23.10 Colon Cancer

The incidence and prevalence of colon cancer increases with age, and most cases occur in patients over age 65. There are several points that are worth reviewing regarding screening. Colon cancer is one of the best understood malignancies in terms of the mechanism of transition from normal tissue to cancer, and there is strong evidence that screening and removal of pre-cancerous growths decreases subsequent colon cancers in older patients. The controversy in screening is primarily based on what techniques to use and how long to continue. Several recent consensus statements indicate that screening should start at age 50 and continuing as long as patients have a life expectancy greater than 10 years. Life tables incorporating morbidity and functional status suggest that the utility of colon cancer screening is low after age 80–85 years (Table 23.9).

23.11 Constipation and Fecal Incontinence

Constipation is very common in older patients due to changes in colonic motility with age and superimposed risks such as immobility and medication use [24]. Constipation is a risk for fecal impaction and resultant fecal incontinence and can contribute to other conditions such as urinary retention and urine infections in elderly patients. Constipation and fecal impaction has also been associated with increased agitation and behavioral changes in patients with dementia who cannot indicate their need to toilet (Table 23.10).

Table 23.9 Indications for colonoscopy in older patients

Screening at age 50 and every 10 years afterward (if no lesions identified)
Stop screening around age 80–85 or earlier if less than 5 years of life expectancy
Shorter frequency of surveillance if risk factors:
First-degree family member with colon cancer
Personal history of colon cancer, colonic polyps, inflammatory bowel disease
History of breast cancer
Diagnostic colonoscopy if alarm symptoms present:
Hemoccult positive stool on routine screening
New change in bowel habits
Anemia secondary to blood loss from the gastrointestinal tract
Hematochezia
Unintentional weight loss and other causes less likely
New unexplained abdominal pain

Acute and chronic fecal incontinence (FI) occur commonly in older patients with comorbid conditions. Fecal incontinence is socially embarrassing, incapacitating [25, 26], and under-reported. Up to 7 % of the older population are incontinent of solid or liquid stool at least weekly. The prevalence is nearly 50 % in patients in long-term care and is the second leading precipitant of nursing home placement of patients with underlying physical or cognitive impairment in the USA. Fecal incontinence is closely associated with urinary incontinence and constipation. Because overflow of liquid stool is a complication of constipation, the latter should always be considered in the workup. A difficult aspect of treating overflow fecal incontinence is convincing the patient and/or family that constipation is actually the problem, not diarrhea.

Evaluation of constipation and FI should include evaluation of cognitive status, a history of the circumstances of the incontinence episodes, abdominal, neurological, and rectal examinations. Hard stool in the rectal vault suggests a fecal

Table 23.10 Common causes of constipation

Motility disorders	
Slow colonic transit	
Pelvic floor dysfunction (anismus, persistent puborectalis contraction)	
Constipation-predominant irritable bowel syndrome (abdominal pain relieved by defecation)	
Medication-induced	
Opiates	Anticholinergics
Calcium channel blockers	Tricyclic antidepressants
Antipsychotics	Ganglion-blocking agents
Mechanical obstruction	
Cancer	Large rectocele
Volvulus	Intussusception
Stricture	Anal fissure
Extrinsic compression	
Descending perineum syndrome	
Neurological disorders	
Parkinson's disease	Prior colon surgery
Spinal cord or sacral root tumors	Spinal cord injury
Multiple sclerosis	
Systemic disorders	
Hypothyroidism	Amyloid
Diabetes mellitus	Connective tissue disorders
Congestive heart failure	
Metabolic disorders	
Hypokalemia	Uremia
Hypophosphatemia	Hypercalcemia
Hypomagnesemia	
Miscellaneous	
Dehydration	
Immobility	
Cognitive impairment	
Autonomic neuropathy	
Diminished rectal sensation	

impaction, however a negative rectal examination does not exclude a proximal fecal impaction, fecal masses, or stool back-up. Mental status examination identifies the patient with dementia or delirium who may have lost self-toileting capacity. Absence of anal sphincter tone or anal wink suggests denervation of the pudendal nerve (S2–4) from a local or spinal cord lesion. An abdominal plain film to assess fecal load is helpful when fecal impaction is suspected. Acute onset of incontinence should prompt examination for fecal impaction and spinal imaging to rule out cord compression. For patients not responding to empiric treatment, consider referral to a group specializing in anorectal motility disorders for additional testing such as anorectal manometry. This measures the resting pressure of the anal canal (predominantly from the IAS), tone and contractile pressures of the EAS, and sensation within the anorectal area. Pudendal nerve testing may be required in some patients. Candidates for referral to a bowel disorders program are generally ambulatory and cognitively intact, as interventions include biofeedback and maneuvers requiring patient participation. These studies are not usually feasible in bed-bound or debilitated patients, and often the focus in the latter is detecting fecal impaction and reviewing medications for those that may cause diarrhea or constipation [27]. The treatment of constipation and fecal impaction include dis-impaction, bowel cleansing, modification of risk factors, and a maintenance regimen. Dis-impaction should start with manual removal of stool and/or enemas, before administering oral polyethylene glycol. Warm tap water enemas of 1–2 L may be needed. Milk and molasses (1 cup each) enemas are both osmotic and mildly stimulating, are often effective when tap water enemas are not, and can be safely administered in the hospital or long-term care setting. Avoid magnesium citrate solutions and Fleet Phospho-soda enemas in patients with underlying cardiac or renal disease due to risk of fluid overload or phosphate nephropathy. Soapsuds enemas may precipitate ischemic colitis and should probably be avoided. Preventing constipation and recurrent impaction involves risk factor modification including mobilization, adequate hydration and nutrition, and minimizing constipating medications. Scheduled toileting after breakfast may be helpful for patients with cognitive impairment. Add fiber supplements when bowel function has been regularized. Regular use of a stimulant laxative such as senna or bisacodyl, or polyethylene glycol (PEG) or lactulose may prevent impaction in high risk patients. Intermittent use of glycerin or bisacodyl suppositories is warranted if patients have infrequent episodes of constipation, but if used more than once a week, the entire bowel regimen should be reviewed and adjusted. The role of lubiprostone or probiotics is not clear; however, these are an alternative in patients unable to take other laxatives. Lubiprostone increases stool frequency in patients aged 70–75 but older patients also respond to much

Table 23.11 Treatment of constipation

Initial management—occasional mild constipation
Increase fluid intake (only effective if dehydrated)
Exercise
Bowel training regimen (try to toilet when gastro-colic reflex active after meals)
Second-line therapy—active otherwise healthy older adults
Bulking agents (avoid as initial therapy in Parkinson's disease and severe constipation)
Stool softeners
Glycerin suppositories
Third-line therapy—consider first if history of chronic constipation or starting narcotic medications
Osmotic agents (milk of magnesia, lactulose, sorbitol)
PEG solutions (Miralax)
Stimulating agents (Senna, bisacodyl)
Fourth-line therapy—start first if no bowel movement in several days
Bisacodyl suppository
Tap water enema or milk and molasses enema (1/2 cup molasses: 1 l milk)
Fifth-line therapy
Misoprostol, colchicine
Other prescription laxatives (lubiprostone)
Methylnaltrexone (if on opiates and failed stimulant/osmotic laxatives)
Agents to avoid
Prokinetics (erythromycin, metoclopramide, cisapride)
Lubricating agents (oral mineral oil because of aspiration)
Routine use of enemas (increased risk of rectal perforation in the elderly)
Phosphate laxatives in renal disease (phosphate nephropathy)
Soapsuds enemas (increased risk of ischemic or chemical colitis)

PEG polyethylene glycol

cheaper alternatives such as senna and PEG solution (Table 23.11).

23.12 Colonic Ischemia

The colon is more commonly affected by ischemia than the small bowel, due to silent occlusion of the inferior mesenteric artery (IMA) in older patients (present in up to 10 % of autopsies > age 80) [28, 29]. The causes of this (CI) include acute and chronic mesenteric ischemia from IMA thrombus or embolus; hypoperfusion (CHF, cardiac arrhythmias, shock, and vasculitis), hematological disorders infections, medications (NSAIDs, digitalis, vasopressin, pseudoephedrine, sumatriptan, cocaine, amphetamines, gold), constipation, surgery, and trauma. The usual site of ischemia is the splenic flexure (so-called watershed area) of the colon primarily supplied by the IMA. Most colonic ischemia is precipitated by hypotension. The extent of injury ranges from mild, reversible mucosal damage to gangrene or fulminant colitis. Abdominal aortic aneurysm repair is a risk for acute CI, with 3 % of elective and 14 % of emergent repairs developing CI, from SMA occlusion. This can also result in small bowel ischemia, which has a very high mortality. Rapid recognition and reversal of the ischemia is essential in treating severe ischemic colitis or small bowel infarction. Patients with acute CI usually present with cramping lower left quadrant pain and loose, bloody stools. GI blood loss sufficient to cause hemodynamic instability is atypical and suggests other diagnoses. Physical examination often reveals tenderness over the affected portion of bowel. Peritoneal signs may be present and persistence of these signs for several hours suggests transmural infarction necessitating rapid surgical exploration. Strictures, chronic colitis, gangrene resulting in perforation, and intra-abdominal sepsis are complications of CI. Chronic CI, which is probably more common than previously thought, may present with diarrhea, left-sided abdominal cramps, and gas or bloating due to postprandial dysmotility caused by the mismatch of blood supply to demand. Symptoms usually occur after meals, can be slowly progressive and insidious, and patients have often been investigated extensively for other causes. Endoscopy may show mild inflammation in the left colon near the splenic flexure, but the mucosa can appear relatively normal if the ischemia is progressing slowly because slow IMA occlusion allows collateral blood supply to develop.

Even if CI is suspected, stool cultures should be obtained to exclude infectious colitis. The patient with suspected CI who does not have peritoneal signs should have CT or MR angiography and possibly careful sigmoidoscopy within 48 h of symptom onset. Patients with peritoneal signs should undergo urgent/emergent CT or MR angiography and surgical exploration. CT scans are normal in up to 66 % of patients with chronic or slowly progressive CI but may show colonic thickening, mucosal edema, or peri-colonic fluid and/or stranding suggestive of inflammation. Evaluation of the intestinal blood flow using Doppler ultrasound may indicate an SMA occlusion; however, more invasive procedures such as MR angiogram or interventional angiography are often required. The latter allows treatment with thrombolytics or angioplasty. The greatest difficulty is early recognition before development of an acute abdomen or hypotension. If no signs of peritonitis or perforation are present, treatment includes fluids, bowel rest, and broad-spectrum antibiotics. Hypotension should be aggressively reversed, CHF or cardiac arrhythmias treated, and vasoconstricting medications stopped. The persistence of peritoneal signs should prompt surgical exploration. Recurrence of CI occurs in only 3–10 % of elderly patients. Congenital or acquired thrombophilic states account for a significant percentage of ambulatory younger patients presenting with colonic ischemia, and, though less likely, should be tested in the elderly (Table 23.12) [30].

Table 23.12 Practice tips for mesenteric ischemia in the elderly

- Mesenteric ischemia is primarily a disease of the elderly, particularly those with underlying cardiovascular disorders
- Acute mesenteric ischemia presents with pain out of proportion to physical findings and may be caused by an embolus, thrombus, or hypoperfusion state
- Mesenteric artery angiography is required for diagnosis and, often, for treatment
- Chronic mesenteric ischemia presents with postprandial pain (intestinal angina) and weight loss. It is seen in elderly patients with arteriosclerotic changes in the mesenteric circulation
- Colonic ischemia presents with left lower quadrant pain and loose bloody stools. It is diagnosed by colonoscopy, but the findings may mimic infectious or inflammatory colitis
- Most patients with colonic ischemia recover with bowel rest, fluids, and IV antibiotics and do not require surgery

23.13 Viral Hepatitis

Hepatitis A (HAV) is less frequent in older than younger populations, but older people may have a more severe course, and higher risk of fulminant liver failure and death. International travel to endemic areas is the main risk factor. Comorbidities and a decreased likelihood of liver transplantation due to age contribute to the lower survival of older patients with fulminant disease. Older patients planning travel should be tested for HAV antibody, and vaccinated if negative 2–3 months prior to travel. A second vaccination may be required in older patients due to decreased immune responsiveness.

Acute hepatitis B virus (HBV) infection is uncommon in the older population and often runs a mild and subclinical course. Symptoms, when present, include fever, malaise, arthralgias, myalgias, nausea, vomiting, abdominal pain, and jaundice [31]. Chronic hepatitis B is endemic in sub-Saharan Africa and the Far East, and patients from high risk areas should be screened as should patients with risk factors for acquisition (IV drug use, sexual exposure, and transfusions or blood products prior to 1980). PEG interferon-α, used to treat chronic HBV in patients with decompensated liver disease, may cause more side effects in the elderly. Other viral suppressive agents such as entecavir and tenofovir are well tolerated by older patients. Patients diagnosed with chronic viral hepatitis should be referred to a hepatologist, and undergo a liver ultrasound to determine whether they have cirrhosis or hepatocellular carcinoma. A non-invasive fibroscan may demonstrate fibrosis. Liver biopsy is recommended for patients with significant elevation in liver enzymes or evidence of active viral replication.

Hepatitis C (HCV) is becoming more common in patients over age 65, due to exposure to IV drugs or blood products before 1990. Most patients with chronic hepatitis C are asymptomatic, and diagnosed when routine laboratory studies reveal elevated aminotransferase levels. Acute HCV symptoms are similar to those seen in acute HBV. Those who acquire HCV infection at an older age are at increased risk of cirrhosis and mortality [32, 33]. Daily alcohol use worsens the prognosis. Because of the increasing prevalence of chronic Hepatitis C in the older population, all patients born between 1945 and 1965 should have one-time screening for HCV antibody. PEG interferon-α with ribavirin has been the standard treatment for chronic HCV infection. Heart disease is a relative contraindication to ribavirin therapy. Several new interferon-free treatments demonstrate significant improvement in viral clearance compared to ribavirin alone and are better tolerated. Decisions concerning screening and treatment of chronic viral hepatitis in the elderly should take into account life expectancy, likelihood of progression to cirrhosis, and the treatment side effects.

23.14 Drug-Induced Liver Disease

Polypharmacy and altered pharmacodynamics accounts for the increased incidence of drug-related hepatotoxicity in the elderly. Many drugs are liver toxic and a reliable information can be found on the NIH LiverTox website (http://livertox.nih.gov/). NSAIDs, amiodarone, hydroxymethylglutaryl coenzyme A reductase inhibitors, and antituberculosis medications may cause hepatotoxicity [34]. LFTs should be monitored in patients receiving these medications. Several herbal medications cause liver injury, including kava, chaparral, black cohosh, and germander. A list of herbal medications should be elicited from all older patients. Statin drugs often cause modest elevation in transaminases, and if these remain $<2 \times$ normal, studies indicate a low risk of liver damage and favorable risk–benefit ratio in patients with hyperlipidemia, cardiac disease, diabetes, or metabolic syndrome.

23.15 Hepatic Ischemia

Patients of any age can develop steep elevations in aminotransferase levels after a hemodynamic insult. Older patients are at increased risk due to comorbidities that cause hypoperfusion (acute myocardial infarction, CHF, valvular heart disease, cardiac arrhythmias, cardiomyopathy, sepsis, trauma, and burns). The magnitude of the aminotransferase elevation does not correlate with the extent of liver injury and does not predict outcome. Most patients recover after correction of hemodynamic instability and abnormal coagulation, with normalization of aminotransferase levels within 10 days.

23.16 Primary Biliary Cirrhosis

Up to 40 % of patients with primary biliary cirrhosis (PBC) are elderly, and women outnumber men by 6:1. Patients present with fatigue, pruritus, and elevated alkaline phosphatase (ALP) levels. As osteoporosis can also elevate ALP, patients should be monitored for progressive elevation, and the ALP fractionated if over 200 units/L. Diagnosis is suggested by the presence of antimitochondrial antibody (AMA) and is confirmed by liver biopsy. Treatment with ursodeoxycholic acid improves survival and delays need for liver transplantation. As with all patients with cirrhosis, patients with PBC should avoid NSAIDs and alcohol. Doses of hepatically excreted drugs should be adjusted in patients with significant cholestatsis to avoid toxicity.

23.17 Hepatocellular Carcinoma

More than 50 % of patients with hepatocellular carcinoma (HCC) in the USA are elderly and survival rates are significantly lower in patients diagnosed with HCC >age 65. Cirrhosis from chronic HCV or HBV infection and alcoholic liver disease are the most frequent causes of HCC. HCC can present with acute onset of right upper quadrant pain, elevated alpha-fetoprotein (AFP) levels or incidental mass on imaging. Patients with cirrhosis should be screened with ultrasonography every 6 months for early detection of HCC. A CT scan of the abdomen is recommended every 1–2 years. Surgical resection is the treatment of choice if the tumor is small and there is no vascular invasion. Liver transplantation is indicated for patients with one tumor <5 cm, or up to three tumors <3 cm without vascular invasion. Unfortunately the mortality of liver transplantation increases over age 70, and 5-year survival is lower. Older patients who are poor surgical candidates may be treated with transarterial chemo-embolization (TACE), mechanical ablation, or systemic chemotherapy, however only survival benefit for TACE has been reported (Table 23.13) [35].

23.18 Cholelithiasis

Age-related increases in cholesterol secretion in bile, combined with decreased bile acid secretion, leads to increased cholesterol saturation and increased bile lithogenicity. Cholelithiasis is twice as common in women as in men, often asymptomatic and discovered during radiological studies performed for unrelated reasons. Ten to twenty-five percent of patients with asymptomatic gallstones will become symp-

Table 23.13 Liver disease in older patients

- Elderly patients should be vaccinated against Hepatitis A prior to international travel
- Screen patients who have immigrated from endemic areas for chronic Hepatitis B
- Screen all patients born between 1945 and 1965 for Hepatitis C (if expected life span >5 years and do not have end-stage liver disease)
- Non-alcoholic fatty liver disease (NAFLD) is the most common cause of elevated liver enzymes, and can progress to fibrosis and cirrhosis in 20 % of patients
- Alcohol is an underdiagnosed cause of liver disease in the elderly
- Both prescription and OTC/herbal drugs can cause elevated liver enzymes and liver damage: withdraw any culprit drug and monitor until enzymes normal
- Check fractionated alkaline phosphatase (ALP) in patients with total ALP >200
- Best candidates for treatment of hepatocellular carcinoma by surgical resection or liver transplantation have small tumors without vascular invasion, no portal hypertension, and normal liver function
- Consider gallstones in patients with acute RUQ pain and fever. Laparoscopic cholecystectomy is well tolerated by stable older patients. Unstable patients should have cholecystotomy drainage followed by delayed cholecystectomy

tomatic each decade [36]. Symptomatic gallstones typically presents with RUQ pain, nausea, and vomiting. Diagnosis is suggested in the appropriate clinical setting by elevated alkaline phosphatase and bilirubin levels and is confirmed by ultrasonography. Diagnosis of gallstones in the biliary ducts is made using ultrasound, or magnetic resonance cholangio-pancreaticogram (MRCP). The sensitivity of MRCP is lower in patients with biliary obstruction and cholestasis, therefore a negative test in a patient strongly suspected to have biliary stones should precipitate consideration of ERCP for diagnosis and treatment. Laparoscopic cholecystectomy is the treatment of choice for symptomatic cholelithiasis in the elderly; postoperative mortality and morbidity in selected elderly patients are comparable to that for younger patients if the patient is hemodynamically stable. Poor surgical candidates may be treated with ERCP with sphincterotomy or ursodeoxycholic acid. Patients with Charcot's Triad (RUQ pain, fever, jaundice) likely have cholangitis, and should undergo emergency ERCP to decompress the biliary system. Asymptomatic cholelithiasis should not be treated.

23.19 Cholecystitis

Symptoms of gallbladder inflammation (cholecystitis) such as epigastric or RUQ pain, nausea, and vomiting may less severe in older patients or mistaken for other disease processes. Elevations in serum bilirubin, alkaline phosphatase, aminotransferases, and white blood cell counts are characteristic. The diagnosis is made clinically and confirmed with RUQ ultrasound. Complications such as necrosis of the gallbladder and cholangitis are more common in the elderly and are associated with increased morbidity and mortality. Treatment of cholecystitis consists of stabilization with intravenous fluids, bowel rest, pain control, and broad-spectrum antibiotics followed by cholecystectomy. Older patients with acute cholecystitis frequently have significant comorbidities that increase risk of complications and death with emergent cholecystectomy. Immediate percutaneous cholecystostomy followed several weeks later by definitive surgery or ERCP has less morbidity and mortality compared to urgent surgery [37]. Gallbladder carcinoma is rare in the USA. Gallstone disease, female gender, and smoking are risk factors. The diagnosis is often made incidentally at surgery. The prognosis is poor.

23.20 Acute Pancreatitis

Gallstones, medications, and cancer account for a higher proportion of acute pancreatitis in older compared with younger patients. Alcohol is a common precipitating factor in both age groups [38, 39]. Typical presenting symptoms include epigastric pain radiating to the back along with nausea and vomiting. The diagnosis is made by elevations in amylase and lipase levels. Elevations in alkaline phosphatase and bilirubin suggest gallstone pancreatitis, which can be confirmed by ultrasonography or CT. Patients with altered mental status, hemodynamic instability, BUN over 25, or those meeting three or more of Ranson's criteria (Table 23.14) should undergo a dynamic CT scan to rule out pancreatic necrosis. Patients with elevated BUN should be considered for ICU admission, as this predicts increased mortality. Bowel rest, intravenous hydration, and pain control are the cornerstones of therapy. Patients with pancreatic necrosis need broad-spectrum antibiotics, and CT-guided aspiration of necrotic areas to check for abscess should be considered if symptoms do not improve after 5–7 days. Surgical or endoscopic debridement should be considered if necrotic tissue is infected. Morbity and mortality of elective laparoscopic cholecystectomy with preoperative ERCP or intraoperative cholangiography is comparable to that for younger individuals. In patients who are poor surgical candidates, ERCP with sphincterotomy decreases the risk for recurrent gallstone pancreatitis. Drug-induced pancreatitis can be caused by azathioprine, 6-mercaptopurine, estrogen, mesalamine, furosemide, and angiotensin-converting enzyme inhibitors. Suspected medications should be stopped when pancreatitis is diagnosed. Other causes of pancreatitis, such as hyperlipidemia or hypercalcemia, should be sought and treated.

Table 23.14 Ranson's criteria in acute pancreatitis

On admission
1. Age >55 years
2. WBC count >16,000/μL
3. Serum glucose >200 mg/dL
4. Serum LDH >350 units/L
5. Serum AST >250 units/L
Over the first 48 h
1. Increase in BUN exceeding 5 mg/dL
2. Arterial PO_2 <60 mmHg
3. Hematocrit drop >10 percentage points
4. Serum calcium <8 mg/dL
5. Base deficit >4 mEq/L
6. Fluid sequestration exceeding 6 L

Presence of 3 or more on admission predicts severe course with a sensitivity of 60–80 %

WBC white blood cell, *LDH* lactate dehydrogenase, *AST* aspartate aminotransferase, *BUN* blood urea nitrogen, *PO2* partial pressure of oxygen

23.21 Chronic Pancreatitis

The diagnosis of chronic pancreatitis in elderly patients is difficult. Structural changes associated with chronic pancreatitis (ductal irregularity or dilation, calcification, abnormal echogenicity) are also observed in aging patients without pancreatitis. Because pancreatic function is maintained in the elderly, functional testing demonstrating enzyme insufficiency may aid in diagnosis. Patients should also be screened for fat-soluble vitamin deficiencies; vitamin D as malabsorption is common in chronic pancreatitis. Treatment consists of pain management, pancreatic enzyme, and vitamin replacement and avoidance of alcohol.

23.22 Pancreatic Cysts in the Elderly

Pancreatic cysts are often found incidentally during cross-sectional imaging. The incidence of pancreatic cysts in the USA is between 3 and 15 % and increases with age; 0.5 % those <40 years old, 25 % in those 70–79 years old, and 37 % in those >80 years old. The debate of what to do with pancreatic cysts is ongoing. Many are benign and the major consequence for patients is stress and anxiety. The risk of a pancreatic cysts being malignant at time of diagnosis is only 0.017 %. The overall risk of any cyst developing into a cancer over a 20-year period is about 1 % [40]. Cystic lesions of the pancreas can be divided into non-neoplastic and neoplastic lesions. Pancreatic cysts can be isolated or found in conditions such as von Hippel–Lindau or polycystic kidney disease. Historically, pseudocysts (inflammatory cysts) represented the majority of benign cysts. These cysts are often found in those who have already been diagnosed with chronic pancreatitis or with a history of trauma. However, if a cyst is associated with new acute pancreatitis, there is more concern for malignancy. Non-neoplastic cysts include retention cysts, mucinous non-neoplastic cysts, and lymphoepithelial cysts. Cystic neoplasms include (descending order of frequency) intraductal papillary mucinous neoplasm (IPMNs) (38%), mucinous cystic neoplasms (23%), serous cystic tumor (16%), and solid pseudopapillary neoplasm (SPNs) (5%), which usually occur in the younger population. Mucinous cysts are exclusively found in women [41]. The initial approach is to determine if the patient is experiencing symptoms from the cysts, which can include abdominal pain, pancreatitis or rarely biliary obstruction, and review previous imaging to assess the timing and growth of the cyst. If a cyst is <1 cm, lacks concerning features on imaging (i.e., dilated pancreatic duct), then it is reasonable to reassess with imaging in 1 year. The likelihood ratio of a cyst being malignant increases to 2.97 for cysts >3 cm, 2.38 for dilated pancreatic duct, and 7.73 if the cyst has a solid component. Based on this, the American Gastroenterological Association (AGA) recommends that if the cyst is <3 cm, lacks a solid component, and has no associated pancreatic duct dilation to repeat an MRI in 1 year and then every 2 years for 5 years [42]. If no changes in characteristics have occurred after 5 years, surveillance can be stopped. If any concerning findings are found, then consider performing an endoscopic ultrasound and fine needle aspiration. Surgery is generally indicated for lesions with malignant potential, which include mucinous cystic neoplasms, main duct IPMNs and solid pseudopapillary neoplasms. Pancreatic surgery often carries a high risk of morbidity and mortality. Decisions should be made in a multiple disciplinary approach with patient preferences and life expectancy in mind [40].

23.23 Pancreatic Cancer

Pancreatic cancer accounts for 5 % of all cancer deaths in the USA, and the majority of cases occur in patients >45 years increasing in incidence from 1/100,000 at age 44 to 100/100,000 at age 85. Painless jaundice, pruritus, and weight loss are common presenting symptoms but usually occur late in the disease. Elevated CA 19-9 levels suggest the diagnosis. The diagnosis is confirmed with abdominal imaging or demonstration of extrinsic compression of the bile duct during ERCP and/or a mass on endoscopic ultrasound (EUS). Pancreaticoduodenectomy (Whipple Procedure) is the only treatment with demonstrated benefit and should be offered to selected older patients with high overall fitness and low comorbidity. The prognosis of pancreatic cancer remains grim as most patients are not surgical candidates.

23.24 Management of Malnutrition and Weight Loss in Older Patients

While not specific for GI disease, weight loss is a common finding in older patients. Unintentional loss of 5 % or more of usual body weight in the past month or 10 % in the past 6 months is associated with increased morbidity and mortality in older patients [43] even after excluding other causes such as underlying malignancy. Weight change during an individual's lifetime is characterized by a gradual increase in weight that peaks in the fourth to fifth decade of life, followed by a period of stable weight and a gradual decline in weight after the sixth to seventh decades. Major indicators of poor nutritional status include weight loss over time, low weight for height (body mass index of 18.5 kg/m^2 or less), a loss of independence in two basic activities of daily living (e.g., bathing and dressing), midarm circumference or triceps skinfold thickness less than the 10th percentile of ideal, and the presence of nutrition-related disorders (e.g., osteoporosis, vitamin B$_{12}$ deficiency, or folate deficiency). A serum albumin level below 3.5 g/dL is generally the most reliable, although nonspecific, indicator of chronic malnutrition. After excluding other causes of weight loss, the major need is to increase calorie intake. If the gastrointestinal tract is functional, enteral is preferred over parenteral nutrition as it is safer, and enteric food provides trophic stimulus to the gastrointestinal tract [44, 45]. Patients who have the cognitive ability to participate in a discussion about tube feeding and are unable to swallow or who cannot eat sufficient calories to maintain adequate nutrition are the best candidates for tube feeding. Nasogastric tubes are a short-term alternative, however percutaneous gastrostomy tube placement is preferred when tube feeding is anticipated for weeks to months, or for palliative care in cases of irreversible bowel obstruction. Aspiration precautions (elevating the head of the bed, checking residuals) should be carefully observed because gastrostomy tube feeding does not prevent aspiration. Gastrostomy tube feedings are not recommended for patients with severe dementia, given the absence of data to show that tube feedings improve quality of life and survival. In older patients with other irreversible causes of dysphagia (stroke, Parkinson's disease), particularly those who cannot make their own decisions, it is important to have a thoughtful discussion with the patient and/or their decision-maker about the risks of feeding tubes, and overall goals of care prior to insertion of a tube. Total parenteral nutrition (TPN) is appropriate only in carefully selected older patients whose GI tract cannot be used. Complications of parenteral feeding include catheter-related thrombosis and sepsis. Older patients have a higher mortality on TPN than younger patients (Table 23.15).

Table 23.15 Practice tips for malnutrition and weight loss in older patients

- Malnutrition is a common problem in older patients and is often multifactorial
- A detailed diet history is very helpful to determine whether the patient is unable to eat, or is unwilling or disinterested in eating
- Depression is a common cause of involuntary weight loss in the elderly, as is cognitive impairment
- Low albumin/prealbumin and vitamin deficiencies are indicators of malnutrition
- In addition to treating diseases associated with weight loss, interventions may need to address social isolation, ability to obtain and prepare meals, and cognitive impairment
- The decision to place a percutaneous gastrostomy tube should take into account the cognitive status and quality of life of the patient. Patients with advanced dementia, while at risk for weight loss, do not benefit from feeding tubes

References

1. Becher A, Dent J. Systematic review: aging and gastro-oesophageal reflux disease symptoms, oesophageal function and reflux oesophagitis. Aliment Pharmacol Ther. 2011;33:442–54.
2. Morganstern B, Anandasabapathy S. GERD and Barrett's esophagus: diagnostic and management strategies in the geriatric population. Geriatrics. 2009;64:9–12.
3. Desilets AR, Asal NJ, Dunican KC. Considerations for the use of proton pump inhibitors in older adults. Consult Pharm. 2012;27:114–20.
4. Heidelbaugh JJ, Inadomi JM. Magnitude and economic impact of inappropriate use of stress ulcer prophylaxis in non-ICU hospitalized patients. Am J Gastroenterol. 2006;101:2200–5.
5. Firth M, Prather C. Gastrointestinal motility problems in the elderly patient. Gastroenterology. 2002;122:1688–700.
6. Lee J, Anggiansah A, Anggiansah R, et al. Effects of age on the gastroesophageal junction, esophageal motility, and reflux disease. Clin Gastroenterol Hepatol. 2007;5:1392–8.
7. Maradey-Romero C, Prakash R, Lewis S, Perzynski A, Fass R. The 2011–2014 prevalence of eosinophilic oesophagitis in the elderly amongst 10 million patients in the United States. Aliment Pharmacol Ther. 2015;41:1016–22.
8. Esfandyari T, Potter JW, Vaezi MF. Dysphagia: a cost analysis of the diagnostic approach. Am J Gastroenterol. 2002;97:2733–7.
9. Pasha S, Acosta R, Chandrasekhara V, et al. The role of endoscopy in the evaluation and management of dysphagia. Gastrointest Endosc. 2014;79:191–201.
10. Griffin MR. Epidemiology of nonsteroidal anti-inflammatory drug-associated gastrointestinal injury. Am J Med. 1998;104:23S.
11. Rosen AM. Gastrointestinal bleeding in the elderly. Clin Geriatr Med. 1999;15:511.
12. Farrell JJ, Friedman LS. Gastrointestinal bleeding in the elderly. Gastroenterol Clin North Am. 2001;30:377.
13. ILanza FL, Chan FKL, Quigley EMM, Practice Parameters Committee of the American College of Gastroenterology. Prevention of NSAID-induced ulcer complications. Am J Gastroenterol. 2009;104:728–38
14. Chey W, Wong B. American College of Gastroenterology guideline on the management of Helicobacter pylori Infection. Am J Gastroenterol. 2007;102:1808–25.
15. Sperber AD, Drossman DA. Review article: the functional abdominal pain syndrome. Aliment Pharmacol Ther. 2011;33:514–24.

16. Saif MW, Makrilia N, Zalonis A, et al. Gastric cancer in the elderly: an overview. Eur J Surg Oncol. 2010;36:709–17.

17. Huntington CR, Walsh K, Han Y, Salo J, Hill J. National trends in utilization of endoscopic ultrasound for gastric cancer: a SEER-medicare study. J Gastrointest Surg. 2016;20:154–63.

18. Guerrant RL, Van Gilder T, Steiner TS, et al. Practice guidelines for the management of infectious diarrhea. Clin Infect Dis. 2001;32:331–51.

19. Dukowicz A, Lacy B, Levine G. Small intestinal bacterial overgrowth. Gastroenterol Hepatol. 2007;3:112–22.

20. Williams JJ, Beck PL, Andrews CN, et al. Microscopic colitis — a common cause of diarrhoea in older adults. Age Aging. 2010;39:162–8.

21. Wheat C, Strate L. Trends in hospitalization for diverticulitis and diverticular bleeding in the United States from 2000 to 2010. Clin Gastroenterol Hepatol. 2016;14:96–103. doi:10.1016/j.cgh.2015.03.030.

22. Stollman NH et al. Diagnosis and management of diverticular disease of the colon in adults. Am J Gastroenterol. 1999;94:3110.

23. Murad Y, Radi ZA, Murad M, Hall K. Inflammatory bowel disease in the geriatric population. Front Biosci. 2011;3E:945–54.

24. Mertz H et al. Symptoms and physiology in severe chronic constipation. Am J Gastroenterol. 1999;94:131.

25. Soffer EE, Hull T. Fecal incontinence: a practical approach to evaluation and treatment. Am J Gastroenterol. 2000;95:1873.

26. Tariq SH. Fecal incontinence in older adults. Clin Geriatr Med. 2007;23:857.

27. Stevens TK, Palmer RM. Fecal incontinence in long-term care patients. Long-Term Care Interface. 2007;8:35.

28. Brandt LJ, Boley SJ. AGA technical review on intestinal ischemia. Gastroenterology. 2000;118:954.

29. Greenwald DA et al. Ischemic bowel disease in the elderly. Gastroenterol Clin North Am. 2001;30:445.

30. Koutroubakis IE et al. Role of acquired and hereditary thrombotic risk factors in colon ischemia of ambulatory patients. Gastroenterology. 2001;121:561.

31. Befeler AS, Di Bisceglie AM. Infections of the liver: hepatitis B. Infect Dis Clin North Am. 2000;14:617.

32. Minola E. Age at infection affects the long-term outcome of transfusion-associated chronic hepatitis C. Blood. 2002;99:4588–91.

33. Lauer GM, Walker BD. Hepatitis C virus infection. N Engl J Med. 2001;345:41.

34. Regev A, Schiff ER. Liver disease in the elderly. Gastroenterol Clin North Am. 2001;30:547.

35. Nishikawa H, Kimura T, Kita R, Osaki Y. Treatment for hepatocellular carcinoma in elderly patients: a literature review. J Cancer. 2013;4:635–43.

36. Affronti J. Biliary disease in the elderly patient. Clin Geriatr Med. 1999;15:571.

37. Spira RM, Nissan A, Zamir O, et al. Percutaneous transhepatic cholecystostomy and delayed laparoscopic cholecystectomy in critically ill patients with acute cholecystitis. Am J Surg. 2002;183:62–6.

38. Martin SP, Ulrich CD. Pancreatic disease in the elderly. Clin Geriatr Med. 1999;15:579.

39. Ross SO, Forsmark CE. Pancreatic and biliary disorders in the elderly. Gastroenterol Clin North Am. 2001;30:531.

40. Scheiman J, Hwang J, Moayyedi P. American gastroenterological association technical review on the diagnosis and management of asymptomatic neoplastic pancreatic cysts. Gastroenterology. 2015;148:824–48.

41. Valsangkar N, Morales-Oyarvide V, Thayer S, et al. 851 resected cystic tumors of the pancreas: a 33-year experience at the Massachusetts General Hospital. Surgery. 2012;152:S4–12.

42. Vege S, Ziring B, Jain R, Moayyedi P. American gastroenterological association institute guideline on the diagnosis and management of asymptomatic neoplastic pancreatic cysts. Gastroenterology. 2015;148:819–22.

43. Chapman IM. Weight loss in older persons. Med Clin North Am. 2011;95:579–93.

44. Jensen GL et al. Nutrition in the elderly. Gastroenterol Clin North Am. 2001;30:313.

45. Meyyazhagan S, Palmer RM. Nutritional requirements with aging: prevention of disease. Clin Geriatr Med. 2002;18:557.

Infection and Immunity

Kevin P. High

24.1 Clinical Take-Home Points

1. Older adults are at increased risk of infection vs. young adults due to:
   (a) The presence of multiple comorbid illnesses, functional limitations, and frailty
   (b) Waning immune function with age
   (c) More frequent contact with healthcare, which increases the risk of exposure, particularly to antibiotic resistant organisms
   (d) Social/environmental factors such as living in a nursing facility, food insecurity/poor nutritional status
2. Older adults with infection frequently present in "atypical" fashion; they are less likely to develop fever, leukocytosis, and typical symptoms than young adults, and more likely to present with altered behavior (e.g., poor oral intake), decline in functional status, or exacerbation of an underlying chronic illness (e.g., congestive heart failure).
3. Diagnostic tests (e.g., echocardiography, chest X-ray) frequently have poorer sensitivity in seniors than in young adults due to age-related changes in structure and/ or comorbid illness. However, making a specific microbiologic diagnosis is of great import in older adults as narrow, targeted antibiotic therapy can reduce the risk of side effects (e.g., *C. difficile* colitis, renal toxicity) and development of colonization with resistant organisms.
4. Colonization without infection occurs frequently in seniors, particularly skin/nasal colonization with methicillin-resistant *S. aureus* and positive urine cultures without specific urinary symptoms (i.e., asymptomatic bacteriuria). Only those with symptoms or about to undergo surgical procedures should undergo treatment to attempt eradication; otherwise, asymptomatic colonization should NOT be treated, and, in fact, in randomized trials this has been found to be harmful.
5. Specific infectious syndromes (e.g., sepsis, pneumonia) are more common and more severe in seniors than young adults, particularly in those with multiple chronic conditions or frailty. Early, aggressive antibiotic therapy is essential to optimizing outcomes in serious infections.

24.2 Predisposition of Older Adults to Infection

A number of factors increase the risk of infection as one ages into late life. Some risk factors are quite unique and changing as different cohorts enter seniority, while others are more "universal truths" and affect every older cohort. For example, many older individuals have latent infection with *Mycobacterium tuberculosis* (i.e., asymptomatic infection), but the percentage of US seniors harboring TB is declining. Similarly, zoster risk will likely climb for the next several decades, but the risk of zoster in those immunized against varicella is unknown and is likely to be quite different in 30 years. In contrast, age is now, and is likely to remain, the strongest risk factor for chronic illnesses—heart, lung, kidney, GI, and other organ systems as we age. Thus, multiple chronic conditions, diminished reserve, and frailty are likely to continue to plague seniors for the foreseeable future. Further, age itself is associated with substantial waning of immune function and host defense mechanisms, increasing the risk of infection in seniors.

Comorbid conditions (e.g., COPD, diabetes) most often result in reduced innate immunity; nonspecific barriers such as skin integrity, cough, and mucociliary clearance, as well as immune responses triggered by recognition of microbial products without the need for prior exposure such as complement, polymorphonuclear neutrophils, etc. Chronic, comorbid illnesses in elderly individuals with infection can also be an important predictor for worse outcomes.

K.P. High, MD, MS (✉)
Department of Administration, Wake Forest Baptist Health,
Medical Center Boulevard, Winston-Salem, NC 27157, USA
e-mail: khigh@wakehealth.edu

© Springer International Publishing Switzerland 2017
J.R. Burton et al. (eds.), *Geriatrics for Specialists*, DOI 10.1007/978-3-319-31831-8_24

While comorbidities substantially predispose older adults to infection, there are also age-related fundamental changes in the adaptive immune response that may predispose the elderly to infection. This waning of immunity with age is called immune senescence and is not merely a global state of reduced immunity, but a dysregulation of immune responses at multiple levels. Some aspects of immunity are upregulated, including the inflammatory response, which demonstrates constitutive activation in older adults, as evidenced by elevated C-reactive protein and interleukin (IL)-6 blood levels. However, T cell function and development of highly specific and high affinity antibodies after exposure to either an infectious organism or vaccine are markedly impaired with advance age and synergistically reduced when frailty is present.

Poor nutritional status is a major confounder in studies of immunity in the elderly population. Protein-energy malnutrition (PEM) is present in 30–60 % of subjects older than 65 years of age who are admitted to the hospital, and is linked to delayed wound healing, pressure ulcer formation, community-acquired pneumonia, increased risk of nosocomial infection, extended lengths of stay, and increased mortality. In community-dwelling older adults, PEM is associated with poor vaccine responses. Specific micronutrient deficiencies are also common in older adults, and several have been linked to poor immune function (e.g., vitamin B_{12} deficiency and inadequate pneumococcal vaccine responses). Despite the strong evidence that PEM and specific vitamin/mineral deficiencies are common and linked to poor immune responses, the efficacy of nutritional supplements has yet to be conclusively demonstrated.

There is increasing recognition that the health of seniors is not only a function of biomedical variables but also socioeconomic status, environment, and delivery of health care services. This "determinants of health" perspective is probably best illustrated by respiratory tract infection risk in older adults. Population-based studies reveal that lower income is associated with higher rates of community-acquired pneumonia and invasive pneumococcal infections amongst elderly individuals. Lower socioeconomic status may predispose to infection either because of increased exposure to infectious agents (e.g., crowding) or because of increased susceptibility due to common exposures (e.g., tobacco smoke). Long-term care residents emphasize the concept of "multiple determinants of health" as well—this subset of the aging population has a particularly high incidence of respiratory, urinary, gastrointestinal, and skin infections vs. community-dwelling seniors. The close contact residents have with other residents plays a key role in the spread of infections such as influenza; frail residents in a confined setting can lead to severe outbreaks with high mortality rates. The intense use of antibiotics in long-term care facilities can lead to higher rates of antibiotic resistant bacteria such as methicillin-resistant *Staphylococcus aureus* (MRSA), vancomycin-resistant enterococci (VRE), and multidrug resistant gram-negative rods.

24.3 Principles of Diagnosis and Management of Infections in the Elderly Patient

24.3.1 Presentation of Illness

Infectious diseases frequently present with atypical features in older adults. Serious infections may be indicated only by nonspecific declines in functional or mental status, or anorexia with decreased oral intake. Underlying illness (e.g., congestive heart failure [CHF] or diabetes) is often exacerbated as an initial manifestation leading one to seek medical attention. The most common sign that triggers the clinician to look for infection, fever, is often absent in the elderly patient. Several studies show that frail elderly individuals have lower mean baseline body temperatures than the currently accepted normal of 98.6 °F (37 °C) and blunted immune stimulation along with the lower basal temperature makes it less likely that frail, older adults will achieve a body temperature commonly recognized as fever. The importance of a "normal" or reduced temperature in the face of significant infection cannot be overemphasized as poor recognition and delayed diagnosis is likely to delay antimicrobial administration which has been shown to adversely affect outcomes.

Cognitive impairment may also lead to difficulty in diagnosing infection in the elderly when patients are unable to communicate symptoms. Finally, age- and comorbidity-related changes in anatomy and physiology may confound interpretation of diagnostic evaluations. For example, age-related calcium deposition reduces sensitivity of transthoracic echocardiography for detecting vegetations in infectious endocarditis from 85 to 90 % in adults age ≤55 to <50 % for those age 70+ years.

24.3.2 Antibiotic Management

Age and comorbidities markedly alter drug distribution, metabolism, excretion, and interactions. Antibiotic dose reductions or widening of the dosing interval is frequently required in older adults because of changes in renal function or predisposition of the elderly adult to important side effects. In addition, antibiotic interactions are more frequent because most elderly persons are taking multiple medications. These changes and the increased incidence of side effects in the elderly often lead clinicians to the dictum of "start low, go slow" whenever new drugs are started in older adults. However, for antibiotics, this is NOT an appropriate strategy. There are data that suggest early achievement of therapeutic levels of antibiotics is MORE important in seniors than in young adults. The reason for this is not fully known, but may be due to impaired defense mechanisms (described above) rendering the need for antibiotic administration more acute in seniors.

Many ethical dilemmas surround antibiotic use in frail elderly persons and terminally ill patients. The 1998 American Medical Association (AMA) Council of Ethical and Judicial Affairs included antibiotics, along with mechanical ventilation, as "life-sustaining" treatment. Others argue that antibiotics are part of ordinary care, even those who are designated to be receiving "comfort measures only," and their use may be appropriate to alleviate symptoms. While every clinical situation is unique, and no blanket recommendation can be made for the use or nonuse of antibiotics in the terminally ill, it seems prudent to include antibiotic administration in the discussion of advanced directives as a potentially life-sustaining maneuver and to treat it no differently than any other medical intervention such as surgery or mechanical ventilation.

24.4 Unique Aspects of Infections Syndromes in Older Adults

Selected common infections in older adults and their unique aspects vs. young adults are outlined in the following paragraphs.

24.4.1 Bacteremia and Sepsis

Compared to young adults, older patients with bacteremia are more likely to have a gastrointestinal or genitourinary source, and thus, isolation of Gram-negative rods is more frequent in older adults. The risk of bacteremia is also increased by the use of invasive devices (e.g., pacemakers, urinary catheters, artificial joints). Poor outcomes of sepsis are more likely in those with underlying comorbid illness. The prevalence of MRSA and other drug-resistant bacteria increases with age and therefore it is more likely to have a mismatch between the activity of the initial antibiotic selected and the susceptibility of the organism isolated.

24.4.2 Fever of Unknown Origin

The differential diagnosis of FUO in older patients differs from that in younger adults. Roughly a third of older patients with FUO have treatable infections (e.g., intra-abdominal abscess, bacterial endocarditis, tuberculosis, perinephric abscess, or occult osteomyelitis), but only endocarditis and tuberculosis are more common in older adults than in younger patients. Giant cell arteritis (GCA, aka temporal arteritis) and polymyalgia rheumatica (PMR) account for nearly one out of every five cases of FUO in the older populations. Thus, evaluation of FUO in patients age 60 years and over should include a high suspicion for GCA and early temporal artery biopsy, particularly if the erythrocyte sedimentation rate or liver enzymes are elevated. Malignant disease as a cause of FUO occurs with similar frequency in old and young adults. In both young and older adults, non-Hodgkin's lymphoma accounts for the majority of cases of FUO due to malignancy.

24.4.3 Infective Endocarditis

Native valve infective endocarditis (IE) is most often related to degenerative disease which occurs more frequently in seniors. Older adults are much more likely than young adults to have undergone valve replacement surgery and are therefore also at higher risk than young adults for prosthetic valve endocarditis (PVE). Older adults have about a fivefold higher risk for IE than the general population with streptococci and staphylococci isolated in about 80 % of older adults with IE. However, when compared to younger adults, enterococcal and Gram-negative organisms occur more commonly, likely explained by a greater incidence of gastrointestinal and genitourinary sources of bacteremia. Age alone does not impair survival after IE, but comorbid conditions do lead to poorer outcomes.

Valvular vegetations are less common, while intracardiac abscesses and paravalvular complications are relatively more common in older than younger adults. These are often difficult to detect by TTE, and sensitivity of TTE for detecting vegetations is low in older adults. Thus, a low threshold for transesophageal echocardiography (TEE) is warranted in older patients with suspected or proven IE. A negative echocardiogram, either transthoracic or transesophageal, however, does not exclude the diagnosis of IE (sensitivity for TTE in seniors is approximately 70 %, but 90 % for TEE).

24.4.4 HIV Infection

The success of antiretroviral therapy (ART) has turned HIV into a chronic illness and long-term survival is now the rule. Patients infected in their 20s can anticipate a life-expectancy at least into their 70s. This has resulted in a large cohort of patients aging with HIV. Newly acquired infections in seniors are more prevalent than most believe as well. Older Americans typically acquire HIV infection via sexual activity, and subjects >50 years of age account for about 15 % of all new diagnoses of AIDS in the USA. Many older individuals did not grow up in an era when sexually transmitted diseases (STDs) were even discussed, and, of course, pregnancy prevention is not an issue in advanced age. Thus, older adults are the least likely group of adults to practice safe sex. The lack of HIV awareness affects both older patients and their clinician providers. Nonspecific symptoms such as poor appetite and weight loss and specific infections such as zoster, tuberculosis, or frequent pneumonias are often mistaken for symptoms related to aging and fail to trigger HIV testing. Special consideration should be given to HIV as a potentially treatable cause of dementia in those with memory loss.

HIV infection in older adults tends to present at a more advanced stage than in younger adults both due to delayed diagnosis and synergistic immune senescence. Additionally, HIV and/or its treatment are associated with accumulation of multi-morbidity earlier in life than in HIV-negative adults. Further, frailty is more frequent at ages 10–20 years earlier in HIV-infected persons. Classic geriatric syndromes such as falls and fractures also appear to be prevalent at younger ages in those with HIV, and the risk is not predicted by HIV-specific variables, but by risk factors similar to those seen in older adults in the general population.

24.4.5 Community-Acquired Pneumonia

Adults age ≥65 years have hospitalization rates for pneumonia that are sixfold higher than young adults if they reside in the community, and 15-fold higher if they reside in a nursing home. Several prognostic formulas are available to assess severity and determine indications for hospitalization in those with CAP (e.g., Pneumonia Severity Index (PSI), CURB65 (confusion, uremia, respiratory rate, low blood pressure, and age >65)) and have been validated in older adults. However, prediction rules are not intended to override clinical judgment and factors not included may be important (living conditions, underlying psychiatric or cognitive issues, comorbid illness, and overall condition of the patient or home environment). Comorbidity is the strongest predictor of mortality in older patients with CAP, other independent risk factors include severe vital sign abnormalities on admission (temperature <36.1 °F, blood pressure <90 mmHg systolic, or pulse >110 bpm), renal dysfunction (creatinine >1.5 mg/dl), impaired activities of daily living (ADLs), and extreme age (>85 years).

The causative organisms of pneumonia in older adults differ from young adults. *S. pneumoniae* is still the most common, but polymicrobial infection and gram-negative organisms occur more commonly, particularly in patients with COPD or in residents of long-term care facilities. *S. aureus* and respiratory viruses are also common causes of CAP in nursing home residents. Tuberculosis is more common in older adults since they are more likely to have been exposed to *M. tuberculosis* as previously noted. Treatment for CAP in older adults follows usual guidelines. However, the risk of MRSA and gram-negative organisms should be taken into account for patients who reside in nursing homes.

Prevention of pneumonia is a complex issue in older adults. Immunization for influenza and pneumococcus are important preventive strategies (see below). Some data suggest use of angiotensin converting enzyme inhibitors when indicated for hypertension or other comorbid illness may reduce the risk pneumonia vs. use of other anti-hypertensive agents presumably due to stimulating cough reflexes. A number of interventions (e.g., positioning, dietary changes, drugs, oral hygiene, tube feeding) have been proposed to reduce the risk of aspiration, especially in older adults with stroke or other illness that impair swallowing, but to date, none has been clearly shown to be effective.

24.4.6 Prosthetic Device Infections

Implanted prosthetic devices (e.g., artificial joints, pacemakers, vascular grafts) are much more commonly used in aged vs. young adults. Infected prosthetic devices are typically coated by microbial biofilms that reduce antibiotic penetration and promote organisms resistant to usual antibiotic concentrations. Thus, the use of bactericidal antibiotics in high doses is preferred. A second agent that penetrates biofilms well (e.g., rifampin for staphylococci) has been associated with improved outcomes, but drug–drug interactions are important to consider. Two-stage procedures with device removal, prolonged antibiotic administration, and subsequent re-implantation are usually considered the gold-standard of therapy. However, comorbidities and poor functional status may alter the risk/benefit ratio; the resulting prolonged immobility may be relatively contraindicated in some and cure infeasible in others. Return to pre-morbid functional status or preservation of current status may be more relevant and achievable with long-term antibiotic suppression in the absence of microbe eradication.

24.4.7 Urinary Tract Infection

UTI is the most common infectious illness in older adults with an incidence of nearly 10 % in women and 5 % in men over the age of 80. Typical pathogens still predominate, but resistant isolates such as *Pseudomonas aeruginosa* and enterococci (*E. faecalis* and *E. faecium*) occur more commonly in seniors vs. young adults.

Asymptomatic bacteriuria occurs in many older women in the community (about 10–15 %) and particularly those residing in nursing homes (up to 50 %). Rates in men are about half those in women. In both genders, rates approach 100% with the use of chronic catheters. Numerous studies show NO clinical benefit when asymptomatic bacteriuria is treated, but treatment can lead to significant side effects, expense, and potential for selection of resistant organisms. Thus, treatment is not recommended, even in the presence of white blood cells in the urine. Clinical guidelines for evaluation for UTI in older adults advise that urinalysis and urine cultures should not be ordered for asymptomatic individuals; diagnostic testing should be reserved for those with fever, dysuria, gross hematuria, worsening incontinence, or suspected bacteremia. The dilemma clinicians face is to determine what defines "symptomatic" in frail, often cognitively impaired seniors. Infections often present in subtle fashion in older adults. Diagnosis of a UTI in an elderly patient relies on clinical signs (e.g., delirium) and symptoms, supported by laboratory data. Symptomatic UTI in older women (aged 65 years or older) be defined by at least two of the following criteria: fever, urinary symptoms (frequency, urgency, dysuria, suprapubic tenderness, or costovertebral angle pain), a positive urine culture of at least 10^5 colony-forming units/mL with no more than two species present, and pyuria (≥ 10 white blood cells/mm^3 of unspun urine). Therapeutic antibiotic 'trials' are not recommended, to avoid possible drug toxicity, drug–drug interaction, and antimicrobial resistance. When the diagnosis of UTI is in doubt, a reasonable management strategy is to withhold antibiotics for 1 week with follow-up since 25–50% of older women with UTI symptoms will improve without therapy in this time frame.

24.5 Immunizations

General recommendations to improve immunization rates — In the USA, only about half of eligible older adults receive pneumococcal or annual influenza vaccine. Many unvaccinated elderly adults diagnosed with invasive pneumococcal disease have had contact with the medical system within the prior 6–12 months. Thus vaccines remain underutilized despite clear opportunities for immunization. Importantly, influenza and pneumococcal vaccine can be administered simultaneously at different anatomic sites, as can influenza and zoster vaccine or pneumococcal and zoster vaccine.

The CDC has recommended a multi-pronged strategy for improving vaccine administration rates in adults to include: (1) Review of immunizations in all persons at age 50 with immunization of those with an indication for vaccination; (2) Standing orders for hospitals and doctor's offices — routine administration in elderly and at-risk patients by nursing personnel without requiring individual orders for each patient; (3) Community-based strategies with public health promotions in undeserved populations and community outreach programs (senior centers, civic organizations, etc.); (4) Physician-reminder systems (chart checklists, computer-assisted flags, pre-hospital discharge, etc.) and, (5) simultaneous immunizations with >1 vaccine in the combinations outlined in the prior paragraph.

24.5.1 Tetanus/Diphtheria and Pertussis

Older adults represent the group most "at risk" for tetanus. Older women are less likely than older men to have antibody levels above those considered protective (>0.01 units per ml) as they are less likely to have received boosters than men (military service and trauma lead to more boosters in men). If there is no documentation of an older adult having received a complete tetanus vaccine series, a series of three injections is indicated. A single dose of tetanus/diphtheria/acellular pertussis (Tdap) should be substituted for one of the Td doses in the 3-dose series. Booster doses of Td should be given at 10-year intervals, but at least once Tdap should be substituted for Td. Since 2012 the US Advisory Committee on Immunization Practices (ACIP) has recommended Tdap for all persons aged 65 and older — older adults are often part of pertussis outbreaks even though the disease is recognized primarily in children. The diagnosis of pertussis in older adults is difficult due to the atypical presentation (usually just chronic cough, not "whooping" cough) and low index of suspicion by providers.

24.5.2 Pneumococcal Vaccine

Pneumococcal vaccine is indicated for all persons 65 years or older and many persons under age 65 with comorbid conditions. Two vaccines are available: a 23-valent polysaccharide vaccine (PPSV23) and a 13-valent pneumococcal conjugate vaccine (PCV13). In 2014, ACIP recommendations for pneumococcal vaccination in older adults were revised; it is now recommended that both PCV13 and PPSV23 be given sequentially to all adults aged ≥ 65 years with PCV13 administered first and PPSV23 given at least 8 weeks later. If a PPSV23 has already been given, repeat immunization with PCV13 should be administered at age 65 years or older as long as at least 1 year has past since PPSV23 was administered. Another dose of PPSV23 dose should then follow 6–12 months later. However, a minimum interval of 5 years between PPSV23 doses should be maintained. When the pneumococcal immunization history is unknown, the PCV13 vaccine should be administered followed by PPSV23 6–12 months later. Once the PCV13-PPSV23 sequence is completed and the patient is age 65 or older, no additional boosters are recommended.

24.5.3 Seasonal Influenza

Annual influenza vaccine is recommended for all older adults. A high-dose inactivated influenza vaccine is available and the vaccine of choice for individuals ≥65 years of age based on data showing increased immunogenicity a 24 % additional benefit for preventing disease in seniors vs. the standard-dose vaccine. Mild to moderate local reactions are more common with the high-dose vaccine than with standard-dose vaccine, but the incidence of serious adverse events is similar.

Many evaluations of influenza vaccine's efficacy have been performed; while protection is incomplete, the vaccine markedly reduces the severity of disease and subsequent rates of respiratory illness, hospitalization, and mortality in elderly adults with estimated efficacy rates of 50–80 %. Despite these findings, there is controversy as to whether the influenza vaccine is truly effective in those ≥70 years of age due to residual bias in case–control studies. Nevertheless, until the controversy is settled or compelling evidence invokes recommendations for alternate strategies, essentially all experts agree there is little risk and immunization should be given to all older adults. In addition, immunization of medical personnel and caregivers for high-risk patients has also demonstrated protection for older adults in their care.

Treatment with antiviral therapy (neuraminidase inhibitors) reduces the duration of illness by about 1–1.5 days if started within 24 h of symptom onset and may lower the risk of hospitalization in older adults. In outbreak situations, chemoprophylaxis may be required, particularly in nursing home settings, and is effective in reducing intra-facility transmission.

24.5.4 Zoster

Zoster vaccine (ZV) was first recommended for the prevention of shingles in adults aged 60 years or older in 2006. The risk of zoster in unvaccinated adults is about 50 % for those who reach age 85 years. Zoster vaccine reduces the risk of developing zoster by half and the risk of post-herpetic neuralgia by two-thirds. It is recommended that adults over the age of 60 receive one dose of zoster vaccine, regardless of whether they have had an episode of herpes zoster. There is no contraindication to vaccination for individuals with common chronic medical conditions, but it is not recommended for those with marked immune compromise (e.g., transplant recipients, active chemotherapy recipients).

Suggested Readings

Brothers TD, Kirkland S, Guaraldi G, Falutz J, Theou O, Johnston BL, Rockwood K. Frailty in people aging with human immunodeficiency virus (HIV) infection. J Infect Dis. 2014;210(8):1170–9. doi:10.1093/infdis/jiu258.

El-Solh AA. Nursing home acquired pneumonia: approach to management. Curr Opin Infect Dis. 2011;24(2):148–51. doi:10.1097/QCO.0b013e328343b6cc.

Kline KA, Bowdish DM. Infection in an aging population. Curr Opin Microbiol. 2015;29:63–7. doi:10.1016/j.mib.2015.11.003.

Mody L, Juthani-Mehta M. Urinary tract infections in older women: a clinical review. JAMA. 2014;311(8):844–54. doi:10.1001/jama.2014.303.

Jump RL. Clostridium difficile infection in older adults. Aging Health. 2013;9(4):403–14.

Morrill HJ, Caffrey AR, Jump RL, Dosa D, LaPlante KL. Antimicrobial stewardship in long-term care facilities: a call to action. J Am Med Dir Assoc. 2016;17(2):183.e1-183.e16. doi:10.1016/j.jamda.2015.11.013.

Zapata HJ, Quagliarello VJ. The microbiota and microbiome in aging: potential implications in health and age-related diseases. J Am Geriatr Soc. 2015;63(4):776–81. doi:10.1111/jgs.13310.

Kidney Disease

25

C. Barrett Bowling and Rasheeda K. Hall

25.1 Introduction

Chronic kidney disease (CKD) is common among older adults and associated with mortality, cardiovascular disease, and increased heath care utilization [1]. Despite the high burden of CKD at older ages, the general approach to kidney disease is based on evidence from young and middle-aged adults and may not apply to older adults with CKD. At younger ages, CKD is often a progressive disorder and the prevention of kidney failure is a key goal. Older patients with CKD may face different challenges [2]. The very old with CKD are 10–20 times more likely to die before progressing to kidney failure [3]. Older adults with CKD often have multiple chronic conditions and may be at increased risk for functional decline, cognitive impairment, and frailty. For the small proportion, but growing absolute number, of older adults who have CKD progression, initiation of dialysis is associated with a poor prognosis and high burden of functional impairment [4, 5].

The purpose of this chapter is to identify the unique aspects of caring for older adults from early stages of CKD through kidney failure and end-of-life. We describe an approach to older adults with CKD that recognizes the impact of non-CKD factors on the lives of CKD patients and recommends geriatric assessment to facilitate the development of individualized care plans. For background, we describe age-related changes in kidney structure and function, provide definitions of CKD, kidney failure, and related disorders, and report on the prevalence of kidney disease among older adults. Next we describe the limitations of a disease-oriented approach to kidney disease in older adults and propose an alternative approach that focuses on providing individualized, patient-centered care. Additionally, we provide detailed descriptions of the unique challenges that arise in older patients with acute kidney injury (AKI), early stages of CKD, and among those with kidney failure. In the final two sections of this chapter we describe kidney disease in special patient populations and end-of-life considerations.

25.2 The Aging Kidney

Structural and functional changes in the kidney have been described with aging. Structural changes include a decrease in overall kidney mass with autopsy studies showing a decrease from 400 g at age 40 to less than 300 g at age 90 [6]. This decrease in mass has been shown to be primarily due to a decrease in the renal cortices with sparing of the renal medulla. While reductions in glomerular number have also been shown, there is a large amount of variability in glomerular number from one older adult to another. Additionally, the incidence of glomerular sclerosis increases with older age with sclerosis present in <5 % of the glomeruli of those 40 years old compared to 30 % of glomeruli exhibiting evidence of sclerosis at age 80 [6]. The contribution of age-related increase in collagen production in the glomerulus versus disease-related pathology remains poorly understood [7].

Declines in kidney function at older ages including reduced glomerular filtration rate (GFR) have also been shown. Cross sectional studies have shown a lower median estimated GFR (eGFR) at older ages, but do not provide information about changes in kidney function within individual patients [6]. In one longitudinal study, declines in creatinine clearance, a maker of GFR, were shown to decrease on average by 0.75 ml/min/year among health aging study participants [8]. However, one third of participants without hypertension or urological disease experienced no decline in

C.B. Bowling, MD, MSPH (✉)
Atlanta VA Medical Center, Birmingham/Atlanta VA Geriatric Research, Education and Clinical Center,
1670 Clairmont Road (11B), Decatur, GA 30033, USA
e-mail: christopher.barrett.bowling@emory.edu

R.K. Hall, MD, MBA, MHS
Medicine, Duke University Medical Center,
DUMC BOX 2747, 2424 Erwin Road, Suite 605, Durham, NC 27705, USA

© Springer International Publishing Switzerland 2017
J.R. Burton et al. (eds.), *Geriatrics for Specialists*, DOI 10.1007/978-3-319-31831-8_25

kidney function, raising the question of whether or not decrease in GFR is inevitable with aging [8]. The decrease in GFR with age has been attributed in part to increasing glomerular sclerosis with age. However, one analysis of kidney biopsies from renal transplant donors that included older adults reported poor correlation between level of GFR and the amount of sclerosis [9]. Therefore, the burden of sclerosis may not predict the level of kidney function. The relationship between aging, disease-related pathology, response mechanisms to increase glomerular filtration, and clinical markers of kidney function is complex and many of the biological processes remain unknown.

25.3 Kidney Disease Terminology and Epidemiology

25.3.1 Kidney Disease Definitions

CKD is defined as abnormalities in kidney structure or function that persist for at least 3 months and have implications for health [10]. Markers of kidney damage include the abnormal presence of protein (proteinuria) or albumin (albuminuria) in the urine. Kidney function is assessed using GFR. Because measuring GFR is rarely available in the clinical setting, definitions of CKD rely on eGFR from formulas that use serum creatinine, age, and race. Decreased eGFR is defined as <60 ml/min/1.73 m². In Sect. 25.6 below, we discuss the challenges and controversies for identifying CKD in older populations using this cut-point to define CKD.

Current CKD clinical practice guidelines use these biomarkers of abnormal kidney function (i.e., eGFR and albuminuria) to both define CKD and stage the disease based on prognosis for CKD-related outcomes. Guidelines recommend a classification and staging system that is based on (1) cause, (2) GFR category, and (3) albuminuria category (ACR) (Table 25.1). While hypertension and diabetes are the most common causes of CKD among older adults, other causes include renal vascular disease, chronic urinary obstruction, systemic vasculitis, multiple myeloma or intrinsic kidney disorders such as glomerulonephritis or nephrotic syndrome. As with many multifactorial geriatric syndromes, for older adults, kidney disease may have more than one cause (e.g., renal vascular disease with chronic urinary obstruction). Clinical practice guidelines recommend categorizing kidney stage by both eGFR level and ACR level because of the improved risk stratification for mortality, kidney failure, AKI, and progressive CKD when eGFR and ACR are considered together. As an example, a patient with CKD related to diabetes with an eGFR of 32 ml/min/1.73 m² and ACR of 150 mg/g would be classified as diabetic CKD, G3b, A2.

As CKD progresses, patients may develop kidney failure defined as an eGFR <15 ml/min/1.73 m² or the need to initiate renal replacement therapy (RRT; hemodialysis or peritoneal dialysis) or kidney transplant [10]. End-stage renal disease (ESRD) is a related administrative term based on the payment for health care by the Medicare ESRD Program. ESRD is used to identify those receiving RRT or who have received a kidney transplant, regardless of eGFR level [11]. In Sect. 25.7 below, we describe the treatment of advanced kidney disease in older populations including dialysis, kidney transplant, and conservative management.

In contrast to CKD and kidney failure, which are considered chronic conditions, AKI is a sudden worsening in kidney function. The term AKI has replaced the diagnosis of acute renal failure to reflect that even small changes in kidney function may impact long-term kidney function and to emphasize the broad spectrum of kidney injury [12]. Current classification of AKI includes three stages based on both serum creatinine and urine output (UOP) (Table 25.2) [13]. In Sect. 25.5 below, we describe risk factors that predispose older adults to AKI and the impact of AKI on CKD progression.

25.3.2 Burden of Kidney Disease Among Older Adults

The overall prevalence of CKD has been reported to be 13.1 % in the adult US population. However, the prevalence of kidney disease increases markedly with age [1]. Nearly half of those with CKD are 70 years of age or older, and there

Table 25.1 Classification of CKD by cause, GFR, and albuminuria

Cause
Common causes in older adults:
Hypertension
Diabetes mellitus
Renal vascular disease
Chronic urinary obstruction
Systemic vasculitis
Multiple myeloma
Glomerulonephritis
Nephrotic syndrome
Multifactorial etiology (e.g., renal vascular disease with chronic urinary obstruction)

GFR	
Category	eGFR, ml/min/1.73 m²
G1	≥90
G2	60–89
G3a	45–59
G3b	30–44
G4	15–29
G5	<15

Albuminuria	
Category	ACR, mg/g
A1	<30
A2	30–300
A3	>300

is a graded increase in the prevalence of CKD at older ages. Among US adults, the prevalence of CKD, defined as an eGFR <60 ml/min/1.73 m^2 was reported to be 0.9, 7.5, 26.5, and 51.1 % among those aged <60, 60–69, 70–79, and ≥80 years old. A similar, but less dramatic, increase in the prevalence of albuminuria, defined as an ACR >30 mg/g, of 6.8, 14.2, 21.3, and 32.7 % at ages 60–69, 70–79 and ≥80 years, respectively, has been reported.

An increase in the prevalence of CKD over the past 2 decades has also been reported in the general US population, especially among older adults [14, 15]. For example, the prevalence of decreased eGFR (<60 ml/min/1.73 m^2) in the US population ≥80 years was examined during three time periods: 1988–1994, 1999–2004, and 2005–2010. The prevalence of decreased eGFR was 40.5, 49.9, and 51.2 % during these time periods. A disproportionate increase in the prevalence of more severe CKD (eGFR <45 ml/min/1.73 m^2) was found from 14.3 % to 18.6 % and 21.7 % in 1988–1994, 1999–2004, and 2005–2010, respectively. These findings were not completely explained by an increase in the prevalence of diabetes and hypertension in the older population during this time. Assuming that the prevalence of CKD remains stable in this age group, with the aging of the US population, the number of US adults ≥80 years old with eGFR <60 ml/min/1.73 m^2 is estimated to increase from 4.6

million in 2005–2010 to 9.9 million and 15.8 million in 2030 and 2050, respectively (Fig. 25.1) [15].

While the prevalence of CKD defined as an eGFR <60 ml/min/1.73 m^2 is highest at older age, older adults are much less likely to progress to kidney failure. The very old with CKD may be 10–20 times more likely to die before progressing to kidney failure. The competing risk of death has been examined by determining at what eGFR level is the risk of requiring RRT greater than the risk of death for different age groups. For example, among younger adults the risk of kidney failure requiring RRT is greater than the risk of death at an eGFR level of 45 ml/min/1.73 m^2 and below [3]. For adults 65–84 years old, the risk of kidney failure requiring RRT is only greater than the risk of death at an eGFR of 15 ml/min/1.73 m^2 and below. For those 85 years and older, the risk of death has been shown to exceeded the risk of kidney failure requiring RRT at any eGFR level.

In addition to the competing risk of death before reaching kidney failure, there are other possible explanations for the age difference in risk of kidney failure including a slower decline in kidney function among older adults. Additionally older adults may be less like to be offered or chose treatment with dialysis or transplantation in the face of kidney failure. For example, when kidney failure is categorized as treated (eGFR <15 ml/min/1.73 m^2 and dialysis or kidney transplant) or untreated (eGFR <15 ml/min/1.73 m^2, but no dialysis or kidney transplant), overall kidney failure is more common at older ages. However, at younger ages, treated kidney failure is more common than untreated kidney failure [16]. At older ages untreated kidney failure is much more common.

Although only a small proportion of older adults with CKD progress to kidney failure and receive RRT, the absolute number of older adults with ESRD (i.e., requiring RRT or kidney transplant regardless of eGFR) has increased over the past 20 years. Through 2010, the fastest growing group with

Table 25.2 Stages for acute kidney injury based on increase in serum creatinine from baseline or level of urine output (UOP)

Stage	Serum creatinine increase from baseline	UOP
1	1.5 to 1.9-fold, or Increase ≥0.3 mg/dL	<0.5 mL/kg per hour for at least 6 h
2	2 to 2.9-fold	<0.5 mL/kg per hour for at least 12 h
3	3-fold or greater, or Increase to ≥4.0 mg/dL	<0.3 mL/kg per hour for 24 h, or No UOP (anuria) for at least 12 h

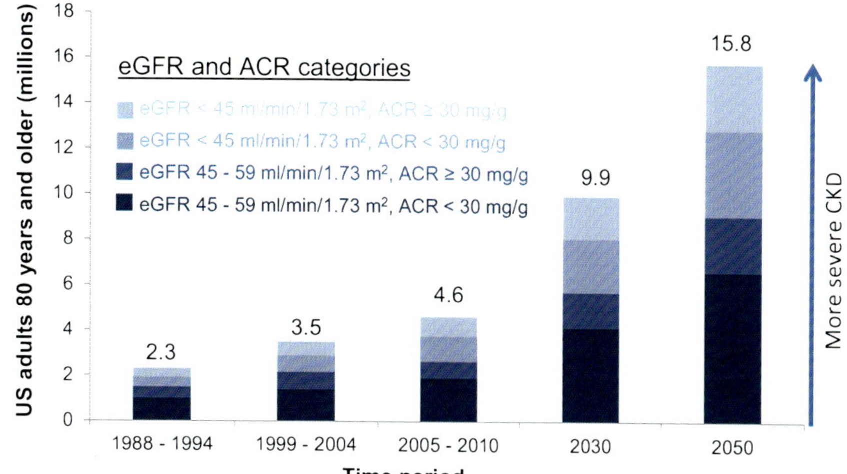

Fig. 25.1 The number of US adults ≥80 years old with CKD has doubled in the past 2 decades and will continue to increase with the aging of the populations. There has been a disproportionate increase in the prevalence of more severe CKD. *eGFR* estimated glomerular filtration rate, *ACR* albumin-to-creatinine ratio

ESRD was those 70 years and older [17]. Several factors may be contributing to the increased incidence of ESRD among older adults. This may be due in part to the increase in CKD prevalence among older adults, the aging US population, as well as an increase in the use of dialysis among older adults.

A similar pattern of graded increase in the incidence of AKI at older ages has been shown. Among hospitalized adults, the incidence of AKI among those 85 years and older is approximately 40 cases compared to 20 cases per 1000 discharges among those <65 years old [12]. The incidence of AKIs has been reported to have increased over the last 2 decades and has been explained by an increase in AKI risk factors, the aging population, as well as improvements in recognition of AKI.

25.4 Disease-Oriented Versus Patient-Centered Approach

25.4.1 Disease-Oriented Approach

The disease-oriented model of care is the prevailing clinical paradigm for the diagnosis and treatment of chronic conditions. This approach emphasizes the prevention, diagnosis, and treatment of individual disease processes [2, 18]. In the disease-oriented approach a direct causal relationship between clinical signs and symptoms and specific disease pathology is assumed. Treatments target the underlying pathophysiology and symptoms are thought to be best treated by interventions that impact the disease course, rather than as a target for intervention themselves. Treatment priorities are often determined by the availability of clinical trial evidence.

There are several strengths to this approach when applied to individual chronic conditions. The development and dissemination of CKD clinical practice guidelines have standardized CKD terminology and improved recognition and treatment of CKD. The disease-oriented approach provides a systemic framework for evidence-based management. Additionally, this approach is well suited for applying quality performance measurement and outcome tracking. Below, we describe the disease-oriented approach to CKD. Next, we describe limitations when applied specifically to older adults with CKD.

Existing CKD practice guidelines follow the disease-oriented model that assumes a direct and linear relationship between underlying kidney pathology with CKD progression, the development of concurrent CKD complications, kidney failure and ultimately death from CKD. Management strategies target the underlying risk factors for CKD and disease-specific biomarkers are used to track the progression of CKD. Clinical trials to prevent CKD progression are considered to provide the highest quality of evidence and are used to make recommendation for CKD treatment. Outcomes of interest are specific to CKD (e.g., kidney failure, mortality).

There are three main categories for CKD management: (1) slowing the progression of CKD to prevent kidney failure, (2) recognition and treatment of concurrent CKD complications, and (3) preparation for RRT [10]. Slowing the progression of CKD is considered a key goal. Approaches to slowing the progression include blood pressure (BP) control for all patients with CKD. For those with albuminuria, renin-angiotensin-aldosterone system (RAAS) interruption with angiotensin-converting enzyme inhibitors (ACE-Is) or angiotensin receptor blockers (ARBs) are recommended. Currently recommended BP goals for CKD patients are $\leq$140/90 for those with an ACR <30 mg/g and $\leq$130/80 for those with diabetes or ACR $\geq$30 mg/g. However, these recommendations are subject to change given findings from a recent clinical trial showing better outcomes among older adults who acheive lower BP targets. [19]. Guidelines also provide recommendations for protein intake, glycemic control, salt intake, and physical activity to prevent CKD progression.

The second category for CKD management is the recognition and treatment of concurrent CKD complications including anemia, metabolic bone disease, acidosis, and cardiovascular disease. Guidelines provide specific drug and lifestyle recommendations to manage these complications. In CKD, anemia is related to reduced erythropoietin and defined as <13.0 g/dL for men and <12.0 g/dL for women. Guidelines encourage evaluation for other causes of anemia and when erythropoietin stimulation agents are used, increasing hemoglobin concentrations to levels above 11.5 g/dL should be avoided. CKD metabolic bone disease includes abnormalities of calcium, phosphate, and parathyroid hormone (PTH) and is associated with increased risk of fractures. Current recommendations include dietary phosphate restriction or using oral binder to maintain serum phosphate within the normal range. Targets for treatment of hyperparathyroidism are more controversial. While clinical trials provide evidence that treatment to reduce PTH improves biomarkers of metabolic bone disease, the impact of these intermediate outcomes on clinically important outcomes such as fractures is limited. Guidelines also recommend treatment with oral bicarbonate supplementation for patients with serum bicarbonate levels <22 mmol/L with the goal to maintain bicarbonate within the normal range.

Lastly, guidelines provide recommendations for referral to nephrologists and preparation and time of RRT. Referral to nephrology is recommended, even if dialysis or transplantation is not a consideration in the presence of: AKI, eGFR <30 ml/min/1.73 m^2, significant albuminuria (ACR >300 mg/g), progression of CKD, urinary red cell casts, hypertension refractory to treatment with four medications, persistent elevated serum potassium, recurrent nephrolithiasis, and hereditary kidney disease. Planning for RRT is based on the risk for progression to kidney failure. Recent studies have shown that the trajectory of CKD progression is often nonlinear and difficult to predict for older adults. Timing of

RRT initiation is determined by the presence of kidney failure symptoms including serositis, acid–base or electrolyte abnormalities, pruritis, inability to control volume status or BP, progressive deterioration in nutritional status or cognitive impairment due to uremia. Recent studies have shown a trend towards initiation of RRT at higher levels of eGFR; however, evidence suggests no benefit or an increased risk for mortality among those with earlier initiation of dialysis in the course of CKD progression.

25.4.1.1 Limitations of the Disease-Oriented Approach

Despite the acceptance of the disease-oriented approach, there are several limitations of this approach when applied to older adults. Here, we describe four characteristics of older populations that may limit the relevance of the disease-oriented approach to CKD management [2]. These include (1) limited life expectancy, (2) a high burden of multimorbidity, and (3) heterogeneity in health goals and treatment preferences, and (4) exclusion from clinical trials.

Limited life expectancy is a key factor to consider for any disease-specific treatment plan for older adults. Both patients and providers recognize that there is a reduction in the years remaining in life expectancy at older ages and this has been shown in CKD. For example, a 70-year-old man with an eGFR 30–44 ml/min/1.73 m^2 and $\geq$2+ dipstick proteinuria may expect on average to live 5 more years. In contrast, an 85-year-old with the same level of kidney function may live on average 2.6 additional years [20]. However, reports of average survival do not capture the remarkable heterogeneity in life expectancy and complexity estimating survival in older adults. One approach to determine the heterogeneity in life expectancy is to calculate not only the median survival, but also the interquartile range (IQR) for survival defined as the 25th percentile to 75th percentile. The IQR for survival is 2.3–8.6 years for the 70-year-old man described above and 1.2–4.5 years for the 85 year old. This means that the highest 75th percentile of surviving 85 year olds may expect to live 4.5 year or longer. This suggests that many 85 year olds will live as long as or longer than the average 70 year old. Similar findings have been shown among older ESRD patients. The median survival for an 80-year-old incident ESRD patient is 1.3 years, however the interquartile range is 5 months to 3 years. Therefore, applying uniform recommendations to all older adults, some of whom may expect to live many more years and benefit from preventive treatments and others who are nearing end of life, is not appropriate.

Among older adults, CKD almost universally occurs in individuals with other chronic medical conditions. While multimorbidity, defined as the presence of two or more chronic conditions is common among older adults with CKD, existing clinical practice guidelines follow a "single disease" framework and do not account for the presence of other chronic conditions. As described above, the disease-oriented approach relies on CKD biomarkers (i.e., eGFR, ACR) to guide treatment decisions and focuses on preventing CKD-related outcomes. However, for older adults with multimorbidity, the application of multiple "single-disease" guidelines may lead to treatment recommendations that are complex and often contradictory or of limited benefit.

In addition to having multiple chronic conditions such as hypertension and diabetes, older adults with CKD have been shown to be at risk for co-occurring geriatric conditions. In the CKD population, the risk for mortality, hospitalizations, and emergency department (ED) visits increases at higher number of these problems. For example, among older adults with eGFR <60 more than two-thirds have 2 or more of 6 geriatric conditions (cognitive impairment, depressive symptoms, exhaustion, impaired mobility, falls, and polypharmacy) [21]. Compared to those with none of these problems, those with three or more experience twice the risk of dying, being hospitalized or requiring an ED visit. This "geriatric" multimorbidity is not considered in the disease-oriented clinical practice guidelines that only focus on CKD.

A third characteristic of older populations that may limit the relevance of the disease-oriented approach is heterogeneity in health goals and treatment preferences reported by older adults [2]. While CKD clinical practice guidelines prioritize the reduction of mortality and prevention of CKD related outcomes such as kidney failure, older adults often frame their health goals in terms of their overall health and maintaining functional independence. Universal health outcomes such as quality of life and functional independence may be viewed as more important than disease-specific outcomes. While a shift in health goals and preferences has been shown among older adults, it is important to recognize the variability in goals and preferences between older adults. The narrow focus on outcomes that are defined by the underlying disease pathology in the disease-oriented model often fails to address what is most important to an individual patient. Disease-oriented clinical practice guidelines lack the flexibility to allow providers to adapt the goals and treatment plans to the individual patient's needs.

Lastly, older adults with complex multimorbidity or limited life expectancy are often excluded from clinical trials. This is often done because the magnitude of treatment effects for a given intervention is often larger in homogenous populations (i.e., smaller variability results in larger treatment effect) [18]. Exclusion of older adults limits the generalizability of individual studies to older adults and the clinical practice guidelines that generate recommendations based on these studies. For example, most of the trials underpinning the guideline recommendations for the use of ACE-Is and ARBs have been conducted in high risk populations and did not enroll participants older than 70. Because ACE-Is and ARBs may be most effective in those at highest risk for progression (e.g., among those with albuminuria), findings from these studies of a number needed to treat (NNT) to prevent one case of ESRD ranging from 9 to 25 may not be generalizable to older adults. In fact, one recent simulation study using a real-world cohort of older adults with CKD showed large differences in the NNT based on the estimated baseline risk for ESRD. For older adults with the lowest risk of ESRD, they reported an NNT to prevent one case of ESRD to be 2500 [22].

25.4.2 Individualized, Patient-Centered Approach

There is an increasing awareness that a "one size fits all" approach to CKD management may not be appropriate. For example, the most recent CKD guidelines have added suggestions to tailor BP targets. However, approaches for how to individualize goals are not provided. Given the limitations of disease-oriented models of care in older populations, geriatricians often favor a more individualized patient-centered approach. The patient-centered approach embraces the complexity and acknowledges the importance of patient health goals and preferences for developing treatment plans. The patient-centered approach recognizes that existing evidence may not be relevant for individual patients. Symptoms are considered important targets for intervention, regardless of the underlying cause.

One approach to implementing a patient-centered approach to CKD is to include geriatric assessment as part of the clinical evaluation of CKD patients. Routine geriatric assessment could be used to identify contextual information (e.g., cognitive impairment, poor social support, markers of frailty, and limited life expectancy) to guide clinical care. It has been suggested that the recognition of geriatric conditions including functional impairment, frailty, mobility impairment, cognitive impairment, and depressive symptoms could be used to signal for the provider to consider a transition from the traditional disease-oriented approach to CKD care to a more individualized, patient-centered approach. For example, recognition of mild cognitive impairment and low social support may be used to tailor management goals such as glucose control in a patient with CKD and diabetes to reduce the risk for hypoglycemia. Recognition of these problems may also facilitate a shared decision-making approach to discussions about RRT. In these discussions, providers can address prognostic markers associated with poor survival on dialysis (e.g., non-ambulatory status, frailty) to help patients make an informed decision regarding dialysis versus conservative management. Eliciting goals of both the individual patient and family and caregivers can be used to prioritize outcomes beyond those reported in the CKD guidelines. In this approach, the CKD-specific diagnosis and management is not abandoned completely and may be incorporated into individualized treatment plans, depending on the extent to which disease-based recommendations are aligned with the preferences and goals of the patient. In Table 25.3, we highlight several components of geriatric assessment, their implications for CKD, and how these might be used to facilitate a patient-centered approach to CKD management.

Table 25.3 Geriatric assessment[a] facilitates individualized, patient-centered approach to the management of CKD in older adults

Assessment	Relevance to CKD	Examples of how geriatric assessment facilitates a patient-centered approach
Functional status	Functional impairment increases at lower levels of kidney function. At dialysis initiation 50 % of older adults are dependent in ADLs	Use a shared decision-making approach that considers prognosis Anticipate and plan for increased functional assistance after dialysis initiation
Cognition	The prevalence and incidence of cognitive impairment increases at lower eGFR. Cognitive impairment is common among older adults with kidney failure	Simplify CKD self-management tasks Include family or caregivers in decision-making
Mobility	CKD is associated with declines in community mobility	Recognize patient and family goals related to maintaining community mobility and social participation
Falls	Falls are common among older adults with CKD and kidney failure. Older adults with CKD mineral bone disease may be at increased risk for fractures	Individualize BP goals to prevent hypotension Limit polypharmacy Evaluate for CKD mineral bone disease
Depression	Depressive symptoms are associated with prevalent CKD, worsening kidney function and kidney failure. In kidney failure, depression is associated with worse outcomes	Address depression to improve quality of life
Frailty	The prevalence of frailty increases at lower eGFR and is very common in kidney failure. Frailty is associated with increased mortality and surgical complications among older adults receiving a kidney transplant	Incorporate prognostic information from frailty assessment into discussion about kidney failure treatment options
Multimorbidity	CKD occurs in patients with complex multiple chronic conditions	Recommend alternative treatment options when discordance in treatment recommendations occurs as in patients with CKD and arthritis

CKD chronic kidney disease, *ADLs* activities of daily living, *eGFR* estimated glomerular filtration rate
[a]See also Chap. 8, Office Tools for Geriatric Assessment

25.5 Acute Kidney Injury

Older adults are vulnerable to AKI due to factors that are both intrinsic and extrinsic to the kidney. While several intrinsic factors underlying this increased risk have been proposed including age-related stress-induced cellular senescence, a key component of AKI risk in older adults is susceptibility to kidney injury from extrinsic factors. Older adults may have decreased physiologic reserve in the face of physiologic stressors. AKI in the older population may be thought of as multifactorial and explained by the presence of chronic predisposing factors and acute precipitating factors, analogous to the current conceptualization of geriatric syndromes such as delirium and falls [12]. Predisposing factors include age-related structural changes including vascular sclerosis, age-related kidney function decline, chronic inflammation, and the presence of underlying CKD. Furthermore, the prevalence of multimorbidity increases at older ages and older patients often need multiple medications or diagnostic tests and procedures. For example, in an older patient with both CKD and arthritis, the addition of NSAIDs to a medication regimen that includes an ACE-I can precipitate AKI. Other medications that have been linked to AKI include diuretics, ARBs, and antibiotics. The co-occurrence of CKD and cardiovascular disease is also common and these patients may be at increased risk for contrast induced nephropathy. Therefore, benefits of cardiac catheterization for diagnosing coronary artery disease must be balanced with the risk for AKI. Older adults may also be at risk for volume depletion due to renal sodium wasting, reduced renal response to antidiuretic hormone and diminished thirst, putting those with vascular kidney disease at higher risk for AKI [23]. Older adults may also be at increased risk for infection and sepsis is a leading cause of AKI. In the older population, prevention of AKI may require improved recognition of both predisposing and precipitating factors, rather than addressing only factors intrinsic to kidneys.

As described above, a disease-oriented approach that focuses only on preventing kidney outcomes may not always be appropriate. Considering a patient's health goals and preferences may be necessary, especially when discordant recommendations arise in the setting of multimorbidity. For example, some older adults with arthritis pain may accept a small increase risk in AKI when taking NSAIDs in order to improve pain control and maintain functional independence.

When older adults have AKI they may be less likely to recover kidney function compared to younger adults. There is also growing recognition that the course of kidney disease progression is often not a predictable, linear decline towards kidney failure. For many older adults, kidney disease progression may result from repeated episodes of AKI. In these cases, it may be more effective to recognize AKI risk factors and prevent or lessen the impact of AKI to prevent progression to kidney failure, rather than management strategies such as BP and glucose control.

25.6 Chronic Kidney Disease

25.6.1 Disease Versus Normal Aging

Although the presence of CKD defined as an eGFR <60 ml/min/1.73 m^2 has been shown to be associated with mortality, CVD, concurrent CKD complications and functional decline, even in older populations, the current CKD definitions remain controversial. Current guidelines define CKD based on eGFR or ACR cut-points regardless of age and disagreement remains regarding CKD definition in older populations. Those in favor of changing the CKD definition to require age calibration for the diagnosis of CKD argue that the current approach labels many millions of older adults with a disease which may actually be age-related decline in kidney function due to organ senescence. Those against changing the guidelines argue for the need of clear and simple definitions regardless of age [1].

25.6.2 Challenges Estimating GFR

A related controversy exists over the estimation of GFR in older adults. Measuring GFR in the clinical setting is not practically possible [1]. Estimation of GFR relies on formulas that use age, race, and sex along with serum creatinine. Because creatinine comes from the breakdown of muscle, it has been argued that these equations may not accurately account for age-related changes in muscle mass that result in lower serum creatinine. Very few research studies have a large number of very old participants and available data on measured GFR; therefore existing estimation equations were developed and validated in studies conducted primarily in the middle-aged and young-old. More recent studies have attempted to develop and validate estimating equations in the very old. However, these studies have been limited to white, European populations and questions remain about the equations' validity in African American older adults [24]. Novel biomarkers such as cystatin-C can be used to estimate GFR and have been shown to be strong predictors of mortality [25]. However, GFR estimating equations that use cystatin-C identify CKD in an even large proportion of older than creatinine based equations [24]. For these reasons, an approach to diagnosis of CKD in older patients that takes into consideration the trajectory of renal function over time (e.g., stable versus declining), the presence of albuminuria, and the co-occurrence of conditions that worsen kidney function such as hypertension and diabetes may be more appropriate than relying on a single estimation of GFR to identify CKD.

25.7   Kidney Failure

25.7.1   Life Expectancy

Progression to kidney failure marks a significant decline in remaining life for older adults. Life expectancy for older adults who require RRT for kidney failure is approximately 25% less than the life expectancy of older adults without **kidney failure** [26]. Survival after kidney failure is typically better for older adults who initiate RRT compared to those who decline RRT (2-year survival rate 76% vs. 47%) [26]. This survival benefit is not only due to RRT itself. Older adults who initiate RRT tend to have fewer comorbid conditions and less functional impairment than those who decline RRT, confounding the association between treatment option and survival.

Among older adults who initiate RRT, life expectancy ranges from less than 3 months to 4.5 years [27]. Prognosis is worse as comorbidity burden, functional limitations, and age increases. Other factors that contribute to prognosis after dialysis initiation are shown in Table 25.4. These factors can be used to calculate risk scores to estimate the probability of death after initiating dialysis [26]. Although evaluated in a cohort of prevalent dialysis patients, the "surprise" question is an additional tool for prognostication. By answering the following question yourself: "Would I be surprised if this patient died in the next 12 months?", clinicians directly use their clinical judgment for prognostication. This clinical judgment is important for informing decisions for both initiation and withdrawal of RRT.

25.7.2   Shared Decision-Making

Because life expectancy is limited in older adults with kidney failure, it is essential to use shared decision-making for clinical decision-making for all medical procedures and intensive therapies (e.g., major surgery, chemotherapy).

Table 25.4 Risk factors for early mortality among older adults receiving hemodialysis[a]

Active malignancy
Body mass index <18.5 kg/m^2
Congestive heart failure
Dementia
Diabetes mellitus
Dysrythmia
Peripheral vascular disease
Severe behavioral disorder
Serum albumin
Would I be surprised if this patient died in the next 12 months?
Total dependence for transfers
Unplanned dialysis initiation

[a]Factors can be used to calculate risk of death after initiating dialysis [17]

Most older adults make RRT decisions based on their personal preferences and consideration of the challenges of adjusting to life with RRT. Therefore, shared decision-making allows patients and their caregivers to communicate their preferences to the clinician. In turn, the clinician using a risk benefit analysis is able to guide the patient towards a decision that addresses the patient's health goals.

For frail older adults, the SPIRES communication framework is an ideal approach to the shared decision-making process [28]. SPIRES involves the following six steps: Setup, Perceptions and Perspectives, Invitation, Recommendation, Empathize, and Summarize and Strategize (Table 25.5). Through this process, the clinician combines prognostic information from the patient's medical records with patient perspectives to develop a recommendation in favor of or against RRT initiation. The clinician develops an individualized treatment plan that involves monitoring for signs or symptoms that RRT is meeting the patient's expectations. This monitoring allows the SPIRES shared decision-making framework to be cyclical. If the patient experiences worsening health status, the clinician can use this new prognostic information (and potentially new patient preferences) to develop a new recommendation regarding continuation of RRT. Thus, SPIRES would facilitate discussions about dialysis withdrawal and end-of-life care.

25.7.3 Treatment Options

Central to dialysis decision-making is consideration of treatment options [e.g., RRT (hemodialysis and peritoneal dialysis), transplantation, and conservative management] for managing ESRD. To provide a recommendation, the clinician should first determine if the patient has any contraindications to specific treatment options. Then, the clinician should determine the patient's preferences and psychosocial status to determine the potential challenges of each treatment option to the individual patient (Table 25.6).

25.7.4 Renal Replacement Therapy

Although RRT is the most common treatment option for older adults approaching kidney failure, it is not the most appropriate treatment option for all older adults. Age is not a contraindication to RRT. However, nephrologists may choose not to initiate RRT in older adults if the risks outweigh the benefits. The benefit of RRT is lower in older adults who have severe cognitive impairment lacking ability to follow commands or respond to their environment. Also, older adults with a terminal illness, aside from kidney failure, would also have low benefit from RRT (unless it is palliative) and are likely be advised to forgo RRT [29].

Table 25.5 The "SPIRES" communication tool provides a helpful framework dialysis decision-making

Step	Description	Specific considerations for dialysis decision-making in older adults
Setup	Review medical records to understand patient's overall clinical picture; Encourage patient to invite loved ones to the discussion	Evaluate for contextual factors including functional decline, cognitive impairment, frailty multimorbidity, and social support. Review rate of decline of kidney function and prior nephrology referral. Consider where the decision is being made—acute setting (e.g., sepsis) versus progressive CKD.
Perceptions and perspectives	Identify patient values, concerns, and desires	Assess patients' understanding of kidney failure treatment options. Elicit past experience with dialysis (e.g., family members with ESRD).
Invitation	Ask patient if they want a recommendation	
Recommendation	Provide a recommendation based on patient values and clinical picture	Incorporate information from geriatric assessment.
Empathize	Acknowledge strong emotions that may arise during the conversation	Studies have shown that patients report regret, uncertainty, and anxiety when making decision about dialysis.
Summarize and strategize	Provide an individualized treatment plan that can be reassessed if health worsens	For patients unfamiliar with dialysis, treatment options may be complex and patients and family may need more information over multiple visits.

CKD chronic kidney disease, *ESRD* end-stage renal disease

Table 25.6 Treatment options for kidney failure and potential challenges for older adults

Treatment option	Potential challenges
Hemodialysis	Vascular access procedures Transportation to/from dialysis clinic Post-dialysis fatigue
Peritoneal dialysis	Functional limitations Home environment Inadequate ultrafiltration and waste removal Peritonitis
Transplantation	Functional limitations Multimorbidity Wait-list interval Diagnostic testing for referral process Infections and malignancies from immunosuppression

Timing of preparation for RRT can be challenging for older adults. Early preparation for RRT involves dialysis access placement for hemodialysis or peritoneal dialysis (e.g., arteriovenous access, central venous catheter (CVC), Tenckhoff catheter). However, it is not clear if an individual patient will progress to kidney failure or die before there is a need for RRT. This uncertainty is challenging for both patients and clinicians when deciding the appropriate timing for dialysis access placement. Early access placement, although recommended, can create physical and emotional burdens on a patient who may not ever initiate RRT.

Hemodialysis access placement is an additional potential challenge for older adults. Clinical guidelines recommend arteriovenous fistula (AVF) as hemodialysis access for all dialysis patients. However, AVF maturation time is approximately 6 months, and less than 50 % of older adults have mature AVFs because of vascular calcifications and reduced vascular elasticity [26]. Compared to younger patients, older adults tend to undergo more procedures to create and maintain patency of AVF. Because of the maturation time and recurrent procedures, AVFs may be less ideal for older adults

who have limited life expectancy (i.e., less than 2 years) [27]. Arteriovenous grafts (AVG) and CVCs are more likely to be successfully placed after a single procedure; however, these alternative accesses are associated with greater risks of infection and long-term patency issues. Thus, AVGs and CVCs are more appropriate for older adults with limited life expectancy and/or unsuccessful AVF maturation. Importantly, AVG should be attempted prior to CVC placement because of higher risk of mortality associated with CVC use. Still, some older adults prefer CVC because it allows avoidance of needles and recurrent procedures.

The benefits of RRT are similar with peritoneal dialysis and hemodialysis; however, some older adults may not be able to receive peritoneal dialysis. Peritoneal dialysis is typically conducted in the home by the patient and/or caregiver after intensive training in sterile technique and equipment use. Therefore, older adults who would have difficulty with peritoneal dialysis include those who do not live in a home with dedicated space for equipment and those with functional limitations (e.g., visual impairment, cognitive impairment, ADL dependence, or mobility disability) and no caregivers available to conduct their treatments. Some older adults who receive peritoneal dialysis can encounter new challenges that require transition from peritoneal dialysis to hemodialysis. Such challenges can be recognized by recurrent peritonitis, inadequate ultrafiltration, or waste removal despite adjustments to the treatment regimen. Also, some older adults may develop functional limitations or experience loss of their social support that makes it difficult to continue peritoneal dialysis.

25.7.5 Transplantation

Renal transplantation provides better survival benefit and quality of life than RRT and is not contraindicated in older adults [26]. However, individual transplant centers have age limits for transplant listing. For transplant listing, older adults may find it burdensome to undergo multiple diagnostic tests (e.g., cardiac stress test, CT scans). These tests may identify abnormalities or yield false positive results that can lead to emotional distress [27]. Still, transplantation can be an ideal option for ESRD for older adults who are not frail and have minimal comorbidities and functional limitations. These patients are more likely to be able to survive their wait-list interval, withstand the physical stress of the surgery, and be adherent to the extensive immunosuppression medication regimen. Clinical trajectories can change over time; therefore, reassessment of comorbidity burden and functional status during the wait-list interval is important to ensure the patient remains to be an eligible transplant candidate. After transplantation, older adults may develop problems with drug interactions between chronic medications and immunosuppression medications, as well as an increased risk of infections and malignancies.

25.7.6 Conservative Management

For many older adults with kidney failure, RRT or transplantation may not be appropriate. Aside from apparent contraindications to RRT described above, some older adults decline RRT because they value quality over quantity of life and prefer to not spend significant time in dialysis sessions during their remaining lifetime [28]. Traditionally, it was thought that there was little to offer these patients. However, there is growing appreciation that older adults who decline RRT benefit from active treatment. This "conservative management" involves routine outpatient visits that focus on CKD management and symptom management as kidney failure progresses. These patients may also receive hospice care. Existing observational studies also suggest that patients who receive conservative management experience fewer hospitalizations and more palliative care services than those who receive RRT [26]. Increasing use of shared decision-making and prognostication of patient's life expectancy may yield an increase in the proportion of older adults receiving conservative management.

25.8 Kidney Failure in Special Patient Populations

25.8.1 Hospital Patients

Older adults receiving dialysis often require hospitalizations and are admitted on average twice per year. Additionally, the majority of older adults who start dialysis do so during an inpatient hospitalization. These patients often require prolonged hospitalization and receive high intensity health care during this time despite an overall poor prognosis. For exam-

ple, among older Medicare beneficiaries more than 20 % require hospitalization for ≥2 weeks at dialysis initiation and over 15 % of those require one or more intensive procedures including mechanical ventilation, feeding tube placement or cardiopulmonary resuscitation [30]. Higher intensity care during the hospitalization is associated with an increased risk for death. Among those 80 years and older who require ≥2 weeks in the hospital at dialysis initiation, median survival is only 1 year or less and 10–20 % of their remaining days of life are spent hospitalized. These reports may suggest the need for earlier involvement of palliative care in the treatment of hospitalized ESRD patients.

Rehospitalizations are also common among older adults with ESRD. More than one in three older dialysis patients who are discharged from the hospital return within 30 days [31]. The high rates of rehospitalization have been reported to contribute to or parallel the high mortality, low quality of life and increasing health care costs in this population. Data are limited on interventions to reduce rehospitalizations specifically for older adults with kidney failure. However, one analysis that used a quasi-experimental approach showed that more frequent provider visits in the month following hospitalization was associated with a decreased risk for readmission. Whether or not inpatient models of care that focus on improving outcomes for hospitalized older adults such as Acute Care of the Elderly (ACE) units in combination with care transition support and more frequent disease-specific follow-up with nephrology providers would reduce readmissions in this high risk population needs to be determined. Chapter 7 provides detailed suggestions in caring for hospitalized seniors.

25.8.2 Post-Acute and Long-Term Care Patients

Because the majority of older adults initiating dialysis do so during a hospitalization these patients are often eligible for post-acute care services in a skilled nursing facility (SNF). These patients may also be eligible for post-acute care services following hospitalizations not related to the initiation of dialysis. The Medicare SNF benefit is provided on a short-term basis after a hospitalization for patients who have skilled nursing or rehabilitation needs. The goal of this program is to improve the patient's condition within predetermined time period or to prevent the condition from worsening. However, because older ESRD patients are medically complex and three times a week dialysis may interfere with daily physical therapy treatments, they may experience worsening health and be less likely to return home or achieve functional independence. For patients who are discharged from an SNF, there are high rates of hospitalization or ED visits within 30 days of returning home [32].

Those requiring long-term nursing home care are a particularly high risk group, however this population has not been well studied. While utilization of nursing home care is common among older adults initiating dialysis, it is poorly recognized by nephrologists. For example, 28% of the 27,913 U.S. older adults who started dialysis in 2006 required nursing home care at the time of initiation. However, only 33% of these patients were accurately identified by their dialysis providers as receiving nursing home care [33]. Older nursing home residents initiating dialysis also face a high burden of functional decline. One analysis of long-term nursing home residents found that initiation of dialysis was associated with a significant and sustained functional decline. In this patient group, mortality rates were 24, 41, 51, and 58%, at 3, 6, 9, and 12 months, respectively [4].

25.9 End-of-Life Considerations

25.9.1 Symptom Burden

Older adults with kidney failure may experience a high burden of symptoms, especially at the end-of-life. For example, in the last month of life older adults with kidney failure treated with conservative management more than half of all patients reported: lack of energy, drowsiness, dyspnea, poor concentration, poor appetite, swelling of the arms or legs, dry mouth, constipation, and nausea [34]. A similar burden of symptoms has been reported among those who receive dialysis as well, suggesting that dialysis alone may not mitigate these symptoms.

25.9.2 Role of Palliative and Supportive Care

Palliative and supportive care is an important resource for older adults with kidney failure. While traditionally palliative care has been reserved for end-of-life or those who decline dialysis, the role of palliative care across the spectrum of kidney disease is increasing. Evaluation by palliative care specialist can provide prognostic information, help elicit patient and family health goals, and support advanced care planning and shared decision-making about dialysis. Palliative care support can also improve the recognition and treatment of complex symptoms. See Chap. 6. Palliative Care and End of Life Issues.

25.10 Summary

Clinical specialists caring for older patients will increasingly encounter those with CKD and/or AKI. While clinical practice guidelines exist for the diagnosis and management of CKD, providers should be prepared to recognize the limitations of these disease-oriented recommendations and the unique aspects of caring for older adults with CKD. We recommend an approach that considers a patient's health goals, life expectancy, and presence of multimorbidity and geriatric conditions, to help tailor treatment plans. Furthermore, clinicians should understand the challenges and controversies for using eGFR to define CKD in this population. For older adults, kidney failure carries a poor prognosis and a shared decision-making approach to RRT is necessary.

References

1. Bowling CB, Muntner P. Epidemiology of chronic kidney disease among older adults: a focus on the oldest old. J Gerontol Ser A Biol Med Sci. 2012;67(12):1379–86.
2. Bowling CB, O'Hare AM. Managing older adults with CKD: individualized versus disease-based approaches. Am J Kidney Dis. 2012;59(2):293–302. Pubmed Central PMCID: 3261354.
3. O'Hare AM, Choi AI, Bertenthal D, Bacchetti P, Garg AX, Kaufman JS, et al. Age Affects outcomes in chronic kidney disease. J Am Soc Nephrol. 2007;18(10):2758–65.
4. Kurella Tamura M, Covinsky KE, Chertow GM, Yaffe K, Landefeld CS, McCulloch CE. Functional status of elderly adults before and after initiation of dialysis. N Engl J Med. 2009;361(16):1539–47. Pubmed Central PMCID: 2789552.
5. Kutner NG, Zhang R, Allman RM, Bowling CB. Correlates of ADL difficulty in a large hemodialysis cohort. Hemodial Int. 2014;18(1):70–7. Pubmed Central PMCID: 3887518.
6. Weinstein JR, Anderson S. The aging kidney: physiological changes. Adv Chronic Kidney Dis. 2010;17(4):302–7. Pubmed Central PMCID: 2901622.
7. Anderson S, Halter JB, Hazzard WR, Himmelfarb J, Horne FM, Kaysen GA, et al. Prediction, progression, and outcomes of chronic kidney disease in older adults. J Am Soc Nephrol. 2009;20(6):1199–209.
8. Lindeman RD, Tobin J, Shock NW. Longitudinal studies on the rate of decline in renal function with age. J Am Geriatr Soc. 1985;33(4):278–85.
9. Rule AD, Amer H, Cornell LD, Taler SJ, Cosio FG, Kremers WK, et al. The association between age and nephrosclerosis on renal biopsy among healthy adults. Ann Intern Med. 2010;152(9):561–7. Pubmed Central PMCID: 2864956.
10. Kidney Disease: Improving Global Outcomes (KDIGO) CKD Work Group. KDIGO 2012 clinical practice guideline for the evaluation and management of chronic kidney disease. Kidney Int. 2013;3:1–150
11. National Kidney Foundation. K/DOQI clinical practice guidelines for chronic kidney disease: evaluation, classification, and stratification. American J Kidney Dis. 2002;39(2 Suppl 1):S1–266. Epub 2002/03/21. eng.
12. Anderson S, Eldadah B, Halter JB, Hazzard WR, Himmelfarb J, Horne FM, et al. Acute kidney injury in older adults. J Am Soc Nephrol. 2011;22(1):28–38.
13. Kidney Disease: Improving Global Outcomes (KDIGO) Acute Kidney Injury Work Group. KDIGO clinical practice guideline for acute kidney injury. Kidney Int. 2012;2:1–138.
14. Bowling CB, Sharma P, Fox CS, O'Hare AM, Muntner P. Prevalence of reduced estimated glomerular filtration rate among the oldest old from 1988-1994 through 2005-2010. JAMA. 2013;310(12):1284–6. Pubmed Central PMCID: 4406347.
15. Bowling CB, Sharma P, Muntner P. Prevalence, trends and functional impairment associated with reduced estimated glomerular

filtration rate and albuminuria among the oldest-old U.S. adults. Am J Med Sci. 2014;348(2):115–20. Pubmed Central PMCID: 4406350.

16. Hemmelgarn BR, James MT, Manns BJ, O'Hare AM, Muntner P, Ravani P, et al. Rates of treated and untreated kidney failure in older vs younger adults. JAMA. 2012;307(23):2507–15.

17. United Stages Renal Data System. USRDS 2013 Annual Data Report: Atlas of Chronic Kidney Disease and End-Stage Renal Disease in the United States Bethesda, MD: National Institution of Health, National Institute of Diabetes and Digestive and Kidney Diseases; 2013.

18. O'Hare AM, Rodriguez RA, Bowling CB. Caring for patients with kidney disease: shifting the paradigm from evidence-based medicine to patient-centered care. Nephrol Dial Transplant. 2015;31: 368–75.

19. Group SR, Wright Jr JT, Williamson JD, Whelton PK, Snyder JK, Sink KM, et al. A randomized trial of intensive versus standard blood-pressure control. N Engl J Med. 2015;373(22):2103–16.

20. Bowling CB, Batten A, O'Hare AM. Distribution of survival times in a real-world cohort of older adults with chronic kidney disease: the median may not be the message. J Am Geriatr Soc. 2015;63(5):1033–5. Pubmed Central PMCID: 4591036.

21. Bowling CB, Booth 3rd JN, Gutierrez OM, Kurella Tamura M, Huang L, Kilgore M, et al. Nondisease-specific problems and all-cause mortality among older adults with CKD: the REGARDS Study. Clin J Am Soc Nephrol. 2014;9(10):1737–45. Pubmed Central PMCID: 4186504.

22. O'Hare AM, Hotchkiss JR, Kurella Tamura M, Larson EB, Hemmelgarn BR, Batten A, et al. Interpreting treatment effects from clinical trials in the context of real-world risk information: end-stage renal disease prevention in older adults. JAMA Intern Med. 2014;174(3):391–7.

23. Phillips PA, Rolls BJ, Ledingham JG, Forsling ML, Morton JJ, Crowe MJ, et al. Reduced thirst after water deprivation in healthy elderly men. N Engl J Med. 1984;311(12):753–9.

24. Schaeffner ES, Ebert N, Delanaye P, Frei U, Gaedeke J, Jakob O, et al. Two novel equations to estimate kidney function in persons aged 70 years or older. Ann Intern Med. 2012;157(7):471–81.

25. Shlipak MG, Matsushita K, Arnlov J, Inker LA, Katz R, Polkinghorne KR, et al. Cystatin C versus creatinine in determining risk based on kidney function. N Engl J Med. 2013;369(10):932–43. Pubmed Central PMCID: 3993094.

26. Berger JR, Hedayati SS. Renal replacement therapy in the elderly population. Clin J Am Soc Nephrol. 2012;7(6):1039–46. Pubmed Central PMCID: 3362311, Epub 2012/04/21. eng.

27. Tamura MK, Tan JC, O'Hare AM. Optimizing renal replacement therapy in older adults: a framework for making individualized decisions. Kidney Int. 2012;82(3):261–9. Pubmed Central PMCID: 3396777, Epub 2011/11/18. eng.

28. Schell JO, Cohen RA. A communication framework for dialysis decision-making for frail elderly patients. Clin J Am Soc Nephrol. 2014;9(11):2014–21. Pubmed Central PMCID: Pmc4220751, Epub 2014/06/28. eng.

29. Moss AH. Shared decision-making in dialysis: the new RPA/ASN guideline on appropriate initiation and withdrawal of treatment. Am J Kidney Dis. 2001;37(5):1081–91. Epub 2001/04/28. eng.

30. Wong SP, Kreuter W, O'Hare AM. Healthcare intensity at initiation of chronic dialysis among older adults. J Am Soc Nephrol. 2014;25(1):143–9. Pubmed Central PMCID: 3871783.

31. Erickson KF, Winkelmayer WC, Chertow GM, Bhattacharya J. Physician visits and 30-day hospital readmissions in patients receiving hemodialysis. J Am Soc Nephrol. 2014;25(9):2079–87. Pubmed Central PMCID: 4147977.

32. Hall RK, Toles M, Massing M, Jackson E, Peacock-Hinton S, O'Hare AM, et al. Utilization of acute care among patients with ESRD discharged home from skilled nursing facilities. Clin J Am Soc Nephrol. 2015;10(3):428–34. Pubmed Central PMCID: 4348677.

33. Bowling CB, Zhang R, Franch H, Huang Y, Mirk A, McClellan WM, et al. Underreporting of nursing home utilization on the CMS-2728 in older incident dialysis patients and implications for assessing mortality risk. BMC Nephrol. 2015;16:32. Pubmed Central PMCID: 4408561.

34. Murtagh FE, Addington-Hall J, Edmonds P, Donohoe P, Carey I, Jenkins K, et al. Symptoms in the month before death for stage 5 chronic kidney disease patients managed without dialysis. J Pain Symptom Manag. 2010;40(3):342–52.

Evaluation and Management of Older Adults with Multimorbidity and Cancer: A Geriatric Perspective on Oncology Care

Thuy T. Koll and William Dale

26.1 Cancer Incidence and Prevalence: A Demographic Shift

Cancer is primarily a disease of older adults. The number of adults 65 years and older is expected to increase from 35 million in 2000 to 72 million by 2030 [1]. The incidence of all cancer types is predicted to increase by 50 % in this age group [2]. Soon, nearly two thirds of all cancer survivors will be aged 65 years and over [3]. The rapidly growing population of older adults with cancer adds significant complexity to cancer care, increasing the clinical challenges for an already difficult clinical scenario. The recent Institute of Medicine (IOM) Report, "Delivering High Quality Cancer Care: Charting a Course for a System in Crisis" emphasizes the unique needs of older patients with cancer and outlines recommendations to improve quality of cancer care in this vulnerable population [4]. Quality cancer care must address the unique needs of older adults through geriatric assessments, shared decision-making, and age-appropriate disease management [5].

26.2 Considerations for Cancer Care in Older Adults

26.2.1 Aging Physiology

A hallmark of aging is the gradual decline of physiological reserve in essentially all organ systems resulting in general loss of functional reserve. This loss is variable across organ

T.T. Koll, MD
Geriatric Medicine, University of Nebraska Medical Center,
986155 Nebraska Medical Center, Omaha, NE 68198-6155, USA

W. Dale, MD, PhD (✉)
Section of Geriatrics and Palliative Medicine, Specialized
Oncology Care & Research in the Elderly (SOCARE) Clinic,
University of Chicago Medicine,
5841 S. Maryland Ave., MC6098, Chicago, IL 60637, USA
e-mail: wdale@medicine.bsd.uchicago.edu

systems in a given individual and between individual older patients. Age-related physiological changes, cancer, and cancer treatments all influence treatment tolerance and risk for toxicity [6]. An understanding of these changes helps tailor treatments and monitor for side effects. Table 26.1 highlights significant age-related organ system changes and potential implications for older patients with cancer.

26.2.2 Multimorbidity and Polypharmacy

The likelihood of multiple chronic health conditions, referred to as multimorbidity, increases with age [7]. Comorbidity burden affects life expectancy, risk of functional decline, and hospitalization risk [8–11]. Increasing multimorbidity impacts survival and treatment tolerance in older adults with cancer [12–14]. The Charlson Comorbidity Index (CCI) is widely used in geriatric oncology research to characterize comorbidity burden. The CCI weights 19 diseases from one to six points based on relative risk of death at 1 year [15]. Higher overall mortality is associated with CCI score of 3 or more in patients with lung, colorectal, and prostate cancer who are 70 years and older [16].

There are also potential interactions between existing chronic diseases, a new diagnosis of cancer, and treatment. For example, the risk of falls with chemotherapy such as taxanes is higher in patients with pre-existing diabetes or peripheral neuropathy [17]. With a diagnosis of cancer, older patients are at higher risk for drug–drug interactions as the number of medication increases to treat the disease and manage symptoms [18]. Potential complications and side effects of treatment should be anticipated to make appropriate adjustment to current medications. For example, blood pressure medications, especially diuretics, may need to be reduced or held during periods of poor nutrition and dehydration due to nausea and vomiting. A careful review of medications for all patients at the beginning of treatment and periodic medication reconciliation is a practical approach to polypharmacy in the oncology setting [18]. The Beers

© Springer International Publishing Switzerland 2017
J.R. Burton et al. (eds.), *Geriatrics for Specialists*, DOI 10.1007/978-3-319-31831-8_26

Table 26.1 Age-related organ system changes and implications for oncology

Organ system	Age-associated physiologic changes	Implications
Cardiovascular	Decrease in maximal heart and ventricular compliance and increase in vascular stiffness	Increase risk of heart failure during stress and increase risk of drug-induced cardiomyopathy
Gastrointestinal	Alteration in mucosal protective mechanisms. Reduced colonic motility Decline in hepatic drug metabolism	Susceptibility to mucositis leading to compromised nutrition Increase risk of constipation Variable absorption of drugs Susceptibility to adverse drug reactions
Pulmonary	Increase in lung compliance Increase in stiffness of chest wall Diminished cough reflex Diminished function of the mucociliary escalator	Decrease in pulmonary reserve Increase risk of aspiration Increased susceptibility to pulmonary infections
Renal	Decrease in glomerular filtration rate Decrease in renal blood flow; reduced response to ADH; sodium wasting Decrease in tubular function and hyporeninemic hypoaldosteronism	Nephrotoxicity from renally excreted drugs Increase risk of volume depletion Increase risk of electrolyte disturbances
Nervous/Cerebrovascular	Decrease in number of neurons Impairment in vision, hearing and olfaction Increase incidence of peripheral neuropathy Impairment in response to postural change in arterial pressure and cerebral blood flow	Increase risk of impairment in memory and cognition Increase risk of anorexia due to decrease in olfaction Increase risk of delirium due to impairment in cognition, hearing, and vision Increase risk of developing peripheral neuropathy or worsening of existing neuropathy Increase susceptibility falls due to orthostatic hypotension and neuropathy
Hematologic	Decrease in bone marrow reserve	Increase risk of developing anemia, thrombocytopenia, and febrile neutropenia
Endocrine	Increase in osteoclast over osteoblast function Altered temperature regulation	Increase risk of falls and fractures Decrease in febrile response to infection
Musculoskeletal	Loss of muscle mass and strength	Loss of mobility Impairment in gait and balance increasing fall risk

From Sawhney R, Sehl M, Naeim A. Physiologic aspects of aging: impact on cancer management and decision making, part I. Cancer J 2005 Nov-Dec;11(6):449–460, and Sehl M, Sawhney R, Naeim A. Physiologic aspects of aging: impact on cancer management and decision making, part II. Cancer J 2005 Nov-Dec;11(6):461–473

Criteria lists potentially inappropriate medications for older adults. Other screening tools that are increasingly used in geriatric oncology to appraise medications for older patients are the STOPP (Screening Tool of Older Persons' Prescriptions) and START (Screening Tool to Alert doctors to Right Treatment). (Chapter 5 provides details on the Beers Criteria and STOPP/START).

26.2.3 Functional Impairment/Malnutrition/Falls: Implications for Cancer Care

Functional impairment (limitations in ADL and IADL), frailty, and geriatric syndromes are common in older adults with cancer [19]. Impairments in IADL predict survival in older patients with cancer [20]. Patients with impairment in IADLs should be further assessed for impairments in cognition, physical performance, and activities of daily living (ADL). Weight loss and malnutrition are associated with chemotherapy toxicity and decreased survival [21–23]. Treatment side effects such as nausea, vomiting, and mucositis can lead

to dehydration and further weight loss. Fatigue can impair the ability to shop, prepare, and enjoy food. One third of patients 65 years and older fall at least once a year and up to half of those who fall have recurrent falls [24]. Treatment side effects such as neuropathy and advanced cancer stage increases the risk of falls in older patients with cancer [25]. Patients should be asked about falls or near falls in the last 6 months. (Further assessment for falls is described in the *Assessment Chap.* 8).

26.2.4 Geriatric Syndromes and Their Interplay with Cancer

Geriatric syndromes are common health conditions in older adults. The etiology is characteristically multifactorial, with shared risk factors including older age, comorbidity burden, cognitive decline, functional impairment, and impaired mobility [26]. In geriatric oncology, the most relevant syndromes are frailty, falls, dementia, depression, and delirium [27]. (Chapter 1 provides a full description of frailty and validated assessment tools.)

Cancer treatment decisions are complex, especially for older patients. The treatment program typically involves multiple office visits and complex medication regimens. The assessment of cognition informs the provider of a patient's decisional capacity, reliability of history, ability to understand and manage complex treatment plans and the insight to report toxicities [28]. Patients with cognitive impairment need close monitoring for toxicities, such as febrile neutropenia. The prevalence of depression in older cancer patients ranges from 17 to 25 % [29]. Depression is under-recognized and under-treated, in part due to the overlap of symptoms of cancer and cancer treatment (fatigue and anorexia) and the signs and symptoms of depression. Delirium is also common in patients with cancer, with risk factors including polypharmacy, fevers, anemia, fatigue, pain, and electrolyte disturbances. (Chapter 2 provides a full description of this syndrome and the Chap. 8 Tools for *Assessment* provides details on assessment using the Confusion Assessment Method.)

26.2.5 Geriatric Assessment: Evaluating the Older Patient with Cancer

There is heterogeneity in physiological reserve, comorbidities, functional abilities, and presence of geriatric syndromes among older individuals, adding complexity to estimation of life expectancy and treatment management decisions. Geriatric assessment (GA) is a multidimensional assessment of an older patient's health, fitness, and capabilities using validated tools. Potential components of GA include the following health domains: (1) *medical*: evaluation of comorbidity, polypharmacy, and nutritional status; (2) *mental health*: evaluation of cognition, depression, and delirium; (3) *functional status*: assessment of activities of daily living (ADL), instrumental activities of daily living (IADL), mobility (physical performance), and falls; (4) *social*: evaluation of environment, resources, and social support/network. There is a growing body of evidence on the utility of GA in oncology practice [30]. Many studies in geriatric oncology propose the use of GA in patients older than 70 years with cancer [30]. The ultimate goal of GA is to guide treatment management decisions and the design of a treatment plan that balances benefits and remaining life expectancy, anticipates complications and care needs, and implements targeted interventions to optimize outcomes and improve quality of life.

GA can be applied to help with clinical decision-making in various clinical scenarios including: (1) prior to cancer surgery to assess for risks and potential post-operative complications such as functional impairment, (2) to estimate life expectancy in the context of competing comorbidities and functional status, particularly in the setting of adjuvant chemotherapy, (3) to evaluate the risks and benefits of treatment options, (4) and to monitor for development of deficits as a result of cancer treatment during and post treatment [31]. Chapter 8, Tools for Assessment, describes validated tools to assess geriatric domains. Table 26.2 summarizes the assessment tools of value in older patients with cancer.

Table 26.2 Summary of geriatric assessment tools important in oncology

Assessment domain	Tools
Comorbidity	Charlson comorbidity index (CCI)
Polypharmacy	Medication reconciliation prior to treatment and periodic review Review of high risk medications based on BEERS Criteria and STOPP/START
Nutrition	Mini-Nutritional Assessment (MNA)
Cognition	Mini Cog Mini-mental state examination (MMSE) Montreal cognitive assessment (MoCA)
Depression	Patient health questionnaire-2 (PHQ-2)
Delirium	Confusion assessment method (CAM)
Function	Katz index of activities of daily living (Katz ADL Index) Lawton instrumental activities of daily living (Lawton IADL Index)
Mobility/Falls	Timed up and go test (TUG) Gait speed
Social	Assess socioeconomic status, family care system, environment and advanced care planning

26.2.6 Geriatric Assessment: Impact on Cancer Care

26.2.6.1 Detection of Important Geriatric Problems

Traditional oncology assessments miss important problems in older patients with cancer. For example, over half of older patients with an Eastern Cooperative Oncology Group Performance Score (ECOG PS) who are classified as "fit" (scores of 0–1) still have impairments of instrumental activities of daily living (IADL) [32]. GA detects impairments in greater than 50 % of older patients with cancer ($n=1967$, Median age 76 years); the most frequent problems are impairment in function, nutrition, and fatigue [33].

26.2.6.2 Prediction of Chemotherapy Toxicity

There are two chemotherapy toxicity risk models for older adults with cancer. The Cancer and Aging Research Group (CARG) (based on 500 subjects with mean age 73 years) model found 11 factors that were predictive of Grade 3–5 chemotherapy toxicity [34]. GA assessment variables in this model were: hearing impairment, history of falls, needing assistance with medication management, limited ability to walk one block, and a decrease in social activities due to health status. CARG model allows risk stratification dividing patients into low (0–5 points), intermediate (6–9 points), or high risk (10–19 points) of chemotherapy toxicity [34]. Similarly, the Chemotherapy Risk Assessment Scale for High-Age Patients (CRASH) model predicts severe hematologic (Grade 4) and non-hematologic toxicity (Grade 3/4) in older cancer patients. In this model, IADL dependence predicts hematologic toxicity while self-rated health status, Mini-Mental State Exam score, and Mini-Nutritional Assessment score predicts non-hematologic toxicity [23].

26.2.6.3 Prediction of Survival

There are currently no life-expectancy prognostic models in geriatric oncology, although there are several such models based on GA variables available for general geriatric patients (Available on Eprognosis.com). These models estimate remaining life expectancy in the context of competing comorbidities and geriatric specific factors. Studies have demonstrated prognostic value of GA domains in specific oncology settings. For example, poor nutritional status on Mini-Nutritional Assessment and abnormal Timed Up and Go scores predict early death in older patients with various cancer types ($n = 384$) [35]. Similarly, poor nutritional status, impaired function, and comorbidity also predict interruption of chemotherapy and mortality in patients with solid malignancies receiving chemotherapy [36]. All-cause and breast cancer-specific death rate at 5 and 10 years are doubled in women with greater than three GA deficits ($n = 660$, stage I to IIIa breast cancer) [37]. Measures of physical performance predicted overall survival and 2-year progression to disability or death in older patients with cancer [38].

26.2.6.4 Estimating the Impact of Treatment on Older Adults

Side effects from treatment may potentiate geriatric problems. For example, anemia and fatigue, which are common in older patients without cancer [39, 40], are more likely to occur during cancer treatment [41]. Fatigue often impairs the ability to complete tasks of daily living (cooking, preparing food, shopping, and taking medications) and increase the risk for cognitive impairment and functional dependence [40, 42, 43]. Continued assessment of physical and cognitive function during and following treatment is important to continue to optimize outcomes.

26.2.7 Geriatric Assessment-Guided Interventions

To be effective, GA must be followed by appropriate interventions to address deficits. Unfortunately, data on the impact of GA-driven interventions in older patients with cancer is limited. However, studies in community-dwelling older patients without cancer have demonstrated effectiveness in improving outcomes [44]. Table 26.3 outlines potential interventions to address deficits identified during GA.

Table 26.3 Geriatric assessment-guided interventions

Geriatric assessment identified problems	Interventions
Functional impairment	Assess social support and implement visiting nurse and home health services Evaluate cognition Referral to physical and occupational therapy Medication review, address vision impairment, Vitamin D status, and home safety evaluation
Nutrition risk	Referral to dietician for nutritional assessment and recommendations Assess for depression, access to food and social isolation Consider home delivered meals
Cognitive impairment	Review medications—minimize medications with higher risk of delirium Assess and treat depression and anxiety Assess ADL and IADL, medications, and driver safety Evaluate for cause of impairment including Vitamin B12, thyroid function, and brain imaging Identify healthcare proxy Delirium risk counseling Social work involvement for caregiver education
Depression	Treatment with medication Consider counseling Suicide risk assessment
Social support	Elicit support from caregivers or implement services such as transportation assistance, home health care, and home delivered meals Monitor caregiver stress
Comorbidity/Polypharmacy	Pharmacy review of medications Consider drug–drug and drug–disease interactions Diabetes—avoid neurotoxic agents Heart failure—closely monitor volume status Kidney disease—avoid nephrotoxic agents

26.2.8 Using Screening Tools to Target Patients for GA

Three screening tools have been proposed to identify patients most likely to benefit from GA. The data supporting the use of screening tools have primarily focused on predicting deficits during Comprehensive GA (CGA) which is considered the "gold standard" for detecting problems in vulnerable older people. The Vulnerable Elders Survey-13 (VES-13) is a 13-item survey including age, self-rated health, and functional status, and is scored from 0 to 13, with 13 being the worst. A score of greater than 3 identified vulnerable older adults at risk for mortality, morbidity, and hospitalization. Higher VES-13 scores predict death and functional decline in vulnerable community-dwelling older adults [45, 46]. VES-13 demonstrates high predictive value for having greater than two deficits on CGA in older patients with prostate cancer [47]. Another tool, the Geriatric-8 (G8) screening tool, includes age, self-rated health, nutrition, cognition, mobility, and polypharmacy, and is scored from 0 to 17, with 17 indicating better function. A score of 14 or less predicts at least one deficit on CGA domains in adults 70 years and older [48]. Finally, the National Cancer Network Guideline recommends using the Fried Frailty score to identify older patients in need of further assessment. See Chap. 1, for further discussion of this syndrome in older patients.

26.2.9 Integration of GA in an Oncology Clinic: A Proposal

Not all older patients with cancer require a CGA. The following is a framework to incorporate GA in an oncology clinic. All patients 70 years and older undergo screening using one of the above described tools (VES-13, G8 and Fried Frailty score). Vulnerable patients identified on screening should be referred for CGA. In addition, patients with normal screening should have additional screening for cognitive impairment (i.e., Mini-Mental State Exam or Montreal Cognitive Assessment) and a fall risk assessment (ask about falls or near falls within the last 6 months) [27]. Patients with a positive screen for cognitive impairment would complete CGA while those with falls would complete gait assessment and referral to physical therapy when needed. CGA is likely not warranted in patients who do not have impairments in any of the proposed screening steps.

26.2.10 Models of Care in Geriatric Oncology

An interprofessional team, led by a geriatrician or geriatric oncologist, is best equipped to provide geriatric oncology care. The interprofessional team may include a nurse, social worker, nutritionist, occupational therapist, physical therapist, and pharmacist. There are three major models for incorporating geriatric principles in oncology care: a consultative model, an "embedded" model, and a dually -trained physician model. In the consultative model, the team makes recommendations prior to treatment and the final care decisions are made by the primary oncologist. Patients are typically not followed during treatment by the geriatrics team. The second model consists of a geriatrician or a geriatric-trained nurse practitioner "embedded" in an oncology clinic where they are part of the team, including oncology. Patients are followed throughout the course of treatment, and the team provides care for geriatric-related issues. Finally, in the third model, patients are cared for by a geriatric oncologist who is dual-trained in geriatrics and hematology and medical oncology [31].

The Specialized Oncology Care and Research in the Elderly (SOCARE) clinics at the University of Rochester and University of Chicago combines a consultative geriatric oncology assessment clinic with an embedded model.

Patients aged 65 and older are referred from surgical, medical, and radiation oncologists. New patients are mailed a questionnaire packet 1 week prior to a scheduled appointment. Assistance is available for patients who require further assistance on the day of the visit. A clinic coordinator completes a physical performance and cognitive assessment. Weight loss and low body mass index is followed by Mini-Nutritional Assessment. Cancer-specific information and proposed treatment plan from the primary oncologist are reviewed. The team then suggest potential modifications and recommend a comprehensive treatment plan that anticipates and addresses the specific needs of the patient. These patients are often followed by the team, in conjunction with the primary oncology team.

26.3 Cancer Treatment Management: A Framework for Shared Decision-Making and Age-Appropriate Management

Cancer management decisions for older adults involve a series of considerations that include assessing: remaining life expectancy, age-specific cancer mortality (with and without treatment), care goals of the patient, values and preferences, risks and benefits according to those treatment goals, and the feasibility and burden of available treatments. Establishing the patient's (and family's) overall treatment goal(s) is the central consideration for decision making—those goals drive the choices made given the options. After decisional capacity is established, the patient's goals and priorities should be carefully elicited. Possible care goals include life prolongation (i.e., maximum survival), functional independence, quality of life, and symptom control. The next step is a careful, data-driven evaluation of the patient's prognosis and the potential benefits of available cancer treatment (cure of disease, symptoms relief) compared with the risks of possible treatments (functional decline, loss of independence), considered in the context of goals. Knowledge of the patient's physical function, cognitive function, psychological state, symptom burden, and social circumstances obtained through GA help predict whether treatment benefits are likely to exceed risks; whether treatment is likely to be tolerated; and determine feasibility and potential burden to the patient. After a shared, informed decision is made, interventions for anticipated needs should be implemented. Over the course of treatment, providers should continue to evaluate feasibility, adherence, and patient preferences.

The following is a recommended step-by-step guide for prioritizing decisions and managing the care of older patients with multimorbidity and cancer adapted from The American of Geriatrics Society Expert Panel on the Care of Older Adults with Multimorbidity [49].

26.3.1 Step 1: Assessment of Decisional Capacity

The capacity to make medical decisions includes the abilities to communicate a choice, comprehend information related to the diagnostic or treatment choice, have an understanding of the current medical situation and personal values, and understand the consequences of a decision [50]. A positive screen for a cognitive deficit can alert clinicians to possible limits on decision capacity, but should not be the *only* criteria to determine decisional capacity, but it is a part of an overall clinical cognitive assessment. Studies of medical decision-making capacity find incapacity in 2% of healthy older adults, 20% in those with mild cognitive impairment and 54% in patients with Alzheimer disease [51]. A potential approach is to use the Mini-Mental State Exam (MMSE) to assess current cognition and further assess capacity in patients with low (MMSE <20) or intermediate scores (MMSE 20–24) [51]. The Aid to Capacity Evaluation (ACE) is a possible capacity assessment tool using a patient's own medical situation and diagnosis or treatment decision [52]. ACE is a short assessment tool that can be administered and scored in 5–10 min (Available at: http://www.utoronto.ca/jcb/_ace). If a patient lacks capacity, decisions about care should be directed to an identified proxy, preferably the documented health care power of attorney. Decision making is situational and specific to a particular decision. For example, during an acute illness, a patient experiencing hypoxia and metabolic disturbances will not have capacity but may regain capacity when the illness is resolved. Patients with dementia may have capacity to make low risk and low complexity decisions. For example, a person with mild to moderate Alzheimer dementia may understand the need for antibiotic in treatment for pneumonia but may not be able to communicate the overall risks and benefits of cancer treatment.

26.3.2 Step 2: Determining Treatment Goals

Knowing a patient's overall treatment goal(s) is key to appropriate decision making. Prior to recommending a management plan, physicians should work with older patients to identify and prioritize a set of treatment goals and evaluate the effect of potential treatment options on these goals [53]. Management decisions should focus on which available treatment option will best address the patient's most important goal(s), and prioritize treatments accordingly. Patient's preferences are dynamic and should be revisited as their health changes [54].

One possible approach for eliciting preferences is to use open-ended questions asking about life goals, important priorities, and concerns about a patients' current and future quality of life. For example, some possible questions to ask include: "At this stage, what is most important to you?"; "In your current situation, what are you most hopeful for or what are you most worried about?"; "Can you imagine a way of living for you that would be worse than death?", or "Can you identify a point in your treatment when you would prefer comfort over life extension?" [55]. These questions help clarify the overall goals toward which treatments should be targeted.

26.3.3 Step 3: Establishing Prognosis

For older adults with cancer and multimorbidity, two related but separate types of prognosis estimates are important: remaining life expectancy based on cancer (stage, grade, location) and subsequent treatment possibilities (from the literature) and remaining life expectancy based on non-cancer-related health status [56]. Prognostic indices incorporating (minimally) age, gender, comorbidities, and functional measures can be utilized to reasonably estimate mortality in older patients. There are six indices for community-dwelling older adults with various time-frame ranging from 1 year to 5 years [57]. (Available at: http://www.eprognosis.org.) Physicians should help reconcile patient's cancer and non-cancer prognosis, the potential benefits of cancer treatment (cure of disease, symptoms relief) versus the risks (functional decline, death) and patient's treatment goals. Taken together, this provides a framework for assessing various management options available for patients.

26.3.4 Step 4: Feasibility and Optimization of Potential Treatments

The feasibility of the proposed treatment option should follow determination of patient preferences and prognosis. Cancer treatments can be complex and burdensome for patients and caregivers (multiple clinic visits, financial stress, and caregiver burdens). Knowledge and understanding of the patient's physical, cognitive, and psychologic function and available social support help determine feasibility. Patients with poor social support and/or cognitive impairment need treatment plans that are realistic and ensure appropriate supportive care throughout the process. Close collaboration and communication between primary care physicians and oncologists are important to ensure feasibility, minimize burden and provide close monitoring of toxicity. Treatment optimization entails implementing interventions for areas of concerns identified on GA (strength and balance training, nutritional supplements, delirium prevention), optimizing medication regimen to minimize adverse drug reactions and optimizing adherence to essential medications and cancer treatment and anticipation of complications and care needs.

26.3.5 A Case Example

Ms. A is a 73-year-old female with diabetes, hypertension, and depression, recently diagnosed with metastatic breast cancer. Based on her treatment goals, she would like to pursue treatment. She lives alone and her daughter assists her with medication management (an IADL). She has fallen 2 times over the last 3 months. Prior to initiation of treatment, her care can be optimized by interventions to increase social support, ensure adequate treatment of depression, nutritional consultation, thorough evaluation of medications, considerations for home delivered meals, visiting nurse to monitor for toxicity, physical therapy evaluation for falls, home safety assessment, and initiation of a medical alert system. Care plan will also consist of continued assessment of falls, nutrition, cognition, and function during the course of treatment or when concerns arise.

26.4 Conclusion and Future Directions

Optimal care for older patients with cancer should assess the age-associated physiologic changes, geriatric syndromes, functional and cognitive limitations, comorbidities and social support. Management decisions should reflect the patient's preferences and goals, prognosis, unique geriatric problems, consideration of interactions between treatment with coexisting conditions and feasibility of a treatment option(s), and the degree of social support available. Once an informed decision is made, implementation of appropriate support and close monitoring using validated GA tools is crucial to help with treatment adherence and tolerance.

Currently, the clinical evidence base for management decisions is limited by the common exclusion of older adults with multimorbidity in clinical trials and exclusion of outcomes that are most relevant to this population such as decline in function and cognition and quality of life [58]. There is a need for a GA to be part of clinical trials to better characterize older patients and develop evidence for benefits and risks. Because maintaining function, independence and quality of life is so important to this population, outcomes other than survival should be regularly included in trials. Finally, longitudinal studies including GA are needed to understand the impact of cancer and treatment on the older population [58].

References

1. Vincent GK, Velkoff VA. The next four decades: the older population in the United States: 2010 to 2050. US Department of Commerce, Economics and Statistics Administration, US Census Bureau; 2010.
2. Smith BD, Smith GL, Hurria A, Hortobagyi GN, Buchholz TA. Future of cancer incidence in the United States: burdens upon an aging, changing nation. J Clin Oncol. 2009;27(17):2758–65.
3. Jemal A, Siegel R, Xu J, Ward E. Cancer statistics, 2010. CA Cancer J Clin. 2010;60(5):277–300.
4. Levit L, Balogh E, Nass S, Ganz PA. Delivering high-quality cancer care: charting a new course for a system in crisis. Washington: National Academies Press; 2013.
5. Hurria A, Naylor M, Cohen HJ. Improving the quality of cancer care in an aging population: recommendations from an IOM report. JAMA. 2013;310(17):1795–6.
6. Yancik R. Cancer burden in the aged. Cancer. 1997;80(7):1273–83.
7. Anderson G. Chronic care: making the case for ongoing care. 2010. Princeton: Robert Wood Johnson Foundation; 2012. p. 43.
8. Klein BE, Klein R, Knudtson MD, Lee KE. Frailty, morbidity and survival. Arch Gerontol Geriatr. 2005;41(2):141–9.
9. Inouye SK, Peduzzi PN, Robison JT, Hughes JS, Horwitz RI, Concato J. Importance of functional measures in predicting mortality among older hospitalized patients. JAMA. 1998;279(15):1187–93.
10. Walter LC, Covinsky KE. Cancer screening in elderly patients: a framework for individualized decision making. JAMA. 2001;285(21):2750–6.
11. Lee SJ, Lindquist K, Segal MR, Covinsky KE. Development and validation of a prognostic index for 4-year mortality in older adults. JAMA. 2006;295(7):801–8.
12. Gross CP, Guo Z, McAvay GJ, Allore HG, Young M, Tinetti ME. Multimorbidity and survival in older persons with colorectal cancer. J Am Geriatr Soc. 2006;54(12):1898–904.
13. Piccirillo JF, Tierney RM, Costas I, Grove L, Spitznagel Jr EL. Prognostic importance of comorbidity in a hospital-based cancer registry. JAMA. 2004;291(20):2441–7.
14. Zauderer M, Patil S, Hurria A. Feasibility and toxicity of dose-dense adjuvant chemotherapy in older women with breast cancer. Breast Cancer Res Treat. 2009;117(1):205–10.
15. Charlson ME, Pompei P, Ales KL, MacKenzie CR. A new method of classifying prognostic comorbidity in longitudinal studies: development and validation. J Chronic Dis. 1987;40(5):373–83.
16. Jorgensen TL, Hallas J, Friis S, Herrstedt J. Comorbidity in elderly cancer patients in relation to overall and cancer-specific mortality. Br J Cancer. 2012;106(7):1353–60.
17. Gewandter J, Fan L, Magnuson A, Mustian K, Peppone L, Heckler C, et al. Falls and functional impairments in cancer survivors with chemotherapy-induced peripheral neuropathy (CIPN): a University of Rochester CCOP study. Support Care Cancer. 2013;21(7):2059–66.
18. Balducci L, Goetz-Parten D, Steinman MA. Polypharmacy and the management of the older cancer patient. Ann Oncol. 2013;24 (Suppl 7):vii36–40.
19. Mohile SG, Xian Y, Dale W, Fisher SG, Rodin M, Morrow GR, et al. Association of a cancer diagnosis with vulnerability and frailty in older Medicare beneficiaries. J Natl Cancer Inst. 2009;101(17):1206–15.
20. Wedding U, Röhrig B, Klippstein A, Pientka L, Höffken K. Age, severe comorbidity and functional impairment independently contribute to poor survival in cancer patients. J Cancer Res Clin Oncol. 2007;133(12):945–50.
21. Dewys WD, Begg C, Lavin PT, Band PR, Bennett JM, Bertino JR, et al. Prognostic effect of weight loss prior tochemotherapy in cancer patients. Am J Med. 1980;69(4):491–7.
22. Aaldriks AA, van der Geest LG, Lydia GM, Giltay EJ, le Cessie S, Portielje JE, Tanis BC, et al. Frailty and malnutrition predictive of mortality risk in older patients with advanced colorectal cancer receiving chemotherapy. J Geriatr Oncol. 2013;4(3):218–26.
23. Extermann M, Boler I, Reich RR, Lyman GH, Brown RH, DeFelice J, et al. Predicting the risk of chemotherapy toxicity in older patients: the chemotherapy risk assessment scale for high-age patients (CRASH) score. Cancer. 2012;118(13):3377–86.

24. Rubenstein LZ. Falls in older people: epidemiology, risk factors and strategies for prevention. Age Ageing. 2006;35(Suppl 2):ii37–ii41.

25. Ward PR, Wong MD, Moore R, Naeim A. Fall-related injuries in elderly cancer patients treated with neurotoxic chemotherapy: a retrospective cohort study. J Geriatr Oncol. 2014;5(1):57–64.

26. Inouye SK, Studenski S, Tinetti ME, Kuchel GA. Geriatric syndromes: clinical, research, and policy implications of a core geriatric concept. J Am Geriatr Soc. 2007;55(5):780–91.

27. Rodin MB, Mohile SG. A practical approach to geriatric assessment in oncology. J Clin Oncol. 2007;25(14):1936–44.

28. McKoy JM, Burhenn PS, Browner IS, Loeser KL, Tulas KM, Oden MR, et al. Assessing cognitive function and capacity in older adults with cancer. J Natl Compr Canc Netw. 2014;12(1):138–44.

29. Massie MJ. Prevalence of depression in patients with cancer. J Natl Cancer Inst Monogr. 2004;32:57–71.

30. Wildiers H, Heeren P, Puts M, Topinkova E, Janssen-Heijnen ML, Extermann M, et al. International Society of Geriatric Oncology consensus on geriatric assessment in older patients with cancer. J Clin Oncol. 2014;32(24):2595–603.

31. Magnuson A, Dale W, Mohile S. Models of care in geriatric oncology. Curr Geriatr Rep. 2014;3(3):182–9.

32. Extermann M, Hurria A. Comprehensive geriatric assessment for older patients with cancer. J Clin Oncol. 2007; 25(14):1824–31.

33. Kenis C, Bron D, Libert Y, Decoster L, Van Puyvelde K, Scalliet P, et al. Relevance of a systematic geriatric screening and assessment in older patients with cancer: results of a prospective multicentric study. Ann Oncol. 2013;24(5):1306–12.

34. Hurria A, Togawa K, Mohile SG, Owusu C, Klepin HD, Gross CP, et al. Predicting chemotherapy toxicity in older adults with cancer: a prospective multicenter study. J Clin Oncol. 2011;29(25): 3457–65.

35. Soubeyran P, Fonck M, Blanc-Bisson C, Blanc JF, Ceccaldi J, Mertens C, et al. Predictors of early death risk in older patients treated with first-line chemotherapy for cancer. J Clin Oncol. 2012;30(15):1829–34.

36. Versteeg KS, Konings IR, Lagaay AM, van de Loosdrecht AA, Verheul HM. Prediction of treatment-related toxicity and outcome with geriatric assessment in elderly patients with solid malignancies treated with chemotherapy: a systematic review. Ann Oncol. 2014;25(10):1914–8.

37. Clough-Gorr KM, Stuck AE, Thwin SS, Silliman RA. Older breast cancer survivors: geriatric assessment domains are associated with poor tolerance of treatment adverse effects and predict mortality over 7 years of follow-up. J Clin Oncol. 2010;28(3):380–6.

38. Klepin HD, Geiger AM, Tooze JA, Newman AB, Colbert LH, Bauer DC, et al. Physical performance and subsequent disability and survival in older adults with malignancy: results from the health, aging and body composition study. J Am Geriatr Soc. 2010;58(1):76–82.

39. Ferrucci L, Balducci L. Anemia of aging: the role of chronic inflammation and cancer. Semin Hematol. 2008;45(4):242–9.

40. Alexander NB, Taffet GE, Horne FM, Eldadah BA, Ferrucci L, Nayfield S, et al. Bedside-to-Bench conference: research agenda for idiopathic fatigue and aging. J Am Geriatr Soc. 2010;58(5): 967–75.

41. Naeim A, Aapro M, Subbarao R, Balducci L. Supportive care considerations for older adults with cancer. J Clin Oncol. 2014;32(24):2627–34.

42. Penninx BW, Pahor M, Cesari M, Corsi AM, Woodman RC, Bandinelli S, et al. Anemia is associated with disability and decreased physical performance and muscle strength in the elderly. J Am Geriatr Soc. 2004;52(5):719–24.

43. Hong CH, Falvey C, Harris TB, Simonsick EM, Satterfield S, Ferrucci L, et al. Anemia and risk of dementia in older adults: findings from the Health ABC study. Neurology. 2013;81(6):528–33.

44. Gill TM, Baker DI, Gottschalk M, Peduzzi PN, Allore H, Byers A. A program to prevent functional decline in physically frail, elderly persons who live at home. N Engl J Med. 2002;347(14):1068–74.

45. Min LC, Elliott MN, Wenger NS, Saliba D. Higher vulnerable elders survey scores predict death and functional decline in vulnerable older people. J Am Geriatr Soc. 2006;54(3):507–11.

46. Min L, Yoon W, Mariano J, Wenger NS, Elliott MN, Kamberg C, et al. The vulnerable elders-13 survey predicts 5-year functional decline and mortality outcomes in older ambulatory care patients. J Am Geriatr Soc. 2009;57(11):2070–6.

47. Mohile SG, Bylow K, Dale W, Dignam J, Martin K, Petrylak DP, et al. A pilot study of the vulnerable elders survey-13 compared with the comprehensive geriatric assessment for identifying disability in older patients with prostate cancer who receive androgen ablation. Cancer. 2007;109(4):802–10.

48. Soubeyran P, Bellera C, Goyard J, Heitz D, Cure H, Rousselot H, et al. Validation of the G8 screening tool in geriatric oncology: the ONCODAGE Project. J Clin Oncol 2011;29:(suppl; abstr 9001) http://meetinglibrary.asco.org/content/82003-102.

49. Boyd C, McNabney M, Brandt N. Guiding principles for the care of older adults with multimorbidity: an approach for clinicians: American Geriatrics Society Expert Panel on the Care of Older Adults with Multimorbidity. J Am Geriatr Soc. 2012;60(10):E1–25.

50. Appelbaum PS, Grisso T. Assessing patients' capacities to consent to treatment. N Engl J Med. 1988;319(25):1635–8.

51. Sessums LL, Zembrzuska H, Jackson JL. Does this patient have medical decision-making capacity? JAMA. 2011;306(4):420–7.

52. Etchells E, Darzins P, Silberfeld M, Singer PA, McKenny J, Naglie G, et al. Assessment of patient capacity to consent to treatment. J Gen Intern Med. 1999;14(1):27–34.

53. Fried TR, Tinetti M, Agostini J, Iannone L, Towle V. Health outcome prioritization to elicit preferences of older persons with multiple health conditions. Patient Educ Couns. 2011;83(2):278–82.

54. Fried TR, Byers AL, Gallo WT, Van Ness PH, Towle VR, O'Leary JR, et al. Prospective study of health status preferences and changes in preferences over time in older adults. Arch Intern Med. 2006;166(8):890–5.

55. Sudore RL, Fried TR. Redefining the "planning" in advance care planning: preparing for end-of-life decision making. Ann Intern Med. 2010;153(4):256–61.

56. Repetto L, Comandini D, Mammoliti S. Life expectancy, comorbidity and quality of life: the treatment equation in the older cancer patients. Crit Rev Oncol Hematol. 2001;37(2):147–52.

57. Yourman LC, Lee SJ, Schonberg MA, Widera EW, Smith AK. Prognostic indices for older adults: a systematic review. JAMA. 2012;307(2):182–92.

58. Mohile S, Dale W, Hurria A. Geriatric oncology research to improve clinical care. Nat Rev Clin Oncol. 2012;9(10):571–8.

Derek A. Kruse and Kristina L. Bailey

27.1 Pulmonary

27.1.1 Changes in Pulmonary Physiology with Aging

Pulmonary physiology changes slowly and steadily becoming dramatic in old age. The natural aging process leads to a decline in lung function as well as structural changes in the lung parenchyma. A change in lung function that is found in an aging population is the loss of elastic recoil in the lung parenchyma [1], which results in expiratory flow limitation and can mimic obstructive lung disease. FEV_1 and FVC both continuously decrease at a rate between 25 and 30 mL with each year of life after about age 20 years [2]. Common structural changes include alveolar enlargement, without destruction of the alveolar walls, and distal duct ectasia [3]. The lack of alveolar wall destruction is important because it delineates the aging process from emphysema-related destruction [4]. These structural and functional changes associated with aging, and the long-standing inflammation endured by the lungs throughout life, contribute to the increased prevalence of non-reversible airflow limitation in older patients (Table 27.1).

27.1.2 Chronic Obstructive Pulmonary Disease

Chronic obstructive pulmonary disease (COPD), including chronic bronchitis and emphysema, is characterized by non-reversible airflow limitation. It can be associated with cough, dyspnea, and chronic sputum production. COPD is a common lung disease that occurs more frequently in older people. In fact, the prevalence of COPD is 2.6 times greater in patients 65 years of age or older when compared to people age 45–64 years [11]. Worldwide, the prevalence of the Global Initiative for Chronic Obstructive Lung Disease (GOLD) stage II (moderate) COPD is 10.1 % of people over the age of 40 years [12]. Given the relatively high prevalence of the disease, its chronic nature and the possibility of frequent exacerbations necessitating hospitalization, COPD has a significant morbidity and mortality burden in older patients.

One reason that COPD is more common in older people is that COPD takes time to develop. Lung function naturally declines with age as noted previously, and even when cigarette smoking accelerates the process, it takes years to result in clinically evident disease [5]. A patient might smoke cigarettes for over 25 years prior to developing COPD [13]. In addition, there are pathophysiological changes observed in COPD patients that are similar to those seen with aging alone. For instance, COPD is marked by chronic inflammation of the lungs that is similar to the effects of aging and has been referred to as an "accelerated aging of the lungs" [5]. Both the natural aging process and the pathophysiology of COPD share a common theme of chronic inflammation, the production of reactive oxygen species, DNA damage and telomere shortening, processes that underlie the accelerated cellular senescence in COPD [5].

27.1.2.1 Diagnosis

Given the aforementioned lung changes with aging, it is not surprising that the diagnosis of COPD in older patients can be difficult. In a patient with a compatible clinical presentation, COPD is diagnosed by spirometry before and after bronchodilator therapy. Traditionally, a fixed FEV_1/FVC ratio of <0.70 was used to diagnose COPD. This was based on the guidelines created by the GOLD criteria [14]. With time, concern grew regarding the over diagnosis of obstructive lung disease in older patients. Given the natural decline in the FEV_1/FVC ratio with aging [15], an FEV_1/FVC ratio <0.70 is not necessarily pathological in older patients.

D.A. Kruse, MD • K.L. Bailey, MD (✉)
Pulmonary, Critical Care, Sleep, and Allergy Division, Department of Internal Medicine, University of Nebraska Medical Center, 985910 Nebraska Medical Center, Omaha, NE 68198-5910, USA
e-mail: kbailey@unmc.edu

J.R. Burton et al. (eds.), *Geriatrics for Specialists*, DOI 10.1007/978-3-319-31831-8_27

Table 27.1 Changes in physiological parameters with aging and various disease states

Parameter	Normal aging	COPD	Asthma	Pulmonary hypertension	Idiopathic pulmonary fibrosis
Lung tissue neutrophil concentration	Mildly increased [5]	Moderately increased	NA	NA	NA
Presence of reactive oxygen species in lungs	Mildly increased [5]	Moderately increased [5]	NA	NA	NA
DNA damage and oxidation	Mildly increased [5]	Moderately increased [5]	NA	NA	NA
Destruction of alveoli	Absent [3]	Present [4]	Absent	Absent	Absent
Enlargement of alveoli	Present [3]	Present	Absent	Absent	Absent
Elastic recoil of lung	Decreased [1]	Decreased	No change	No change	Increased
Forced expiratory volume in 1 second	Decreased-fixed [1, 2] FEV1 decline of approximately 20 ml/year [5]	Decreased with no to minimal response to bronchodilator FEV1 decline of 50–100 ml/year [5]	Intermittently decreased with exacerbations. Obstruction reversible with bronchodilators early but can become fixed and non-reversible in older patients	No change	No change or increased
DLCO	Decreased (although not to a clinically significant degree)	Deceased	Normal	Decreased	Decreased
Pulmonary artery pressure	Mildly increased [6, 7]	Mildly increased	No change	Moderate to severely elevated	Mild to moderately elevated
Respiratory muscle strength	Decreased [8]	Decreased [9]	No change	No change	No change
Mucocilliary clearance	Decreased [10]	Normal clearance but increased mucous production	Normal clearance but increased mucous production	No change	Increased mucous production clearance may be reduced

In fact, Hardie et al. demonstrated that approximately 35 % of healthy patients over the age of 70 years had an FEV_1/FVC ratio of less than 0.70 [16]. In 2005, the American Thoracic Society (ATS) and the European Respiratory Society (ERS) released a guideline recommending the use of a fifth percentile lower limit of normal (LLN) for the FEV_1/FVC ratio as a cutoff value to diagnose obstructive lung disease [17]. Large population studies have been used to determine "normal" lung function for patients from each of many different demographic groups. This method limits the over diagnosis of obstructive lung disease in older patients by taking into account the natural decline in the FEV_1/FVC ratio in aging [18]. Given the accumulation of co-morbid illnesses with aging, it is important to carefully evaluate all causes of dyspnea and avoid simply ascribing shortness of breath to COPD in all older patients with an FEV1/FVC of <0.70.

COPD has become more accurately recognized as a systemic disease in both young and older patients [19]. Patients with COPD are at risk of extra-pulmonary comorbidities, including: coronary artery disease, lung cancer, peripheral skeletal muscle dysfunction, malnutrition, osteoporosis, hypertension, diabetes, depression, stroke, and obesity [20].

These comorbidities lead to increased morbidity and mortality in COPD [21]. This underscores the importance of recognizing and treating COPD as a systemic disease involving multiple organ systems. The approach to treatment therefore must be multifaceted and address co-morbid malnutrition, depression, muscle wasting, and loss of exercise capacity. An important component of this multifaceted approach is pulmonary rehabilitation, which can include aerobic exercise and/or resistance training. A monitored regimen of either type of exercise has been proven to be successful at improving older patient's functional status, depression scores, and subjective measures of quality of life at all stages of COPD [22, 23].

27.1.2.2 Treatment

The pharmacotherapy for COPD in an aging population requires special considerations. The volume of distribution for medications can change significantly with age, as can the rate of metabolism, especially in patients with co-morbid renal or liver disease [24]. Maintaining vigilance to avoid adverse effects associated with medical therapy is an important part of alleviating patients' symptoms and improving quality of life. Provider familiarity with common adverse effects is paramount in avoiding harm when prescribing medical therapy. Anticholinergic medications are commonly used in the treatment of patients with COPD and adverse effects of these medications can be significant, especially in an older population. The two most prominent adverse effects with this drug class include urinary retention and mucosal dryness [25], both of which can contribute to significant morbidity in older patients. Beta-agonists are associated with tremors, anxiety, palpitations, and cardiac arrhythmias [25]. Finally, corticosteroids have significant adverse effects of their own. Inhaled steroids, although seemingly less likely to cause significant adverse effects than systemic steroids, do cause thrush and dysphonia and are associated with pneumonia [25]. Oral steroids are associated with hypertension, glaucoma, diabetes, bruising, myopathy, gastritis, adrenal insufficiency, and osteoporosis [25]. Considering the above, it is important to evaluate patients for adverse effects at each clinic visit. Something as simple as assuring patient understanding of proper inhaler technique can improve patient adherence, increase efficacy, and decrease morbidity associated with their therapy. There are three basic types of inhaler devices available including a dry powder inhaler (DPI), a metered dose inhaler (MDI), and a nebulized delivery of the therapy. Although studies have failed to establish a greater efficacy with one type of inhaler device over another [26], individualized therapy is recommended [26]. Individualized therapy can be based on several considerations including: the patient's cognitive function and ability to follow instructions, their hand strength and dexterity to manipulate the inhaler device, whether they can generate an inspiratory flow rate sufficient to properly inhale dry powders, the drug availability in a given inhaler device and the cost of a given inhaled therapy [27]. Older patients who have developed mild cognitive impairment or who have deficits in their coordination may benefit from the use of DPI devices. DPI devices require less coordination than MDI devices, which require the patient to actuate the inhaler and inhale nearly simultaneously. Manual dexterity and hand strength are also important when it comes to actuating either MDI or DPI devices. Rheumatoid arthritis, Parkinson's disease, and loss of hand strength can all contribute to difficulties for older patients when it comes to using inhalers. When cognitive function and manual dexterity limit a patient's ability to use either MDI or DPI inhalers, nebulized drug delivery can be more effective than either of these alternatives.

27.1.3 Asthma

For many years, asthma has been thought of as a disease of younger people. Asthma, however, is not uncommon in older patients, a population where asthma has a predicted prevalence between 4 and 6 % [28–30]. This is a population that

has been shown to have a higher hospitalization rate [31, 32] and a higher mortality rate than other age groups with asthma [33]. Patients older than 65 years of age have a significantly increased mortality rate when compared to patients of the same age who do not carry this diagnosis [34]. More than 50 % of all deaths from asthma are in patients age 65 years or older [33]. Despite these facts, asthma is underappreciated in older patients and often the diagnosis is delayed [35]. Extrapolation of population data suggests that nearly a quarter of all older patients with asthma are currently undiagnosed [28]. This may be related to the often-atypical presentation of asthma in this patient population. Older patients with reversible airway obstruction most frequently present with cough rather than dyspnea, wheezing, or other typical symptoms of asthma [35]. Older patients may also not perceive chest tightness related to bronchospasm [36] and tend to decrease activity, masking exertional symptoms [28]. As a result, older patients tend to present later in the course of the disease process with fixed obstruction [29], and are commonly misdiagnosed with COPD [37].

In addition to the difficulties in diagnosing asthma in older patients, the data suggests that this population is also undertreated. A large, cross-sectional study revealed that the treatment of asthma in older patients was not congruent with the National Asthma Education and Prevention Program's treatment guidelines [38]. Older patients were less likely to be on a controller therapy, a long-acting beta-agonist or a short acting beta-agonist rescue inhaler when compared to younger patients with asthma [38]. These studies demonstrate an opportunity for improvements to both the recognition and treatment of asthma in older patients.

27.1.4 Pulmonary Hypertension

Pulmonary hypertension (PH) is a pathological state marked by a mean pulmonary artery pressure of 25 mmHg or greater [39] and is becoming a more frequent diagnosis in older patients [40]. PH is a diagnosis that includes a broad array of pathophysiological processes, hemodynamic characteristics, and treatment options [41]. It is traditionally divided into five sub-groups based on their characteristics [41]. We will focus the discussion on group 1 pulmonary hypertension (PH), also known as pulmonary arterial hypertension (PAH), because it is a group where PH-targeted medical therapy has been demonstrated to be effective as a treatment option. Idiopathic pulmonary arterial hypertension is a sub-group of PAH where no identifiable cause of an elevated pulmonary artery pressure can be identified.

The incidence of PAH is increasing in older patients [42]. The reasons underlying this increase remain unknown, but hypotheses suggest it may be related to the increasing life expectancy in this country and a greater awareness of the disease [43]. As the awareness of PAH increases, clinicians must remain vigilant of the pitfalls in making the diagnosis of PAH in older patients because pulmonary artery systolic pressure increases with healthy aging patients [6, 7]. Two of the physiologic changes of aging that contribute to an elevated pulmonary artery pressure include a decline in the pulmonary capillary volume [44] and vascular stiffening of the pulmonary arteries [45]. Several disease processes that are common in older patients also increase pulmonary artery pressures including: COPD [11], idiopathic pulmonary fibrosis [46], valvular heart disease, and systolic and diastolic heart failure [43]. These relatively common comorbidities can make the diagnosis of PAH in older patients more difficult.

The multitude of causes for an elevated pulmonary artery pressure in older patients underscores the need for a thorough diagnostic evaluation. The diagnosis of PAH deserves special consideration. The diagnosis is based on a mean pulmonary artery pressure on right heart catheterization to be 25 mmHg or greater and the pulmonary capillary wedge pressure to be 15 mmHg or less [47]. Transthoracic echocardiography is becoming a much more commonly used diagnostic tool, which has likely contributed to the increase in incidence of PAH in older patients. Noteworthy, echocardiography can be used as a screening tool for PAH, but concern for PAH warrants a right heart catheterization. A diagnosis of PAH should not be made without right heart catheterization, nor should the treatment for PAH [48]. During right heart catheterization vasoreactivity testing should be performed to assess for the likelihood of a long-term response to oral calcium blockers [49]. Positive vasoreactivity testing is defined as a drop in the mean pulmonary artery pressure (PAP) by at least 10 mmHg and achieving an absolute value for the mean PAP of 40 mmHg or less [49]. A complete and detailed evaluation is vital, as the specialized medical therapy is not efficacious for treatment outside this group.

General treatment considerations for PAH include supplemental oxygen as needed to maintain a patient's oxygen saturation >88 %. Additionally, anticoagulation is generally recommended in patients with idiopathic PAH, familial PAH, drug-induced PAH and chronic thromboembolic pulmonary hypertension. Diuretics are used as needed for symptomatic right heart failure. Routine vaccinations and regular aerobic exercise are also encouraged for all patients with PAH. Advanced therapies for treatment of PAH include intravenous, sub-cutaneous, inhaled, and oral pulmonary vasculature vasodilators. Consensus guidelines recommend treatment be started when patients develop at least WHO class 2 symptoms and have group 1 PAH based on a right heart catheterization, a thorough clinical history, physical exam, imaging and laboratory testing [50]. Therapy generally starts with oral agents, but additional oral, inhaled, and intravenous agents can be added for lack of clinical response

or worsening of a patient's symptoms [50]. The efficacy of these therapies has yet to be established in an older population and has been less well studied as compared to younger patients. Results from the COMPERA registry suggest older patients are less likely to be prescribed these therapies and those who are prescribed an advanced therapy are less likely to experience clinical improvement when compared to younger patients [51]. Given the increasing prevalence of PAH in older patients, further efforts to establish the most efficacious treatment regimen for this population are warranted.

Older patients are more likely to present with NYHA class 3 or 4 functional limitation as compared to younger patients [40]. Despite the lower functional status, older patients are more likely to have lower pulmonary artery systolic pressures and to have lower levels of pulmonary vascular resistance [40]. This is likely secondary to co-morbid conditions including a general decline in conditioning with aging. Finally, older patients are less likely to have a significant clinical response to therapy [40, 51]. As new therapies for the treatment of PAH are developed, a focus on diagnostic accuracy and establishing the most efficacious treatment regimen for an older population is of great clinical importance.

27.1.5 Pneumonia

Older patients are four times more likely to develop pneumonia than younger age groups [52] and nearly 90 % of deaths due to pneumonia occur in those 65 or older [53, 54]. The mortality rate of pneumonia also increases exponentially with age, from 1.3 % in those younger than 45 to 26 % in those over 65 [55, 56]. The increase in incidence and mortality with age has been associated with the presence of multiple comorbidities in this population including chronic respiratory and cardiovascular diseases, cerebrovascular disease, Parkinson's disease, epilepsy, dementia, dysphagia, and chronic renal or liver disease [57]. However, age itself is an independent risk factor for pneumonia [58]. Likely contributing to this is the myriad of changes with aging that impair pulmonary innate immunity. Mucociliary function is impaired with aging [10], leading to inefficient clearance of pathogens, including bacteria. There is also diminished function of natural killer cells, macrophages, and neutrophils in normal aging [59].

The diagnosis of pneumonia in older patients is complicated by the fact that they have fewer symptoms. Older patients are less likely than younger patients to report cough, pleuritic chest pain, fever, and chills. They are more likely, however, to present with tachypnea [60]. They are also more likely to present with confusion or delirium [61]. Despite these differences in clinical presentation, there are similarities in regard to the causative pathogens in patients both younger and older than

65 years of age. Steptococcus pneumoniae is still the most frequent cause of community acquired pneumonia (CAP) in all patients 65 years of age or older [62], but polymicrobial infection and gram-negative organisms occur more frequently in older patients, especially if they have COPD or reside in a long-term care facility [55].

27.1.6 Idiopathic Pulmonary Fibrosis

27.1.6.1 Epidemiology

Idiopathic pulmonary fibrosis (IPF) occurs nearly exclusively in patients over the age of 65. It is a chronic and progressive disease marked by interstitial fibrosis of the lungs and usual interstitial pneumonia (UIP) on histology [63]. The incidence of IPF is estimated to be between 6.8 and 16.3 cases per 100,000 persons each year in the USA, while the population prevalence is estimated to be between 14.0 and 42.7 cases per 100,000 persons [64]. Both the incidence and prevalence are highest in males over the age of 65 years [64]. For example, in people age 75 years and older, the prevalence is 227.2 per 100,000 persons [59].

27.1.6.2 Pathogenesis

The pathogenesis of IPF is complex and poorly understood. The current understanding suggests that the pathogenesis of IPF is based on multiple factors including a genetic predisposition, environmental factors, and accumulation of gene mutations with aging that lead to abnormal epithelial cell growth and fibrosis [65]. Genetic mutations in epithelial cell–associated proteins predispose to the development of lung fibrosis by leading to the development of short telomeres or endoplasmic reticulum (ER) stress [65]. Environmental factors suspected to play a role in the pathogenesis include tobacco smoke [66], occupational exposures [67], and viral infections [68, 69], among others.

27.1.6.3 Diagnosis

The clinical diagnosis of IPF in older patients needs to balance making a confident diagnosis with the risk associated with testing. Typical presenting symptoms include the insidious onset of dyspnea on exertion and a dry cough, which are non-specific findings, but when considering an IPF diagnosis, the patient's age alone is predictive [70]. The older the patient, the more likely they are to have IPF and not another type of idiopathic interstitial pneumonia [70]. The diagnosis of UIP, a histological component of IPF, can be made confidently in older patients with a compatible clinical presentation by radiographic evidence of a definite UIP pattern on high resolution CT imaging (HRCT). A definite UIP pattern consists of sub-pleural, basilar reticular changes with honeycombing, with or without traction bronchiectasis [71]. In cases with definite UIP on imaging, a lung biopsy is not necessary. HRCT findings consistent with "Possible UIP" or "Inconsistent with UIP" require further evaluation with surgical lung biopsy for diagnosis [72]. The patient's age, frailty, and comorbidities should be considered when discussing the option of a surgical procedure.

27.1.6.4 Treatment

The treatment of IPF has focused on treating the complications of the disease and not the disease process itself, until the recent release of two anti-fibrotic medications, pirfenidone and nintedanib. Although nintedanib and pirfenidone have been shown to reduce the rate of decline in FVC in patients with IPF, they have a relatively modest effect on the clinical outcomes [73–75]. Supportive measures that improve outcomes include: oxygen therapy to maintain oxygen saturations >88 %, pulmonary rehabilitation [76], and treatment of asymptomatic esophageal reflux [77]. Lung transplantation may also be considered in patients felt able to tolerate the surgery [72].

Unfortunately, IPF has a relatively poor prognosis. The median time of survival for patients diagnosed with IPF has been estimated at approximately 3–4 years [78]. It is uncertain if the new anti-fibrotic medications will significantly change that prognosis.

27.1.7 Lung Cancer

It has been estimated that by the year 2030, 70 % of all cancers will be diagnosed in patients 65 years of age or older [79]. This includes an expectation for a significant increase in the incidence of lung cancer in this population, the majority of which will be the non-small cell type [79]. Lung cancer is currently the most common cancer diagnosis in all people, as well as the most common cause of death from cancer [80]. Despite lung cancer typically being a cancer of older patients, lung cancer treatment for older patients is frequently extrapolated from the treatment of younger patients [81]. This raises concern regarding the safety of these treatments in an older population, where comorbidities and frailty are more prevalent. In older patients with lung cancer, clinicians should consider a comprehensive geriatric assessment (CGA) to determine the patient's fitness for a given cancer treatment regimen [81]. A comprehensive geriatric assessment (CGA) is a multidisciplinary assessment of a patient's medical, psychosocial, functional, and environmental problems [82]. The CGA's can help establish the most appropriate treatment plan and follow-up for each older patient diagnosed with lung cancer [82]. Utilization of a CGA can lead to improvements in mortality as well as improvement in patient's cognitive and physical functional status [82]. See Chap. 26 Geriatric Oncology for additional information on CGA.

27.2 Critical Care Medicine for the Older Patient

Physiological changes of aging alter the most common ICU admission diagnoses, and the optimal treatment for these disease processes. In patients 65–85 years of age there is an increasing incidence of ICU admission for heart failure, cardiac arrhythmias, and valvular heart disease [83]. At the same time, there is a decreasing rate of ICU admissions related to complications of diabetes, alcohol abuse, COPD, and liver failure [83]. No matter the admitting diagnosis, an age greater than 74 is considered an independent risk factor for 30-day and 1-year mortality [83]. One of the causes of this increased mortality may be the higher rate of delirium.

27.2.1 Delirium

Delirium is a frequent co-morbid condition in older patients in the ICU ranging between 31 and 79 % of all older patients [84, 85]. Increasing age and APACHE II scores are both independent risk factors for ICU delirium [86]. Studies suggest a mean time to onset of approximately 2.6 days after admission and the mean duration of signs and symptoms of 3.4 days [87]. The duration of delirium is directly related to the ICU and hospital length of stay [87] and the 1-year post-admission mortality [88]. Delirium at any point during hospitalization is an independent risk factor for mortality [85]. For these reasons, there have been continued efforts to prevent delirium when possible, to improve early recognition when it occurs and optimize treatment.

Reducing the incidence of delirium is the first priority, although up to 72 % of patients 60 years of age and older present for admission to the ICU with delirium [88]. Eliminating new cases of delirium and shortening the duration of delirium when present are both important and have a similar approach.

One important factor in preventing new cases of delirium is to avoid medications that are known to precipitate it. See also Chap. 5. Medication Management. The list of medications associated with delirium is extensive, but the most frequent offenders are: sedatives, analgesics, and anticholinergic medications. In an unadjusted comparison, patients who received benzodiazepines or opioids had an average ICU delirium duration of 5.79 days for each week at risk, compared to 3.08 days for patients who did not receive benzodiazepines or opioids [89]. Given this data, benzodiazepines should be avoided, especially in an older population. Avoiding opioid analgesics is difficult due to the prevalence of severe pain in this population, but minimizing use, and age-adjusting doses is warranted. Anticholinergic medications including antihistamine receptor-2 antagonists (used for gastric ulcer prophylaxis) [90] are associated with delirium in hospitalized older patients [91].

In a critical care population, anticholinergic bronchodilators are commonly used but should be avoided if possible.

Antipsychotic medications are not effective in preventing delirium. Haloperidol actually increases the risk of delirium in the 24 h following administration [92] and has been shown to increase the duration of delirium [89]. All antipsychotics carry a black-box warning for increased mortality in older patients with dementia.

Environmental disturbances in the ICU that likely contribute to the development of delirium include: the absence of visible daylight, transfer to another hospital unit and use of physical restraints [93]. Noise is an established cause of fragmented and poor quality sleep in ICU patients [94]. Patient questionnaires upon discharge from an ICU suggest that diagnostic testing and interactions with medical staff are also significant contributors to sleep deprivation [95]. Sleep deprivation is hypothesized to contribute to the development of delirium [96] Therefore, promoting an appropriate sleep–wake cycle by dimming the lights at night, avoiding excessive noise in patient rooms (such as loud TVs, radios, and conversations), avoiding stimulating the patient at night when possible and promoting wakefulness during the day are all advocated. A lack of sensory input can be disorienting as well [97]. Patients with visual and hearing impairment benefit from having their hearing aids and glasses on whenever possible. Similarly, patients benefit from being able to read calendars and clocks, which help keep them oriented to time [97].

There has also been work toward preventing ICU delirium with tools such as the ABCDE bundle [98] into daily practice in the ICU (Table 27.3). While this approach is designed to prevent delirium, it should also be viewed as the appropriate approach for patients with delirium in an effort to correct the factors that precipitated the episode of delirium. The ABCDE acronym is broken into three parts, which will be described separately. The "ABC" portion of the acronym stands for "Awakening and Breathing trial Coordination," the "D" stands for "Delirium Assessment," and the "E" stands for "Early Mobility." The purpose of the "ABC" portion of the bundle is to limit unnecessary sedation, support early liberation from mechanical ventilation, and coordinate an interprofessional effort to achieve these goals. This consists of a daily weaning of sedation and a spontaneous breathing trial for all mechanically ventilated patients deemed appropriate. Studies have shown that this can significantly reduce the number of days of mechanical ventilation, as well as complications of mechanical ventilation [99]. Again, the "D" in the acronym stands for "Delirium Assessment." This portion of the bundle focuses on the assessment for pain, agitation and delirium. The routine assessment of pain with an observational pain assessment instrument can decrease the ICU length of stay and decrease the duration of mechanical ventilation [100]. There are multiple pain assessment tools available, including: the Pain Assessment and Intervention Notation (PAIN) algorithm, the

Table 27.2 Critical care pain assessment tool[a]

Behavioral Parameter	Description	Score
Facial expression	No muscle tension in face-Relaxed	0
	Frowning, tightening of orbit-Tense	1
	Eyelid tightly closed-Grimacing	2
Body movements	No movement	0
	Slow cautious movements	1
	Restless, agitated, trying to sit up	2
Muscle tension (passive flexion and extension of upper extremities)	Relaxed-No resistance to movements	0
	Some resistance to movements	1
	Strong resistance-Inability to complete movements	2
Compliance with ventilator/intubated patients	No ventilator alarms-Easy to ventilate	0
	Intermittent ventilator alarms-Coughing	1
	Frequent ventilator alarms-Difficult to ventilate	2
Or		
Vocalization-Non-intubated patients	Not talking or talking in a normal fashion	0
	Sighing or moaning	1
	Crying out	2

[a]A CPOT score >2 is considered a positive test for pain

Table 27.3 ABCDE Bundle: For delirium prevention and morbidity reduction

Components	Description
"A" awake	Promoting sedation weaning on appropriate patients daily
"B" breathe	Daily spontaneous breathing trials on appropriate patients to promote early liberation from mechanical ventilation
"C" coordination of care	Coordinating patient care to involve the respiratory, nursing, physical therapy, and physician teams in the daily plan
"D" delirium assessment	Monitor delirium, pain and agitation using validated bedside screening tools like the CAM-ICU, CPOT, and RASS
"E" early mobility	Involving the nursing staff, respiratory therapist, physical therapist, and physician in promoting early mobility

Nonverbal Pain Assessment Tool (NPAT), the Adult Nonverbal Pain Scale (NVPS), the Behavioral Pain Scale (BPS), and the Critical-Care Pain Observation Tool (CPOT; Table 27.2) [100]. Of these pain assessment tools, the CPOT has superior validity and reliability when used in nonverbal, critically ill adults [100] (Table 27.3). The treatment of pain must be balanced with the treatment of agitation and delirium. Agitation, treated after adequate pain control is assured, can also be assessed using multiple different assessment tools. The Richmond Agitation-Sedation Scale (RASS) is a validated assessment tool for the detection of changes in sedation

Table 27.4 Confusion assessment methodology for the ICU

Components	Description
1) Altered mental status or abnormal behavior	Acute change in mental status, or fluctuating changes in mental status or behavior over the last 24 h
2) Inattention	Difficulty focusing attention based on abnormal results from either the auditory or visual Attention Screening Examination (ASE)
3) Altered level of consciousness	RASS not equal to 0, so either agitated or sedated. Ex. Hyperalert, drowsy, difficult to arouse, unarousable, etc.
4) Disorganized thinking	Ask to follow simple commands or answer simple questions ex. "Hold up four fingers" "Will a rock float on water?"

Patients are considered to have delirium if 1 and 2 are present and either 3 or 4 is present [102]

status over consecutive days of ICU care, which is compared against constructs of level of consciousness and delirium, and correlated with the administered dose of sedative and analgesic medications [101]. The evaluation for delirium is an extremely important part of daily assessments in ICU patients. The CAM-ICU delirium assessment tool is a rapidly administered, highly reproducible, sensitive, and specific tool for diagnosing delirium in ventilated and non-ventilated ICU patients (Table 27.4) [102]. The final portion of the bundle focuses on "Early Mobility." The literature suggests that not only is early mobility in ICU patients possible, but it also enhances the recovery of functional exercise capacity, self-perceived functional status, and muscle strength at hospital discharge [103]. The use of the "ABCDE" bundle in the ICU has been shown to significantly decrease the number of days a patient spends mechanically ventilated, to significantly decrease the incidence of delirium and to increase the number of patients who are ambulating prior to ICU discharge [104].

27.2.2 Treatment of Agitation in ICU Delirium

Environmental factors and the ABCDE approach described above should be the initial approach to agitation. Pharmacotherapy for agitation is a subject of ongoing debate, but current opinion favors avoiding benzodiazepine sedatives. Conventional and atypical antipsychotics should be avoided unless agitation in delirium is a danger to the patient or others. Currently, there are no pharmacological interventions that are recommended for the treatment of agitated delirium [105]. When antipsychotics are used that should be at the lowest dose and for the shortest duration possible. If haloperidol is to be used, an EKG must be checked for Qt prolongation which is a contraindication to use of this drug. The reader is referred to Chap. 2, for additional information on the definition, diagnostic criteria, clinical presentation, risk factors, and evaluation for this important ICU condition.

27.2.3 Invasive Mechanical Ventilation and Non-Invasive Positive Pressure Ventilation

A common reason for ICU admission is respiratory failure requiring invasive or non-invasive mechanical ventilation. Aging is associated with multiple anatomical and physiological changes in the lungs that are associated with an increased susceptibility to respiratory failure [2]. There are a few special considerations in respiratory failure in the older patient.

A common cause of respiratory failure in older patients is COPD exacerbations. Outcomes are improved when acute exacerbations of COPD, resulting in acute or acute on chronic hypercarbic respiratory failure, are treated with bi-level NIPPV, compared to patients treated with medical therapy alone [106, 107]. Medical therapy consists of systemic steroids, bronchodilators and antibiotics where indicated. NIPPV therapy also decreases the likelihood of intubation and lead to shorter hospital stays as well as a lower mortality during the hospitalization and up to 1 year later [106, 107]. This evidence strongly supports the use of NIPPV in the treatment of COPD exacerbations, but careful consideration should be given to selecting the correct therapy for each individual patient. Contraindications to NIPPV include: the inability to clear secretions, the inability to cooperate with the medical staff, and the inability to protect their airway [108]. Delirium is also considered a relative contraindication to NIPPV. It can lead to poor patient-device synchrony, difficulty in keeping an acceptable seal with the mask, and a greater likelihood of needing sedation to achieve adherence with therapies. Concerns for aerophagia, vomiting, and aspiration exist as well. Combined, these factors can make using NIPPV in older patients difficult and leave the patient at an increased risk for complications. Despite this, older patients suffering acute or acute on chronic hypercarbic respiratory failure associated with COPD exacerbations are more likely to be treated with NIPPV as compared to younger patients [109] although these same patients are also more likely to fail to respond to NIPPV, necessitating intubation and mechanical ventilation [109]. Unfortunately, failure of NIPPV requiring IMV is associated with a doubling of the in-hospital mortality rate [109]. Providers should remain cognizant of the fact that use of NIPPV, despite contraindications, may result in an untoward increase in mortality.

Increasing age is independently associated with a significant increase in ICU mortality in mechanically ventilated patients [110]. The increased mortality in older patients is multifactorial. Delirium contributes to this mortality [85, 86, 88], but the patient's severity of illness and the use of vasopressors are also associated with an increased mortality in older patients who require mechanical ventilation [111]. Age is also an independent risk factor for ventilator-associated pneumonia (VAP) [112], which is associated with a 10 % attributable mortality rate [113]. Measures to prevent VAP in the elderly are similar to those described for younger patients. Considerations include: elevation of the head of the bed, daily sedation vacations to assess patient readiness for ventilator weaning, peptic ulcer disease prophylaxis, and daily oral hygiene with chlorhexidine. There is evidence that early tracheostomy, performed less than 7 days after intubation, results in fewer VAPs in the elderly, shorter hospital stays and a trend toward a mortality benefit [114]. This concept requires further study, but is a worthwhile consideration in older patients that are experiencing difficulty in being liberated from the ventilator.

Certain patient populations require special consideration when approaching spontaneous breathing trials (SBT) to assess for readiness for extubation. Patients at high risk for re-intubation include: those with significant heart disease, chronic lung disease, and older patients. A standard 30-minute SBT may not be as accurate at predicting the re-intubation rate in older patients because the studies testing it did not include high-risk patients [115]. Older patients are more likely to have co-morbid heart disease and chronic lung disease, which puts them at higher risk for re-intubation [116]. Although data supporting longer SBTs in older patients are limited, it has recently been proposed that a 2-hour SBT would reduce the need for re-intubation in high-risk patients [116]. This study also proposed performing an SBT using less ventilatory support, such as using a T-piece for elderly patients, as this would also reduce the need for re-intubation as compared to a pressure support mode of ventilation [116]. In summary, this study suggests that older patients would benefit from a more stringent SBT to avoid early re-intubation. Adjunctive testing may also help improve ventilator liberation in older patients. Further study including randomized and controlled studies would be helpful as, at this point, these recommendations are based on expert opinion.

27.2.4 Venous Thromboembolic Disease

Venous thromboembolic disease (VTE), including deep vein thrombosis (DVT) and pulmonary embolus (PE), is a common cause of preventable in-hospital morbidity and mortality. Approximately 1 out of every 1000 people in the USA will develop VTE each year [117]. The incidence of both DVT and PE increases with age, e.g., there is a 2.5 fold increase in DVT/PE in patients older than 80 compared to those 60–69 [118]. The increase in incidence with age is attributed to both increased prevalence of co-morbid disease and age as an independent risk factor [118]. Not only is age a risk factor for VTE, it is also a risk factor for death secondary to VTE. A large population-based cohort study demonstrated a 1-year mortality from PE with or without DVT to be 47.7 % and age was an independent risk factor for mortality [119].

Diagnosing DVT/PE in older patients can be more difficult, because the clinical presentation may be more subtle than in younger patients. Nearly one quarter of all older patients with PE present with collapse, a significantly greater proportion when compared to younger patients [120]. There are also limitations to our standard testing in older patients. D-dimer is more likely to be elevated in older patients and an age-adjusted D-dimer cutoff value improves specificity without sacrificing sensitivity [121]. The formula for upper limit of D-dimer $\leq$ age $\times$ 100 is used. Renal impairment in older patients is more likely to limit the use of contrast enhanced CT scan. Ventilation/perfusion scans (VQ) may also be limited due to underlying lung disease in the elderly [122].

Because patients over the age of 75 already have one major risk factor for VTE, age, they only need one additional acute medical condition to consider VTE prophylaxis [123]. Older patients have a higher risk of bleeding complications [124–126], which can complicate the choice of VTE prophylaxis. Enoxaparin has been specifically studied in patients >75 years old, and it reduced VTE by 78 % and did not have more adverse events than placebo [127]. Likewise, dalteparin has been shown to be safe and effective in older patients [128].

27.2.5 Sepsis

Every year there is an estimated 750,000 hospital admissions for severe sepsis and more than half of these patients require ICU admission [129]. The incidence of sepsis is the lowest in young adults and climbs slowly throughout adulthood, achieving a rate of 5.3/1000 persons by the age of 65 years [129]. The incidence then sharply increases to an estimated rate of 26.2/1000 persons by the age of 85 years [129]. Not only is age associated with an increasing incidence, it is also associated with an increasing mortality rate [129]. The overall hospital mortality rate for severe sepsis is 28.6 %, which represents 215,000 deaths annually [129]. When controlling for comorbidities, age is an independent risk factor for mortality [129, 130].

The cause of the increasing incidence of sepsis in older patients is likely multifactorial. The acquisition of resistant and virulent organisms by residence in long-term care facilities and recurrent hospital admissions [131], along with a general decline in homeostatic processes and immunological defense mechanisms in older patients [132] likely contribute. As an example, patients in this age group are at an increased risk for gram-negative sepsis, especially from pneumonia [129, 130]. Specific organ dysfunction with aging includes the decrease in mucocilliary clearance noted [112], a weaker cough and the anatomical and physiological changes noted in lung parenchyma [2], which may contribute to the high incidence of sepsis in pneumonia. The incidence of urinary tract infection (UTI) and asymptomatic bacteriuria increases with age and UTI is the second leading cause of infection in community dwelling older patients [133]. Other co-morbid conditions leading to placement of indwelling devices such

as pacemakers, artificial valves, chronic indwelling intravascular catheters and urinary catheters all contribute to the increase rate of sepsis in this population.

The approach to making a diagnosis of sepsis in older patients warrants special consideration. Studies suggest the typical signs of sepsis may be absent in this patient population. In one study, 13 % of bacteremic patients with an age >65 years were afebrile while only 4 % of those <65 years were afebrile [134]. Tachycardia and hypoxemia are also less common in patients >75 years of age [135]. Lactic acidosis, tachypnea, and delirium are more commonly present in these patients [135]. Remaining cognizant of these differences is necessary to institute appropriate therapy in a timely manner.

Given the high rate of sepsis in older patient populations, there are studies and evidence suggesting improved outcomes in older patients when a "sepsis bundle" is instituted [136]. The bundle assures early and aggressive fluid administration, early antibiotic therapy, if needed, after fluid resuscitation and steroids in those with septic shock that do not respond to fluids and vasopressor therapy The Society of Critical Care Medicine supports the use of steroids in this setting, without the need to assess the patient's response to adrenal stimulation testing prior to starting steroids [137]. In one study, the absolute risk reduction in the 28-day mortality was 16 % compared to a retrospectively, matched, control group [136]. A specific consideration is the treatment of anemia. In septic older patients, anemia should prompt transfusion to maintain a hemoglobin concentration of 7–9 g/dl [138]. In this study, maintaining a hemoglobin concentration greater than 10 g/dl did not result in improved outcomes [138]. In a separate study, older patients who developed myocardial infarction had an improved mortality when their hemoglobin concentration is kept >10 g/dl [139]. These data suggest that in the scenario of concomitant sepsis and myocardial infarction, the goal hemoglobin concentration should be >10 g/dl, although a recent pilot study enrolling patients >55 years with critical illness and randomizing to restrictive (Hgb 7–9) vs liberal (Hgb 9–11) did not show any differences in outcomes [140]. Likewise, another study did not show any improvement in delirium with liberal (Hgb >10) transfusions [141].

The reader is also referred to Chap. 24, Infection and Immunity in Older Adults, for additional information.

27.3 CPR Outcomes/Palliative Care and Hospice

Cardiac arrest in the elderly is often a difficult experience for providers and families. Questions regarding the patient's wishes, adverse effects associated with treatment, and expected outcomes must be answered quickly. The first and most difficult question to be answered is "what is the probability of this patient surviving and if so, will their quality of life be acceptable to them?" This can be difficult to answer, but retrospective studies suggest that age is not an independent risk factor for the inability to achieve a return of spontaneous circulation (ROSC) or for in-hospital mortality after out-of-hospital arrest [142]. This is possibly because of the overall poor prognosis associated with out-of-hospital arrest, for which survival to hospital discharge is only 4–5 %, no matter the age of the patient [142]. The prognosis was driven by the initial cardiac rhythm and out-of-hospital life support [142]. Studies assessing in-hospital cardiac arrest in the elderly report that only 18.3 % of patients experiencing in-hospital cardiac arrest survived to discharge [143]. Male gender, increasing age, a greater number of co-morbid illnesses, and admission from a nursing home were all predictors of a worse prognosis [143, 144].

Another consideration not addressed by these statistics is the cognitive function, physical function and quality of life for the patients surviving to discharge. Age and length of hospitalization prior to cardiac arrest are both predictors of a worse functional status after CPR and also death prior to hospital discharge [144].

Palliative care and hospice programs facilitate advanced care planning in older patients and improve end of life care and family satisfaction. It also reduces stress, anxiety, and depression in family members [145]. With the poor outcomes in older patients suffering cardiac arrest and severe sepsis, and those with end-stage lung disease, the benefit to discussing available services and utilizing palliative treatments in these settings is warranted. The reader is referred to Chap. 6, for further information.

References

1. Turner JM, Mead J, Wohl ME. Elasticity of human lungs in relation to age. J Appl Physiol. 1968;25(6):664–71.
2. Janssens J, Pache J, Nicod L. Physiological changes in respiratory function associated with ageing. Eur Respir J. 1999;13(1):197–205.
3. Fukuchi Y. The aging lung and chronic obstructive pulmonary disease: similarity and difference. Proc Am Thorac Soc. 2009;6(7):570–2.
4. Snider GL, Kleinerman J, Thurlbeck WM, Bengali ZH. The definition of emphysema: Report of a National Heart, Lung, and Blood Institute, Division of Lung Diseases Workshop 1. Am Rev Respir Dis. 1985;132(1):182–5.
5. Ito K, Barnes PJ. COPD as a disease of accelerated lung aging. Chest. 2009;135(1):173–80.
6. Lam CS, Borlaug BA, Kane GC, Enders FT, Rodeheffer RJ, Redfield MM. Age-associated increases in pulmonary artery systolic pressure in the general population. Circulation. 2009;119(20):2663–70.
7. Davidson WR, Fee EC. Influence of aging on pulmonary hemodynamics in a population free of coronary artery disease. Am J Cardiol. 1990;65(22):1454–8.
8. Tolep K, Higgins N, Muza S, Criner G, Kelsen SG. Comparison of diaphragm strength between healthy adult elderly and young men. Am J Respir Crit Care Med. 1995;152(2):677–82.
9. Barreiro E, Gea J. Respiratory and limb muscle dysfunction in COPD. COPD. 2015;12:413–26.
10. Ho JC, Chan KN, Hu WH, Lam WK, Zheng L, Tipoe GL, et al. The effect of aging on nasal mucociliary clearance, beat frequency, and ultrastructure of respiratory cilia. Am J Respir Crit Care Med. 2001;163(4):983–8.
11. Tuder RM. Aging and cigarette smoke: fueling the fire. Am J Respir Crit Care Med. 2006;174(5):490–1.
12. Buist AS, McBurnie MA, Vollmer WM, Gillespie S, Burney P, Mannino DM, et al. International variation in the prevalence of COPD (the BOLD Study): a population-based prevalence study. Lancet. 2007;370(9589):741–50.
13. Lokke A, Lange P, Scharling H, Fabricius P, Vestbo J. Developing COPD: a 25 year follow up study of the general population. Thorax. 2006;61(11):935–9.
14. Pauwels RA, Buist AS, Calverley PM, Jenkins CR, Hurd SS. Global strategy for the diagnosis, management, and prevention of chronic obstructive pulmonary disease. Am J Respir and Crit Care Med. 2001;163(5):1256–76.
15. Hansen JE, Sun X, Wasserman K. Discriminating measures and normal values for expiratory obstruction*. Chest. 2006;129(2):369–77.
16. Hardie JA, Buist AS, Vollmer WM, Ellingsen I, Bakke PS, Morkve O. Risk of over-diagnosis of COPD in asymptomatic elderly never-smokers. Eur Respir J. 2002;20(5):1117–22.
17. Swanney MP, Ruppel G, Enright PL, Pedersen OF, Crapo RO, Miller MR, et al. Using the lower limit of normal for the FEV1/FVC ratio reduces the misclassification of airway obstruction. Thorax. 2008;63(12):1046–51.
18. Schermer TR, Smeele IJ, Thoonen BP, Lucas AE, Grootens JG, van Boxem TJ, et al. Current clinical guideline definitions of airflow obstruction and COPD overdiagnosis in primary care. Eur Respir J. 2008;32(4):945–52.
19. Nussbaumer-Ochsner Y, Rabe KF. Systemic manifestations of COPD. Chest. 2011;139(1):165–73.
20. Agusti A, Noguera A, Sauleda J, Sala E, Pons J, Busquets X. Systemic effects of chronic obstructive pulmonary disease. Eur Respir J. 2003;21(2):347–60.
21. Divo M, Cote C, de Torres JP, Casanova C, Marin JM, Pinto-Plata V, et al. Comorbidities and risk of mortality in patients with chronic obstructive pulmonary disease. Am J Respir Crit Care Med. 2012;186(2):155–61.
22. Spruit MA, Gosselink R, Troosters T, De Paepe K, Decramer M. Resistance versus endurance training in patients with COPD and peripheral muscle weakness. Eur Respir J. 2002;19(6):1072–8.
23. Paz-Díaz H, De Oca MM, López JM, Celli BR. Pulmonary rehabilitation improves depression, anxiety, dyspnea and health status in patients with COPD. Am J Phys Med Rehabil. 2007;86(1):30–6.
24. Majid H, Sharafkhaneh A. The pharmacotherapy of chronic obstructive pulmonary disease in the elderly: an update. Clin Med Insights Ther. 2011;3:339.
25. Grosser T, Smyth E, FitzGerald G. Anti-inflammatory, antipyretic and analgesic agents; pharmacotherapy of gout. In: Bruton L, Chabner B, Knollman B, editors. Goodman and Gilman's the pharmacological basis of therapeutics. 12th ed. New York: McGraw-Hill; 2011. p. 973.
26. Dolovich MB, Ahrens RC, Hess DR, Anderson P, Dhand R, Rau JL, et al. Device selection and outcomes of aerosol therapy: evidence-based guidelines: American College of Chest Physicians/American College of Asthma, Allergy, and Immunology. Chest. 2005;127(1):335–71.
27. Barrons R, Pegram A, Borries A. Inhaler device selection: special considerations in elderly patients with chronic obstructive pulmonary disease. Am J Health Syst Pharm. 2011;68(13):1221–32.

28. Enright PL, McClelland RL, Newman AB, Gottlieb DJ, Lebowitz MD. Underdiagnosis and undertreatment of asthma in the elderly. Chest. 1999;116(3):603–13.

29. Stupka E. Asthma in seniors. Part 1. Evidence for underdiagnosis, undertreatment, and increasing morbidity and mortality. Am J Med. 2009;122(1):6–11.

30. Burrows B, Barbee R, Cline M, Knudson R, Lebowitz M. Characteristics of asthma among elderly adults in a sample of the general population. Chest. 1991;100(4):935–42.

31. Moorman JE. National surveillance for asthma--United States, 1980-2004. Department of Health and Human Services, Centers for Disease Control and Prevention Atlanta, GA; 2007.

32. Hanania NA, King MJ, Braman SS, Saltoun C, Wise RA, Enright P, et al. Asthma in the elderly: current understanding and future research needs—a report of a National Institute on Aging (NIA) workshop. J Allergy Clin Immunol. 2011;128(3):S4–24.

33. Moorman JE, Moorman J, Mannino DM. Increasing US asthma mortality rates: who is really dying? J Asthma. 2001;38(1):65–71.

34. Bellia V, Pedone C, Catalano F, Zito A, Davì E, Palange S, et al. Asthma in the elderly: mortality rate and associated risk factors for mortality. Chest. 2007;132(4):1175–82.

35. Banerjee D, Lee G, Malik S, Daly S. Underdiagnosis of asthma in the elderly. Br J Dis Chest. 1987;81:23–9.

36. Connolly MJ, Crowley JJ, Charan NB, Nielson CP, Vestal RE. Reduced subjective awareness of bronchoconstriction provoked by methacholine in elderly asthmatic and normal subjects as measured on a simple awareness scale. Thorax. 1992;47(6):410–3.

37. Bellia V, Battaglia S, Catalano F, Scichilone N, Incalzi RA, Imperiale C, et al. Aging and disability affect misdiagnosis of COPD in elderly asthmatics: the SARA study. Chest. 2003;123(4):1066–72.

38. Navaratnam P, Jayawant SS, Pedersen CA, Balkrishnan R. Asthma pharmacotherapy prescribing in the ambulatory population of the United States: evidence of nonadherence to national guidelines and implications for elderly people. J Am Geriatr Soc. 2008;56(7):1312–7.

39. Galie N, Hoeper MM, Humbert M, Torbicki A, Vachiery JL, Barbera JA, et al. Guidelines for the diagnosis and treatment of pulmonary hypertension: the Task Force for the Diagnosis and Treatment of Pulmonary Hypertension of the European Society of Cardiology (ESC) and the European Respiratory Society (ERS), endorsed by the International Society of Heart and Lung Transplantation (ISHLT). Eur Heart J. 2009;30(20):2493–537.

40. Minai O, Cleveland J, Tonelli A, Rose J. Impact of age on pulmonary arterial hypertension studies. Am J Respir Crit Care Med. 2015;191:A5502.

41. Simonneau G, Gatzoulis MA, Adatia I, Celermajer D, Denton C, Ghofrani A, et al. Updated clinical classification of pulmonary hypertension. J Am Coll Cardiol. 2013;62(25):D34–41.

42. Ling Y, Johnson MK, Kiely DG, Condliffe R, Elliot CA, Gibbs JSR, et al. Changing demographics, epidemiology, and survival of incident pulmonary arterial hypertension: results from the pulmonary hypertension registry of the United Kingdom and Ireland. Am J Respir Crit Care Med. 2012;186(8):790–6.

43. Lador F, Herve P. A practical approach of pulmonary hypertension in the elderly. Semin Respir Crit Care Med. 2013;34(5):654–64.

44. Aguilaniu B, Maitre J, Glenet S, Gegout-Petit A, Guenard H. European reference equations for CO and NO lung transfer. Eur Respir J. 2008;31(5):1091–7.

45. Mackay EH, Banks J, Sykes B, Lee G. Structural basis for the changing physical properties of human pulmonary vessels with age. Thorax. 1978;33(3):335–44.

46. Lettieri CJ, Nathan SD, Barnett SD, Ahmad S, Shorr AF. Prevalence and outcomes of pulmonary arterial hypertension in advanced idiopathic pulmonary fibrosis. Chest. 2006;129(3):746–52.

47. Badesch DB, Champion HC, Sanchez MAG, Hoeper MM, Loyd JE, Manes A, et al. Diagnosis and assessment of pulmonary arterial hypertension. J Am Coll Cardiol. 2009;54 Suppl 1:S55–66.

48. McGoon M, Gutterman D, Steen V, Barst R, McCrory DC, Fortin TA, et al. Screening, early detection, and diagnosis of pulmonary arterial hypertension: ACCP evidence-based clinical practice guidelines. Chest. 2004;126 Suppl 1:14S–34.

49. Sitbon O, Humbert M, Jais X, Ioos V, Hamid AM, Provencher S, et al. Long-term response to calcium channel blockers in idiopathic pulmonary arterial hypertension. Circulation. 2005;111(23):3105–11.

50. Galiè N, Corris PA, Frost A, Girgis RE, Granton J, Jing ZC, et al. Updated treatment algorithm of pulmonary arterial hypertension. J Am Coll Cardiol. 2013;62 Suppl 25:D60–72.

51. Hoeper MM, Huscher D, Ghofrani HA, Delcroix M, Distler O, Schweiger C, et al. Elderly patients diagnosed with idiopathic pulmonary arterial hypertension: results from the COMPERA registry. Int J Cardiol. 2013;168(2):871–80.

52. Janssens J, Krause K. Pneumonia in the very old. Lancet Infect Dis. 2004;4(2):112–24.

53. Krajcik S, Haniskova T, Mikus P. Pneumonia in older people. Rev Clin Gerontol. 2011;21(1):16–27.

54. Hoyert DL, Heron MP, Murphy SL, Kung H. Deaths: final data for 2003. Natl Vital Stat Rep. 2006;54(13):1–120.

55. El-Solh AA, Sikka P, Ramadan F, Davies J. Etiology of severe pneumonia in the very elderly. Am J Respir Crit Care Med. 2001;163(3):645–51.

56. Naucler P, Darenberg J, Morfeldt E, Ortqvist A, Henriques Normark B. Contribution of host, bacterial factors and antibiotic treatment to mortality in adult patients with bacteraemic pneumococcal pneumonia. Thorax. 2013;68(6):571–9.

57. Torres A, Peetermans WE, Viegi G, Blasi F. Risk factors for community-acquired pneumonia in adults in Europe: a literature review. Thorax. 2013;68(11):1057–65.

58. Farr B, Woodhead M, Macfarlane J, Bartlett C, McCracken J, Wadsworth J, et al. Risk factors for community-acquired pneumonia diagnosed by general practitioners in the community. Respir Med. 2000;94(5):422–7.

59. Sansoni P, Cossarizza A, Brianti V, Fagnoni F, Snelli G, Monti D, et al. Lymphocyte subsets and natural killer cell activity in healthy old people and centenarians. Blood. 1993;82(9):2767–73.

60. Metlay JP, Schulz R, Li Y, Singer DE, Marrie TJ, Coley CM, et al. Influence of age on symptoms at presentation in patients with community-acquired pneumonia. Arch Intern Med. 1997;157(13):1453–9.

61. Riquelme R, Torres A, El-Ebiary M, Mensa J, Estruch R, Ruiz M, et al. Community-acquired pneumonia in the elderly: clinical and nutritional aspects. Am J Respir Crit Care Med. 1997;156(6):1908–14.

62. Cillóniz C, Polverino E, Ewig S, Aliberti S, Gabarrús A, Menéndez R, et al. Impact of age and comorbidity on cause and outcome in community-acquired pneumonia. Chest. 2013;144(3):999–1007.

63. Raghu G, Collard HR, Egan JJ, Martinez FJ, Behr J, Brown KK, et al. An official ATS/ERS/JRS/ALAT statement: idiopathic pulmonary fibrosis: evidence-based guidelines for diagnosis and management. Am J Respir Crit Care Med. 2011;183(6):788–824.

64. Raghu G, Weycker D, Edelsberg J, Bradford WZ, Oster G. Incidence and prevalence of idiopathic pulmonary fibrosis. Am J Respir Crit Care Med. 2006;174(7):810–6.

65. Wolters PJ, Collard HR, Jones KD. Pathogenesis of idiopathic pulmonary fibrosis. Annu Rev Pathol. 2014;9:157–79.

66. Baumgartner KB, Samet JM, Stidley CA, Colby TV, Waldron JA. Cigarette smoking: a risk factor for idiopathic pulmonary fibrosis. Am J Respir Crit Care Med. 1997;155(1):242–8.

67. Lee SH, Kim DS, Kim YW, Chung MP, Uh ST, Park CS, et al. Association between occupational dust exposure and prognosis of idiopathic pulmonary fibrosis. Chest. 2015;147(2):465–74.

68. Lawson WE, Crossno PF, Polosukhin VV, Roldan J, Cheng DS, Lane KB, et al. Endoplasmic reticulum stress in alveolar epithelial cells is prominent in IPF: association with altered surfactant protein processing and herpesvirus infection. Am J Physiol Lung Cell Mol Physiol. 2008;294(6):L1119–26.

69. Kelly BG, Lok SS, Hasleton PS, Egan JJ, Stewart JP. A rearranged form of Epstein–Barr virus DNA is associated with idiopathic pulmonary fibrosis. Am J Respir Crit Care Med. 2002;166(4):510–3.

70. Fell CD, Martinez FJ, Liu LX, Murray S, Han MK, Kazerooni EA, et al. Clinical predictors of a diagnosis of idiopathic pulmonary fibrosis. Am J Respir Crit Care Med. 2010;181(8):832–7.

71. Meyer KC, Danoff SK, Lancaster LH, Nathan SD. management of idiopathic pulmonary fibrosis in the elderly patient: addressing key questions. Chest. 2015;148(1):242–52.

72. Raghu G. Idiopathic pulmonary fibrosis: guidelines for diagnosis and clinical management have advanced from consensus-based in 2000 to evidence-based in 2011. Eur Respir J. 2011;37(4):743–6.

73. Noble PW, Albera C, Bradford WZ, Costabel U, Glassberg MK, Kardatzke D, et al. Pirfenidone in patients with idiopathic pulmonary fibrosis (CAPACITY): two randomised trials. Lancet. 2011;377(9779):1760–9.

74. King Jr TE, Bradford WZ, Castro-Bernardini S, Fagan EA, Glaspole I, Glassberg MK, et al. A phase 3 trial of pirfenidone in patients with idiopathic pulmonary fibrosis. N Engl J Med. 2014;370(22):2083–92.

75. Richeldi L, du Bois RM, Raghu G, Azuma A, Brown KK, Costabel U, et al. Efficacy and safety of nintedanib in idiopathic pulmonary fibrosis. N Engl J Med. 2014;370(22):2071–82.

76. Nishiyama O, Kondoh Y, Kimura T, Kato K, Kataoka K, Ogawa T, et al. Effects of pulmonary rehabilitation in patients with idiopathic pulmonary fibrosis. Respirology. 2008;13(3):394–9.

77. Lee JS, Ryu JH, Elicker BM, Lydell CP, Jones KD, Wolters PJ, et al. Gastroesophageal reflux therapy is associated with longer survival in patients with idiopathic pulmonary fibrosis. Am J Respir Crit Care Med. 2011;184(12):1390–4.

78. Pérez ERF, Daniels CE, Schroeder DR, Sauver JS, Hartman TE, Bartholmai BJ, et al. Incidence, prevalence, and clinical course of idiopathic pulmonary fibrosis: a population-based study. Chest. 2010;137(1):129–37.

79. Smith BD, Smith GL, Hurria A, Hortobagyi GN, Buchholz TA. Future of cancer incidence in the United States: burdens upon an aging, changing nation. J Clin Oncol. 2009;27(17):2758–65.

80. Ferlay J, Shin H, Bray F, Forman D, Mathers C, Parkin DM. Estimates of worldwide burden of cancer in 2008: GLOBOCAN 2008. Int J Cancer. 2010;127(12):2893–917.

81. Ganti AK, deShazo M, Weir 3rd AB, Hurria A. Treatment of non-small cell lung cancer in the older patient. J Natl Compr Canc Netw. 2012;10(2):230–9.

82. Stuck AE, Siu AL, Wieland GD, Rubenstein L, Adams J. Comprehensive geriatric assessment: a meta-analysis of controlled trials. Lancet. 1993;342(8878):1032–6.

83. Fuchs L, Chronaki CE, Park S, Novack V, Baumfeld Y, Scott D, et al. ICU admission characteristics and mortality rates among elderly and very elderly patients. Intensive Care Med. 2012;38(10):1654–61.

84. McNicoll L, Pisani MA, Zhang Y, Ely E, Siegel MD, Inouye SK. Delirium in the intensive care unit: occurrence and clinical course in older patients. J Am Geriatr Soc. 2003;51(5):591–8.

85. Lin S, Liu C, Wang C, Lin H, Huang C, Huang P, et al. The impact of delirium on the survival of mechanically ventilated patients*. Crit Care Med. 2004;32(11):2254–9.

86. Thomason JW, Shintani A, Peterson JF, Pun BT, Jackson JC, Ely EW. Intensive care unit delirium is an independent predictor of longer hospital stay: a prospective analysis of 261 non-ventilated patients. Crit Care. 2005;9(4):R375–81.

87. Ely EW, Gautam S, Margolin R, Francis J, May L, Speroff T, et al. The impact of delirium in the intensive care unit on hospital length of stay. Intensive Care Med. 2001;27(12):1892–900.

88. Pisani MA, Kong SY, Kasl SV, Murphy TE, Araujo KL, Van Ness PH. Days of delirium are associated with 1-year mortality in an older intensive care unit population. Am J Respir Crit Care Med. 2009;180(11):1092–7.

89. Pisani MA, Murphy TE, Araujo KL, Slattum P, Van Ness PH, Inouye SK. Benzodiazepine and opioid use and the duration of intensive care unit delirium in an older population. Crit Care Med. 2009;37(1):177–83.

90. Fujii S, Tanimukai H, Kashiwagi Y. Comparison and analysis of delirium induced by histamine h(2) receptor antagonists and proton pump inhibitors in cancer patients. Case Rep Oncol. 2012;5(2):409–12.

91. Han L, McCusker J, Cole M, Abrahamowicz M, Primeau F, Elie M. Use of medications with anticholinergic effect predicts clinical severity of delirium symptoms in older medical inpatients. Arch Intern Med. 2001;161(8):1099–105.

92. Pisani MA, Araujo KL, Murphy TE. Association of cumulative dose of haloperidol with next-day delirium in older medical ICU patients. Crit Care Med. 2015;43(5):996–1002.

93. Van Rompaey B, Elseviers MM, Schuurmans MJ, Shortridge-Baggett LM, Truijen S, Bossaert L. Risk factors for delirium in intensive care patients: a prospective cohort study. Crit Care. 2009;13(3):R77.

94. Freedman NS, Gazendam J, Levan L, Pack AI, Schwab RJ. Abnormal sleep/wake cycles and the effect of environmental noise on sleep disruption in the intensive care unit. Am J Respir Crit Care Med. 2001;163(2):451–7.

95. Freedman NS, Kotzer N, Schwab RJ. Patient perception of sleep quality and etiology of sleep disruption in the intensive care unit. Am J Respir Crit Care Med. 1999;159(4):1155–62.

96. Weinhouse GL, Schwab RJ, Watson PL, Patil N, Vaccaro B, Pandharipande P, et al. Bench-to-bedside review: delirium in ICU patients - importance of sleep deprivation. Crit Care. 2009;13(6):234.

97. McCusker J, Cole M, Abrahamowicz M, Han L, Podoba JE, Ramman-Haddad L. Environmental risk factors for delirium in hospitalized older people. J Am Geriatr Soc. 2001;49(10):1327–34.

98. Pandharipande P, Banerjee A, McGrane S, Ely EW. Liberation and animation for ventilated ICU patients: the ABCDE bundle for the back-end of critical care. Crit Care. 2010;14(3):157.

99. Ely EW, Baker AM, Dunagan DP, Burke HL, Smith AC, Kelly PT, et al. Effect on the duration of mechanical ventilation of identifying patients capable of breathing spontaneously. N Engl J Med. 1996;335(25):1864–9.

100. Stites M. Observational pain scales in critically ill adults. Crit Care Nurse. 2013;33(3):68–78.

101. Ely EW, Truman B, Shintani A, Thomason JW, Wheeler AP, Gordon S, et al. Monitoring sedation status over time in ICU patients: reliability and validity of the Richmond Agitation-Sedation Scale (RASS). JAMA. 2003;289(22):2983–91.

102. Ely EW, Inouye SK, Bernard GR, Gordon S, Francis J, May L, et al. Delirium in mechanically ventilated patients: validity and reliability of the confusion assessment method for the intensive care unit (CAM-ICU). JAMA. 2001;286(21):2703–10.

103. Burtin C, Clerckx B, Robbeets C, Ferdinande P, Langer D, Troosters T, et al. Early exercise in critically ill patients enhances short-term functional recovery. Crit Care Med. 2009;37(9):2499–505.

104. Balas MC, Vasilevskis EE, Olsen KM, Schmid KK, Shostrom V, Cohen MZ, et al. Effectiveness and safety of the awakening and breathing coordination, delirium monitoring/management, and early exercise/mobility bundle. Crit Care Med. 2014;42(5):1024–36.

105. Inouye SK, Westendorp RG, Saczynski JS. Delirium in elderly people. Lancet. 2014;383(9920):911–22.

106. Confalonieri M, Parigi P, Scartabellati A, Aiolfi S, Scorsetti S, Nava S, et al. Noninvasive mechanical ventilation improves the immediate and long-term outcome of COPD patients with acute respiratory failure. Eur Respir J. 1996;9(3):422–30.

107. Brochard L, Mancebo J, Wysocki M, Lofaso F, Conti G, Rauss A, et al. Noninvasive ventilation for acute exacerbations of chronic obstructive pulmonary disease. N Engl J Med. 1995;333(13):817–22.

108. Evans TW. International Consensus Conferences in Intensive Care Medicine: non-invasive positive pressure ventilation in acute respiratory failure. Intensive Care Med. 2001;27(1):166–78.

109. Chandra D, Ramos R, Taylor B, Mannino D, Krishnan JA, Holguin F. Patterns and outcomes of non-invasive positive-pressure ventilation for acute exacerbations of COPD in the US. Am J Respir Crit Care Med. 2011;183:A4574.

110. Esteban A, Anzueto A, Frutos F, Alia I, Brochard L, Stewart TE, et al. Characteristics and outcomes in adult patients receiving mechanical ventilation: a 28-day international study. JAMA. 2002;287(3):345–55.

111. Sudarsanam TD, Jeyaseelan L, Thomas K, John G. Predictors of mortality in mechanically ventilated patients. Postgrad Med J. 2005;81(962):780–3.

112. Bauer TT, Ferrer R, Angrill J, Schultze-Werninghaus G, Torres A. Ventilator-associated pneumonia: incidence, risk factors, and microbiology. Semin Respir Infect. 2000;15(4):272–9.

113. Melsen WG, Rovers MM, Koeman M, Bonten MJ. Estimating the attributable mortality of ventilator-associated pneumonia from randomized prevention studies. Crit Care Med. 2011;39(12): 2736–42.

114. Schneider GT, Christensen N, Doerr TD. Early tracheotomy in elderly patients results in less ventilator-associated pneumonia. Otolaryngol Head Neck Surg. 2009;140(2):250–5.

115. Perren A, Domenighetti G, Mauri S, Genini F, Vizzardi N. Protocol-directed weaning from mechanical ventilation: clinical outcome in patients randomized for a 30-min or 120-min trial with pressure support ventilation. Intensive Care Med. 2002;28(8): 1058–63.

116. Jeganathan N, Kaplan CA, Balk RA. Ventilator liberation for high-risk-for-failure patients: improving value of the spontaneous breathing trial. Respir Care. 2015;60(2):290–6.

117. White RH. The epidemiology of venous thromboembolism. Circulation. 2003;107(23 Suppl 1):I4–8.

118. Anderson FA, Wheeler HB, Goldberg RJ, Hosmer DW, Patwardhan NA, Jovanovic B, et al. A population-based perspective of the hospital incidence and case-fatality rates of deep vein thrombosis and pulmonary embolism: the Worcester DVT Study. Arch Intern Med. 1991;151(5):933–8.

119. Heit JA, Silverstein MD, Mohr DN, Petterson TM, O'Fallon WM, Melton LJ. Predictors of survival after deep vein thrombosis and pulmonary embolism: a population-based, cohort study. Arch Intern Med. 1999;159(5):445–53.

120. Timmons S, Kingston M, Hussain M, Kelly H, Liston R. Pulmonary embolism: differences in presentation between older and younger patients. Age Ageing. 2003;32(6):601–5.

121. Schouten HJ, Geersing GJ, Koek HL, Zuithoff NP, Janssen KJ, Douma RA, et al. Diagnostic accuracy of conventional or age adjusted D-dimer cut-off values in older patients with suspected venous thromboembolism: systematic review and meta-analysis. BMJ. 2013;346:f2492.

122. Righini M, Goehring C, Bounameaux H, Perrier A. Effects of age on the performance of common diagnostic tests for pulmonary embolism. Am J Med. 2000;109(5):357–61.

123. Cohen AT, Alikhan R, Arcelus JI, Bergmann J, Haas S, Merli GJ, et al. Assessment of venous thromboembolism risk and the benefits of thromboprophylaxis in medical patients. Thromb Haemost. 2005;94(4):750.

124. Landefeld CS, Beyth RJ. Anticoagulant-related bleeding: clinical epidemiology, prediction, and prevention. Am J Med. 1993;95(3):315–28.

125. White RH, Beyth RJ, Zhou H, Romano PS. Major bleeding after hospitalization for deep-venous thrombosis. Am J Med. 1999;107(5):414–24.

126. Levine MN, Raskob G, Landefeld S, Kearon C. Hemorrhagic complications of anticoagulant treatment. Chest. 2001;119 Suppl 1:108S–21.

127. Alikhan R, Cohen AT, Combe S, Samama MM, Desjardins L, Eldor A, et al. Prevention of venous thromboembolism in medical patients with enoxaparin: a subgroup analysis of the MEDENOX study. Blood Coagul Fibrinolysis. 2003;14(4):341–6.

128. Kucher N, Leizorovicz A, Vaitkus PT, Cohen AT, Turpie AG, Olsson C, et al. Efficacy and safety of fixed low-dose dalteparin in preventing venous thromboembolism among obese or elderly hospitalized patients: a subgroup analysis of the PREVENT trial. Arch Intern Med. 2005;165(3):341–5.

129. Angus DC, Linde-Zwirble WT, Lidicker J, Clermont G, Carcillo J, Pinsky MR. Epidemiology of severe sepsis in the United States: analysis of incidence, outcome, and associated costs of care. Crit Care Med. 2001;29(7):1303–10.

130. Martin GS, Mannino DM, Moss M. The effect of age on the development and outcome of adult sepsis*. Crit Care Med. 2006;34(1):15–21.

131. Bonomo RA. Multiple antibiotic-resistant bacteria in long-term-care facilities: an emerging problem in the practice of infectious diseases. Clin Infect Dis. 2000;31(6):1414–22.

132. Opal SM, Girard TD, Ely EW. The immunopathogenesis of sepsis in elderly patients. Clin Infect Dis. 2005;41 Suppl 7:S504–12.

133. Foxman B. Epidemiology of urinary tract infections: incidence, morbidity, and economic costs. Am J Med. 2002;113(1):5–13.

134. Gleckman R, Hibert D. Afebrile bacteremia: a phenomenon in geriatric patients. JAMA. 1982;248(12):1478–81.

135. Iberti TJ, Bone RC, Balk R, Fein A, Perl TM, Wenzel RP. Are the criteria used to determine sepsis applicable for patients <75 years Of age? Crit Care Med. 1993;21(4):S130.

136. El Solh AA, Akinnusi ME, Alsawalha LN, Pineda LA. Outcome of septic shock in older adults after implementation of the sepsis "bundle". J Am Geriatr Soc. 2008;56(2):272–8.

137. Marik PE, Pastores SM, Annane D, Meduri GU, Sprung CL, Arlt W, et al. Recommendations for the diagnosis and management of corticosteroid insufficiency in critically ill adult patients: consensus statements from an international task force by the American College of Critical Care Medicine. Crit Care Med. 2008;36(6):1937–49.

138. Hébert PC, Wells G, Blajchman MA, Marshall J, Martin C, Pagliarello G, et al. A multicenter, randomized, controlled clinical trial of transfusion requirements in critical care. N Engl J Med. 1999;340(6):409–17.

139. Wu W, Rathore SS, Wang Y, Radford MJ, Krumholz HM. Blood transfusion in elderly patients with acute myocardial infarction. N Engl J Med. 2001;345(17):1230–6.

140. Walsh TS, Boyd JA, Watson D, Hope D, Lewis S, Krishan A, et al. Restrictive versus liberal transfusion strategies for older mechanically ventilated critically ill patients: a randomized pilot trial. Crit Care Med. 2013;41(10):2354–63.

141. Gruber-Baldini AL, Marcantonio E, Orwig D, Magaziner J, Terrin M, Barr E, et al. Delirium outcomes in a randomized trial of blood transfusion thresholds in hospitalized older adults with hip fracture. J Am Geriatr Soc. 2013;61(8):1286–95.

142. Wuerz RC, Holliman CJ, Meador SA, Swope GE, Balogh R. Effect of age on prehospital cardiac resuscitation outcome. Am J Emerg Med. 1995;13(4):389–91.

143. Ehlenbach WJ, Barnato AE, Curtis JR, Kreuter W, Koepsell TD, Deyo RA, et al. Epidemiologic study of in-hospital cardiopulmonary resuscitation in the elderly. N Engl J Med. 2009; 361(1):22–31.

144. van Gijn MS, Frijns D, van de Glind EM, C van Munster B, Hamaker ME. The chance of survival and the functional outcome after in-hospital cardiopulmonary resuscitation in older people: a systematic review. Age Ageing 2014;43(4):456–63.

145. Detering KM, Hancock AD, Reade MC, Silvester W. The impact of advance care planning on end of life care in elderly patients: randomised controlled trial. BMJ. 2010;340:c1345.

Index

© Springer International Publishing Switzerland 2017

J.R. Burton et al. (eds.), *Geriatrics for Specialists*, DOI 10.1007/978-3-319-31831-8